T0202100

OXFORD MEDICAL PUBLICATIONS

Oxford Handbook of Paediatrics

Published and forthcoming Oxford Handbooks

OXFORD HANDBOOK OF
Paediatrics

THIRD EDITION

EDITED BY

Robert C. Tasker

Professor of Anaesthesia (Pediatrics),
Harvard Medical School; First Chair of Neurocritical Care,
Boston Children's Hospital, Boston,
USA

Carlo L. Acerini

University Senior Lecturer,
Cambridge University Clinical School,
Cambridge, UK

WITH

Edward Holloway

Consultant Paediatrician,
Croydon University Hospital, London,
UK

Asma Shah

Consultant Paediatrician, Lead for Shared Care, Paediatric
Oncology,
St Richard's Hospital, Western Sussex NHS Foundation Trust,
Chichester,
UK

Peter Lillitos

Paediatric Cardiology Registrar,
Leeds Teaching Hospitals NHS Trust, UK

OXFORD
UNIVERSITY PRESS

OXFORD
UNIVERSITY PRESS

Great Clarendon Street, Oxford, OX2 6DP,
United Kingdom

Oxford University Press is a department of the University of Oxford.
It furthers the University's objective of excellence in research, scholarship,
and education by publishing worldwide. Oxford is a registered trade mark of
Oxford University Press in the UK and in certain other countries

© Oxford University Press 2021

The moral rights of the authors have been asserted

First Edition published 2008
Second Edition published 2013
Third Edition published 2021

Impression: 3

Published in the United States of America by Oxford University Press
198 Madison Avenue, New York, NY 10016, United States of America

British Library Cataloguing in Publication Data
Data available

Library of Congress Control Number: 2020931222

ISBN 978–0–19–878988–8

Printed and bound in China by
C&C Offset Printing Co., Ltd.

Foreword to the first edition

Textbooks have been the mainstay of medical education for centuries. Clearly, the development of the information superhighway via the Internet has changed how we learn, find information, and communicate. What does yet another paediatric textbook add to the current long list of titles?

Drs Tasker, McClure, and Acerini have conceived of and edited a new book. It is a handbook of paediatrics that joins a stable of similar publications from Oxford University Press. There are 23 contributing editors. Using a well-tested format for presentation, the handbook consists of 31 chapters, ranging from sections on epidemiology, evidence, and practice, through the more traditional topics, such as nephrology and neurology, and concluding with international health and travel, and paediatrics, ethics, and the law. Each chapter follows the same format, 5–40 sections, followed by bulleted points. Both signs and symptoms of illness, as well as specific diseases are covered. Virtually all topics are limited to 1–2 pages of important information. Tables are carefully inserted, and complement the text. Doses of important drugs are included in the text and/or the tables. There are a limited number of figures, but like the tables, they supplement the text and have been carefully chosen to add clarity.

The *Oxford Handbook of Paediatrics* is a worthy addition to your library. It will be particularly appealing to medical students and younger physicians, who have learned to digest a great deal of information quickly and in an abbreviated format. Its availability on a CD-ROM is an added and necessary benefit. Drs Tasker, McClure, and Acerini have done a wonderful job in ensuring consistency, clarity, and completeness.

Professor Howard Bauchner,
Boston University School of Medicine/Boston Medical Center,
Vice-Chair, Academic Affairs,
Editor in Chief, *Archives of Disease in Childhood*,
January 2008

Preface

The first 'boke' of paediatrics printed in English was written by Thomas Phaire (1510–1560), a man from East Anglia who studied medicine at Oxford University. The 56-page book covered:

' . . . innumerable passions & diseases, whereunto the bodye of man is subjecte, and as well moste commonly the tender age of children is chefely vexed and greued with these diseases folowyng. Apostume of the brayne, swellyng of the head . . . '[1]

In 1553, the 'innumerable passions & diseases' came to 39 presenting clinical problems. The first and second editions of the *Oxford Handbook of Paediatrics* grew out of a commitment that Carlo Acerini and I had to teaching medical students in the heart of East Anglia (Cambridge University) and the similarity with Thomas Phaire's book did not escape us, particularly as we saw the importance of concentrating on common presenting clinical problems.

This third edition still aims to provide a compact source of information and clinical thinking that can be used in the clinic or hospital ward, at a time when the child is being seen. The challenge therefore was to distil content, sift out important facts crucial to clinical practice, and be contemporary. Key to this task has been the inclusion of three new editors for the *Oxford Handbook of Paediatrics*—Ed Holloway, Peter Lillotos, and Asma Shah. These are outstanding young Consultants who have maintained our tradition of harnessing text that we believe is vital from the start of one's education in paediatrics, through higher general training in the field, and—here we hope to spark a lifelong interest—beyond. Above all, we hope that the handbook will give you confidence to manage paediatric clinical problems effectively and safely.

Lastly, it is with a heavy heart and sadness that I have to report that Carlo passed away in May 2019.[2] Oxford University Press have been most supportive through this time, and this edition is dedicated in Carlo's memory, and his commitment to friendship, colleagues, and his family.

RCT
EH, PL, AS
CLA (posthumous)
April 2020

References

1. Phaire T. (1553). *The Boke of Chyldren*. Reprint edited by Naeale AV, Wallis HRE. E&S Livingstone Ltd, Edinburgh; 1965.
2. Dunger D, Cameron F. Obituary: Carlo Acerini—raging against the dying of the light. *Diabet Med* 2019; 36: 1187–8.

Authors' disclaimer

All reasonable efforts have been undertaken in order to ensure the accuracy of drug doses in this book. UK readers are advised to also consult the *British National Formulary for Children* (National Institute for Health and Care Excellence) (℅ https://bnfc.nice.org.uk), which is free online in the UK and was last updated on 30 September 2019. Other readers should refer to their own regional or national guidelines. The authors cannot be held responsible for any errors herein.

Acknowledgements

We thank all of the previous contributors to the 1e and 2e of the *Oxford Handbook of Paediatrics*. We now extend our thanks and gratitude to new and old contributors for all of their hard work in updating the text. We are especially grateful to Michael Hawkes, Karen Moore, and Elizabeth Reeve at OUP for their help and assistance, and for their patience with us. Finally, but not least, a special thanks goes to our respective families for their encouragement, support, sacrifice, and understanding throughout the preparation of this book.

The editors and OUP would like to acknowledge Professor Robert McClure for his contribution as an original co-editor of the first and second editions.

Robert C. Tasker
Edward Holloway
Peter Lillotos
Asma Shah

Contents

Contributors

Dr David Albert
Senior Paediatric ENT Consultant, Great Ormond Street Hospital, London, UK

Dr Louise Allen
Consultant Paediatric Ophthalmologist, Cambridge University Hospitals NHS Foundation Trust; Associate Lecturer, University of Cambridge, Cambridge, UK

Dr Cherry Alviani
Paediatric Allergy Registrar, University Hospital Southampton, Southampton, UK

Professor Yogesh Bajaj
ENT Consultant, Royal London Hospital, London; Visiting Professor of ENT, Canterbury University, Canterbury, UK

Professor Imti Choonara
Emeritus Professor in Child Health, University of Nottingham, The Medical School, Derby, UK

Professor David Coghill
Developmental Mental Health, Royal Children's Hospital, Melbourne, Australia

Dr Rachael Foster
Consultant Paediatric Dermatologist, Perth Children's Hospital, Nedlands, Australia

Dr Dionysios Grigoratos
Consultant Paediatrician, Special Interest in Epilepsy (SPIN 2017), King's College Hospital NHS Foundation Trust, London UK

Dr Christopher Hands
PICU Fellow, Guy's and St Thomas' NHS Foundation Trust, London, UK

Dr David James
Consultant in Paediatric Emergency Medicine, University Hospital Southampton NHS Foundation Trust, Southampton, UK

Dr Hugh Lemonde
Consultant in Paediatric Inherited Metabolic Disease, Evelina London Children's Hospital, London, UK

Dr Elaine Lewis
Consultant Community Paediatrician, Cambridgeshire Community Services NHS Trust, Cambridge, UK

Dr Georgina Malakounides
Consultant Paediatric Surgeon, Addenbrookes Hospital, Cambridge University Hospitals NHS Foundation Trust, Cambridge, UK

Dr Rob McClure
Consultant Neonatologist and Paediatrician, Consultant Anatomical Pathologist, Fiona Stanley Hospital, Associate Professor of Anatomical Pathology, Murdoch University, Perth, Western Australia, Australia

Dr Frances Nelson
Specialty Registrar, Paediatrics with SPIN Diabetes, East of England Deanery, UK

Dr Roddy O'Donnell
Consultant in Paediatric Intensive Care, Cambridge University Hospitals NHS Foundation Trust, Cambridge, UK

Dr Catherine O'Sullivan
Paediatric Immunology and Infectious Diseases Registrar, Great Ormond Street Hospital, London, UK

Dr Trisha Radia
Consultant Paediatrician, Croydon
University Hospital NHS Trust,
London, UK

Dr Willie Reardon
Consultant Clinical Geneticist,
Department of Clinical Genetics,
Our Lady's Hospital for Sick
Children, Dublin, Ireland

Professor Lesley Rees
Consultant Paediatric Nephrologist,
Great Ormond Street Hospital for
Children NHS Trust, London, UK

Dr Praveen Saroey
Infection Prevention and Control
Fellow, McMaster Children's
Hospital, McMaster University,
Hamilton, Canada

Dr Nick Wilkinson
Consultant Paediatric
Rheumatologist, Evelina London
Children's Hospital, London, UK

Ben Fisher
ST3 and academic clinical fellow in
paediatrics and neonatology
Addenbrooke's Hospital,
Cambridge, UK

Symbols and abbreviations

☞	controversial topic
⮀	cross-reference
ℛ	website address
↑	increased
↓	decreased
→	leading to
↔	normal
~	approximately
♂	male
♀	female
±	with or without
>	greater than
<	less than
≥	equal to or greater than
≤	equal to or less than
°	degree
°C	degree Celsius
α	alpha
β	beta
δ	delta
γ	gamma
®	registered
™	trademark
+ve	positive
–ve	negative
1,25-OHD	1,25-dihydroxyvitamin D3
25-OHD	25-hydroxyvitamin D3
6MP	6-mercaptopurine
AA	amyloid A
AABR	automatic auditory brainstem response
AAP	American Academy of Pediatrics
AASA	α-aminoadipic semialdehyde
ABC	airway, breathing, circulation
ABCD	airway, breathing, circulation, disability
ABG	arterial blood gas
ABPM	ambulatory blood pressure monitoring
AC	activated charcoal
ACE	angiotensin-converting enzyme
ACh	acetylcholine
ACR	American College of Rheumatology

ACTH	adrenocorticotrophic hormone
AD	autosomal dominant
ADEM	acute disseminated encephalomyelitis
ADH	antidiuretic hormone
ADHD	attention-deficit/hyperactivity disorder
ADP	adenosine diphosphate
ADPKD	autosomal dominant polycystic kidney disease
ADR	adverse drug reaction
A&E	accident and emergency (department)
AED	antiepileptic drug
aEEG	amplitude-integrated electroencephalography
AFP	α-fetoprotein
AG	anion gap
aHUS	atypical haemolytic uraemic syndrome
AIDS	acquired immune deficiency syndrome
AIS	androgen insensitivity syndrome; autoinflammatory syndrome
AKI	acute kidney injury
ALCL	anaplastic large cell lymphoma
ALG	anti-lymphocyte globulin
ALI	acute lung injury
ALL	acute lymphoblastic leukaemia
ALP	alkaline phosphatase
ALPS	autoimmune lymphoproliferative syndrome
ALT	alanine aminotransferase
AMH	anti-Müllerian hormone
AMR	antimicrobial resistance
ANA	antinuclear antibodies
ANCA	antineutrophil cytoplasmic antibodies
AP	antero-posterior
APC	activated protein C
APECED	autoimmune polyendocrinopathy, candidiasis, ectodermal dystrophia
APH	antepartum haemorrhage

APS	antiphospholipid antibody syndrome
APTT	activated partial thromboplastin time
AR	autosomal recessive; aortic regurgitation; allergic rhinitis
araC	cytarabine
ARB	angiotensin II receptor blocker
ARDS	acute respiratory distress syndrome
ARF	acute renal failure; acute rheumatic fever
ARM	artificial rupture of membranes
ARPKD	autosomal recessive polycystic kidney disease
AS	Angelman syndrome; aortic stenosis
ASA	5-aminosalicylic acid
ASCA	anti-*Saccharomyces cerevisiae* antibodies
ASD	atrial septal defect
ASIS	anterior superior iliac spine
ASM	antiseizure medication
ASO	anti-streptolysin O
ASOT	anti-streptolysin O titre
ASP	antimicrobial stewardship programme
AST	aspartate aminotransferase
AT	ataxia telangiectasia
ATN	acute tubular necrosis
ATP	adenosine triphosphate
AV	atrioventricular
AVM	arteriovenous malformation
AVP	arginine vasopressin
AVSD	atrioventricular septal defect
AXR	abdominal X-ray
BAL	broncho-alveolar lavage
BBS	Bardet–Biedl syndrome
BCG	bacille Calmette–Guérin
bd	twice a day
BECTS	benign epilepsy with centro-temporal spikes
BLCL	Burkitt's large B-cell lymphoma
BMD	Becker muscular dystrophy; bone mineral density
BMI	body mass index
BMT	bone marrow transplantation
BNF	*British National Formulary*
BP	blood pressure
BPD	bronchopulmonary dysplasia

BSA	body surface area
BSI	bloodstream infection
BSS	Bernard–Soulier syndrome
BT	Blalock–Taussig (shunt)
BWS	Beckwith–Wiedemann syndrome
BXO	balanitis xerotica obliterans
Ca^{2+}	calcium
CA	choanal atresia
CAD	coronary artery disease
CAE	childhood absence epilepsy
CAH	congenital adrenal hyperplasia
CAMHS	Child and Adolescent Mental Health Services
CAMPS	CARD-14-mediated pustular psoriasis
CAP	community-acquired pneumonia
CAPS	cryopyrin-associated periodic syndrome
CBF	ciliary beat frequency
CBP	ciliary beat pattern
CBT	cognitive behavioural therapy
CCAM	congenital cystic adenomatoid malformation
CCNU	lomustine
CCPD	continuous cycling automated peritoneal dialysis
CD	Crohn's disease
CDC	Centers for Disease Control and Prevention
CDD	conduct disorder
CDGP	constitutional delay in growth and puberty
CDH	congenital diaphragmatic hernia
cEDS	classical Ehlers–Danlos syndrome
CF	cystic fibrosis
CFAM	cerebral function analysis monitoring
CFRD	cystic fibrosis-related diabetes
CFS	chronic fatigue syndrome
CFTR	cystic fibrosis transmembrane receptor
CGA	corrected gestational age
CGD	chronic granulomatous disease
CGM	continuous glucose monitoring
CGMS	continuous glucose monitoring system
CH	cystic hygroma

CHARGE	coloboma, heart defects, choanal atresia, retarded growth, genital anomalies, ear abnormalities
CHC	choriocarcinoma
CHD	congenital heart disease
CHEOPS	Children's Hospital of Eastern Ontario Pain Scale
CHO	carbohydrate
CK	creatine kinase
CKD	chronic kidney disease
CKD-MBD	chronic kidney disease, mineral and bone disorder
CLD	chronic lung disease
CLE	congenital lobar emphysema
cm	centimetre
CMG	congenital myasthenia gravis
cmH_2O	centimetre of water
CML	chronic myeloid leukaemia
CMV	cytomegalovirus
CN	cranial nerve
CNS	central nervous system
CO	carbon monoxide
CO_2	carbon dioxide
CoA	coarctation of the aorta
CoRF	corticotrophin-releasing factor
CP	cerebral palsy
CPAM	congenital pulmonary airway malformation
cPAN	cutaneous polyarteritis nodosa
CPAP	continuous positive airway pressure
CPH	chronic paroxysmal hemicrania
CPK	creatine phosphokinase
CRF	chronic renal failure
CRMO	chronic recurrent multifocal osteomyelitis
CRP	C-reactive protein
CRPS	complex regional pain syndrome
CRT	capillary refill time
CS	Caesarean section
CSE	child sexual exploitation
CSF	cerebrospinal fluid
CSII	continuous subcutaneous insulin infusion
CT	computerized tomography
CTA	computerized tomography angiography
CTG	cardiotocogram
CVH	combined ventricular hypertrophy
CVL	central venous line
CVP	central venous pressure
CVS	cardiovascular system
CWP	chronic widespread pain
CXR	chest X-ray
CYP	cytochrome P450
D	dioptre
dB	decibel
dBP	diastolic blood pressure
DC	direct current
DCD	developmental coordination disorder
DCT	direct Coombs' test
DDAVP	deamino-8-d-arginine vasopressin (desmopressin)
DDH	developmental dysplasia of the hip
DEND	developmental delay, epilepsy, and neonatal diabetes
DEXA	dual-energy X-ray absorptiometry
DHEAS	dehydroepiandrosterone sulfate
DI	diabetes insipidus
DIC	disseminated intravascular coagulation
DIDMOAD	diabetes insipidus, diabetes mellitus, optic atrophy, deafness
DIRA	deficiency of the IL-1 receptor antagonist
DJF	duodenojejunal flexure
DKA	diabetic ketoacidosis
dL	decilitre
DMARD	disease-modifying antirheumatic drug
DMD	Duchenne muscular dystrophy
DMSA	dimercaptosuccinic acid
DNA	deoxyribonucleic acid
DPG	2,3-diphosphoglycerate
DPP-4	dipeptidyl peptidase 4
DPT	diphtheria, pertussis, tetanus
DRESS	drug reaction with eosinophilia and systemic symptoms
dsDNA	double-stranded deoxyribonucleic acid
DSM	*Diagnostic and Statistical Manual of Mental Disorders*

DTM&H	diploma in tropical medicine and health
DVM	delayed visual maturation
DVT	deep vein thrombosis
EAC	Ethics Advisory Committee
EBM	expressed breast milk
EBV	Epstein–Barr virus
EC	embryonal carcinoma
ECG	electrocardiogram
ECLS	extracorporeal life support
ECMO	extracorporeal membrane oxygenation
ED	emergency department
EDS	Ehlers–Danlos syndrome
EDTA	ethylenediaminetetraacetic acid
EEG	electroencephalogram
eGPA	eosinophilic granulomatosis with polyangiitis
EJV	external jugular vein
ELBW	extremely low birthweight
ELISA	enzyme-linked immunosorbent assay
EM	electron microscopy; erythema migrans
EMA	endomysial antibody
EMDR	eye movement desensitization and reprocessing
EMG	electromyogram
EMU	early morning urine
EN	enteral nutrition
eNO	exhaled nitric oxide
ENT	ear, nose, and throat
EPO	emergency protection order
ERA	enthesitis-related arthritis
ERCP	endoscopic retrograde cholangiopancreatography
ES	Ewing's sarcoma
ESES	electrical status in slow-wave sleep
ESKD	end-stage kidney disease
ESR	erythrocyte sedimentation rate
ESRF	end-stage renal failure
ET	exchange transfusion
ETAT	Emergency Triage, Assessment, and Treatment
EtCO$_2$	end-tidal carbon dioxide
ETT	endotracheal tube
EVW	episodic viral wheeze
FA	Fanconi's anaemia

factor VIIIC	factor VIII procoagulant
FAOD	fatty acid oxidation defect
FAST	Face, Arms, Speech Time
FB	foreign body
FBC	full blood count
FDG	18F-fludeoxyglucose
FDP	fibrin/fibrinogen degradation products
FEL	familial erythrophagocytic lymphohistiocytosis
FeNa	fractional excretion of sodium
FeNO	fractional exhaled nitric oxide
FEV$_1$	forced expiratory volume in 1 second
FFP	fresh frozen plasma
FGF23	fibroblast growth factor 23
FHL	familial haemophagocytic lymphohistiocytosis
FiO$_2$	fractional inspired oxygen
FISH	fluorescence *in situ* hybridization
FIX	factor IX
FLACC	Face, Legs, Activity, Cry, Consolability (scale)
FNA	fine-needle aspiration
FPIES	food protein-induced enterocolitis syndrome
Fr	French
FRAXA	fragile X syndrome
FRC	functional residual capacity
FS	febrile seizure
FSGS	focal segmental glomerulosclerosis
FSH	follicle-stimulating hormone
FTT	failure to thrive
FVC	forced vital capacity
FVIII	factor VIII
FVL	factor V Leiden
g	gram
G	gauge
GA	general anaesthesia
GA1	glutaric aciduria type 1
GAA	guanidinoacetate
GAD	generalized anxiety disorder; glutamic acid decarboxylase
Gal-1-PUT	galactose-1-phosphate uridyl transferase
GAS	group A *Streptococcus*
GBS	group B *Streptococcus*
G-BS	Guillain–Barré syndrome

GCS	Glasgow coma scale
G-CSF	granulocyte colony-stimulating factor
GCT	germ cell tumour
GDAP	ganglioside-induced differentiation-associated protein
GDD	global developmental delay
GFR	glomerular filtration rate
GGT	gamma-glutamyl transferase
GH	growth hormone
GI	gastrointestinal
GIR	glucose infusion rate
GIST	gastrointestinal stromal tumour
GLP-1	glucagon-like peptide 1
GLUT1	glucose transporter type 1
GMC	General Medical Council
GN	glomerulonephritis
GnRH	gonadotrophin-releasing hormone
GOR	gastro-oesophageal reflux
GORD	gastro-oesophageal reflux disease
GP	general practitioner
GPA	granulomatosis with polyangiitis
G6PD	glucose-6-phosphate dehydrogenase
GPI	glycosyl phosphatidylinositol
GSD	glycogen storage disease
GTC	generalized tonic–clonic
GU	genitourinary
GVHD	graft-versus-host disease
h	hour
HAV	hepatitis A virus
Hb	haemoglobin
HbA1c	glycated haemoglobin index
HBL	hepatoblastoma
HbO$_2$	oxyhaemoglobin
HBsAg	hepatitis B surface antigen
HBV	hepatitis B virus
HCC	hepatocellular carcinoma
hCG	human chorionic gonadotrophin
HCO$_3$	bicarbonate
Hct	haematocrit
HCV	hepatitis C virus
HD	haemodialysis
HE	hereditary elliptocytosis

HELLP	haemolytic anaemia, elevated liver enzymes, low platelet count
HFOV	high-frequency oscillatory ventilation
HH	hypogonadotrophic hypogonadism
HHNFC	humidified high-flow nasal cannula
HHS	hyperosmolar hyperglycaemic state
HHV6	human herpesvirus 6
HHV7	human herpesvirus 7
HiB	*Haemophilus influenzae* type B
HIDA	hepato-iminodiacetic acid
HIDS	hyperIgD syndrome
HIE	hypoxic–ischaemic encephalopathy
HIH	hiatus hernia
HIT	heparin-induced thrombocytopenia
HIV	human immunodeficiency virus
HL	Hodgkin's lymphoma
HLA	human leucocyte antigen
HLH	haemophagocytic lymphohistiocytosis
HLHS	hypoplastic left heart syndrome
HOCM	hypertrophic obstructive cardiomyopathy
HONK	hyperosmolar non-ketotic
HPA	human platelet antigen
HPC	history of presenting complaint
HPLC	high-performance liquid chromatography
HPV	human papillomavirus
HR	heart rate
HRCT	high-resolution computerized tomography
HS	hereditary spherocytosis
HSD	Hirschsprung's disease; hypermobility spectrum disorders
HSP	Henoch–Schönlein purpura
HSV	herpes simplex virus
HUS	haemolytic uraemic syndrome
HVA	homovanillic acid
Hz	oscillation frequency per second (hertz)
HZV	herpes zoster virus
IA-2	islet cell antigen 2

IAP	intrapartum antibiotic prophylaxis	IUT	intrauterine blood transfusion
IAS	intra-articular steroids	IV	intravenous
IBD	inflammatory bowel disease	IVC	inferior vena cava
IBS	irritable bowel syndrome	IVGT	intravenous glucose tolerance test
IC1	imprinting centre 1	IVH	intraventricular haemorrhage
ICD	International Classification of Diseases	IVI	intravenous infusion
ICP	intracranial pressure	IVIG	intravenous immunoglobulin
ICS	intercostal space	J	joule
ICU	intensive care unit	JAE	juvenile absence epilepsy
IDDM	insulin-dependent diabetes mellitus	JAS	juvenile ankylosing spondylitis
IDM	infant of diabetic mother	JDM	juvenile dermatomyositis
IEM	inborn errors of metabolism	JIA	juvenile idiopathic arthritis
IgA	immunoglobulin A	JPM	juvenile polymyositis
IgE	immunoglobulin E	JPsA	juvenile psoriatic arthritis
IGF	insulin-like growth factor	J-SLE	juvenile systemic lupus erythematosus
IGFBP1	insulin-like growth factor-binding protein 1	jSSC	juvenile systemic sclerosis
IgG	immunoglobulin G	JVP	jugular venous pressure
IgM	immunoglobulin M	K^+	potassium
IGRA	interferon-gamma release assay	kb	kilobase
IGT	impaired glucose tolerance	KCl	potassium chloride
IHPS	idiopathic hypertrophic pyloric stenosis	KD	Kawasaki disease
		kg	kilogram
IIH	idiopathic intracranial hypertension	KH	ketotic hypoglycaemia
		kPa	kilopascal
IL-1	interleukin 1	KS	Kallmann syndrome
IL-6	interleukin 6	L	litre
IM	intramuscular	LA	local anaesthetic
IMCI	Integrated Management of Childhood Illness	LAD	left axis deviation
		LAH	left atrial hypertrophy
IMD	inherited metabolic disease	LBP	low back pain
INR	international normalized ratio	LBW	low birthweight
IO	intraosseous	LCH	Langerhans cell histiocytosis
IPEX	immune dysregulation, polyendocrinopathy, enteropathy, X-linked (syndrome)	LCHADD	long-chain 3-hydroxyacyl-CoA dehydrogenase deficiency
		lcSSc	limited cutaneous systemic sclerosis
IPPV	intermittent positive pressure ventilation	LDH	lactate dehydrogenase
		LDL	low-density lipoprotein
IQ	intelligence quotient	LFT	liver function test
IRT	immunoreactive trypsinogen	LGA	large for gestational age
IT	intrathecal	LGBTQ	lesbian, gay, bisexual, transgender, and questioning
ITP	idiopathic thrombocytopenic purpura	LH	luteinizing hormone
		LHRH	luteinizing hormone-releasing hormone
IU	international unit	LIP	lymphoid interstitial pneumonitis
IUGR	intrauterine growth restriction/retardation		

LIPN1	lipin-1
LKS	Landau–Kleffner syndrome
LM	lymphatic malformation
LMW	low molecular weight
LOC	level of consciousness
LOS	lower oesophageal sphincter
LP	lumbar puncture
LQTS	long QT syndrome
LRTI	lower respiratory tract infection
LS	localized scleroderma
LSCS	lower-segment Caesarean section
LTBI	latent tuberculosis infection
LVH	left ventricular hypertrophy
m	metre
MA	microalbuminuria
MAC	*Mycobacterium avium* complex
MAHA	microangiopathic haemolytic anaemia
MAOI	monoamine oxidase inhibitor
MARD	mean absolute relative difference
MART	maintenance and reliever therapy
MAS	meconium aspiration syndrome; macrophage activation syndrome
Mb	megabase
MCADD	medium-chain acyl-coenzyme A dehydrogenase deficiency
McAS	McCune–Albright syndrome
MCD	minimal change disease
MCDK	multicystic dysplastic kidney
mcg	microgram
MCH	mean cell haemoglobin
MCHC	mean corpuscular haemoglobin concentration
MCI	meconium ileus
MC&S	microscopy, culture, and sensitivity
MCTD	mixed connective tissue disease
MCUG	micturating cystourethrography
MCV	mean cell volume
MDG	Millenium Development Goal
MDI	metered-dose inhaler; multi-dose injection
MDS	myelodysplastic syndrome
MDT	multidisciplinary team

MELAS	mitochondrial encephalopathy, lactic acidosis, and stroke-like episodes (syndrome)
MEN	multiple endocrine neoplasia
MERFF	myoclonic epilepsy with ragged red fibres
MFS	Marfan's syndrome
mg	milligram
Mg^{2+}	magnesium
MIBG	meta-iodo-benzylguanidine
min	minute
mL	millilitre
mm	millimetre
MMF	mycophenolate mofetil
mmHg	millimetre of mercury
mmol	millimole
MMR	measles, mumps, and rubella (vaccination)
MODY	maturity-onset diabetes of the young
mOsm	milliosmole
MPA	main pulmonary artery; microscopic polyangiitis
MPH	mid-parental height
MPS	mucopolysaccharidosis
MR	mitral regurgitation
MRD	minimal residual disease
MRI	magnetic resonance imaging
MRSA	meticillin-resistant *Staphylococcus aureus*
MRV	magnetic resonance venography
MS	mitral stenosis; multiple sclerosis
MSK	musculoskeletal
MSU	midstream urine
MSUD	maple syrup urine disease
mth	month
MTHFR	methyltetrahydrofolate reductase
MTX	methotrexate
MTV	multi-trigger wheeze
mV	millivolt
MV	mechanical ventilation
Na^+	sodium
$NAHCO_3$	sodium bicarbonate
NAHI	non-accidental head injury
NAI	non-accidental injury
NAIT	neonatal alloimmune thrombocytopenia
NAT	non-accidental trauma

NC-O_2	nasal cannula oxygen
NDI	nephrogenic diabetes insipidus
NEC	necrotizing enterocolitis
NEE	neonatal epileptic encephalopathy
NeOProM	Neonatal Oxygenation Prospective Meta-analysis
NF	neurofibromatosis (NF1, NF2)
NFCS	Neonatal Facial Coding Scale
ng	nanogram
NG	nasogastric
NGT	nasogastric tube
nHF	nasal high flow
NHL	non-Hodgkin's lymphoma
NHS	National Health Service
NHSBT	NHS Blood and Transplant
NICE	National Institute for Health and Care Excellence
NICU	neonatal intensive care unit
NIPE	newborn and infant physical examination
NIPS	Neonatal and Infant Pain Scale
NIV	non-invasive ventilation
NJT	nasojejunal tube
NLS	Newborn Life Support
NMJ	neuromuscular junction
nmol	nanomole
NO_2	nitrogen dioxide
NS	normal saline; Noonan's syndrome
NSAID	non-steroidal anti-inflammatory drug
NSPCC	National Society for the Prevention of Cruelty to Children
NTM	non-tuberculous mycobacteria
NT-proBNP	N-terminal pro-B type natriuretic peptide
O_2	oxygen
OA	oesophageal atresia; organic acidaemia
OAE	otoacoustic emission
OAS	oral allergy syndrome
OCD	obsessive–compulsive disorder
od	once daily
ODD	oppositional defiant disorder
OFC	occipitofrontal circumference
OGT	orogastric tube
OGTT	oral glucose tolerance test
OI	osteogenesis imperfecta; oxygenation index

OS	osteosarcoma
OSA	obstructive sleep apnoea
OSAS	obstructive sleep apnoea syndrome
OT	occupational therapy
OTC	ornithine transcarbamylase
PA	postero-anterior
$PaCO_2$	arterial partial pressure of carbon dioxide
PAN	polyarteritis nodosa
p-ANCA	perinuclear antineutrophil cytoplasmic antibody
PANDAS	paediatric autoimmune neuropsychiatric disorder associated with *Streptococcus*
PaO_2	arterial partial pressure of oxygen
PAPA	pyoderma gangrenosum, cystic acne and pyogenic sterile arthritis
P_{aw}	mean airway pressure
PBB	persistent bacterial bronchitis
PBSCT	peripheral blood stem cell transplant
PCA	patient-controlled analgesia
PCD	primary ciliary dyskinesia
PCH	paroxysmal cold haemoglobinuria
PCKD	polycystic kidney disease
pCO_2	partial pressure of carbon dioxide
PCOS	polycystic ovarian syndrome
PCP	pneumocystis pneumonia
PCR	polymerase chain reaction
PCV	packed cell volume
PD	peritoneal dialysis
PDA	patent ductus arteriosus
PDPE	psychologically determined paroxysmal events
PE	pulmonary embolism
PEEP	positive end-expiratory pressure
PEFR	peak expiratory flow rate
PEG	polyethylene glycol
PELVIS	perineal haemangioma, external genital anomalies, lipomyelomeningocele, vesicorenal abnormalities, imperforate anus, and skin tags
PEM	protein–energy malnutrition
PET	positron emission tomography

PFA	platelet function assay		PPV	positive predictive value
PFO	patent foramen ovale		PR	rectally, per rectum; pulmonary regurgitation
PFV	persistent intra-ocular fetal vasculature		PrAP-A	pregnancy-associated protein-A
pGALS	paediatric Gait Arms Legs Spine		pREMS	paediatric regional examination of the musculoskeletal system
PGE	prostaglandin E		PResp	parental responsibility
PGE1	prostaglandin E1		PRICE	Pressure dressing, Ice (bag of frozen peas), Rest (non-weight-bearing), Compress (cold if possible), Elevation of limb
PHACES	posterior fossa abnormalities, haemangioma, arterial anomalies, cardiac anomalies, eye abnormalities, sternal cleft or supra-umbilical raphe			
			PROM	prolonged rupture of membranes
PHVD	post-haemorrhagic ventricular dilatation		PS	pulmonary stenosis
PICU	paediatric intensive care unit		PT	prothrombin time; physiotherapy
PIE	pulmonary interstitial emphysema		PTH	parathyroid hormone
PIP	peak/positive/proximal peak inspiratory pressure		PTSD	post-traumatic stress disorder
			PTT	partial thromboplastin time
PIPP	Premature Infant Pain Profile		PTV	patient-triggered ventilation
PJP	Pneumocystis jiroveci pneumonia		PUJ	pelviureteric junction
			PUO	pyrexia of unknown origin
PK	pyruvate kinase		PUV	posterior urethral valve
PKU	phenylketonuria		PV	processus vaginalis
PLEVA	pityriasis lichenoides et varioliformis acuta		PVH	periventricular haemorrhage
PMDI	propellant metered-dose inhaler		PVL	periventricular leucomalacia
			PVNS	pigmented villonodular synovitis
pmol	picomole		PVR	pulmonary vascular resistance
PN	parenteral nutrition		PWS	Prader–Willi syndrome
PNDM	permanent neonatal diabetes mellitus		qds	four times a day
			RA	rheumatoid arthritis
PNET	primitive neuroectodermal tumour		RAD	right axis deviation
			RAH	right atrial hypertrophy
PNH	paroxysmal nocturnal haemoglobinuria		RAST	radioallergosorbent test
			RBC	red blood cell
PNPO	pyridoxamine-5'-phosphate oxidase		RCC	red cell count
			RCM	red blood cell mass
PO	orally/by mouth		RCPCH	Royal College of Paediatrics and Child Health
POCUS	point-of-care ultrasound			
POTS	post-orthostatic tachycardia syndrome		RCT	randomized controlled trial
			RDS	respiratory distress syndrome
PP	precocious puberty		REM	rapid eye movement
ppb	parts per billion		RF	rheumatoid factor
PPD	purified protein derivative		Rh	rhesus
PPE	personal protective equipment		rhGH	recombinant human growth hormone
PPHN	persistent pulmonary hypertension of the newborn			
PPI	proton pump inhibitor		RIF	right iliac fossa
ppm	parts per million		RMS	rhabdomyosarcoma
PPROM	preterm prolonged rupture of membranes		ROP	retinopathy of prematurity

RP	retinitis pigmentosa
RR	respiratory rate
RSV	respiratory syncytial virus
RT	renal tubule
RTA	renal tubular acidosis
RTH	resistance to thyroid hormone
RV	residual volume; right ventricular
RVH	right ventricular hypertrophy
s	second
SAA	severe aplastic anaemia
SAD	separation anxiety disorder
SAM	severe acute malnutrition
SAPHO	synovitis, acne, pustulosis, hyperostosis, and osteitis
sBP	systolic blood pressure
SBR	serum bilirubin
SC	subcutaneous
SCD	sickle-cell disease
SCID	severe combined immunodeficiency
SD	standard deviation
SDG	Sustainable Development Goal
SDH	subdural haemorrhage; succinate dehydrogenase
SE	status epilepticus; significant event
SENCO	special educational needs coordinator
SGA	small for gestational age
SGLT-2	sodium–glucose co-transporter 2
SHBG	sex hormone-binding globulin
sHLH	secondary haemophagocytic lymphohistiocytosis
SIADH	syndrome of inappropriate antidiuretic hormone
SIDS	sudden infant death syndrome
sIgE	specific immunoglobulin E
SIMV	synchronized intermittent mandatory ventilation
SIPPV	synchronized intermittent positive pressure ventilation
SIRS	systemic inflammatory response syndrome
SJS	Stevens–Johnson syndrome
SLE	systemic lupus erythematosus
SLICC	Systemic Lupus International Collaborating Clinics (SLICC)
SMA	spinal muscular atrophy
SMN	survival motor neuron
SN	sensorineural
SNRPN	small nuclear ribonucleoprotein polypeptide N
SOB	shortness of breath
SoJIA	systemic-onset juvenile idiopathic arthritis
SPA	suprapubic aspiration
SpO_2	pulse oximetry measurement of oxyhaemoglobin saturation
spp.	species
SPT	skin prick test
SSPE	subacute sclerosing panencephalitis
SSRI	selective serotonin reuptake inhibitor
STI	sexually transmitted infection
SUDEP	sudden unexpected death in epilepsy
SUFE	slipped upper femoral epiphysis
SUI	serious untoward incident
SVC	superior vena cava
SVT	supraventricular tachycardia
T3	triiodothyronine
T4	thyroxine
TA	tricuspid atresia; Takayasu arteritis
TaGVHD	transfusion-associated graft-versus-host disease
TAPVD	total anomalous pulmonary venous drainage
TAR	thrombocytopenia-absent radius (syndrome)
TB	tuberculosis
TBM	tuberculous meningitis
TCA	tricyclic antidepressant
TCD	transcranial Doppler
TcO_2	transcutaneous oxygen pressure
TCPC	total caval pulmonary circulation
TCPL	time-cycled, pressure-limited
TDC	thyroglossal duct cyst
TDD	total daily dose (of insulin)
T1DM	type 1 diabetes mellitus
T2DM	type 2 diabetes mellitus
tds	three times a day
TdT	terminal deoxynucleotidyl transferase
TE	expiratory time

TEM	transmission electron microscopy	UK	United Kingdom
TEWL	transepidermal water loss	U_{Na}	urinary sodium
TFT	thyroid function test	UNHS	universal newborn hearing screening
TGA	transposition of the great arteries	UPr:UCr	urinary protein-to-urinary creatinine (ratio)
TH	therapeutic hypothermia	Urbp:Ucr	urine retinol-binding protein-to-creatinine (ratio)
Ti	inspiratory time	URTI	upper respiratory tract infection
TIBC	total iron-binding capacity	US	ultrasound
TLC	total lung capacity	USS	ultrasound scan
TNDM	transient neonatal diabetes mellitus	UTI	urinary tract infection
TNF	tumour necrosis factor	UV	umbilical vein
ToF	tetralogy of Fallot	UVC	umbilical venous catheter
TOF	tracheo-oesophageal fistula	VA	visual acuity
TORCH	toxoplasmosis, others, rubella, cytomegalovirus, herpes virus II	VATER	vertebral defects, anal atresia, tracheo-oesophageal fistula, renal defects
TPA	tissue plasminogen activator	VACTERL	vertebral anomalies, anal atresia, cardiac malformations, tracheo-oesophageal fistula, renal and limb anomalies
TPN	total parenteral nutrition		
TPPPS	Toddler—Preschooler Postoperative Pain Scale		
TRAB	TSH receptor antibody	V_d	volume of distribution
TRALI	transfusion-related acute lung injury	VDDR	vitamin D-dependent rickets
TRAPS	tumour necrosis factor receptor-associated periodic syndrome	VDRL	Venereal Disease Research Laboratory (test)
		vEDS	vascular Ehlers–Danlos syndrome
TS	tricuspid stenosis; tuberous sclerosis	VEGF	vascular endothelial growth factor
TSC	tuberous sclerosis complex	VF	ventricular fibrillation
TSH	thyroid-stimulating hormone	VHF	viral haemorrhagic fever
TSS	toxic shock syndrome	VHL	von Hippel–Lindau (disease)
TST	tuberculin skin test	VIP	vasoactive intestinal polypeptide
TT	thrombin time		
TTG	tissue transglutaminase IgA antibody	VLBW	very low birthweight
TTN	transient tachypnoea of the newborn	VLCFA	very long-chain fatty acid
		VLDL	very low-density lipoprotein
TTP	thrombotic thrombocytopenic purpura	VMA	vanillylmandelic acid
		VOD	vaso-occlusive disease
U	unit	VSAA	very severe aplastic anaemia
UAC	umbilical arterial catheter	VSD	ventricular septal defect
UAO	upper airway obstruction	V_T	tidal volume
Ua:Ucr	urine albumin-to-creatinine (ratio)	VT	ventricular tachycardia
UC	ulcerative colitis	VUJ	vesicoureteric junction
UCa	urinary calcium	VUR	vesicoureteric reflux
UCD	urea cycle defect	vWD	von Willebrand's disease
UCr	urinary creatinine	vWF	von Willebrand's factor
U&E	urea and electrolytes	VZIG	varicella-zoster immunoglobulin

VZV	varicella-zoster virus
WAGR	Wilms', aniridia, gonadal dysplasia, and retardation
WBC	white blood cell
WCC	white cell count
WES	whole exome sequencing
WHO	World Health Organization
wk	week

WPW	Wolff–Parkinson–White
WS	Williams syndrome
y	year
YST	yolk sac tumour
ZIG	zoster immunoglobulin
Zp	airway pressure difference around mean airway pressure

Practising paediatrics

Professional attitudes in paediatrics

Stepping from adult medicine into paediatrics is daunting for everyone. Medical education is weighted towards care of adults, and it is of no surprise that young clinicians, after becoming competent and self-sufficient in adult practice, are frustrated when they have to ask their 'Paeds Reg' about everything, including how to take blood! Starting in paediatrics is 'like learning to walk all over again', but rest assured that every reasonable senior paediatrician is expecting you to ask for help (and will be worried if you do not) and support—our duty is patient safety, and asking for help and a senior opinion is all part of that.

Four key pointers to success in *Paediatrics and Child Health* include:

1. *Learn to enjoy working with kids.* If you're reading this, you're going to be spending a lot of time with young people—whether it is in a hospital-based emergency department (ED) or primary care clinic. If you 'don't do kids', take our advice and either learn it quickly or give up now and change career path. This may sound flippant, but there's a really important basis to the above statements—it flows something like this:
   a. If you like kids, there's a much better chance that they'll like you.
   b. If they like you, there's a good chance that they'll give you an accurate history and let you examine them without resistance.
   c. If they do this, you've got a better chance of making the right diagnosis and management plan.
   d. If you get it right, you'll enjoy your job more.
   e. If you enjoy the job more, you'll like children more and get better and better at taking histories and examining them, etc.
   f. Unfortunately, the converse is also true—if you start from a point of not liking kids, they won't like you and you'll spend a career avoiding them, and you will not to be a good clinician for it.

2. *Learn how to communicate with children.* On most paediatric wards, there is a range in age, cultural background, languages, etc. Age is the biggest variable—how you talk to a toddler is very different to how you talk to a 16y old. Go to the clinic waiting room and spend time with parents and/or the play therapist—it's well spent.

3. *Learn the power of observation.* While you're in the play room or the clinic waiting room … , learn to spot clinical signs from a child's behaviour—you'll soon develop an instinct for developmental milestones and signs of serious illness. Before long, you'll be spotting the patient that needs admission as they enter the ED.

4. *Follow up your patients.* In the world of shift work, there is little opportunity to find out if you got it right—it is a pointless educational experience if you do not find out the final diagnosis and outcome in your patient. It will improve your clinical skills.

Challenges in paediatric training

Child health is changing worldwide. Access to primary care, improvements in sanitation, and universal immunization programmes mean the spectrum of infectious diseases is changing. However, as neonatal care improves and long-term conditions are increasingly survived, the burden of chronic disease in childhood is increasing. The Internet and social media also give parents pre-formed ideas of what they think is wrong with their child and what they expect you to do about it!

Professional approach in paediatrics

If you are a novice, the skills needed to excel in paediatrics are initially daunting. Take heart. Your senior colleagues all had to learn those skills. Here are some basic attitudes that you need early on in your experience, in order to maximize your progress:

- *Open your eyes and ears at all times:* your powers of observation are critical to developing an understanding of normal child behaviour, so that you will spot the really sick child when you meet one.
- *Listen to carers and families:* their concerns contain the clues to the diagnosis; ignore them at your peril.
- *Learn to be a team player:* answer your bleep promptly; make friends with ward colleagues across all disciplines—their experience may be invaluable and you'll learn much from listening to them.
- *Know your limitations:* and ask for help if you're uncertain.
- *Follow up your patients:* reflect on the outcome of your assessments and management—it will help embed good practice and you will learn from any mistakes you make along the way.
- *Learn core knowledge:* also know where to look for more advanced knowledge (e.g. favourite apps, textbook, and local guidelines).
- *Take a broader perspective:* understand more about the upbringing and health of children in society, and in our different communities.

As you scan through this handbook, you will see that the chapters cover varying aspects of these points. Enjoy the read and personalize the text with your own annotations.

Taking a paediatric history

History taking in paediatrics is no different in aim to any other branch of medicine. The art lies not so much in knowing what questions to ask, but in what to do with the answers you receive:

1. *Timekeeping*: there are always more questions you can ask. The clock runs quickly in the ED, not much slower in an outpatient clinic, so it is important to know when to stop asking and move on.

2. *A 'focused history'*: this implies a relevant one, e.g. perinatal history is important if seeing a 2wk old with fever but is unlikely relevant when seeing a teenager with suicidal ideation. When you start out in paediatrics, you'll likely be following a set pattern (see below). After you take the history, ask yourself which questions weren't relevant in this case. You'll soon find yourself trimming down to relevant questions and mastering the art of a 'focused history'.

3. *Schematic for a paediatric history*:
   a. *Presenting complaint*: 'What brought you to hospital today?' or 'Tell me the story of what's been happening.'
   b. *History of presenting complaint (HPC)*:
      • Take each symptom of presenting complaint, and consider: when did it start? How did it start? Has anything helped? For example, if presenting with fever, how many days present, did it start suddenly, is there a response to antipyretics?
      • Are there associated symptoms or signs that you'd expect? For example, if there's a fever, is there a rash?
      • What have you done to try to alleviate the symptoms so far? For example, giving paracetamol to a febrile child.
   c. *Past medical history*:
      • Known conditions.
      • Previous hospital admissions.
      • Names of paediatricians involved in longer-term care and when they last saw the child. When is the next appointment?
   d. *Perinatal history*:
      • Gestation.
      • Need for resuscitation/neonatal unit admission.
      • Need for respiratory support—type and duration.
   e. *Medication (drug) history, including allergies*:
      • Regular medications.
      • Medications taken during this acute illness.
      • Any adverse reactions and details of what happened.
   f. *Immunization history*:
      • See the Department of Health's *'Green Guide'* for up-to-date immunization schedule for the United Kingdom (UK). Wide variance worldwide.

g. *Developmental history:*
  • Start by screening with a few memorable milestones, e.g. 'At what age did the child start to walk?', 'At what age did they say their first words?'. If your screening picks up a delay, then proceed to more detailed developmental questioning.
h. *Family history:*
  • Any childhood or young adult diseases in the family?
  • Ask if the parents are related [known as consanguinity—there is an ↑ risk of autosomal recessive (AR) conditions].
i. *Social history:*
  • Who else lives in the household?
  • Does the child/family have a social worker? If so, what is their name and contact details?
  • Sensitively, ask about domestic violence, school absences, etc.
j. *Review of systems:*
  • Not generally a part of the paediatric history, as you'll have asked most questions when taking the HPC, but worth finishing with some open questions: 'Does your child have any other symptoms you have noticed?', 'Is there anything else we haven't covered that you'd like to mention?'

Physical examination in paediatrics

Details of the clinical signs in each system are covered in the chapters that follow. Paediatric examination follows the same stages of inspection, palpation, percussion, and auscultation for each body system used in other medical examination. However, the order and which part of the body is examined vary. The choice you make of where to start and finish may be critical to successfully completing your examination. *An upset and crying child does not make it easy for you to hear a subtle heart murmur!* For this reason, you'll see paediatricians often leave the ear, nose, and throat (ENT) examination until last.

1. The *environment* in which you examine the child (e.g. ED) will be unfamiliar to them. Most children will be wary, some terrified, so you're at a disadvantage before you've introduced yourself. Cuddly toys and pictures on the walls may take the edge off a child's fears, enough to allow you to auscultate their chest. Some suggestions:
   a. *Use distraction:* tools such as mobile phones, your pen torch, an ID badge on a lanyard, and even the cardiac monitor to which the child is attached can keep the smaller child interested long enough to allow you to examine them before they realize what's happening.
   b. *Warm your hands and your stethoscope before you examine a child:* keep your stethoscope head in your hand while you're taking the history. Then clean them (hands and stethoscope!) between patients . . .
   c. *Try to avoid a noisy environment:* when auscultating a child's chest, you may find that you need quiet from bleeping monitors and ED voice intercom messages. It can be a challenge to differentiate transmitted upper airway sounds, breath sounds, and rapid heart sounds versus fine crepitations in the left lower lobe.
   d. *Keep practising:* remember that history and inspection will already have you on the right track. If you're thinking an infant has bronchiolitis, but auscultation is a struggle, try closing your eyes to block the visual sense; mentally filter out other noises until you are focused on the end of inspiration to the exclusion of all else . . . and hear the sound of fine inspiratory crepitations that clinches the diagnosis you suspected, which you confidently pronounce to your colleagues and the family.
2. *Inspection:* if a good history should give you 95% of the diagnosis, then inspection should give you 95% of the examination findings. Children and young people rarely masquerade or hide clinical signs. If they have pain in their leg, they limp. If they have an itchy eye, they rub it. Spotting the signs requires familiarity with children and your skill at observation. *Inspection starts from the moment a child enters the room.* Develop the habit of inspection, while taking the history from a parent—often this is the time the child will be most relaxed. By the

time you brandish a tendon hammer and approach the child, fear may have entered the equation and fear is the paediatrician's worst enemy for successful physical examination.

   a. *Environment:* look around you—the toys with which the child is playing (clues to developmental stage of the child), medical equipment (therapy, monitoring), feeds (high-energy/low-energy).

   b. *Appearance of the child:* scars, vascular devices, feeding tubes, birthmarks, jaundice, cyanosis, pallor, rashes.

   c. *Behaviours:* interaction between child and parent—is it consistent with the context? Is there something amiss?

3. *Palpation:* how do you tell if a 500g 24wk premature baby (whose tiny body fits almost in the palm of your hand) has abdominal tenderness confirming necrotizing enterocolitis (NEC)?

   a. Abdominal palpation is notoriously tricky to the inexperienced—but enters the realm of fine art when undertaken with care. Children don't like strangers pushing on their abdomen! Start gently, start slowly, get down on your knees to be at the child's level. Use your powers of distraction and watch the child's face. Know where your hands were when the child flinched in the middle of a discussion of their favourite TV show. More importantly, you'll know nothing—the pain was real.

   b. Palpation of other body parts is often overlooked in the name of 'efficiency', but don't—rashes must be palpated, murmurs may have thrills, chest expansion is often unequal in pneumonia, etc.

4. *Percussion:* percussion has limited uses in paediatric examination—detecting 'stony' dullness for pleural effusions and percussing out the liver edge are good examples of when it is useful and the technique varies little from examination of an adult. Tell the child what you're going to do, and you'll find children rarely resist . . . and may even find it amusing when you 'make a sound like a drum!'

5. *Auscultation:* in the public's mind, the doctor is almost obliged to use a stethoscope to make diagnoses, but generally you should have a clear idea of the diagnosis without relying on this skill. Clinical signs are similar to those of adult examination, although the interpretation and pathophysiology may be different. Use the correctly sized stethoscope diaphragm for each age. Audible signs on auscultation are dealt with in the systems-based chapters that follow.

Practical procedures

Capillary blood sampling

Capillary blood sampling is used when small volumes of blood are necessary for analysis, e.g. full blood count (FBC), blood gas, and blood glucose.

It is generally a procedure best suited to neonatal feet but can be used in older children (e.g. from fingers) if venepuncture is not possible.

Equipment

- Alcohol-impregnated swab.
- Automated device is preferred over sterile lancet because it causes less pain and reduces risk of bone damage or infection.
- Petroleum jelly.
- Appropriate sample bottles or capillary tubes.
- Cotton wool or gauze swab.

Site

- Plantar heel surface outside the medial and lateral limits of calcaneous bone in the young infant (see Fig. 2.1).
- Finger or toe in the older child.

Procedure

- Warm the site to encourage vasodilatation and good perfusion.
- In the case of foot sampling, hold dorsiflexed.
- Clean with an alcohol-impregnated swab.
- Gently massage the area, and occlude venous blood drainage using your fingers as a tourniquet.
- Apply a tiny amount of white soft paraffin—this encourages droplet formation, rather than smearing of the blood.
- Puncture the skin and collect drops of blood in sample containers.
- Avoid excessive squeezing, since it leads to falsely high serum potassium (K^+) and haematocrit (Hct) levels, as well as bruising.
- Once the sample has been collected, stop any residual bleeding by local pressure with a cotton wool ball or gauze swab.

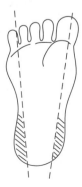

Fig. 2.1 Site for capillary blood sampling on the plantar surface of the foot. The sampling area is indicated by the shaded area.

Venepuncture

Venepuncture is preferable to capillary blood sampling when a reduced risk of haemolysis is needed and when sterility of sample is important, e.g. blood culture.

Equipment

- In older children, as in adults, a 21–23G needle and syringe or a vacuum tube should be used.
- In infants and small children, use either a 23G butterfly needle and syringe or a 21–23G butterfly needle without the normal tubing.
- A standard 21G needle will also suffice if sterility of sample is not required (blood droplets must be collected).
- Tourniquet (or assistant to restrain child and use hand as tourniquet).
- A sterilizing swab.
- Appropriate sample bottles or capillary tubes.
- Cotton wool or an occlusive plaster.

Procedure

- Suitable sites include: antecubital fossa, dorsum of the hand, and dorsum of the foot. Sometimes, other sites are used such as the scalp, particularly in infants.
- Identify a suitable vein and warm the limb, if necessary.
- Topical local anaesthetic (LA) cream under an occlusive dressing for 30–60min reduces pain and may be used in young children.
- Apply a tourniquet proximal to the venepuncture site. In infants, use your gloved fingers or ask an assistant to squeeze the limb. Also, use your fingers to stretch the overlying skin to stabilize the vein. In a young child, an assistant may need to keep the child's limb steady.
- Clean the overlying skin with a sterilizing skin swab.
- Along the line of the vein and in a proximal direction, insert the needle through the overlying skin at 20–30° into the vein until blood 'flashes' back into the needle.
- Stabilize the needle/butterfly with your fingers and then aspirate into the syringe or, if using a needle with no tubing, allow blood to drip into sample bottles. Repeated gentle release and re-tightening of tourniquet may assist blood flow.
- Once blood has been collected, release the tourniquet; remove the needle and then apply gentle pressure to the puncture site for a few minutes with cotton wool.
- Once bleeding has stopped, an occlusive plaster is optional but is often appreciated!

Intravenous cannulation

Intravenous (IV) cannulation is used for infusion of fluids or drugs. Blood sampling may also be done at the time of IV insertion. This 'combined' technique will save puncturing the child twice.

Equipment

- A sterilizing skin swab. Tourniquet or assistant's hand.
- IV cannula: sized for vein diameter, but beware small cannulae for large-volume administration. Use: 24G in newborns, 22G in children >1y old, 20G in >5y old, 16–18G in adolescents.
- IV giving set; 3-way tap, Luer lock flushed with 0.9% normal saline (NS).
- Fixing tape or transparent occlusive dressing to fix cannula in site.

Procedure

This procedure is difficult to master, particularly in newborns. Do not be afraid to ask for senior help if unsuccessful after two attempts.

- Find a suitable vein: dorsum of the hand or foot or antecubital fossa are ideal. Other sites: anatomical snuffbox, volar aspect of forearm, great saphenous vein at medial malleolus or knee. Scalp veins can be used, but shave the hair. *Tip:* transillumination of the hand or foot with 'cold' light can show 'hidden' veins in the newborn. You may need to scour the whole body and use any vein that you can find!
- 45min of LA cream (under an occlusive dressing) is needed for an effect, and remove the cream before starting.
- Ensure good vein perfusion, e.g. warm extremity before cannulation.
- If needed, ask an assistant to help with keeping the child's limb steady, which may require wrapping a young child in a sheet.
- In older children, apply a tourniquet proximal to the vein. In infants, in the hand dorsum: apply compression and immobilize by flexing the wrist; then grasp with the index and middle fingers over the dorsum, while the thumb is placed over the child's fingers.
- Clean the site with a sterilizing skin swab.
- Insert a cannula at an angle of 10–15° to the skin, with the bevel upright, just distal to, and along the line of, the vein.
- When the stylet tip penetrates into the vein, blood will flash back (unless significant circulatory collapse).
- Once the vein lumen is entered: advance 1–2mm into the vein, and then advance the cannula over the stylet into the vein.
- Remove the stylet; collect blood required from the cannula hub.
- Attach the extension set and flush the cannula with NS to confirm IV placement (should infuse without resistance) and to prevent clotting.
- Secure the cannula with adhesive tape or dressing, leaving the skin over the cannula tip visible, so that extravasation can be observed.
- Splint and bandage the extremity to prevent the cannula from being kinked by movement, or accidental displacement/removal.

Peripheral arterial blood sampling

Used for determination of arterial blood gases (ABGs), acid–base, or when large blood volumes are required and IV access is difficult.

Equipment

- As for venepuncture (see ➲ Venepuncture, p. 11).
- Point-of-care ultrasound (POCUS), if available.
- Heparinized ABG syringe or capillary tube, if analysis intended.

Procedure

- In descending order of appropriateness, the suitable sites are: radial artery (perform Allen's test and only proceed if adequate ulnar artery hand perfusion), posterior tibial artery (in newborns), dorsalis pedis artery (newborns), and ulnar artery (only if Allen's test confirms a patent adjacent radial artery). NOT the brachial artery.
- Identify artery by pulse, 'cold' light, or POCUS.
- Partially extend limb (e.g. extend wrist for radial artery sampling), and with a finger, stretch skin over artery to stabilize its position.
- Clean overlying skin using a sterilizing skin swab.
- Insert needle through skin at 15–30° into artery until blood flashes back; if no flash, withdraw slowly as blood may then appear.
- Collect blood by aspirating into the syringe/collecting from hub.
- Remove needle, and apply pressure with cotton wool or gauze swab to puncture wound for at least 5min and until bleeding has stopped.

Peripheral arterial cannulation

This procedure is indicated when repeated arterial blood sampling or invasive arterial blood pressure (BP) monitoring is required.

Equipment

As for IV cannula (see ➲ Intravenous cannulation, p. 12).

Procedure

- Identify selected artery by method described in ➲ Peripheral artery blood sampling, p. 13, and follow the procedure described, but use a cannula instead of a needle.
- When blood flashes back into the hub, advance the cannula smoothly over the stylet and into the artery.
- Remove the stylet and immediately stop the bleeding by applying pressure over the artery and the tip of the catheter with your finger.
- Connect a 3-way tap, previously flushed with heparinized NS (1U heparin/mL), and samples can be obtained from unused ports.
- Flush the arterial line with heparinized NS, and connect to an infusion pump at 1–2mL/h (1U heparin/mL).
- Connect to pressure transducer for continuous BP monitoring.

Assess perfusion distal to the cannula straight after the procedure and at regular intervals; remove the cannula if perfusion is compromised.

Umbilical arterial catheter

An umbilical arterial catheter (UAC) can be used in newborns up to 48h old for invasive BP monitoring, continuous ABG monitoring, blood sampling, fluid infusion, and/or exchange transfusion.

Site

To avoid the origins of the coeliac, mesenteric, and renal arteries, the tip of the UAC should be positioned in the aorta above the diaphragm at the T6–T10 vertebral level or in the distal aorta at the L3–L5 level.

Equipment

- Antiseptic solution, e.g. 0.5% chlorhexidine.
- Sterile surgical instruments: fine forceps, blunt-ended dilator probe, scalpel, artery forceps, scissors, suture forceps, sutures.
- Sterile drapes, gown, gauze swabs, and gloves.
- Umbilical catheters: 3.5Fr if birthweight <1500g; 5.0Fr for newborns ≥1500g. 3-way taps, IV extension sets, syringes, ligatures.
- 5–10mL syringes, one containing heparinized NS (1U/mL).
- BP transducer if monitoring is intended.

Procedure

- During the procedure, monitor the baby, e.g. use pulse oximetry oxyhaemoglobin saturation (SpO_2) monitoring. Have monitor screens in direct line-of-sight, and advise nursing staff that you will not be able to see the baby under the sterile drapes.
- Keep in mind that loss of a few millilitres of blood may cause clinical compromise in very premature or critically ill babies.
- An assistant to hold the baby's legs, with the infant supine.
- Calculate the distance (cm) to insert the UAC from the umbilicus to the aorta at T6–10 level, using the formula:

    Insertion distance $= 3 \times$ weight $(kg) + 9 +$ umbilicus stump length

- To control bleeding, tie a cord ligature around the umbilical stump.
- Catheter insertion should be performed using aseptic technique.
- Wash hands and put on sterile gloves, gown ± surgical mask. Consider double gloves, and dispose of one pair if contaminated.
- Connect a 3-way tap to catheter, and prime with heparinized NS (but do not use heparin if coagulation testing is required).
- Clean cord and periumbilical area with antiseptic solution.
- Surround periumbilical area with sterile towels for sterile field.
- Clamp the umbilical cord horizontally with artery forceps 0.5–1cm above umbilical skin. Using the artery forceps as a guide, cut the umbilical cord horizontally and immediately below with the scalpel.
- Identify the two umbilical arteries and umbilical vein (see Fig. 2.2).
- Dilate the end of one of the arteries with fine forceps or a probe until wide enough for the catheter tip to be easily introduced.

- Gently advance catheter the calculated distance (see formula). If resistance is met, put gentle traction on the umbilicus using artery forceps to ease insertion down the spiral umbilical artery.
- Aspirate blood to confirm position and take required samples. NB: arterial blood should pulsate and still bleed if catheter hub is held above the infant (unlike blood from the umbilical vein).
- Secure UAC with a zinc oxide flag around the catheter and suture to the stump (see Fig. 2.2). Check for bleeding, leaving the ligature for emergency occlusion in case of haemorrhage from the cord stump.
- Connect catheter to 3-way tap and infusion set. BP monitoring can be performed by connecting an appropriate pressure transducer.
- Confirm correct placement with chest (CXR) and abdominal X-ray (AXR). Catheter should loop initially downwards to the pelvis, as it traverses the iliac arteries before ascending up the aorta.
- Check perfusion of the perineum and lower limbs. If ischaemia occurs, it can be corrected with 2mL of NS into the catheter; if ischaemia persists, remove the catheter immediately.
- The abdomen should remain exposed to allow immediate observation of any haemorrhage, e.g. from accidental removal of catheter.

When the catheter is no longer needed, remove it. Cut the surrounding suture, then slowly withdraw the UAC, taking several minutes to remove the final few centimetres. Then apply pressure or suture to limit bleeding.

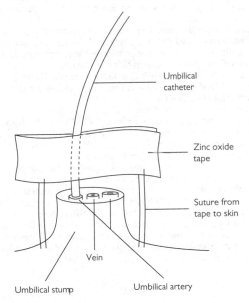

Umbilical catheter

Zinc oxide tape

Suture from tape to skin

Vein

Umbilical stump

Umbilical artery

Fig. 2.2 One method of umbilical catheter fixation.

Umbilical venous catheter

An umbilical venous catheter (UVC) is used in newborns <7 days of age for: emergency vascular access during resuscitation, inotrope or paren-teral nutrition (PN) infusions needing central venous access, or exchange transfusion.

Equipment

- 5 or 6Fr UVC.
- Remaining equipment as for UAC (see ➔ Umbilical arterial catheter, p. 14).

Procedure

- Measure umbilicus to mid-sternum (= insertion distance).
- Catheter insertion under strict aseptic technique.
- Wash hands; put on sterile gloves (consider double-gloving and disposing of one pair if contaminated), gown ± surgical mask.
- Clean, prepare umbilical stump, and create sterile field (see ➔ Umbilical arterial catheter, pp. 14–5).
- Identify umbilical vein (see Fig. 2.2), and then dilate opening with fine forceps or a dilating probe if needed.
- Insert catheter the measured distance (see insertion distance in first bullet point of this section).
- Aspirate blood to confirm insertion. Blood from the umbilical vein should not pulsate.
- If blood does not aspirate, or resistance is felt before the catheter is inserted the measured distance, it is likely the catheter tip has lodged in the hepatic portal veins or sinus. Withdraw the catheter and reinsert as far as it will go while still allowing blood aspiration.
- Flush umbilical catheter with 2mL of heparinized NS (1U/mL).
- Secure UVC and ligate any unused umbilical vessel, using method described for UAC (see Fig. 2.2).
- Remove cord ligature and check for bleeding.
- Confirm correct position in a combined CXR/AXR. UVC should only follow a direct course proximally through the liver (ductus venosus). The tip should lie in the inferior vena cava (IVC), at or just below diaphragm, and must not be in the heart or the liver.
- The catheter can now be used for blood sampling, fluid, or drugs.
- *In an emergency resuscitation*, the procedure is simplified and non-sterile:
  - Cut the umbilical cord with a scalpel blade 1–2cm distal to the umbilical skin, and rapidly insert the UVC until blood is aspirated.
  - Resuscitation drugs and fluids can then be given safely.
  - A cord ligature is good practice, but haemorrhage is unlikely because cardiac output will be minimal or absent in such an emergency! NB: caution is needed as air embolism will occur if a UVC is left open to air for any significant time.

Peripheral central venous 'long line'

For central venous infusion of concentrated IV fluids, drugs, or PN.

Sites

Sites include antecubital fossa veins and long saphenous vein anterior to the medial malleolus or inferior–medial to the knee. Less preferred sites include the axillary or scalp veins.

Equipment

- Sterile surgical instruments, including fine forceps and scissors.
- Sterile gloves, gauze swabs, gown, and drapes.
- Antiseptic solution, e.g. 0.5% chlorhexidine.
- 23 or 27G silastic long-line catheter. 27G should only be used when a 23G line cannot be inserted.
- 2–5mL syringe and heparinized NS (1U/mL).
- Introducer, e.g. 19G butterfly needle, 22G IV cannula.
- Sterile adhesive tape and transparent occlusive dressing.

Procedure

- Measure from insertion to just before the right atrium (RA) (RA catheter tip risks pericardial tamponade): *via arm*—measure from insertion, along the arm, to top of anterior axillary fold, then to sternum, at second intercostal space (ICS); *via leg*—measure from insertion to groin, then diagonally to xiphisternum; *via scalp*—measure from insertion to clavicular head, then to sternum, at second ICS.
- Catheter insertion using strict aseptic technique.
- Wash hands and put on sterile gloves, gown ± surgical mask.
- Prime catheter with sterile or heparinized NS.
- Apply tourniquet proximal to selected insertion point.
- Immobilize relevant limb, then clean insertion site with antiseptic.
- Place sterile drapes around insertion point to create sterile field.
- Insert introducer needle into vein until blood flash; remove stylet.
- Use fine forceps to advance catheter via introducer needle/cannula.
- Continue to advance catheter until desired distance is reached. *Tip:* catheter may meet resistance if it wedges in a kinked vein or valve; proximal finger-milking over the catheter may help here.
- Remove tourniquet and then flush catheter with heparinized NS.
- Once fully inserted, withdraw introducer needle/cannula. Remove from line after unscrewing catheter hub. Reconnect hub to catheter.
- Ensure haemostasis at puncture site by applying gentle pressure with sterile gauze swab. This may take some time!
- Secure line in place with thin strips of sterile adhesive tape and sterile transparent occlusive dressing.
- Start infusion of heparinized NS (1U/mL) to keep line patent.
- Confirm catheter tip with CXR (in very thin catheters, use 0.5mL of contrast). The tip should be just proximal to the RA, not in the heart.

External jugular venous cannulation

Peripheral venous cannulation is usually achieved using veins in the limbs, and less commonly sites in the scalp, abdominal wall, and neck can be used. The external jugular vein (EJV) offers an often easily visible option that can also be used to achieve central venous access, although the internal jugular vein is more commonly chosen for this. The method below assumes the aim is peripheral access, and so a 'clean', rather than 'sterile', procedure.

Equipment

- Sterilizing swabs.
- 22G peripheral cannula.
- Appropriate sample bottles or capillary tubes.
- Cotton wool or gauze swab.

Site

The EJV runs from behind the angle of the jaw, down across the sterno-cleidomastoid muscle, and pierces the fascia above the mid third of the clavicle and then empties into the subclavian vein. It is seen between the angle of the mandible and the mid clavicle.

Procedure

- Restrain patient if required (e.g. with blanket around torso).
- Turn patient's head to opposite side of access.
- A slight 5–10° downward angle of the bed will allow temporary increase in jugular venous pressure (JVP) and may aid EJV visibility.
- Occlude venous return by placing a finger on the external jugular just above the clavicle, may also aid EJV visibility.
- Cleanse the site, starting at the site itself and working outwards.
- Insert the catheter at a 10–30° angle (with bevel up), entering the EJV midway between the angle of the jaw and the mid-clavicular line.
- Advance until you feel the catheter pierce the vein or see blood in the flashback chamber.
- Carefully advance the IV catheter and withdraw the needle.
- Occlude blood flow at the catheter tip; remove the needle, and attach the IV extension set to the catheter.
- Flush the IV catheter, checking distal to the tip to look for signs of swelling that would indicate extravasation or misplacement.
- Secure IV with Steri-Strip® and sterile adhesive dressing.
- Document time of procedure, operator, IV site, and catheter size.
- A plain CXR is not routinely required but may be performed if there is doubt over the position of the cannula tip.

Airway management

Before effective ventilation can take place, the airway must be patent, which can be achieved in various ways, alone or in combination.

- *Head tilt:* tilt the head back gently to a neutral position in newborns, slightly extended in older children.
- *Chin lift:* using one or two fingers, apply forward pressure to just under the chin to pull the tongue forward.
- *Jaw thrust:* apply forward pressure behind one or both angles of the jaw to pull the tongue forward.
- *Oropharyngeal airway:* slip the airway over the tongue until the flange reaches the lips. Be careful not to push the tongue back. To determine the correct size, hold the airway along the line of the jaw, with the flange in the middle of the lips. The end of the correctly sized airway should be level with the angle of the jaw.

Endotracheal intubation

(See ➲ Endotracheal intubation, pp. 22–3.)

Suction

Not routinely required, especially in newborn resuscitation. However, if the methods described above are not successful in obtaining an adequate airway, check that the airway is not obstructed by secretions, vomit, blood, meconium, etc. If there is obstruction on inspection, or it is obvious from the start, suction should be performed using a suction catheter connected to a suction source.

Tracheotomy

Bypasses upper airway obstruction and when oral or nasal endotracheal intubation fails or is contraindicated. Perform only if already trained by a senior doctor. The description of this technique is beyond the scope of this handbook.

Mask ventilation

Mask ventilation is used during resuscitation or for short periods of assisted ventilation. It can be performed using a self-inflating bag and face mask with an appropriately sized reservoir bag. Alternatively, using a mask connected to a 'T-piece' and a continuous supply of gas, as well as a pressure-limiting device. In the latter, a breath is given by occluding the open aperture of the 'T-piece'.

Procedure

- Ensure patent airway (see ➔ Airway management, p. 20).
- Select appropriate-sized mask:
  - It should be big enough to be able to cover the face from the bridge of the nose to below the mouth, but not extend over the edge of the chin or over the orbits.
  - In infants, a round mask, e.g. Laerdal® or Bennett's mask, is most appropriate.
  - In older children, the Laerdal® moulded mask is more suitable.
- Connect face mask to an appropriate self-inflating bag or tubing with a 'T-piece' and then to an oxygen (O_2) or air supply at an adequate flow rate, e.g. 5–8L/min in the newborn.
- In newborns, a pressure-limiting valve should be used and initially be set at 25–30cmH$_2$O.
- Apply mask to face over mouth and nose, and apply enough downward pressure to make an effective seal.
- Give inflation breaths by either compressing self-inflating bag or occluding the open aperture of the 'T-piece'.
- Observe and auscultate chest wall for adequate inflation. Note whether the condition of the child is improving or deteriorating.
- If inflation is poor, or the child is deteriorating, check the airway is not obstructed (use techniques described in ➔ Airway management, p. 20 to ensure patent airway).
- Prolonged mask ventilation is likely to lead to a distended stomach. Insert an orogastric tube with free drainage in order to decompress the stomach and prevent diaphragmatic splinting.

Endotracheal intubation

Indications

Endotracheal tube (ETT) intubation is used in advanced resuscitation, or if non-invasive ventilation (NIV) is ineffective and mechanical ventilation (MV) is needed. ETT placement requires a skilled operator.

Equipment

- *Laryngoscope sizes:* neonatal straight blade sizes 0 (7.5cm long) for preterm infants and size 1 (10cm) for term infants. In older children, use curved blade laryngoscopes (Macintosh).
- *ETT size:* 2–2.5mm (internal diameter) in neonate <1000g; 3mm in 1000–3000g; 3.5mm in >3000g. Over the age of 1y, the formula for ETT diameter is: (age in years/4) + 4
- *Cuffed ETT are used in older children.*
- Use an ETT stylet during emergency intubation, but take great care to ensure the tip does not extend beyond the ETT tip.
- Lubricating jelly if attempting nasal intubation.
- Magill forceps if attempting nasal intubation.
- Suction catheter and tubing connected to suction source.
- End-tidal carbon dioxide ($EtCO_2$) monitoring device.
- Appropriate ETT connection adaptors, tubing, and O_2 source.
- Fixation device and tapes.

Procedure

- Oral ETT intubation is preferred during short-term intubation or resuscitation. Nasal ETTs are better tolerated in prolonged MV.
- Check laryngoscope light, O_2 supply, and suction are all working.
- Connect child to SpO_2 probe and cardiac monitor.
- A nasogastric tube (NGT) should be sited, and the stomach aspirated (unless intubating in a resuscitation emergency).
- Sedation/anaesthesia before elective intubation, e.g.:
  - Ketamine 2mg/kg, fentanyl 2mcg/kg, rocuronium 1mg/kg.
  - In neonates: fentanyl 2–5mcg/kg, suxamethonium 2mg/kg.
  - Use atropine 20mcg/kg if risk of vagal stimulation.
- Pre-oxygenate the child—fractional inspired O_2 (FiO_2) 0.85—for 15–30s before elective intubation.
- Place child supine. with the head neutral and neck slightly extended.
- Open the mouth and use suction to clear visible airway secretions.
- Holding the laryngoscope in the left hand, insert the blade to the right side of the mouth and advance to the base of the tongue.
- Once inserted, move the laryngoscope blade into the centre of the mouth, thereby pushing the tongue to the left.
- Advance the blade until the epiglottis is seen, and then insert blade tip into the vallecula (space between base of tongue and epiglottis).
- Vertically lift up the whole blade, thereby exposing the vocal cords (see Fig. 2.3). Apply cricoid pressure, if needed (e.g. with the little finger of the left hand), to see the vocal cords.

- If the vocal cords cannot be seen after 30s, do not attempt blind intubation. Abandon the attempt; maintain patent airway (see ➜ Airway management, p. 20), and perform mask ventilation (see ➜ Mask ventilation, p. 21), before trying again.
- When the vocal cords are seen, insert the ETT between them. If difficult or nasal intubation, use Magill forceps, with the right hand to advance the ETT tip:
  - If using a straight tube, advance the ETT until the thick black line at the tip is level with the vocal cords.
  - If using a cuffed tube, advance until the cuff is just below the vocal cords. Then inflate the cuff with air using a syringe.
- Once intubation is successful, connect tubing and start MV.
- Check for bilateral chest movement, and auscultate each lung to ensure equal and bilateral air entry. Correct ETT placement gives:
  - An $EtCO_2$ trace, and improving SpO_2 and heart rate (HR).
- Fix ETT in place appropriately following local preference.
- Perform a CXR to confirm ETT position, which should be at the level of T2 vertebra and above the carina.

Causes of intubation failure

- Poor vocal cord visualization due to neck over-extension or laryngoscope too deep; vocal cord spasm (wait, as they will open—do not force ETT, as it will cause tracheal damage); anatomical abnormalities, e.g. laryngeal atresia; vocal cord oedema.
- Conditions that give an impression of failed intubation (little chest movement on MV) include: thoracic pathology, e.g. tension pneumothorax, diaphragmatic hernia; right main bronchus intubation with unequal air entry; and particulate obstruction of airway/ETT.

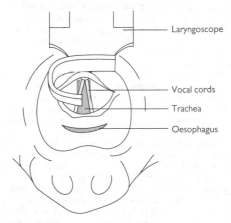

Fig. 2.3 Anatomy of laryngeal intubation.

Needle thoracentesis and chest drain

Indications

A chest drain is used to drain a pneumothorax, pleural effusion, or chylothorax. A haemothorax may need chest drainage, but only with cardiothoracic/surgical support because of risk of further bleeding. In an emergency (most commonly tension pneumothorax), drainage by needle thoracentesis should first be performed by inserting a 21–23G butterfly into the affected side in the mid-clavicular line at the second ICS. The butterfly tubing can be placed under water-seal. Alternatively, use a 3-way tap to allow aspiration with a syringe. Air can be aspirated with the syringe and then expelled through the empty port of the 3-way tap. NB: if pleural fluid is needed only for diagnosis, then use needle aspiration. A chest drain can be inserted, as follows.

Equipment

- Antiseptic solution, e.g. 0.5% chlorhexidine.
- LA, e.g. 1% lidocaine, needle, and 10mL syringe.
- Intercostal drain: 8–12Fr for newborns, up to 18Fr for young adults.
- Straight surgical scalpel blade, artery forceps, and suture.
- Sterile dressing pack, including gauze, gloves, and drapes.
- Underwater drainage system and suction pump.
- Steri-Strips® and plastic transparent dressing, e.g. Tegaderm®.

Procedure

- Child supine, with affected side raised by 30–45° using a towel.
- Raise the arm towards the head.
- Suitable sites are the fourth ICS in the mid-axillary line (be careful to avoid the nipple), and second ICS in the mid-clavicular line.
- Perform chest drain insertion with strict aseptic technique.
- Wash hands and put on sterile gloves, gown ± surgical mask.
- Clean skin over the insertion site with antiseptic solution.
- Prepare sterile field, then infiltrate a small amount of LA into the tissues down to the pleura.
- Wait 1–2min; make a small skin incision with the scalpel just above, and parallel to, rib. NB: blood vessels lie just below each rib.
  - Using artery forceps: blunt dissection to the parietal pleura.
  - Using forceps: clamp the chest drain and then insert into pleural space. Remove the trocar before drain insertion into the cavity.
- Advance the chest drain tip towards the lung apex. In a small pneumothorax, aim the tip towards the pneumothorax, remembering to aim anteriorly (air rises in the ill child lying supine).
- Connect the drain to the underwater drainage system; unclamp the drain; use –ve pressure of 5–10cmH$_2$O. Bubbling should start.
- Use single sutures to close skin wound closely around chest drain. Do not use a purse string suture, as this will increase scarring.
- Apply zinc oxide tape to chest drain and fix to skin using sutures.
- CXR to check drain position and pneumothorax/effusion drainage.

Remove drain when not required (i.e. pneumothorax resolved and no bubbling for >24h). Release holding sutures; rapidly remove drain; immediately
apply pressure, and rub with gauze swab to close underlying tissues. Apply
Steri-Strip® across skin incision to provide air-tight seal. Use CXR to confirm pneumothorax has not re-accumulated.

Pigtail pleural drain

Seldinger technique, instead of trocar:
- Advantages of pigtail drains: less traumatic insertion and fewer
  complications, suitable for very preterm babies.
- Disadvantages: may kink or obstruct due to its softer consistency.

Equipment
- An example of this device is a Cook® Fuhrman pigtail pleural drain,
  which has six side-ports. Sizes are: 6Fr/15cm for >1501g, and 5Fr/
  15cm for <1500g.
- 8G introducer needle with J-wire guide (length 40cm) and dilator.
- Radio-opaque pigtail catheter with 1cm markings (first marker 7cm).
- 3-way tap; multipurpose tubing adapter; 5mL syringe, mosquito artery
  (or similar), and sterile procedure pack.

Procedure
- Preferred site: fourth/fifth ICS; adequate analgesia/sedation; mark
  insertion site with permanent marker pen; and use sterile technique.
- Position the patient supine, with procedure side slightly upwards; identify
  landmark; 0.5–1% lidocaine local infiltration up to 1mL.
- Assemble needle and syringe, and attach mosquito forceps 1–1.5cm
  proximal to needle tip to reduce risk of deep insertion into the chest.
- Slowly insert needle (with forceps 90° to the rib) in upper rib margin
  to avoid the neurovascular bundle. Gently angle anteriorly for
  pneumothorax, aspirating until air is obtained; or if draining a pleural
  effusion, aim posteriorly and aspirate until fluid obtained.
- Remove syringe and advance J wire soft end (via introducer and needle)
  to 5cm in the chest (beware long J-wire, so keep aseptic).
- Slowly withdraw the needle; when tip is seen, hold the J-wire where it
  exits the chest wall in order to avoid accidental J-wire removal.
- Advance dilator over wire by a rotating action to pass through the chest
  wall. Then withdraw the dilator, again securing the J-wire.
- Advance catheter (coiled porthole-end first) over J-wire into chest—to
  first mark in extreme preterms; to second to fourth mark in bigger babies.
- Remove J-wire, and use Steri-Strip® to anchor pigtail to the skin.
- Place Tegaderm® dressing over insertion site.
- Connect catheter to drainage unit using adapter and 3-way tap.
- CXR to confirm position of catheter.

Intraosseous needle insertion

Indication

In an emergency, the intraosseous (IO) needle is used as an alternative to vascular access for resuscitation drugs or fluids, or for blood sampling. It counts as central access, and therefore, drugs usually administered via central venous lines can be given such as inotropes.

Equipment

- 22G IO needle and 5mL syringe.
- Sterilizing skin swab.
- LA, e.g. 1% lidocaine, 2mL syringe, and a small-gauge needle if patient conscious and LA is appropriate.

Sites

Tibial tuberosity, femoral condyle, head of humerus, anterior superior iliac spine (ASIS) of pelvis.

Procedure using trochar IO

- Identify site and inject LA if the patient is conscious.
- Clean skin with an antiseptic swab.
- Insert at 90° to the skin. Advance into bone using a rotary action.
- Advance trocar until bone cortex is reached, when a 'give' will be felt.
- Remove stylet; attach syringe, and aspirate to confirm position. Take blood samples (blood glucose and culture) if needed.
- Flush needle with NS to again confirm position. Swelling outside the bone indicates needle displacement.
- Infuse any required fluids (any IV fluid can be used).
- Obtain vascular access as soon as possible and remove IO needle.

Procedure using a powered device such as EZ-IO

- Landmarks, LA, and aseptic technique as above.
- Choose appropriate needle, and attach to drill—it will fix magnetically.
- Hold the drill and needle at 90° to the skin, and push through the skin without drilling until bone is felt.
- Now drill until there is a loss of resistance—this 'give' indicates penetration of the bone cortex.
- Remove the drill and unscrew the trochar. If clinically appropriate, attempt to aspirate marrow.
- Flush needle with NS to again confirm position. Swelling outside the bone indicates needle displacement.
- Infuse fluids if needed (use any fluid given IV).
- Obtain other vascular access as soon as possible, and then remove IO needle.

Pericardiocentesis

Indications
Drainage of a pericardial effusion or for diagnosis.

Equipment
- Antiseptic swabs and antiseptic solution, e.g. 0.5% chlorhexidine.
- 21G needle or IV cannula and 10–20mL syringe.
- Sterile gloves, drapes, gown, and adhesive plaster.
- Sterile sample containers if pericardial fluid analysis intended.

Procedure
- Lay child on a 30° slope to cause effusion to pool inferiorly.
- Locate insertion site; this lies just below the angle between the sternum and the left costal margin.
- Use sterile gloves and gown. Clean the site with antiseptic and place sterile drapes around insertion site.
- LA infiltration may be appropriate.
- Insert needle with syringe 30° to the skin and advance slowly, aiming at the left shoulder. Gently aspirate the syringe during insertion.
- Stop when pericardial fluid (usually straw-coloured) is aspirated, and remove desired amount as indicated.
- Once drainage is complete, remove needle and apply adhesive plaster.

Abdominal paracentesis

Indications
Drainage is indicated when ascites compromises breathing (e.g. hydrops fetalis) or for diagnostic purposes.

Equipment
As above for pericardiocentesis (see ➔ Pericardiocentesis, p. 27).

Procedure
In infants, the left iliac fossa is the preferred site (which avoids the liver and spleen). In older children, a midline site between the symphysis pubis and the umbilicus is preferred because of less vascularity.
- Lay the child supine, and tilt the infant towards the left side.
- Clean and prepare site (as for pericardiocentesis).
- Attach needle to the syringe and carefully insert at 90° to the skin.
- Aspirate fluid and fill sample containers. If large volumes are to be drained, use an IV cannula. Once inserted, remove stylet, and leave the cannula *in situ* to reduce risk of bowel perforation. If prolonged drainage is needed, attach cannula to skin using tape or stitches.
- Once complete, remove needle and apply sterile plaster to site.
- If a large amount of fluid is withdrawn, drainage should be followed by IV infusion of albumin.

Urethral bladder catheterization

Indications

This procedure is used for bladder decompression, e.g. potential obstruction, accurate measurement of urine output, and collection of urine for bacteriology in suspected urinary tract infection (UTI).

Equipment

- 3–8Fr urinary catheter (depending on child's size).
- Anaesthetic lubricating gel, e.g. 0.1% lidocaine gel.
- Water-based antiseptic solution, e.g. 0.5% chlorhexidine.
- Sterile urine sample container.
- Sterile gloves and adhesive tape.

Procedure

- Lay child in supine position, with hips abducted, with an assistant holding the child.
- Clean penile tip or vulval area with antiseptic solution.
- Use anaesthetic lubricating gel on catheter tip and urethral opening.
- Partially withdraw the foreskin in ♂. Part the labia in ♀.
- Insert and advance catheter into urethra in a posterior manner until urine is obtained, indicating that the bladder has been entered.
- Once in the bladder, inflate the catheter balloon with NS if the catheter is intended to be indwelling.
- Use adhesive tape to secure the catheter to the thigh.
- Connect catheter to collection bag, or aspirate urine for analysis.
- In boys, return foreskin to normal position (if retracted prior).

Suprapubic aspiration of urine

Optimal method for obtaining urine for bacteriology in <2y olds.

Equipment

- 21–23G needle and 2–5mL syringe.
- Antiseptic swabs, cotton wool or gauze swab, and adhesive plaster.
- Sterile urine sample container.

Procedure

- Wait at least 30min from last urination. If in doubt as to whether the bladder contains urine, use POCUS of the bladder to confirm.
- Place child supine (with an assistant holding hips abducted) and then identify site—midline anterior lower abdominal wall, 1cm above the pubic bone.
- Clean site with antiseptic swabs.
- Insert needle connected to the syringe at 90° to the skin, aspirating continuously until urine is obtained.
- Insert to almost the depth of the needle. If no urine is obtained, partially withdraw it before inserting again at a different angle.
- Once the required amount of urine is aspirated, remove the needle; press on puncture site with cotton wool or gauze swab, and then apply an adhesive plaster.
- Place urine in sterile container.
- If unsuccessful, repeat the procedure 30–60min later.

Lumbar puncture

Indications

To obtain cerebrospinal fluid (CSF) sample for laboratory analysis or for therapeutic CSF drainage in communicating hydrocephalus.

Contraindications

Thrombocytopenia or coagulation defect; raised intracranial pressure (ICP); significant cardiorespiratory compromise, as positioning may risk cardiorespiratory arrest; and local skin infection.

Site

L3–L4 intervertebral space (spinal cord can be as low as L2 in neonates).

Equipment

- 24–22G 1.5-inch spinal needle.
- Antiseptic solution, e.g. 0.5% chlorhexidine.
- Sterile dressing pack (including gauze, gloves, drapes).
- Three sterile universal containers for: microscopy, culture, and sensitivity (MC&S); and protein, virology, and glucose (same bottle as blood glucose).
- Adhesive plaster or aerosol plastic dressing spray.
- Manometer and 3-way tap when measuring CSF opening pressure.

Procedure

- Apply topical LA cream to site for 45min under occlusive dressing.
- Place child on their side, with back along the edge of a firm surface.
- Ask an experienced assistant to firmly, but gently, hold the child with the spine maximally flexed. Beware compromising respiration!
- Locate site—L4 spinous process lies on a line joining the iliac crests.
- Using strict aseptic technique, clean the site with antiseptic solution and then create a sterile field by surrounding it with sterile drapes.
- Inject LA into site if child is ≥6mth old.
- Insert spinal needle into intervertebral space slowly at 90° to the skin, and aim in the direction of the umbilicus, i.e. slightly cephalad.
- Slowly advance needle until the 'give', as the dura is penetrated.
- Remove stylet and wait for CSF to drain. If no drainage, advance needle very slowly and withdraw stylet every 1–2mm to check for CSF. If bone struck or needle fully inserted and still no CSF, remove the stylet and withdraw cannula slowly in case CSF appears.
- Allow 3–5 drops of CSF to drain into each sample bottle.
- When measuring CSF pressure, connect 3-way tap before collecting samples and direct fluid into manometer. Once opening pressure is measured, turn 3-way tap to allow CSF to drain.
- If therapeutic CSF drainage is required, drain the amount needed to give target CSF pressure (normal pressure 18–25cmH$_2$O).
- Once drainage is complete, remove the needle and apply a sterile gauze swab with pressure.
- Cover site with an adhesive plaster or aerosol plastic dressing.

Cerebral ventricular tap

Indications

Cerebral ventricular tap is used in non-communicating hydrocephalus, for CSF drainage, to obtain CSF for microbiological testing, e.g. to diagnose ventriculitis, and to administer intraventricular antibiotics.

Equipment

As for lumbar puncture (LP) (see ⊃ Lumbar puncture, p. 30).

Procedure

Before the procedure, cerebral lateral ventriculomegaly must be confirmed by cranial ultrasound (US), then:
- Place the baby supine, with an assistant holding the baby's head.
- Measure the necessary depth required for needle insertion.
- Palpate and locate the lateral corner of the anterior fontanelle on the intended side to drain.
- Shave a small area of scalp, at the needle insertion point if required.
- Set out sample containers ± manometer if needed.
- Full aseptic technique should be used.
- Wash hands and put on sterile gloves, gown, ± surgical mask.
- Clean area with antiseptic solution, and create a sterile field with sterile drapes.
- Insert needle into lateral corner of fontanelle in a direction slightly forward and inward, aiming towards inner canthus of ipsilateral eye.
- After the needle is inserted to the predetermined distance, remove stylet and CSF should drip out.
- When CSF pressure measurement is required, attach manometer and allow it to fill until measurement is complete.
- If CSF drainage or sample is required, then allow CSF to drip spontaneously into containers until the required amount is drained.
- Once required CSF has been drained, remove the needle and then cover with adhesive plaster or spray with plastic dressing to seal.
- The child should lie flat for the next 6h and have hourly neurological observations and BP measurement.

Exchange transfusion

Indications

- Severe or rapidly rising hyperbilirubinaemia, e.g. due to severe rhesus or other neonatal haemolytic disease (see ➲ Rh disease, p. 176).
- Cardiac failure due to severe anaemia (with normal or ↑ plasma volume), e.g. hydrops fetalis in rhesus haemolytic disease.
- Polycythaemia with venous Hct >70% and/or symptomatic: use dilutional exchange (see ➲ Polycythaemia, p. 174).
- Acute poisoning, including that due to metabolic disease.
- Life-threatening sickle-cell sequestration (e.g. chest crisis).

Exchange strategy

Exchange is achieved by sequentially removing 10–15mL of blood from the child and then infusing warmed (37°C), cross-matched, fresh (<72h old), rhesus –ve, cytomegalovirus (CMV) –ve, irradiated or leucocyte-filtered [to prevent graft-versus-host disease (GVHD)], partially packed or whole blood. Exchange transfusion can be performed by:

- Both withdrawing and then infusing blood via a single central venous catheter (e.g. UVC).
- Withdrawing blood via a central catheter (arterial or venous) or a peripheral arterial catheter and returning blood via a second central or peripheral venous catheter.

The blood volume (in millilitres) to remove and then replace (i.e. exchange):

- In severe anaemia with hydrops—requires a single-volume exchange, i.e. 80mL/kg. Perform over a minimum of 1h.
- When removing toxins (e.g. bilirubin or ammonia)—requires a double-volume exchange, i.e. 160mL/kg in newborns. This replaces >90% of total blood volume. Perform over a minimum of 2h.
- When treating polycythaemia, a dilutional exchange transfusion is used, with exchange volume depending on Hct, and calculated as:

$$\text{Volume} = [(\text{actual Hct} - \text{desired Hct}) \times \text{blood volume} (80\text{mL/kg})]/\text{actual Hct}$$

In a dilutional exchange, replace blood with NS and 0.45% albumin.

Equipment

- Venous and arterial catheters, either central or peripheral.
- Two 20mL syringes and 3-way taps.
- Blood administration set, warming coils ± high-flow infusion pump.
- Calibrated waste blood container.
- Appropriately cross-matched blood (see ➲ Indications, p. 32).
- Electrocardiogram (ECG) and BP monitor.
- Sterile dressing pack (gown, gauze swabs, drapes, and gloves).

Procedure

- Insert central or peripheral venous/arterial catheters.
- Start continuous ECG and frequent BP monitoring.

- At baseline, measure serum FBC, urea and electrolytes (U&E), calcium (Ca^{2+}), glucose, and ABG.
- Prime blood administration set and warm blood to 37°C.
- An assistant logs volumes removed and replaced.
- Use full aseptic technique throughout the procedure.
- Wash hands and put on sterile gloves, gown ± surgical mask.
- Connect 3-way taps into the system (exact arrangement depends on choice of method; see the following bullet points).
- If using a single central venous catheter (e.g. UVC), use two sequential 3-way taps to perform the following in order:
  1. Withdraw 5–20mL of blood using a syringe over a few minutes.
  2. Turn first 3-way tap to syringe waste blood into a waste bag.
  3. Turn second 3-way tap to allow 5–20mL of fresh, warmed blood to be drawn from pack.
  4. Turn tap and syringe fresh blood slowly into baby (2–3min).
- If using two catheters together:
  1. Remove 5–20mL aliquots of blood from the central or arterial catheter over 5–10min.
  2. Turn a single 3-way tap to push waste blood into waste bag.
  3. Simultaneously, the same volume of fresh, warmed blood is infused via the venous catheter using a high-flow rate infusion pump.
- A safe volume to remove each turn varies, depending on size of infant. Remove 5mL aliquots for extremely low-birthweight (ELBW) infants, increasing up to 20mL for full-term infants.
- In addition to monitoring pulse, ECG, BP, and temperature, measure every 30–60min ABG, FBC, serum U&E, Ca^{2+}, and glucose.
- Once the procedure is completed, leave catheters in place in case repeat exchange transfusion is required.

Complications of exchange transfusion

- Catheter-induced thrombotic or embolic phenomenon, e.g. portal vein thrombosis or NEC.
- Haemodynamic compromise (e.g. cardiac arrhythmia, hypotension).
- Metabolic: hypoglycaemia (transfused plasma often has low blood glucose due to red cell consumption), hypokalaemia, hypocalcaemia, hypomagnesaemia, acidaemia.
- Coagulopathy or thrombocytopenia.
- Infection: bacteraemia, human immunodeficiency virus (HIV), CMV, hepatitis B or C. Blood must be screened before transfusion.
- GVHD: risk reduced by irradiation or leucocyte filtration.

Further reading

NeoMate app (created by Neonatal Transport Service, London), available on Apple and Google Play.
NICU Tools. A useful web calculator for neonatal procedures and calculations. Available at: ℘ NICUtools.org.

Emergency and high dependency care

Emergency care: a structured approach

A major challenge for clinicians is how to identify children who require urgent treatment and admission and those most at risk of deterioration.

Recognition of the acutely unwell child

Knowledge of normal ranges for observations, normal clinical findings, and normal child behaviour are invaluable. See Table 3.1.

Table 3.1 Warning signs for acute deterioration

Age	Airway obstruction or evidence of tachypnoea (breaths/min)	
Term to 3mth	>60	
4–12mth	>50	
1–4y	>40	
5–12y	>30	
>12y	>30	
Age	Bradycardia (beats/min)	Tachycardia (beats/min)
Term to 3mth	<100	>180
4–12mth	<100	>180
1–4y	<90	>160
5–12y	<80	>140
>12y	<60	>130
Age	Action systolic pressure (mmHg)	
Term to 3mth	<60	
4–12mth	<65	
1–4y	<70	
5–12y	<80	
>12y	<90	

Altered mental state or convulsion

Low pulse oximetry values: <90% in any supplemental oxygen (<60% if cyanotic heart disease).

The structured approach to initial management

Use the 'ABCDE' sequence of assessment in the acutely ill child. Check frequently and reconsider the diagnosis if no improvement.

A—Airway

Assessment

A crying/talking child has a patent airway. Upper airway noises are common; stridor is particularly noteworthy and needs monitoring.

Provide oxygen

Use FiO_2 1.0 (100%)—up to 2L/min via nasal cannulae; up to 15L/min via face mask and non-rebreather bag.

Maintain airway
If obstruction detected, support airway, e.g. with jaw thrust and:
- Suction nasopharynx and mouth, as needed.
- Insert oral or nasopharyngeal airway if tolerated.
- *Maintain patient in position of their choice:* do not force a distressed patient to lie down. Sitting minimizes respiratory effort.

B—Breathing
- Check SpO_2 and aim to keep >92%.
- Assess degree of difficulty in breathing: respiratory rate (RR) and any signs of respiratory distress.
- *Identify the level of respiratory involvement:* treat specific problems appropriately (e.g. bronchodilators for wheeze).
- Consider respiratory support:
  - Non-invasive, e.g. with humidified high-flow nasal cannula O_2 therapy or continuous positive airway presssure (CPAP).
  - Invasive, i.e. ETT intubation and MV if respiratory arrest or signs of respiratory failure despite the above.

C—assess circulation
- Start cardiac monitoring.
- Check HR, BP, central capillary refill time (CRT) (normally <2s).
- Establish vascular access: peripheral cannula or use an IO needle to avoid delay (attempt IO by 2min if there is difficulty).
- *Consider fluid bolus:* if signs of circulatory failure, treat with 10–20mL/kg of IV NS and assess response; repeat as needed.
- *Start inotropes:* if BP low despite adequate fluid resuscitation.
- Monitor fluid status by measuring input and output closely.

D—assess disability
- Assessment of Glasgow coma scale (GCS) score: See ➔ Altered LOC: Glasgow Coma Scale, p. 61.
- Check pupil with a bright light source:
  - Unequal pupils point to focal neurology (e.g. cranial nerve VI palsy).
  - Small pupils are associated with opiate use.
  - Large pupils seen in seizures and fear after atropine administration.
- *DEFG—Don't ever forget glucose:*
  - Hypoglycaemia is common in the younger child.
  - If having seizures, check glucose as an easily treatable cause.

E—exposure
- Visible signs of serious illness/injury are important clues.
- Rashes: See also ➔ Chapter 21.

Respiratory failure

Respiratory failure in children is usually preceded by signs of respiratory distress which must always be looked for. The hallmarks are accessory muscle use and tachypnoea. Respiratory failure can be caused by disorders of gas exchange [O_2 absorption or carbon dioxide (CO_2) elimination], respiratory drive, neuromuscular disease, and infection (see Box 3.1).

Box 3.1 Causes of respiratory failure

Nasopharyngeal obstruction
- *Nose*: choanal atresia or stenosis.
- *Oropharynx*: tonsillar hypertrophy.
- *Tongue*: glossomegaly.
- *Pharynx*: peritonsillar abscess, retropharyngeal abscess, diphtheria.

Upper airway obstruction
- *Larynx*: vocal cord dysfunction, subglottic stenosis or cyst, laryngomalacia, papilloma, haemangioma, croup.
- *Epiglottis*: epiglottitis, FB.

Lower airway obstruction
- *Trachea*: tracheitis, tracheobronchomalacia, FB, pulmonary artery sling.
- *Bronchi*: bronchitis, bronchomalacia.
- *Bronchioles*: asthma, bronchiolitis.

Disordered gas exchange
- Hb: CO poisoning, methaemoglobinaemia, acidosis.
- Ventilation–perfusion mismatch: pulmonary hypertension, pulmonary haemorrhage, pulmonary embolism (PE), sickle chest crisis.
- Dead space ventilation ('air trapping'): asthma, bronchiolitis.
- Reduction in alveolar surface area: pneumonia, pulmonary oedema/effusion, pneumothorax/chylothorax.

Impaired respiratory drive
- Hyperventilation: psychogenic, brainstem tumour.
- Hypoventilation: CNS injury, toxins, acidosis.

Neuromuscular dysfunction
- *Respiratory muscle weakness:* Duchenne muscular dystrophy (DMD), spinal muscle atrophy (SMA), CNS depression.
- *Chest wall injury:* rib fracture, flail chest.

Clinical assessment

Assess the patient for the following:

- *Colour:* pallor or cyanosis.
- *Respiratory drive:* pattern and timing of breathing may reflect a central or brainstem cause.
- *Inspiration and expiration of air at the mouth and nose:*
  - Upper airway obstruction produces stridor.
  - Lower airway obstruction leads to cough, wheeze, and a prolonged expiratory phase.
- *Chest wall movement:* chest and abdominal wall dynamics may indicate flail chest, diaphragmatic palsy, pneumothorax, or foreign body (FB) inhalation (asymmetrical chest wall movement).
- *Position and level of agitation.*
- *Mental state.*
- *HR and perfusion:* these may reflect an impending arrest.

Investigations

- *Non-invasive:* SpO_2.
- *ABG:* assessment of acid–base, arterial partial pressure of O_2 (PaO_2) and CO_2 ($PaCO_2$).
  - A capillary blood sample is a good alternative for pH and pCO_2 if the extremity is warm and blood flows freely.
- *Blood tests:* FBC, U&E, glucose, cultures.
- *CXR:* for diagnosis (e.g. severe pneumonia); for assessment of complications (e.g. pulmonary oedema, pneumothorax) (see Box 3.1).
- *POCUS of thorax:* for diagnosis (e.g. pulmonary effusion).
- *Peak expiratory flow rate (PEFR) or spirometry:* assessment of severity of asthma.

Therapy

The focus of therapy in respiratory failure is the 'B' of the ABCD approach (see ➲ Emergency care: a structured approach, pp. 36–7).

- *First step:* O_2 therapy and ventilatory support.
- *Specific treatment directed at cause,* e.g.:
  - Antibiotics for pneumonia.
  - Bronchodilators for asthma, etc.
- *Fluid therapy:* in acute respiratory failure, without shock, restriction of fluid volumes (e.g. to two-thirds of usual maintenance) is often used because of the risk of the frequent occurrence of syndrome of inappropriate antidiuretic hormone (SIADH) secretion.

Emergency upper airway presentations

Laryngotracheobronchitis (croup)

Typically caused by viral infections (parainfluenza type 3) with sudden onset of loud cough (like seal bark), progressing to stridor—use:

- Steroids [e.g. oral (PO) dexamethasone 0.15mg/kg STAT or 2mg nebulized budesonide] usually sufficient to reduce severity of symptoms.
- If *severe airway obstruction* (hypoxic, visibly tiring): 4mL of 1:1000 adrenaline nebulized (monitor for rebound as effect).
- If *signs of toxicity* and fever: think bacterial tracheitis (rare, but important in the differential) and give antibiotics (e.g. co-amoxiclav).

Foreign body inhalation

FB aspiration is commoner in toddlers and infants, who tend to put objects in their mouths. FBs can be inhaled into the airway or they may get caught in the oesophagus. Common examples include seeds, grapes, parts of toys, batteries, and coins. Many are radiolucent, and therefore not visible on plain CXR.

Symptoms

The symptoms of FB inhalation range from no symptoms to complete airway obstruction. The level and degree of obstruction determine the signs and symptoms. Persistent cough is commonest:

- *Larynx:* hoarseness, cough, dysphonia, haemoptysis, stridor.
- *Trachea and bronchus:* cough, wheeze, may present with recurrent pneumonia in an otherwise healthy child.
- *Oesophagus:* drooling, dysphagia, or vomiting.

Diagnosis

- A monophonic *wheeze or absent breath sounds* are classically described, but infrequently detected.
- CXR and neck *radiographs*, with lateral views, may reveal asymmetry and an area of air trapping, indicating the location of an object. Expiratory films may further reveal the area of hyperinflation if partial obstruction.
- *Bronchoscopy* is required if high degree of suspicion.

Initial treatment

Prioritize good oxygenation (SpO_2 >92%). In the out-of-hospital setting, a spontaneous cough is most effective and should be encouraged:

- If the child is apnoeic, back blows and/or chest thrusts should be used, as per standard paediatric resuscitation protocols.
- As with all upper airway disorders, airway muscle tone is highly sensitive to stress, so keep the child calm (e.g. on parent's lap).
- Definitive treatment with bronchoscopy and removal of FB under direct visualization requires general anaesthesia (GA).
- Consider the most likely type of FB; most cause local inflammation. Button batteries are time-critical, as discharging current erodes nearby soft tissue structures (e.g. trachea, aorta).

Other disorders of the nasopharynx

Epistaxis

Nosebleeds (epistaxis) are common. Usually, no obvious cause, but may be associated with minor nasal trauma; rarely caused by coagulation disorder [e.g. acute lymphoblastic leukaemia (ALL)]. Purulent, unilateral bloody nasal discharge should raise suspicion, and initial care is:

- *Sitting position* with head tilted forwards.
- *Pressure* to cartilaginous part of the nose (finger and thumb for 15min).
- *Refer to ENT:* if simple measures fail to stop bleeding, nasal packing and cauterization under direct visualization are needed.
- *Blood tests:* FBC, clotting screen, blood group testing.

Nasal FB

Children may present with offensive, unilateral nasal discharge. FB removal is urgent because the object may be inhaled. If the patient can cooperate, have them try to blow their nose; alternatively, attempt removal by dislodging with a suitable instrument:

- Use alligator-type forceps to remove cloth, cotton, or paper FBs.
- Pebbles, beans, and other hard FBs are removed by rolling them out and getting behind them with an ear curette or a right-angle hook.
- If these measures are unsuccessful, refer to ENT.

Nasal polyps

Infrequent, but associated with allergic rhinitis or cystic fibrosis (CF). Signs include clear rhinorrhoea, post-nasal drip, and nasal obstruction. Snoring may be a feature. Treat with topical corticosteroids (e.g. fluticasone).

Gingivostomatitis

Gingivostomatitis is characterized by multiple sores and mouth ulcers. Common in preschool children and secondary to viral infection:

- Herpes simplex: cold sores and acute herpetic stomatitis.
- Coxsackie viruses: hand, foot, and mouth disease, and herpangina.

Vesicular lesions may erupt on the lips, gums, tongue, and hard palate. Clinical features range from mild to severe, characterized by:

- Pain on eating and drinking, high fever, bleeding from gums.
- Extensive ulceration of the tongue, palate, and buccal mucosa.
- Cervical lymphadenopathy and dehydration (poor intake).

Investigations

Usually no specific tests are required for the diagnosis. Nevertheless, blood for Coxsackie virus or herpesvirus serology and culture of material obtained from the surface of the sore may identify the viral infection.

Treatment

Use symptomatic and supportive treatment, including:

- *Analgesia:* mouth spray (e.g. benzydamine), oral hygiene mouthwash.
- *Supportive fluids:* may need admission for rehydration with IV.
- *Severe infection:* may need treatment with PO or IV aciclovir.

Status asthmaticus

(See also ➲ Asthma: long-term management, p. 236.)

Status asthmaticus is a severe exacerbation of asthma that does not respond to initial bronchodilator therapy and is a medical emergency.

Symptoms

Acute presentation of asthma is characterized by rapid onset of wheeze and difficulty breathing. Multiple triggers should be looked for in the history [e.g. inhaled smoke, exercise, cold air, pollen, upper respiratory tract infection (URTI)]. *Life-threatening* status asthmaticus has the following characteristics:

- SpO_2 <92%, may be cyanosed *in extremis*.
- PEFR <33% at best or predicted.
- Silent chest and poor respiratory effort.
- Raised $pCO_2/PaCO_2$ hypotension, and exhaustion are end-stage signs.

Initial treatment

- ABCDE assessment: if SpO_2 <94%, use high-flow O_2 via face mask with non-rebreather bag.
- *Life-threatening asthma* requires prompt use of IV bronchodilators and anaesthetic review, as ETT intubation and MV may be needed.
- *Severe asthma attacks* (PEFR 33–50% of best, only speaks short sentences) may respond to inhaled bronchodilators and steroids:
    1. *Inhaled β_2-agonist*: 100mcg salbutamol × 10 puffs via metered-dose inhaler (MDI) and spacer, or 2.5–5mg nebulized if O_2 requirement or non-responder.
    2. *Ipratropium bromide*: 250mcg nebulized and mixed with β_2-agonist if symptoms are refractory to initial β_2-agonist.
    3. *Magnesium sulfate*: 250mcg can be added to each nebulized β_2-agonist and ipratropium in the first hour for children with a short duration of acutely severe asthma symptoms.
    4. *Steroids*: give PO steroids early (prednisolone 10mg for children <2y, 20mg for those aged 2–5y, 30–40mg for children >5y). Children on maintenance treatment should have 2mg/kg prednisolone (maximum 60mg). Repeat dose if child vomits or consider IV hydrocortisone 4mg/kg 6-hourly if life-threatening.
    5. *IV magnesium sulfate*: dose of 40mg/kg for children who respond poorly to first-line treatment.
    6. *IV salbutamol*: consider early bolus dose in life-threatening asthma, when aerosol salbutamol is likely ineffective. Use bolus 15mcg/kg IV over 10min, then an infusion (1mcg/kg/min, with maximum 20mcg/kg/min). Monitor for signs of toxicity (e.g. lactic acidosis, jitteriness, nausea, vomiting, and hypokalaemia).
    7. *IV aminophylline*: if unresponsive to maximum doses of bronchodilators and steroids, use 5mg/kg IV loading, followed by infusion. Monitor signs of toxicity (e.g. headaches, gastric irritation, arrhythmias) and use continuous cardiac monitoring and sampling for plasma theophylline levels every 12h.

Ongoing treatment

Once the patient is stable, the following can be considered:
- *Nebulizers:* if established on IV bronchodilators, there is no additional benefit from continuing nebulized β_2-agonist. Ipratropium bromide nebulizers can be continued 4-hourly.
- *Steroids:* should continue for at least 3 days; duration of treatment can be extended if recovery is slow.
- *ETT intubation:* consider when there is hypoxia or signs of fatigue despite using the treatment outlined above. Do not wait for pCO_2/ $PaCO_2$ retention (late sign). ETT intubation and MV in asthmatics are challenging, so ensure senior staff members (paediatric and anaesthetic) are present. During MV, use slow rate (e.g. 16–20/min) and match intrinsic positive end-expiratory pressure (PEEP) because of the risk of dynamic hyperinflation.

Recovery

- The child can be discharged when stable, with SpO_2 >94% on room air and on 3- to 4-hourly inhaled bronchodilator therapy.
- Follow-up with primary care within 2 days of discharge from hospital, in order to review and reinforce education.
- Follow-up in an asthma clinic is recommended if hospital admission has been required or if there are frequent ED attendances.
- All patients should be given an *asthma action plan* detailing usual medications and actions to take if there is another asthma attack.

Drowning

Drowning is an infrequent, but highly distressing, cause of death in childhood. Usually, only a small volume of water (<22mL/kg) is aspirated; in ≤10%, there is laryngospasm without aspiration. The type of water is of little consequence, but water temperature is important because hypothermia is a factor in the deaths.

Aetiology

Children <3y old and teenagers are most at risk. Ask for the duration of submersion, water temperature, and resuscitation attempts; consider:
• Head and neck injuries from diving.
• Pre-existing cardiac arrhythmia or seizure disorder.
• Drug and alcohol abuse.

Initial treatment

• *A/B:* the neck may be injured, or the airway obstructed by particulate material.
• *C:* poor perfusion occurs in children with severe hypoxic–ischaemic encephalopathy (HIE) or pulmonary oedema. Treat any arrhythmia, but adrenaline and amiodarone may be ineffective and have a prolonged half-life with temperature <32°C. Similarly, direct current (DC) shock may be ineffective until core temperature is >32°C.
• *D—temperature:* remove wet clothing in order to avoid further cooling. Aim to achieve core temperature >35°C (use a heating blanket and warmed IV fluids); invasive methods of warming may be used on the intensive care unit (ICU), e.g. bladder and gastric lavage.

After resuscitation

• *Antibiotics:* broad-spectrum antibiotics should be considered in children after resuscitation. Bacterial risk typically occurs in fresh water and includes Gram –ve infections, anaerobes, and fungi.
• *Neurological:* if there is HIE or brain swelling with raised ICP, so-called neuroprotective measures should be applied in all cases.
• *Respiratory:* at risk of acute lung injury (ALI) and acute respiratory distress syndrome (ARDS); consider whether the child would benefit from extracorporeal membrane oxygenation (ECMO).
• *Metabolic:* at risk of rhabdomyolysis and renal failure on warming, so monitor serum creatine phosphokinase (CPK) and U&E.

Cardiac emergencies

(See also ➜ Chapter 5.)

Cardiogenic shock

Shock is defined as failure to deliver adequate O_2 to the tissues to maintain cell function. Cardiogenic shock occurs in the context of:

- *HR disturbance:* bradycardia, tachyarrhythmias.
- ↓ *stroke volume:* hypovolaemia, poor contractility, obstruction.

In early shock, findings can be subtle and easily missed (see Box 3.2). Many features are shared with other disease presentations and experience counts more than numbers in the recognition of early shock.

> ### Box 3.2 Signs of shock
> *Early shock*
> - *Pulse:* tachycardia.
> - *BP:* normal, but postural drop.
> - *Breathing:* tachypnoea.
> - *Limbs:* cool and mottled.
> - *CNS:* agitated, becoming drowsy.
> - *Laboratory:* metabolic (lactic) acidosis.
>
> *Late shock*
> - *Pulse:* tachycardia and weak pulses; bradycardia when peri-arrest.
> - *BP:* profound hypotension.
> - *Breathing:* bradypnoea suggests peri-arrest.
> - *Limbs:* cool, clammy, and pale or blue.
> - *CNS:* depressed LOC.
> - *Laboratory:* metabolic acidosis, multiorgan dysfunction and failure.

Treatment
Initial therapy includes the following.

- O_2: provide supplemental O_2, FiO_2 1.0. Early ETT intubation and MV will assist left ventricular function.
- *Position:* in congestive heart failure, elevate the head.
- *IV access:* central access is usually required for monitoring central venous pressure (CVP), or mixed venous saturation, and inotropes.
- *Temperature:* control fever with antipyretics.
- *Biochemistry:* correct hypoglycaemia and hypocalcaemia. Use IV magnesium (Mg^{2+}) if arrhythmia (may help to stabilize the myocardium).

Fluid volumes for shock
- If concerned about cardiac cause, reduce IV fluid bolus to increments of 5–10mL/kg NS.
- *Stop fluid volume resuscitation when there is/are:*
  - Clinical improvement.
  - Signs of volume overload: hepatosplenomegaly, JVP distension, gallop rhythm, wheeze, or crackles.

Inotropes for shock
Start inotropes when circulation is unsatisfactory (especially if low BP) despite fluid resuscitation or CXR showing large heart, pulmonary vascular congestion, pulmonary oedema, or effusion (see Box 3.3).

> **Box 3.3 ICU treatments for shock**
>
> *Inotropes*
> • Dopamine: 5–20mcg/kg/min (start at 10mcg/kg/min). Can use peripherally if no CVL available.
> • Adrenaline: 0.05–1mcg/kg/min (start at 0.05–0.10mcg/kg/min).
> • Noradrenaline: 0.05–1mcg/kg/min (start at 0.05–0.10mcg/kg/min).
>
> *Hypotension refractory to volume and single inotrope*
> • Combinations of inotropes may be required.
> • Discuss with paediatric intensive care.
> • Consider steroids, e.g. hydrocortisone 1–2mg/kg qds.
> • Afterload reduction may be helpful adjunct in cardiogenic shock: milrinone 0.5mcg/kg/min.

Congestive heart failure

Usually slower onset than cardiogenic shock above; the patient may have sweating on exertion or feeding, malaise and irritability, or ↓ appetite. The physical findings include:
• *Tachycardia:* gallop rhythm on auscultation.
• *Tachypnoea:* wheeze and crackles on auscultation.
• *Raised JVP:* hepatosplenomegaly and oedema.
• *Pale or mottled and cool extremities; hypotension.*
• *CXR:* cardiomegaly, pulmonary vascular congestion, or oedema.

Treatment
Use fluid restriction and inotropic support after cardiology advice.
• *Diuretics:* furosemide 0.5–1mg/kg three times a day (tds); spironolactone 0.5–1mg/kg twice a day (bd).
• *Angiotensin-converting enzyme (ACE) inhibitors:* e.g. captopril.

Pericarditis

There may be chest pain or features of the underlying cause. Look for:
• Congestive heart failure.
• Friction rub.
• Pulsus paradoxus (>10mmHg).

When cardiac tamponade is present, there are classic signs of:
• Shock.
• Distended jugular veins.
• Heart sounds appearing distant.
• *ECG:* ↓ voltage, elevated ST segment and inverted T-wave.
• *CXR:* the heart will look enlarged if an effusion is present.

Hypertension

Definition

Systolic BP (sBP) or diastolic BP (dBP) >95th percentile for age, height, and sex, using the appropriate-sized cuff. Use standard charts (see ➔ Hypertension, p. 343), but upper limits of normal BP are:

- *<2y*: sBP, 110mmHg; dBP, 65mmHg.
- *3–6y*: sBP, 120mmHg; dBP, 70mmHg.
- *7–10y*: sBP, 130mmHg; dBP, 75mmHg.
- *11–15y*: sBP, 140mmHg; dBP, 80mmHg.

Treatment

(See ➔ Hypertension: management, p. 348.) For severe, symptomatic hypertension, BP should be lowered by 20–25%. Do not aim for normal levels immediately.

- Discuss early with nephrology and ICU teams.
- Hypertensive encephalopathy is an emergency and too rapid lowering of BP may lead to stroke.
- Use short-acting antihypertensives and consider:
  - *Diazoxide*: 1–3mg/kg IV rapid infusion; repeat after 5–15min.
  - *Hydralazine*: 100–500mcg/kg IV over several minutes (maximum dose 20mg). May repeat dose in 20–30min.
  - *Sodium nitroprusside infusion*: starting dose 500ng/kg/min.

Congenital heart disease

(See also ➲ Congenital heart disease, p. 197.) In cyanotic congenital heart disease (CHD) babies, the history and examination can be used to exclude respiratory causes of cyanosis. The assessment includes the hyperoxia test (measurement of PaO_2 after 10min of FiO_2 1.0].

- *PaO_2 <13.3kPa (100mmHg):* possible cyanotic heart disease.
- *PaO_2 13.3–26.7kPa (100–200mmHg):* possible heart disease with complete mixing and ↑ pulmonary blood flow.
- *PaO_2 >33.3kPa (>250mmHg):* cyanotic heart disease unlikely.

Treatment

(See also ➲ Circulatory adaptation at birth, Management, p. 149.) In neonates, consider alprostadil [prostaglandin E1 (PGE1)] infusion if a duct-dependent cardiac lesion is suspected:

- PGE1 dose:
  - 10–50ng/kg/min (start at 5–10ng/kg/min; use 5ng/kg/min increments if response is not adequate).
  - Be aware that apnoea may develop, but if signs of cardiogenic shock, early intubation and ventilation needed anyway.

Dysrhythmias

(See also ➔ Palpitations, p. 196; ➔ Cardiac arrhythmias, p. 220–1.)

Sinus bradycardia and heart block

If there is haemodynamic instability (i.e. hypotension or poor perfusion), significant bradycardia is present if the HR is:

- <80/min in neonates.
- <50/min in infants.
- <40/min in older children.

Do not immediately treat if asymptomatic and consider non-cardiac causes of bradycardia such as raised ICP, acidosis, or hypercapnia. If vagal stimulus is a possible cause, give atropine (10–20mcg/kg IV).

Tachydysrhythmia

These may be:

- *Narrow complex* (QRS normal/<0.12s): supraventricular tachycardia (SVT) and atrial flutter. P waves not visible in SVT.
- *Broad complex* (QRS >0.12s): ventricular tachycardia (VT).

Supraventricular tachycardia

If haemodynamically stable, consider the following:

- *Vagal manoeuvres:* ice bag to face for 15–20s or unilateral carotid massage or Valsalva manoeuvre. Do not compress the orbits.
- *Adenosine:* 50–100mcg/kg as rapid IV push (maximum 500mcg/kg, 300mcg/kg <1mth).
- *DC shock:* synchronized shock 1J/kg should be reserved for the haemodynamically unstable. ETT intubation and appropriate analgesia and sedation are required first.
- *Other:* amiodarone, procainamide, and flecainide, with specialist cardiology advice.
- *If recurrent:* β-blockers (e.g. atenolol) usually commenced; radiofrequency ablation if persistent or Wolff–Parkinson–White (WPW) syndrome.

Ventricular tachycardia

If haemodynamically stable and pulse present, consider the following after advice from cardiology specialist:

- Amiodarone 5mg/kg; synchronized shock if ineffective.
- Pulseless VT is managed as cardiac arrest: DC shock 4J/kg, adrenaline, and amiodarone.

Box 3.4 Differential diagnosis for cyanosis

Alveolar hypoventilation
- *CNS:* seizures; cerebral oedema; haemorrhage; infection; hypoxia/ischaemia; drugs.
- *Hypothermia.*

Ventilation–perfusion inequality
- *Lung:* bronchiolitis, pneumonia, pneumothorax, pleural effusion, respiratory muscle dysfunction [e.g. muscular dystrophy, myasthenia gravis, Guillain–Barré syndrome (G-BS)].
- *Cardiac:* ↓ pulmonary blood flow [tricuspid atresia, pulmonary atresia with intact ventricular septum, critical pulmonary stenosis, tetralogy of Fallot (ToF)]; ↓ systemic perfusion [coarctation of the aorta (CoA), sepsis].

Impairment of oxygen diffusion
- *Lung:* bronchopulmonary dysplasia (BPD), hypoplasia, diaphragmatic hernia.

Right-to-left shunting
- *Cardiac:* CHD, Eisenmenger syndrome, AV fistula—pulmonary or systemic.
- ↓ O_2 *affinity for Hb:*
  - *Methaemoglobinaemia:* measured by blood gas analyser—may be hereditary or toxin-mediated (e.g. aniline dyes, nitrobenzene, azo compounds and nitrites).
  - *Carboxyhaemoglobinaemia:* usually related to smoke inhalation (hyperoxygenate until resolution).

Cyanosis

Cyanosis is the result of deoxygenated haemoglobin (Hb) or abnormal Hb in red blood cells (RBCs). Cyanosis is apparent when there is 4g/dL of reduced Hb or 0.5g/dL of methaemoglobin. Anaemic patients may not become cyanosed, even in the presence of marked SpO_2 desaturation. In light-skinned patients, cyanosis is usually noted with SpO_2 <85%.

Central cyanosis is best seen in the tongue. All peripheral areas (lips, perioral area, fingers, nose) will take on a blue hue in the presence of central cyanosis. However, they are also (and very commonly) sensitive to ambient temperature and/or peripheral vasoconstriction unrelated to deoxygenated Hb levels.

A full assessment of cardiovascular, respiratory, and gastrointestinal (GI) systems will be needed to identify the cause. If a cause is not found, prompt investigation (e.g. analysis of methaemoglobin) is important. Acute cyanosis is often life-threatening.

Clubbing

This sign may be present in the older infant or child and indicates long-standing cyanosis in CHD, but other paediatric causes include:
- Hereditary.
- Idiopathic.
- Cyanotic CHD.
- Infective endocarditis.
- Pulmonary conditions (e.g. CF).
- GI disease [e.g. Crohn's disease (CD), ulcerative colitis (UC), cirrhosis].

Causes of cyanosis

The differential diagnosis of cyanosis is shown in Box 3.4, in which causes can be categorized broadly as:
- *Pulmonary impaired gas exchange:*
  - Alveolar hypoventilation.
  - Ventilation–perfusion inequality.
  - Impairment of O_2 diffusion.
- *Cardiovascular pump misdirection:* right-to-left shunt.
- *Haematological:* ↓ affinity of Hb for O_2.

Anaphylaxis

Anaphylaxis is a life-threatening systemic immune-mediated allergic reaction (see also ➲ Anaphylaxis, p. 524–5).

Symptoms

The reaction includes involvement of:
- *Respiratory system:* acute stridor and/or wheeze.
- *Cardiovascular system (CVS):* hypotension and shock.
- *Associated signs of immunoglobulin E (IgE)-mediated allergic reaction:* lip/eye swelling, urticarial rash, sneezing, abdominal pain, vomiting, diarrhoea.

Aetiology

The symptoms of anaphylaxis are usually abrupt, often within minutes of exposure to an allergen. The triggers include:
- *Drugs:* penicillin, muscle relaxants (in GA).
- *Injections:* radiographic contrast dyes.
- *Stings:* bites and envenomations.
- *Foods:* e.g. peanut, tree nuts, eggs, sesame.
- *Exercise:* rare.

Initial treatment

- *Standard ABCDE resuscitation.*
- *Epinephrine (adrenaline):* give IM 10mcg/kg (0.01mL/kg of 1:1000 adrenaline). Repeat every 15min if required.
- *Antihistamine:* chlorphenamine IV 250mcg/kg.
- *Salbutamol:* if wheezing, give nebulized salbutamol 2.5mg for <4y and 5mg for ≥4y of age, every 15min if required.
- *Steroid:* give IV bolus hydrocortisone 4mg/kg if vomiting or in shock, or PO prednisolone [once daily (od)] for up to 5 days.
- *Hypotension:* adrenaline as slow IV bolus (1mcg/kg or 0.01mL/kg of 1:10 000). Adrenaline IV infusion may be needed, as well as fluid resuscitation to restore normal BP.

Hypovolaemic shock

Shock is characterized by inadequate systemic (major organ) perfusion. The commonest type—hypovolaemic shock—is related to abnormally low circulating blood volume.

Aetiology

Causes of hypovolaemia include:

- Trauma.
- GI bleeding (see ⊃ Gastrointestinal haemorrhage, p. 280).
- Burns.
- Peritonitis.
- Severe gastroenteritis (see ⊃ Gastrointestinal infections, pp. 306–7).

Initial treatment

- *Airway, Breathing, Circulation, Disability (ABCD).*
- *Fluid:* BP and perfusion need to be restored urgently with IV bolus 20mL/kg NS, and repeated as necessary. If >60mL/kg is required, consider ETT intubation, MV, and inotropes.
- *Blood:* in patients with significant blood loss, transfusion will be required and is given in preference to crystalloid in trauma/surgery cases [5mL/kg, with equal aliquots of 5mL/kg of fresh frozen plasma (FFP)]. Also refer to any 'massive transfusion protocol' for administration of blood, platelets, and FFP.
- *Refractory hypotension:* inotropic support (see Box 3.2).

Monitoring the response

- *HR should be watched carefully:* it will typically show temporary improvement with each bolus of IV fluid, and once approaching normal HR range, sufficient fluid has been given.
- Similarly, a *temperature gradient* may be felt on limbs with distal warming as effective fluid resuscitation is given.
- *Non-invasive BP* may not give accurate dBP, but aim for sBP in normal/higher normal range.
- Palpate for *hepatomegaly* (or monitor CVP) and auscultate lungs for signs of pulmonary oedema that suggest fluid overload.

Burns

Most burns in children need referral to a specialist burns unit. There are different forms of thermal injury to the body, including:
• Contact with fire.
• Scalding fluids.
• Chemicals.
• Electricity.
• Inhalation of flame, heated vapour, and toxic fumes.
• Cold freezing injury.

Severity

The severity of the burn is categorized by the depth of skin affected:
• *First-degree:* limited to epidermis; painful and erythematous.
• *Second-degree:* includes epidermis and dermis. Superficial is blistered and painful, and deep is white and painless.
• *Third-degree:* includes epidermis and all of the dermis; painless, pale, and leathery.

Surface area

For the extent of the burn as a proportion of the body surface area (% BSA), see Box 3.5.

Box 3.5 Contribution of different body parts to total body surface area at different ages

	Body part area/total BSA (%) at ages		
Body part	<1y	1–11y	>11y
Head	18	13	9
Trunk (front)	18	18	18
Trunk (back)	18	18	18
Arm	9	9	9
Leg	14	16	18
Genitalia	1	1	1

Symptoms

Symptoms of inhalation in the lung
• Tachypnoea.
• Signs of airway obstruction (wheeze/stridor).
• Black sputum.

Aetiology

You should find out the following about the injury:
- Mechanism and agent(s) causing the burn.
- The duration of exposure.
- Environmental factors (closed or open space).
- Loss of consciousness during the accident.
- Any child safeguarding considerations should be escalated early.

Investigations

Major burns (i.e. >5% BSA) or smoke inhalation or electrocution
- ABG.
- Carboxyhaemoglobin level.
- FBC and cross-match.
- Serum U&E, creatinine, and CPK.

Treatment

Initial approach and standard protocol
- *ABC:* if inhalation injury, request early anaesthetic review and ETT intubation before oedema leads to critical airway obstruction.
  - In smoke inhalation, consider *carbon monoxide (CO) poisoning* and measure carboxyhaemoglobin level. Give humidified FiO_2 1.0.
  - Consider *cyanide exposure and poisoning* if breath smells of almonds, or fire-related accident, or anion gap metabolic acidosis.
  - If >10% BSA affected, consider an IV bolus of NS (20mL/kg). If >25% BSA, use the Parkland's formula (see Box 3.6).
- *Analgesia:* treat pain early (e.g. IV morphine 100mcg/kg)
- *Other injuries:* do a secondary survey of associated traumatic injuries. Assess for cardiac and skeletal muscle injury in electrical accidents. In chemical burn, wash and neutralize the chemical.
- SpO_2 and *cardiac monitoring* are useful, but remember their limitations in CO poisoning.
- *Eyes:* examine the eyes for burn or abrasion.
- Give tetanus *immunoprophylaxis* if required.

Box 3.6 Parkland's formula

0–24h after burn
Crystalloid
- 4mL/kg per 1% BSA burn.
- Use 50% of this volume in the first 8h.

24–48h after burn
Crystalloid + colloid
- Use 50–75% of fluid requirements on day 1.
- Add albumin (1g/kg/day) to maintain serum level >2g/dL.

Box 3.7 Paediatric 'sepsis 6'

1. High-flow O_2

Face mask and reservoir bag at 15L/min: give irrespective of SpO_2.

2. Access

IV or IO access. Do not delay treatment while trying to establish IV access. Resuscitation can start with IO access.

3. Antibiotics

- *When:* do not delay first dose because of tests, but it is worthwhile trying to get a blood culture first.
- *Which:* broad-spectrum antibiotics as per local guidance, IV or IO (e.g. ceftriazone 80mg/kg). In the following instances:
  - Age <8wk: consider group B *Streptococcus* and *Listeria* (e.g. cefotaxime and amoxicillin).
  - Indwelling IV catheter: consider *Staphylococcus aureus* (e.g. anti-staphylococcal cover, teicoplanin).
  - Intra-abdominal pathology: consider gut anaerobe (e.g. metronidazole, gentamicin).
  - Immunosuppressed or oncological: *bacteria*—piperacillin-tazobactam and gentamicin; *fungi*—amphotericin; *herpes simplex or varicella*—aciclovir.
  - TSS, cellulitis, or fasciitis: consider adding clindamycin which has anti-inflammatory effects.

4. Fluid therapy

NS at 20mL/kg unless differential includes cardiac disease—then give in smaller increments of 5–10mL/kg. Repeat boluses of 20mL/kg until normal HR and BP, or signs of cardiac failure (see ➲ Hypovolaemic shock, p. 53).

5. Inotropes

Commence dopamine peripherally at 10mcg/kg/min and add (nor) adrenaline IV once CVL is obtained.

6. Escalate

Ensure senior members of the team are informed (e.g. paediatric and anaesthetic consultants). Escalate to the ICU team early.

Sepsis

Sepsis is 'life-threatening organ dysfunction caused by a dysregulated host response to infection' and is accompanied by signs of systemic toxicity. In this chapter, the recognition and treatments for sepsis are considered. Management of the commonly associated hypovolaemic shock is covered in ➔ Cardiogenic shock, p.45; ➔ Hypovolaemic shock, p. 53; ➔ Bacterial meningitis and septicaemia, pp. 634–5.

Clinical assessment

Fever and tachycardia are hallmarks of infection, but non-specific. Evidence of end-organ dysfunction (lactic acidosis, coagulopathy, confusion, hypotension) are late signs ('septic shock'), leaving a considerable 'grey area' where treatment for sepsis may need to start and then be suspended once there is no progression to shock.

Investigations

All organ systems may be involved in sepsis, so consider these tests:

Blood

- FBC with differential.
- Coagulation state: international normalized ratio (INR), activated partial thromboplastin time (APTT), fibrinogen.
- Serum U&E and creatinine.
- Liver function tests (LFTs): alanine aminotransferase (ALT), aspartate aminotransferase (AST), gamma-glutamyl transferase (GGT).
- Arterial or capillary blood gas (lactate may be raised).
- Inflammatory markers, e.g. C-reactive protein (CRP) and/or erythrocyte sedimentation rate (ESR).

Sepsis screen

- Blood culture.
- Urine culture.
- Stool (viruses and bacterial culture).
- LP for CSF: MC&S, viral PCR, glucose, and protein.
- Other cultures: throat, wound, samples from indwelling catheters.

Monitoring

- Continuous SpO_2.
- Continuous ECG.
- Hourly BP.
- Hourly urine output.

Therapy

Early and timely implementation of the six treatments in Box 3.7 improves outcomes and needs to be prioritized within 1h of recognition of severe sepsis or septic shock.

Altered level of consciousness

The brain can be injured in many ways. Its responses to injury include any combination of:
- Altered level of consciousness (LOC) or agitation.
- Seizures, dystonia, or weakness.
- Impaired respiratory function.
- Loss of cardiovascular autoregulation.
- Cerebral swelling and raised ICP.
- SIADH.

Take a note of:
- When symptoms started and progression (gradual versus sudden).
- Possible ingestion or exposure to medication or toxins.
- Possible recent trauma, illness, or exposure to infection.
- History of previous seizures, LOC.
- Family history and consanguinity.

Aetiology

Infectious causes
- Meningitis, encephalitis (see ➔ Chapter 16).
- Toxic shock.
- Subdural empyema, cerebral abscess.

Autoimmune
- Acute disseminated encephalomyelitis (ADEM) (see ➔ Acute disseminated encephalomyelitis, p. 398)
- *Toxins:* (see ➔ Poisoning, p. 67).
- *Neoplastic causes:* brain tumours (see ➔ Central nervous system tumours, p. 596–7).

Trauma
- *Head injury:* concussion or contusion.
- *Haemorrhage:* epidural, subdural, intracerebral.

Vascular causes
- Arteriovenous malformation (AVM).
- Aneurysm, venous thrombosis.

Metabolic causes
- Hypoglycaemia (see ➔ Hypoglycaemia, p. 78–9).
- Diabetic ketoacidosis (DKA) (see ➔ Diabetic ketoacidosis, p. 80–1).
- Inborn errors of metabolism (IEM), (see ➔ Inborn errors of metabolism, p. 82).
- Hepatic encephalopathy.
- *Endocrine:* thyroid, adrenal, pituitary (see ➔ Chapter 10).
- Uraemic encephalopathy.

Other
- Seizures and post-ictal state.
- Hypertension (see ➔ Hypertension, p. 47).
- Hydrocephalus (see ➔ Hydrocephalus, p. 380).
- Hypoxia–ischaemia.

Initial examination in children with depressed LOC

General examination can provide an explanation for the patient's state. After the ABCD assessment, a focused neurological assessment is then needed (see Box 3.8). Look for evidence of ↑ ICP and potential site of intracranial lesion.

General

- *Vital signs:* make a note of the adequacy, rate, and depth of respiration, HR and rhythm, BP, and body temperature.
- *MedicAlert® bracelet:* search for a bracelet or tag, or other information that may indicate a long-standing medical condition.
- *Skin:* examine for evidence of trauma, rash, petechiae, jaundice, and needle tracks.
- *Breath:* check for odours of alcohol, ketones, or toxins.

Head and neck

- *Head:* if the anterior fontanelle is patent, a tense fontanelle indicates ↑ ICP, whereas a sunken fontanelle suggests dehydration.
- *Nose and ears:* leakage of blood or CSF; 'raccoon eyes' or battle sign suggest basal skull fracture.

Pupils

- *Small (2–3mm) reactive pupils:* suggest metabolic cause of coma.
- *Mid-size (4–5mm) unreactive, mid-position pupils:* suggest midbrain lesion.
- *Pinpoint (1–2 mm) pupils:* indicate a pontine disorder but are also commonly associated with opiates.
- *Unequal pupils with one fixed and dilated:* suggest a brain disorder on the side of the dilated pupil.
- *Bilateral fixed, dilated pupils:* imply a poor prognosis, although similar pupils may be produced by mydriatics (e.g. atropine), barbiturate intoxication, and hypothermia.

Fundi

Examine for evidence of retinal haemorrhages and papilloedema.

Signs of raised ICP

Signs of raised ICP include:
- Abnormal respiratory pattern.
- Unequal or unreactive pupils.
- Impaired or absent oculocephalic or oculovestibular responses.
- Systemic hypertension with bradycardia and apnoea (Cushing's triad).
- Tense fontanelle.
- Abnormal body posture (decerebrate or decorticate) or muscle flaccidity.

Box 3.8 Specific neurological presentations

Pattern of respiration
- *Cheyne–Stokes* (alternating apnoea and hyperpnoea): can be seen with metabolic disturbance, bilateral cerebral hemisphere dysfunction, and insipient temporal lobe herniation.
- *Central neurogenic hyperventilation* (deep rapid respiration): can occur with hypoxia–ischaemia, hypoglycaemia, or lesion between low midbrain and mid pons.
- *Ataxic respiration* (irregular depth and rate): can be caused by abnormality of the medulla and impending respiratory arrest.
- *Apneustic breathing* (gasping, respiratory arrest in inspiration): indicates pontine involvement.

Eye movements
- *Roving eye movements:* seen in light coma without structural brain disease.
- *Absence of movements:* suggests infratentorial disorder or drug intoxication.
- *Abnormality of lateral gaze:* the eyes are deviated towards the side of a destructive cerebral lesion and away from an irritative cerebral lesion. In a brainstem lesion, the eyes are directed away from the side of the lesion.

Lateral eye movement reflexes
Lateral eye movements are mediated by brainstem structures and require an intact midbrain and pons. These are assessed clinically by:
- *Oculocephalic reflex (doll's eye):* sudden turning of the head from one side to the other normally causes conjugate deviation of the eyes in the direction opposite to that in which the head is turned. *Do not test when the neck is unstable.*
- *Oculovestibular reflex (cold caloric):* cold water irrigated into the ear with the head held 30° above the horizontal normally causes conjugate deviation of the eyes towards the side of the irrigation.

Motor function and posture
- *Decorticate rigidity:* the arms are held in flexion and adduction, and the legs in extension. This signifies a lesion in the cerebral white matter, internal capsule, or thalamus.
- *Decerebrate rigidity:* the arms are extended and internally rotated. The legs are extended. Occurs with lesions from the midbrain to mid pons and with bilateral anterior cerebral lesions. Can also be seen with metabolic abnormalities or hypoxia–ischaemia.

Altered LOC: Glasgow Coma Scale

As a summary of the conscious state, the GCS score should be used (see Boxes 3.9 and 3.10). It is also a useful tool for monitoring changes. An alternative, rapid assessment is the AVPU scale for identifying impaired consciousness (Alert, responding to Voice, responding to Pain, Unresponsive).

Box 3.9 GCS: scores for older children

Response	Score
Eye opening (E)	
Spontaneous	4
To verbal stimuli	3
To pain	2
None	1
Best verbal (V)	
Orientated	5
Confused speech	4
Inappropriate words	3
Non-specific sounds	2
None	1
Best motor (M)	
Follows commands	6
Localizes pain	5
Withdraws to pain	4
Flexes to pain	3
Extends to pain	2
None	1

Reproduced from Teasdale G, Jennett B. (1974) Assessment of coma and impaired consciousness. A practical scale. *Lancet* Jul 13; 2(7872): 81–4, with kind permission from Elsevier.

Box 3.10 GCS scores adapted for infants

Response	Score
Eye opening (E)	
Spontaneous	4
To speech	3
To pain	2
None	1
Best verbal (V)	
Coos and babbles	5
Irritable cries	4
Cries to pain	3
Moans to pain	2
None	1
Best motor (M)	
Normal	6
Withdraws to touch	5
Withdraws to pain	4
Abnormal flexion	3
Abnormal extension	2
None	1

Reproduced from Teasdale G, Jennett B. (1974) Assessment of coma and impaired consciousness. A practical scale. *Lancet* Jul 13; 2(7872): 81–4, with kind permission from Elsevier.

Altered LOC management

Investigations where unknown cause

- *Blood:* FBC, coagulation, glucose, U&E, LFTs, ammonia, lactate.
- *Toxicology:*
  - Urine, blood, gastric aspirate for ingestions.
  - Serum lead and free erythrocyte protoporphyrin.
- *Acid–base:* ABG.
- *Microbiology:* blood and urine cultures; viral respiratory PCR.
- *Imaging:*
  - Cranial computerized tomography (CT) scan; brain magnetic resonance imaging (MRI) is better for posterior fossa or white matter lesions.
  - Electroencephalography (EEG).

Lumbar puncture

Defer LP if there are signs of raised ICP, focal neurology, or active bleeding. Examine CSF for MC&S, glucose, protein, and viral PCR.

Bacterial meningitis

- >20 white blood cells (WBCs)/mm³ with a polymorphonuclear neutrophil leucocyte predominance.
- An elevated protein level >100mg/dL.
- Low glucose <2mmol/L (or <50% of plasma level).

Encephalitis

- 20–1000 WBCs/mm³ with lymphocyte predominance.
- CSF protein may be normal or mildly up; viral PCR may be +ve.
- Glucose is usually normal (70% of plasma level).

Monitoring

Monitoring will be dictated by the cause of LOC. When concerned about acute neurological deterioration, use 20min 'neuro observations' (i.e. GCS score, pupil reaction, HR, BP, fluid balance).

Treatment

- *ABC:* the initial priority.
- IV antibiotics (e.g. ceftriaxone and clarithromycin). Add aciclovir if risk of HSV encephalitis.
- Dexamethasone [IV 150mcg/kg, four times/day (qds) for 4 days] if >3mth and pneumococcal meningitis possible cause.

Suspected raised ICP

- *GCS ≤8:* rapid sequence ETT intubation and MV to normocapnia.
- Maintain sBP at upper end of normal range.
- Head of bed elevated to 30°, with head in the midline.
- 3% (hypertonic) saline 3mL/kg over 15min and repeat as necessary. Otherwise mannitol (IV 0.25–1g/kg) can be used.
- Limit maintenance IV fluids to two-thirds of usual maintenance rates.

Status epilepticus

The new International League Against Epilepsy definition for status epilepticus (SE) considers two time points as important:

- T_1, 5min: the time by which antiseizure medication (ASM) should be given for an abnormally prolonged seizure.
- T_2, 30min: the time after which an ongoing seizure will result in brain injury.

Aetiology

The common causes of childhood SE include:

- Known epilepsy ± subtherapeutic anticonvulsant levels.
- Genetic/metabolic abnormalities.
- Fever.
- Symptomatic: central nervous system (CNS) infection, trauma, and poisoning.

Investigations

If the cause of a seizure/SE is clear, then investigation may not be required. When the trigger is unclear:

- Glucose: hypoglycaemia is common and easily treated.
- Brain imaging: CT or MRI.
- EEG.
- LP if safe to do so (see ➔ Lumbar puncture, p. 30; ➔ Lumbar puncture, p. 63; ➔ Diagnostic testing, p. 635).
- *Blood*: Mg^{2+}, U&E, Ca^{2+}, glucose, and creatinine levels.
- ABG.
- *Toxicology*: blood and urine.
- Anticonvulsant levels in those on anticonvulsants.
- FBC and WBC differential.

Initial treatment

Box 3.11 summarizes the ASM treatment according to time after seizure begins. At all stages, reassess ABC and resuscitate, if required.

Once the seizure has stopped

After termination of clinical seizures:

- *Ensure no ongoing seizures* (suspect if persistent tachycardia and abnormal pupillary responses). Intermittent irregular myoclonic jerks are common but do not need further treatment.
- *After prolonged seizures*, the child may have a respiratory arrest and require ETT and MV support.
- *Airway support* (e.g. oropharyngeal or nasopharyngeal airway insertion) may be needed.
- Roll child into *lateral recovery position* to reduce risk of aspiration.
- Continue O_2 *therapy* until breathing pattern has become normal.

Box 3.11 Antiseizure medication in status epilepticus

0–5min: ABC
- Note time.
- Call for help.
- Consider whether it is a genuine epileptic seizure.
- Check glucose.
- Establish IV access.
- Monitor vital signs, especially SpO_2.
- Give 100% O_2 via mask.

5min: start ASM if seizure is ongoing
- Use IV lorazepam (100mcg/kg, up to 4mg), OR
- If no IV/IO access: rectal diazepam (0.5mg/kg) or buccal midazolam (0.5mg/kg).

15min: repeat ASM if seizure is ongoing
- If there is no response, repeat the dose of lorazepam IV or IO.

25min: repeat ASM if seizure ongoing
- Load with IV phenytoin (20mg/kg, over 20min), OR
- IV phenobarbital (20mg/kg, at rate <1mg/kg/min) if already on phenytoin as regular antiepileptic medication.

45min: refractory SE (failure to respond to two ASM classes)
- If seizures persist, ICU care should be initiated because a continuous infusion is needed (practice varies but includes midazolam versus ketamine versus short-acting barbiturate like thiopental).
- ETT intubation and a period of MV will be required until the underlying cause of seizure is treated/resolves.

Box 3.12 Clinical effects: causative drugs or poisons

- *Depressed respiration:* antipsychotics, carbamate pesticides, clonidine, cyclic antidepressants, alcohol, narcotics, nicotine.
- *Tachycardia, high BP:* amphetamines, antihistamines, cocaine.
- *Tachycardia, low BP:* salbutamol, CO, tricyclic antidepressants (TCAs), hydralazine, iron, phenothiazine, theophylline.
- *Bradycardia, high BP:* clonidine, ergotamine, ephedrine.
- *Bradycardia, low BP:* calcium channel blockers, clonidine, digoxin, narcotics, organophosphates, phentolamine, propranolol, sedatives.
- *AV block:* astemizole, β-adrenergic antagonists, calcium channel blockers, clonidine, cyclic antidepressants, digoxin.
- *VT:* amphetamines, anti-arrhythmics (encainamide, flecainide, quinidine, procainamide), carbamazepine, chloral hydrate, chlorinated hydrocarbons, cocaine, TCAs, digoxin, phenothiazine, theophylline.
- *Torsades de pointes:* amantadine, antihistamines (astemizole), cyclic antidepressants, lithium, phenothiazine, quinidine, sotalol.
- *Coma with miosis:* alcohol, barbiturates, bromide, chloral hydrate, clonidine, ketamine, narcotics, organophosphates, phenothiazine.
- *Coma with mydriasis:* atropine, CO, cyanide, cyclic antidepressants, glutethimide.
- *Hypoglycaemia:* alcohol, insulin, oral hypoglycaemic agents, propranolol, salicylates.
- *Seizures:* amphetamines, anticonvulsants (carbamazepine, phenytoin), anticholinergic, antihistamines, camphor, CO, chlorinated hydrocarbons, cocaine, cyanide, TCAs, isoniazid, ketamine, lead, lidocaine, pethidine, phenothiazine, phenylpropanolamine, propranolol, theophylline.
- *High AG ($[Na^+] - [Cl^-] + [HCO_3^-]$) metabolic acidosis:* alcohol, CO, cyanide, ethylene glycol, iron, isoniazid, methanol, salicylate, theophylline.
- *Low AG:* bromide, lithium, hypermagnesaemia, hypercalcaemia.

Odours
- Acetone, alcohol, bitter almonds (cyanide), garlic (heavy metals), oil of wintergreen (methyl salicylates), pears (chloral hydrate), carrots (water hemlock).

Bedside or laboratory tests include:
- *Urine:* dip-tests and toxicology.
- *Blood:* ABG (including carboxyhaemoglobin level); glucose, U&E, LFTs, coagulation profile; suspected drug levels in blood.
- *ECG:* 12-lead for assessment of rhythm and QT interval.
- *X-rays:* AXR to detect radio-opaque tablets (e.g. iron).

Poisoning

Peak incidence of childhood accidental poisoning is 2–3y, with most cases at home. In older children, suspect self-poisoning or self-harm.

Aetiology

Parents usually know the name and amount of material ingested. Obtain the bottle/container of ingestant and get these details:
- *Exact name of the drug* or chemical exposure.
- *Preparation and concentration* of the drug exposure.
- *Probable dose* in mg/kg, as well as maximum possible dose.
- *Time since ingestion or exposure.*
- *Check the national toxicology database (TOXBASE®).*

Symptoms, signs, and testing

Poisoning produces various signs and symptoms. Consider each body system and think of potential causes and tests (see Box 3.12).

Initial treatment of poisoning

Follow the ABCDE resuscitation approach and seek advice early from your regional or national poisons centre (see Box 3.13).

Gastrointestinal decontamination

Rarely recommended because of aspiration risk. Gastric lavage and emesis are not recommended. Consider *activated charcoal* (AC) if:
- Presentation within 1h of ingestion and toxin absorbed by AC.
  - Patient managing and protecting own airway, no LOC, AND
  - Substance is highly toxic and difficult to treat.
- *PO or nasogastric (NG):* 1g/kg is used for possible adsorbed substances.
- DON'T if *risk of aspiration* (e.g. bowel obstruction, ileus, no gag).
- DON'T after alcohol, iron, boric acid, caustics, lithium, electrolyte.

Eyes and skin decontamination

Irrigate eyes with NS until pH <8.0. Wash skin with water.

Urinary alkalinization

- Urinary alkalinization (pH 7–8) helps to eliminate weak acids (salicylates, barbiturates), but beware of electrolyte disturbance.
- Use IV sodium bicarbonate ($NaHCO_3$, 1–2 mmol/kg), followed by ↑ maintenance fluids (1.5–2 times) with added $NaHCO_3$.

Box 3.13 Antidotes/substrates (always consult a toxicologist)

Paracetamol (acetaminophen)
- Children taking >150mg/kg need assessment. Risk of liver damage is likely with doses >250mg/kg.
- Take blood 4h after ingestion and use nomogram. Give acetylcysteine if high or staggered dose. Check LFTs and INR.
- Acetylcysteine: IV load 150mg/kg, then 50mg/kg over 4h, and then 100mg/kg over 16h. Repeat blood level at 24h.

(Continued)

Box 3.13 (Contd.)

Anticholinergics, antihistamines (diphenhydramine), plants (deadly nightshade, jimson weed, henbane), anti-Parkinsonian drugs, dilating eye drops, skeletal muscle relaxants
- *Benzodiazepines:* use if agitation and seizures (avoid phenytoin).
- *Physostigmine:* for anticholinergic syndrome—reverses agitation and seizures. Slow IV 20mcg/kg. Repeat every 5min, but maximum total dose <2mg. Use atropine for cholinergic symptoms.

Benzodiazepines: chlordiazepoxide, clonazepam, diazepam, temazepam
- If ABCs are stable, there is little need to do more than observe.
- *Flumazenil:* reverses lethargy and coma. *NOT* for TCA or chloral hydrate overdose or for child with seizure disorder on benzodiazepines. Give 10mcg/kg over 1min.

β-adrenergic antagonists: atenolol, esmolol, labetalol, propranolol
- *Glucagon:* useful for reversing bradycardia and hypotension. Give 0.05–0.1mg/kg bolus, followed by 0.1mg/kg/h infusion.
- *Atropine, isoprenaline, and amiodarone:* can be used if bradycardia or hypotension persist after glucagon.
- Cardiac pacing may be needed.

Calcium channel blockers: diltiazem, nifedipine, nimodipine, verapamil
- Use glucagon, amrinone, isoprenaline, atropine, and dopamine for hypotension unresponsive to fluids and Ca^{2+}.
- Give calcium chloride (20mg/kg of 10% solution) or calcium gluconate (100mg/kg of 10% solution) for hypotension and bradyarrhythmias. Consider *cardiac pacing*.

Carbon monoxide fire; exhaust from fuel engines, furnaces, or burners; paint remover with methylene chloride
- Ensure ABCs and use FiO_2 1.0.
- Check carboxyhaemoglobin level.
- Also consider cyanide toxicity if smoke inhalation.

Cyanide
- There are special kits for rescue that will be in pharmacy.
- *Sodium nitrate 3%:* dose depends on Hb level, but do not give if CO poisoning as well.
- *Sodium thiosulfate 25%:* dose depends on Hb level.

Digoxin
- Measure serum drug level. Toxicity occurs with level >2ng/mL.
- Check U&E, Mg^{2+}, thyroxine, and Ca^{2+}.
- Correct hypokalaemia.
- If *hyperkalaemic:* give insulin and dextrose, $NaHCO_3$, and Kayexalate®. Do not give calcium chloride or calcium gluconate because these potentiate ventricular arrhythmias.
- *Digoxin-specific antibody (FAB fragments):* give for ventricular dysrhythmias or supraventricular bradyarrhythmias, hyperkalaemia,

Box 3.13 (*Contd.*)

hypotension, heart block. Phenytoin may be used to improve AV conduction. Avoid quinidine, procainamide, isoprenaline, or disopyramide if AV block present.

Ethylene glycol, methanol
- *Fomepizole* (loading 15mg/kg, then 10mg/kg bd for four doses).
- If not available, use ethanol (loading dose 0.6g/kg).
- Other agents: *pyridoxine* 2mg/kg and thiamine 500mcg/kg.
- In the case of methanol, also give *folic acid* (50–100mg over 6h).

Iron
- Measure serum concentration 2–6h after ingestion. A level >350mcg/dL is frequently associated with systemic toxicity. If ingestion <20mg/kg, no treatment needed.
- *Desferrioxamine*: IV infusion 5–15mg/kg/h in all cases of serious poisoning (i.e. based on symptoms, AXR, serum level >500mcg/dL). Continue until symptoms have resolved.

Isoniazid
- For stopping seizure, use *pyridoxine* (vitamin B_6) 3–5g.

Lead
- Immediate intervention for blood level ≥70mcg/dL.
- Oral chelation with dimercaptosuccinic acid (DMSA): 30mg/kg/day divided every 8h.
- Parenteral chelation with British anti-Lewisite (BAL): initial dose 75mg/m² deep IM.

Methaemoglobinaemia: sulfonamides, quinines, phenacetin, nitrates, aniline dyes, naphthalene
- Measure level and if >30%, start treatment.
- *Methylene blue 1%*: 1–2mg/kg (0.1–0.2mL/kg) IV over 5min.
- Beware of methylene blue in glucose-6-phosphate dehydrogenase (G6PD) deficiency.
- Consider exchange transfusion if no response.

Narcotics: codeine, dextromethorphan, propoxyphene, pentazocine, butorphanol, methadone
- *Naloxone*: useful for reversing coma caused by opiates. Response is rapid and repeat doses or infusion can be used.

Organophosphates: pesticides
- *Atropine*: initial dose 20mcg/kg (maximum 2mg) IV.
- *Pralidoxime*: 25–50mg/kg/dose (up to 1g) IV.

Phenothiazines: chlorpromazine
- For extrapyramidal syndrome, use *diphenhydramine*.
- If life-threatening, IV *benzatropine* 20–50mcg/kg/dose.

Fluid and electrolytes

Normal fluid requirements

All children with serious acute illness who are unable to have enteral fluids in hospital are given IV fluids and electrolyte solutions. It is important to match what you prescribe to what the child actually needs. There are a number of ways of calculating daily requirements, but the method commonly used is based on patient weight (see Box 3.14).

> **Box 3.14 Calculating fluid and electrolyte requirements (outside neonatal period)**
>
> *24h fluid requirements*
> - *100mL/kg*: for the first 10kg of weight.
> - *+50mL/kg*: for the second 10kg of weight.
> - *+20mL/kg*: for the remaining weight above 20kg.
>
> *24h electrolyte requirements*
> - *Na⁺*: 2–4mmol/kg.
> - *K⁺*: 1–2mmol/kg.

In the fasting child, the type of fluid given should contain dextrose (usually 5%), sodium chloride, and added potassium chloride (KCl). Outside the neonatal period, use NS with 5% dextrose for IV maintenance.

The volume of fluid administered should be ↑ in dehydration (see ➔ Fluid and electrolytes in dehydration, p. 71–72), and restricted to 50–75% of usual maintenance volume in cases of:
- Risk of SIADH (see ➔ Hyponatraemia, p. 72; ➔ Posterior pituitary: SIADH, p. 430), e.g. cerebral pathology, pneumonia.
- Fluid overload (see ➔ Circulatory overload, p. 583).
- Congestive heart failure (see ➔ Congestive heart failure, p. 46).
- Renal failure with oliguria or anuria (see ➔ Renal insufficiency, p. 76–7).

Fluid and electrolytes in dehydration

Dehydration can lead to shock, severe metabolic acidosis, and death, particularly in infants. Its severity can be assessed using acute changes in body weight or the following physical signs:

	Clinical dehydration (<10% dehydrated)	Hypovolaemic shock (>10% dehydrated)
Skin turgor	↓	↓ (with tenting)
Mucosa	Dry	Dry
Urine output	↓	↓/anuric
HR	↑	↑
BP	Normal	↓
RR	↑	↑
Perfusion	Normal CRT and peripheral pulses	Prolonged CRT and weak peripheral pulses
Extremities	May be cool	Cold and mottled/blue
Eyes	Sunken	Sunken
LOC	Irritable, lethargic	Reduced GCS score/coma

After you have assessed the degree of dehydration in your patient, two problems need to be addressed—water and electrolyte losses (see Box 3.15).

Box 3.15 Water and electrolyte losses in severe dehydration

Losses in severe dehydration

H_2O (mL/kg)	Na^+ (mmol/kg)	K^+ (mmol/kg)	Cl^- (mmol/kg)
Isotonic dehydration (Na^+ 130–150mmol/L)			
100–120	8–10	8–10	8–10
Hyponatraemic dehydration (Na^+ <130mmol/L)			
100–120	10–12	8–10	10–12
Hypernatraemic dehydration (Na^+ >150mmol/L)			
100–120	2–4	0–4	2–6

Isotonic or hyponatraemic dehydration

- First assess the degree of dehydration (use weight change and signs).
- Calculate the fluid deficit (e.g. 10% dehydration when weight is 15kg suggests a 1500mL fluid deficit).
- Check U&E (Na^+, K^+, Ca^{2+}), creatinine, and glucose.

Initial emergency treatment is directed at restoring any haemodynamic compromise with IV boluses of 20mL/kg NS (see ➲ Hypovolaemic shock, p. 53). Monitoring should include: vital signs, losses (urine output, stool, vomitus, or NG), daily weights, and BP. To rehydrate over 24h, take account of the deficit, maintenance requirements, and ongoing losses:

$$\text{Hourly rate (mL/h)} = [(24h \text{ maintenance} + \text{estimated deficit}) - \text{resuscitation fluids}]/24$$

Hypernatraemic dehydration

- Water losses exceed Na^+ loss.
- Cerebral oedema is a risk during rehydration, so correction of the deficit should be achieved slowly and evenly, *over 48h*.
- Emergency treatment of shock using 10–20mL/kg IV NS.
- Monitor as above, but with at least 8-hourly blood U&E.
- Use NS, so that Na^+ correction occurs slowly.

Seizures and cerebral oedema may complicate rehydration in hypernatraemic dehydration. Treat symptomatically and refer to an ICU.

Other fluid and electrolyte abnormalities

Hyponatraemia (<130mmol/L)

Infrequent cause of dehydration; suspect iatrogenic causes.

Sodium depletion

- *Associations:* hypovolaemia and low urine Na^+ (<10mmol/L).
- *Causes:* inadequate Na^+ intake, excessive Na^+ losses.
- *Symptomatic therapy (<120mmol/L):* if there are seizures, serum Na^+ level should be acutely raised by 5–10mmol/L in 1h. Use 3–4mL/kg of 3% saline IV and repeat after 20min if needed.

Dilution

- *Associations:* normovolaemia (occasionally overload), paradoxically high urine Na^+, and sometimes cerebral oedema.
- *Causes:* impaired water excretion; excess water given.
- *Treatment:* correct the volume-overloaded circulation with diuretics (furosemide 0.5–1.0mg/kg IV). Provide O_2 and inotropes if required. Restrict fluids to less than maintenance.
- *SIADH:* there are many causes of SIADH. Features are low urine volume and high urine osmolality in the absence of hypovolaemia, renal disease, and adrenal disease. Urine Na^+ is paradoxically high (20–30mmol/L) in the presence of hyponatraemia due to volume overload (see ➲ Posterior pituitary: SIADH, p. 430).

Hypernatraemia (>150mmol/L)

Besides hypernatraemic dehydration and salt poisoning, hypernatraemia occurs in diabetes insipidus (DI), in which there is excess renal water loss. The urine is 5–10 times the usual volume, with low osmolality (50–100mOsm/L), in the absence of glycosuria.

Antidiuretic hormone (ADH) deficiency (diabetes insipidus)
- *Causes:* severe asphyxia, and CNS trauma, surgery, or infection.
- *Treatment:* use two IV solutions—one for maintenance and replacement of insensible losses, the other for replacing urine losses. Check urine Na^+/K^+, and prepare IV replacement solution to match.
- *Hormone replacement:* DI is sometimes transient and so initial fluid therapy is reasonable. However, if this problem is established, hormonal replacement is needed: nasal DDAVP (desmopressin) 10–40mcg/day in one or two doses; parenteral [intramuscular (IM)/IV] DDAVP (desmopressin) 2–4mcg/day in two doses. You should see a response within 1h.

Hypokalaemia (<3mmol/L)

- *ECG changes:* flattened, prolonged, or inverted T-wave, prominent U wave, ST segment depression, atrioventricular (AV) block.

Symptoms
- *Cardiovascular:* dysrhythmias, hypotension.
- *Neuromuscular:* weakness, hypotonia, hyporeflexia, paraesthesiae.
- *GI:* ileus, constipation.

Correction
- *Urgent:* ECG changes, on digoxin, or serum K^+ <2.5mmol/L.
- *Treatment:* 0.5mmol KCl/kg IV over 1h via central venous line (CVL). The bolus should not exceed 20mmol. Peripheral IV infusions should not be more concentrated than 40mmol/L KCl.
- Monitor continuous ECG and repeat serum K^+ level after 1–2h.

Hyperkalaemia (>5.5mmol/L)

- *ECG changes:* peaked T-wave, widened QRS, depressed ST segment progressing to increasingly aberrant ECG complexes.
- Most commonly false elevation due to haemolysis during/after blood sampling, so repeat recommended to confirm diagnosis.
- *Dysrhythmias:* bradycardia, ventricular tachycardia/fibrillation (VF), cardiac arrest.

Symptomatic treatment (>8.0mmol/L or ECG changes)
- *Protect the myocardium:* calcium gluconate 10% (100mg/kg/dose IV, maximum rate 100mg/min; 1.5–3.3mL/min, 50mg/mL), and monitor for bradycardia and hypotension.
- *Increase intracellular K^+ uptake:* $NaHCO_3$ (1–2mmol/kg IV over 5–10min); insulin/glucose (0.1U/kg IV *with* dextrose 25% 0.5g/kg over 30min).
- *Induce urinary excretion:* nebulized or IV salbutamol infusion.
- *Consider:* furosemide 1mg/kg IV.
- *Decrease total K^+ load:* calcium resonium (polystyrene sulfonate) 125–250mg/kg (maximum 15g) 3–4 times a day PO or per rectum (PR).

Hypocalcaemia (<1.1mmol/L)

(See also ➲ Hypocalcaemia, p. 424–5.) Low ionized values of Ca^{2+} can result in:

- *ECG changes:* prolonged QT, AV block.
- *CNS effects:* seizures, tetany, and weakness.

Symptomatic therapy

- Calcium gluconate 10% for seizures, tetany, hypotension, and arrhythmias.

Refractory hypocalcaemia

- *Check Mg^{2+} level and serum albumin:* if low, correct (25–50mg/kg) with IV magnesium sulfate over 30min.
- If these are normal, with *raised phosphate*, ↓ phosphate intake and use phosphate binders. Check renal function.

Unexplained metabolic acidosis

Metabolic acidosis is a common feature of illness, and often the cause is immediately identified from clinical features (e.g. sepsis, cardiac failure) and corrected by specific therapy (e.g. fluids and antibiotics in sepsis). However, when the cause is unclear, this approach may be helpful.

Calculate the anion gap (AG)

$$AG = [Na^+] - ([HCO_3^-] + [Cl^-])$$

$AG = 10 - 12mmol/L$ (normal range, check with your laboratory)

Increased AG metabolic acidosis

This is due to production of exogenous acid. As an aide-memoire, think of 'a mudpile':

- Alcohol or aspirin.
- Methanol.
- Uraemia.
- DKA.
- Paraldehyde.
- Ingestion or inborn error.
- Lactate.
- Ethylene glycol.

Normal AG metabolic acidosis

This is commonly due to bicarbonate (HCO_3^-) loss from the gut or kidney, or impaired acid secretion by the kidney:

- *Diarrhoea.*
- *Type I (distal) renal tubular acidosis (RTA):* inability to excrete hydrogen ion, urine pH always high (>6.5); caused by medications or inherited; often associated with hypokalaemia and hypercalciuria.
- *Type II (proximal) RTA:* impaired reabsorption of HCO_3^- from proximal tubule, usually associated with other proximal tubular dysfunction such as phosphaturia or glycosuria (Fanconi syndrome).
- *Type IV (hyperkalaemic) RTA:* poor aldosterone production or lack of response to it in acute pyelonephritis or obstructive uropathy.
- *Bicarbonate replacement in RTA:* estimate the deficit as $(20 - [HCO_3^-]) \times$ weight in kg $\times$ 0.5mmol; replace over 24–48h with oral supplements.

Renal insufficiency

(See also ➲ Acute kidney injury, p. 350–3.) Acute renal failure (ARF) is the sudden reduction or cessation of renal function to the point where body fluid homeostasis is compromised, leading to accumulation of nitrogenous waste products, with or without reduced urine output. Children in this state need prompt assessment and transfer to a specialized renal unit. More commonly seen are patients with a degree of renal insufficiency that is complicating an acute illness—either at presentation or evolving during admission.

Clinical assessment

Take a thorough history and do a full examination. Gauge the fluid state, as clinical signs can be conflicting (e.g. peripherally oedematous, but hypovolaemic in the nephrotic state), and look for signs of the aetiology:

- *Fluid state:* BP, HR, CRT, pulse volume, limb temperature gradients; urine output (oliguria <0.5mL/kg/h).
- Evidence of preceding *infection:* throat, *Streptococcus*; gastroenteritis, haemolytic uraemic syndrome (HUS); exposure to drugs/toxins.
- Evidence of *general illness:* pallor, anorexia, oedema, fatigue.
- *Rash:* petechial or purpuric.
- *Organ systems involved:*
  - Cardiovascular: hypertension, signs of heart failure.
  - Respiratory: tachypnoea, cough, or haemoptysis.
  - GI: nausea, vomiting, bleeding, flank mass, or ascites.

Investigations

The following tests are required in acute care:

- *Blood:* FBC with differential.
- *Serum biochemistry:* U&E, creatinine, ABG or capillary gas.
- *Urine:* check for protein, blood, or sediment (red cell casts, tubular cells, WBC casts) or evidence of UTI.
- *Imaging:* CXR, AXR, and abdominal and renal US examination with Doppler studies of renal vessel blood flow.
- *Other tests:* consider taking blood samples for complement levels (C3, C4), serum titres [e.g. anti-streptolysin O (ASO) titres], and antinuclear (ANA) and antineutrophil cytoplasmic antibodies (ANCA).

Monitoring

Generic parameters for monitoring in renal failure include:

- Standard BP monitoring.
- Strict documentation of hourly fluid input, output, and balance.
- Twice-daily weights.

Acute therapy

In the acute setting, first assess the intravascular status and decide whether the patient is hypovolaemic or hypervolaemic. If the patient is uraemic with ↓ LOC, urgent transfer to a renal unit is a priority.

Hypovolaemia
- Administer 20mL/kg of 0.9% NS as IV bolus, and repeat if necessary.
- If the cause of anuria is fluid depletion, fluid resuscitation should restore urine flow within 6h.
- Give blood if necessary, and continue to monitor.
- Acute tubular necrosis (ATN) is likely if no response to the above:
  - Repeat the fluid bolus with furosemide (1–5mg/kg IV), but do not use if obstructive uropathy is suspected—refer to a urologist.
  - If the patient produces urine, expect large amounts (which will need to be replaced) as polyuric renal failure may ensue.
- If the urine output is minimal, then treat as ARF.

Acute renal failure and kidney injury

A child in ARF will need transfer to a renal unit. Hypertension, hyperkalaemia, hyponatraemia, and seizures may occur and need treatment before transfer.

BP
- Hypertension if sBP or dBP >95th centile (see → Hypertension, p. 47; → Hypertension, p. 343).
- Restrict salt intake.
- Consider antihypertensive drugs (e.g. amlodipine 300mcg/kg).

Fluids
- Treat hypovolaemia with NS boluses until stable.
- Then restrict fluids to urine replacement and insensible losses (300–400mL/m²/day).

Electrolytes
- Correct hyponatraemia if causing seizures.
- Correct hypocalcaemia if symptomatic—do this before correcting acidosis.
- Discontinue any potassium administration. Remember that for every 0.1 fall in pH, K^+ will rise by 0.4mmol/L, so you may need to treat acidosis if pH <7.2 and HCO_3^- <10mmol/L.

Diet
- Limit protein intake to 0.5–1.0g/kg/day.

Hypoglycaemia

In infants and children, this emergency is defined as a blood value <2.6mmol/L or <3.0mmol/L if symptomatic.

Aetiology

Hypoglycaemia is a sign of an underlying condition that interferes with carbohydrate intake or absorption, gluconeogenesis, or glycogenolysis. (See also ➲ Acute complications of T1DM, p. 476; ➲ Hypoglycaemia, p. 496–8). Outside the neonatal period, in the acute setting, the causes of hypoglycaemia can be grouped as follows.

Endocrine
- Hyperinsulinism.
- Hypopituitarism.
- Growth hormone (GH) deficiency.
- Hypothyroidism.
- Congenital adrenal hyperplasia (CAH).

Metabolic
- Glycogen storage disease.
- Galactosaemia.
- Organic acidaemia.
- Ketotic hypoglycaemia.
- Carnitine deficiency.
- Acyl CoA dehydrogenase deficiency.

Toxic
- Salicylates.
- Alcohol.
- Insulin.
- Valproate.

Hepatic
- Hepatitis.
- Cirrhosis.
- Reye syndrome.

Systemic
- Starvation.
- Malnutrition.
- Sepsis.
- Malabsorption.

Clinical assessment

Take a thorough history, and identify the timing of hypoglycaemia in relation to feeding and medication. On examination, assess for:
- Short stature (see ➲ Short stature, pp. 440–1).
- Failure to thrive (FTT) (see ➲ Faltering growth, pp. 276–7).
- Hepatomegaly (see ➲ Systems—hepatic, p. 506).
- Features of any generalized metabolic disorder (see ➲ Chapter 12).

Investigation

If possible, during an acute episode, you should try to:
- Save blood and urine for metabolic and endocrine testing.
- Check blood glucose in the laboratory.
- Blood U&E, LFTs, and osmolality.
- ABG.
- Blood ketones.
- Toxicology screen.

Treatment

Asymptomatic child
- PO glucose drink or gel.

Symptomatic child
- *Glucose:* 2mL/kg 10% dextrose IV.
- *Followed by:* continuous infusion of IV dextrose (6–8mg/kg/min), e.g. NS with 5% dextrose at normal maintenance rate.
- If *hypoglycaemia persists*, ↑ input to 10–12mg/kg/min.
- If there is *no response*, consider glucagon, hydrocortisone, or diazoxide (and seek specialist advice).

Diabetic ketoacidosis

(See also ➔ Diabetic ketoacidosis, p. 477.)

DKA is life-threatening (death by cerebral oedema, hypokalaemia, or aspiration). Fluid deficit is difficult to assess because signs are masked by catabolic weight loss. DKA is defined as:

- Acidosis—pH <7.3 or plasma [HCO_3^-] <18mmol/L.
- Ketonaemia (blood β-hydroxybutyrate) >3mmol/L.
- High blood glucose level >11mmol/L.

Mild to moderate DKA

- pH ≥7.1 and assume 5% fluid deficit.

Severe DKA

- pH <7.1 and assume 10% fluid deficit.

Clinical assessment

- Weight, degree of dehydration (e.g. estimates by pH, as above).
- LOC (see ➔ Altered level of consciousness, p. 58).
- Any evidence of cerebral oedema, infection, or GI ileus.

Investigations

- FBC with WBC differential and packed cell volume (PCV).
- Serum U&E and creatinine.
- Glucose.
- LFTs (transaminases) and pancreatic amylase/lipase.
- ABG or capillary gas.
- Lactate and ketone levels.
- Blood culture if signs of infection.
- Brain imaging if concerned about cerebral oedema (may be normal).

Monitoring

- Blood: 1-hourly glucose, 2-hourly ketones.
- CNS: *follow the neurological state. If there is headache or altered LOC, treat as though raised ICP has developed.*
- Continuous: SpO_2 and ECG (*T-wave changes should alert you to hypokalaemia or hyperkalaemia*).
- Intermittent BP, 1-hourly urine output, and daily weight.

DKA treatment

Fluid therapy

Fluid management is different in patients with DKA because of the risk of cerebral oedema in acute illness.

Resuscitation fluid

- Do not give a fluid bolus to patients with mild to moderate DKA.
- If signs of hypovolaemic shock (see ➔ Hypovolaemic shock, p. 53) but give aliquots of 10mL/kg NS.
- Do not use >1 fluid bolus without discussing with a senior.
- If >20mL/kg bolus given, subtract addition volumes from the total fluid replacement to be given in the 48h.

Calculation of deficit and maintenance fluid (reduced volume rules)
- *Deficit:* % deficit by severity of DKA to be restored over 48h.
- *Maintenance by weight:* <10kg, 2mL/kg/h; 10–40kg, 1mL/kg/h; >40kg, fixed volume of 40mL/h.
- *Hourly IV rate:* (deficit/48h) + maintenance.

Type of fluid
Initially use NS with 20mmol KCl in 500mL bag, even if K^+ normal.
- Consider calculated corrected Na^+: falsely low levels are given by the indirect ion-selective electrode measurement in hyperglycaemia.
- Fall in corrected Na^+ is associated with risk of cerebral oedema.
- When glucose is 14mmol/L, add dextrose to the fluid (see ➔ Insulin therapy, p. 81).

Bicarbonate and phosphate
- There is no evidence for using HCO_3^-/phosphate replacement.[1]

Electrolytes
- Check 2-hourly after resuscitation, and then 4-hourly.

Oral fluids
- Initially nil by mouth and use NGT if LOC reduced.
- Juices/rehydration fluid permitted only after substantial clinical improvement and added to the overall calculation of fluid intake.

Insulin therapy
- 1h after rehydration with KCl, start insulin to stop ketogenesis.
- Avoid insulin boluses and use low-dose insulin infusion (50mL soluble insulin in NS at 0.05–0.1U/kg/h).
- When blood glucose <14mmol/L:
  - *Ketones <3.0mmol/L:* change fluid to NS with 5% dextrose and 20mmol/L KCl per 500mL bag; keep fluid rate the same; consider continuing or reducing insulin to 0.05IU/kg/h.
  - *Ketones >3.0mmol/L:* change fluid to NS with 10% dextrose and 20mmol KCl per 500mL bag; keep fluid rate the same; maintain insulin at 0.05–0.1U/kg/h.

Treatment failure
If blood glucose is uncontrolled, or the pH worsens after 4–6h, check IV lines and insulin dose, and consider possible sepsis and add antibiotics.

DKA complications
Of most concern is cerebral oedema, and the warning signs are:
- Headache, behavioural change with restlessness, drowsiness.
- Posturing, cranial nerve III palsy, seizures, unequal pupils or dilation.
- Slowing HR, haemodynamic instability, abnormal breathing pattern.

Once identified
- Start ABC.
- Emergency IV hypertonic saline (3% at 2.5–5mL/kg over 15min) or mannitol (20% 0.5–1.0g/kg over 15–20min).
- Consider head CT scan.
- Transfer to ICU.

Inborn errors of metabolism

IEM are rare; emergencies to consider:
- Child with IEM presenting with acute decompensation (often vomiting or intercurrent infection) (see ➲ Chapter 12).
- Undiagnosed collapsed infant/child with hypoglycaemic metabolic acidosis, seizures, or sepsis, but early recognition of IEM is vital.

Clinical assessment

History
- Perinatal history of unexplained feeding difficulties/hypoglycaemia.
- Assess whether any consanguinity or unexpected deaths.
- Any unexplained episodes of vomiting or sleepiness?
- History of developmental delay.

Examination
- Any dysmorphic features, abnormal odours, or hepatosplenomegaly.
- Check growth and/or developmental delay.
- Other: skin (dermatitis or alopecia), eyes (cataracts), breathing (Kussmaul or central hyperventilation).

Investigations

Rapid tests (if all normal metabolic causes unlikely)
- Blood: glucose, ketones, ammonia, LFTs, U&E, FBC, ABG, lactate.

Delayed laboratory results (but send early)
- Urine organic acids; serum amino acids and acylcarnitine profile.

Therapy

Use supportive treatment directed at metabolic acidosis or hypoglycaemia. Stop protein intake and feeds until diagnosis. Avoid catabolism using glucose infusion 6–8mg/kg/min (see Box 3.16). (See also ➲ Initial management, p. 492–3.)

> ### Box 3.16 Calculation of glucose infusion rate (GIR)
>
> GIR = [infusion rate (mL/h) x % dextrose of fluid)/[weight (kg)×6]
>
> A 5.2kg baby with IV 10% dextrose at 100mL/kg/day ('maintenance') would have GIR = $(21.7 \times 10)/(5.2 \times 6) = 6.97$mg/kg/min.

Supportive care
- Treat underlying or precipitating illness.
- Later, ensure immunizations are up-to-date to prevent future infections.

Acidosis
- Correct and optimize MV and circulation.
- After this, HCO_3^- replacement may be needed.
- For more persistent problems, treat in specialist centres.

Hypoglycaemia
(See ➲ Hypoglycaemia, pp. 78–9.)
- Use dextrose 10% (2mL/kg/dose IV).

Further reading

British Society for Paediatric Endocrinology and Diabetes. Recommended DKA management guidelines (2020). Available at: ℘ https://www.bsped.org.uk/clinical-resources/guidelines/.

Wolfsdorf J, Craig ME, Daneman D, *et al.* Diabetic ketoacidosis in children and adolescents with diabetes. *Pediatr Diabetes* 2009; **10** Suppl 12: 118–33.

For evidence base to the DKA management guidelines, see: Wolfsdorf JI, Glaser N, Agus M, *et al.* *ISPAD Clinical Practice Consensus Guidelines 2018: Diabetic ketoacidosis and the hyperglycemic hyperosmolar state*. Available at: ℘ https://cdn.ymaws.com/www.ispad.org/resource/resmgr/consensus_guidelines_2018_/11.diabetic_ketoacidosis_and.pdf.

Neonatology

Perinatal definitions

- *Gestational age (post-menstrual age):* age measured from the first day of the last menstrual period before conception and expressed in complete weeks or days.
- *Chronological/postnatal age:* time elapsed from birth.
- *Corrected age:* chronological age minus the number of weeks born before 40wk gestation.
- *Spontaneous abortion (miscarriage):* a conceptus born after spontaneous labour without signs of life before 24 completed weeks' gestation.
- *Live birth:* a baby that displays any sign of life (i.e. breathing, heartbeat, cord pulsation, or voluntary movement) after complete delivery from the mother, irrespective of gestation.
- *Stillbirth (late fetal death):* fetal death before complete delivery from the mother after 24 completed weeks' gestation.
- *Perinatal mortality:* includes all stillbirths and neonatal deaths in the first week. UK ~7–8 per 1000 total births.
- *Neonatal mortality:* death amongst live births before 28 days of age (whatever the gestation at birth). UK ~3 per 1000 live births.
- *Neonatal period:* from birth to 28 postnatal days in term infants. If preterm, from birth to 44wk post-menstrual age.
- *Preterm:* birth before 37 completed weeks' gestation; ~8% of births.
- *Term birth:* between 37 and 42 completed weeks' gestation.
- *Post-term (post-mature):* birth after 42 completed weeks' gestation; <5% of births.
- *Low birthweight (LBW):* birthweight <2500g; 7% of births.
- *Very low birthweight (VLBW):* birthweight <1500g; 1.2% of births.
- *Extremely low birthweight (ELBW):* birthweight <1000g.
- *Small for gestational age (SGA):* birthweight <10th centile for gestational age.
- *Large for gestational age (LGA):* birthweight >90th centile for gestational age.

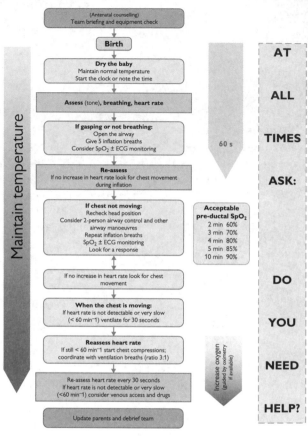

Fig. 4.1 Newborn life support. SpO₂ values are 25th centile for term infants.
Reproduced with kind permission of Resuscitation Council (UK) 2015.

Newborn life support

All who attend deliveries should be proficient in newborn resuscitation, as taught on the *Newborn Life Support* (NLS) or equivalent. The algorithm shown in Fig. 4.1 demonstrates a general approach to resuscitation. Preterm infants require special consideration (see ➔ Prematurity, pp. 94–5).

Before birth
- Check equipment.
- Ask about: gestation, fetal distress, and meconium.

At birth
For uncompromised babies, a delay in cord clamping of at least 1min is recommended. If the baby appears severely compromised, then delayed cord clamping should not delay resuscitation.

Meconium
Vigorous infants born through meconium-stained liquor do NOT require airway suctioning either on the perineum or the Resuscitaire®:
- Pale, floppy, poor respiration, or bradycardia? Inspect oropharynx and perform suction if required.
- Appropriate *expertise*:
  - *Available:* ETT intubation and suction in non-vigorous babies.
  - *Unavailable or ETT intubation attempt prolonged or unsuccessful:* start mask ventilation, particularly if persistent bradycardia.

Lung inflation
Inflation breaths are given initially; use air (FiO$_2$ 0.21):
- 3s each breath, 30cmH$_2$O (term infants)—give in sets of 5.
- Once the chest is moving, ventilation breaths (shorter and gentler) are given at a rate of 30–40/min if required.

Airway manoeuvres
- *Jaw thrust* (2-person technique very useful).
- Direct inspection of oropharynx and airway suction.
- Guedel airway.
- ETT intubation (if competent).

Chest compressions
- Rate >100/min, using two-thumbs technique.
- Three chest compressions per lung inflation (3:1 ratio).
- Reassess infant after each 30s (15 cycles).

Drugs
- Give through UVC or IO.
- High-dose adrenaline via ETT can be considered.
- Drugs are B/A/D (Bicarbonate/Adrenaline/Dextrose 10%).

Small for gestational age

(See also ➔ Small for gestational age, p. 102.)
- *SGA*: birthweight <10th centile for gestational age.
- *Intrauterine growth restriction (IUGR)*: is failure of growth *in utero* that may or may not result in SGA.
- *Symmetric (proportional) SGA*: all growth parameters symmetrically small; suggests fetus affected from early pregnancy, e.g. chromosomal disorder or constitutional.
- *Asymmetric (disproportional) SGA*: weight centile < length and head circumference. Usually because of IUGR due to insult in late pregnancy, e.g. pre-eclampsia. Infants at risk of complications.

Causes

- *Constitutional*, i.e. small parents (commonest).
- *Restricted fetal O_2 or glucose supply*, e.g. placental dysfunction, maternal hypertension, multiple pregnancy, maternal illness.
- *Fetal abnormality*, e.g. chromosomal disorders, congenital anomalies and syndromes, congenital infection.
- *Maternal substance exposure*, e.g. alcohol, smoking, therapeutic, or other drugs.

Complications

- Risk of fetal death or asphyxia: SGA indicates fetal compromise.
- May have congenital infection, or toxoplasmosis, others, rubella, CMV, herpesvirus II (TORCH), or malformation (see ➔ Transplacental (congenital infection), p. 164).
- Hypoglycaemia due to ↓ glycogen stores (see ➔ Inborn errors of metabolism, p. 169).
- Hypothermia.
- Polycythaemia secondary to chronic intrauterine hypoxia (see ➔ Polycythaemia, p. 174).
- NEC or feed intolerance: chronic fetal bowel hypoxia (see ➔ Necrotizing enterocolitis, pp. 160–1).
- Thrombocytopenia, neutropenia, coagulopathy: bone marrow and hepatic compromise (see ➔ Thrombocytopenia, p. 175).
- Meconium aspiration syndrome (MAS) secondary to fetal hypoxia (see ➔ Meconium aspiration syndrome, p. 132).

Management

- Manage on a postnatal ward with ↑ ratio of midwives.
- Routine postnatal care.
- Evaluate clinically for features suggestive of underlying cause.
- Particular attention to thermal care and blood glucose monitoring.
- Observe temperature, HR, and respiration for the first 48h.
- Admit to neonatal ICU (NICU) if birthweight <1800g. Local policies may vary.
- Well infants can be discharged when:
  - Sucking all feeds 3- to 4-hourly.
  - Weight gain is satisfactory (20–30g/day).
  - Body temperature maintained at room temperature.
  - Mother capable of caring for infant.

Prognosis

(See also ➔ Outcome following prematurity, p. 98.)

- Neurodevelopmental impairments commoner in SGA infants.
- Symmetric SGA infants often stay small.
- The Barker hypothesis suggests IUGR infants with a small placenta are at risk in later life of coronary disease, stroke, obesity, and hypertension.

Large for gestational age

(see ➔ Large for gestational age, p. 102)
Defined as birthweight >90th centile for gestational age.

Causes

- Most frequently constitutional, i.e. large parents.
- Infant of a mother with diabetes mellitus.
- Fetal hyperinsulinism, pancreatic islet cell hyperplasia.
- Hydrops fetalis (see ➔ Hydrops fetalis, pp. 118–19).
- Beckwith–Wiedemann syndrome (BWS) (see ➔ Beckwith–Wiedemann syndrome, p. 885).

Complications

- Perinatal asphyxia, nerve palsies, shoulder dystocia, fractures.
- *Hypoglycaemia*, especially if due to maternal diabetes or in BWS.
- Problems associated with the underlying cause of LGA.

Management

- Careful obstetric management to prevent obstetric complications.
- Examine for associated features, e.g. BWS or signs of birth injury.
- Prevent hypoglycaemia (see ➔ Hypoglycaemia, pp. 112–13).

Prognosis

- Generally excellent (unless hydrops fetalis) if managed well.

Infant of a mother with diabetes mellitus

Pathophysiology

- *Maternal hyperglycaemia*: increases fetal glucose, which increases fetal insulin secretion (antenatally has GH function); leads to macrosomia, organomegaly, and polycythaemia.
- Rarely, maternal vascular disease results in *fetal IUGR*.

Associated complications

- 2–4 times risk of *congenital abnormalities*: caudal regression syndrome (sacral and femoral agenesis or hypoplasia); transient hypertrophic cardiomyopathy; small left colon syndrome; neural tube defects.
- *Obstetric complications* (see ➲ Obstetric problems, pp. 102–4): ↑ risk of spontaneous miscarriage, intrauterine fetal death, and prematurity.
- *Hypoglycaemia*: generally resolves as serum insulin level falls.
- *Respiratory disease*: respiratory distress.
- *Polycythaemia*: risk of secondary thrombosis (e.g. renal vein).
- Exaggerated physiological jaundice.
- Hypocalcaemia and hypomagnesaemia.

Management

Optimize maternal glycaemic control during pregnancy (decreases risk of complications, except for congenital abnormalities.

Prognosis

- Normoglycaemia occurs within 48h in vast majority.
- Seven times ↑ risk of diabetes mellitus in later life.
- ↑ risk of later obesity and possibly poor development.

Prematurity

Birth before 37 completed weeks' gestation (8% of all births). Most problems seen in infants born <32 completed weeks (72% of all births).

Predisposing factors

- Idiopathic (40%).
- Previous preterm birth.
- Multiple pregnancy.
- Maternal illness, e.g. chorioamnionitis, polyhydramnios, pre-eclampsia, diabetes mellitus.
- Premature rupture of membranes.
- Uterine malformation or cervical incompetence.
- Placental disease, e.g. dysfunction, antepartum haemorrhage (APH).
- Poor maternal health or socio-economic status.

Associated problems

- *Respiratory:* surfactant deficiency causing respiratory distress syndrome (RDS) (see ➔ Respiratory distress syndrome, pp. 130–1), apnoea of prematurity (see ➔ Apnoea of prematurity, p. 134), chronic lung disease (CLD)/BPD (see ➔ Bronchopulmonary dysplasia, pp. 146–7; ➔ Chronic lung disease of prematurity, pp. 246–7).
- *CNS:* intraventricular haemorrhage, periventricular leukomalacia, retinopathy of prematurity (ROP) (see ➔ Retinopathy of prematurity, pp. 170–1).
- *GI:* NEC (see ➔ Necrotizing enterocolitis, pp. 160–1), inability to suck, and poor milk tolerance.
- *Hypothermia.*
- *Immunocompromise* with ↑ risk/severity of infection.
- Impaired fluid/electrolyte homeostasis (↑ transepidermal water loss, poor renal function).
- *Patent ductus arteriosus* (PDA) (see ➔ Patent ductus arteriosus, p. 150).
- *Anaemia* of prematurity (see ➔ Anaemia, pp. 174–5).
- *Jaundice* (liver enzyme immaturity; see ➔ Neonatal jaundice, pp. 110–11).
- *Birth trauma* (see ➔ Birth trauma, pp. 106–7).
- *Perinatal hypoxia* (see ➔ Hypoxic–ischaemic encephalopathy, pp. 154–5).
- *Later:* adverse neurodevelopmental outcome, behavioural problems, sudden infant death syndrome (SIDS), non-accidental trauma (NAT), and/or parental marriage break-up.

General management

Antenatal

- Delivery should be planned in a centre capable of preterm care.
- If a woman has threatened preterm labour in a centre unable to care for the baby, possible *in utero* transfer should be discussed by both NICU and obstetrics teams. Consider fetal fibronectin screening to aid diagnosis and tocolysis to delay birth before transfer.
- Give the mother IM corticosteroids (two doses, 12–24h apart) of either betamethasone or dexamethasone, if <34wk gestation. Steroids decrease mortality by 40% (↓ severity of RDS, periventricular haemorrhage, and NEC), provided they are given >24h before birth. Benefit persists for at least 7 days. Effect of repeated doses remains unclear—may have adverse impact on later growth.

Postnatal
- Infants need stabilization (support in transition), not resuscitation.
- Senior paediatrician present at birth if very preterm, e.g. <28wk.
- Delay cord clamping for 1min if infant not compromised.
- Immediately after birth, place in food-grade plastic bag and under radiant heater. Cover the head with a woollen hat.
- *Provide respiratory support, NIV or MV*, as required:
  - Use PEEP at 5cmH$_2$O.
  - Start with lower peak inspiratory pressure (PIP) 20cmH$_2$O.
  - Use NIV if adequate effort of breathing, e.g. PEEP/nasal CPAP or nasal high flow.
- *ETT intubation and surfactant* if <27wk gestation and respiratory insufficiency not responding to NIV (the very smallest babies often require elective ETT intubation and surfactant).
- *Monitor SpO$_2$* if available (right wrist = pre-ductal), and target O$_2$ therapy appropriately:
  - Be familiar with normal values.
  - 10% of well preterm infants will have SpO$_2$ <70% at 5min.
  - Resuscitate in air initially and titrate O$_2$ as needed.
- Once stable: well infants >1800g and >35/40 may be transferred to a postnatal ward if midwifery staffing and expertise exist for the additional care. Otherwise admit to a neonatal unit.
- Measure weight and temperature on NICU admission and monitor:
  - <1000g: 37.0–37.5°C.
  - >1000g: 36.5–37.0°C.
- Nurse in *80% humidity* for first 7 days if <30/40.
- *Monitor and maintain blood glucose* with enteral feeds (expressed breast milk), PN, or 10% glucose as appropriate. Encourage ALL mothers to express breast milk from day 1.
- Start *broad-spectrum antibiotics* if any possibility of infection, e.g. benzylpenicillin and gentamicin.
- Start treatment for associated diseases and complications of prematurity, e.g. surfactant for RDS.
- Aim for *minimal handling* of infant, with appropriate levels of noise and cycled lighting in the nursery.
- *Support parents.*

Birth at the limit of viability

The World Health Organization (WHO) defines the perinatal period as starting at 22wk gestation, which is realistically the earliest gestation of viability. In the UK, threshold viability is generally accepted to be when birth is a minimum of 23 completed weeks' gestation.

Management before birth

As gestation falls, the likelihood of mortality and serious long-term disability increases. When preterm birth at the threshold of viability is threatened, there should be close collaboration between the paediatrician, obstetrician, midwife, and family. Unless delivery is precipitated, a senior paediatrician should meet parents before birth to assess and do the following:

- Ascertain whether an estimate of gestation is likely to be reliable.
- Give relevant information.
- Outline potential problems.
- Outline possible management (including option of no resuscitation).
- Describe relevant survival and disability rates.
- Parents should fully participate in any decision about the appropriateness of any later attempted resuscitation.

Management at birth

<23wk gestation

- Rarely suitable for resuscitation, but it may still be beneficial for a senior paediatrician/neonatologist to attend birth to reassure parents and support staff in provision of comfort care.

23–23+6wk gestation

- Senior obstetrician and paediatrician should be present to assess size, maturity, and condition of the newborn and then manage.
- If an infant appears viable, respiratory support should be given.
  - External cardiac massage or resuscitation drugs are not generally considered appropriate.
  - If junior doctors are present alone at such a delivery, full resuscitation should be started and continued until a senior paediatrician arrives and makes an assessment.
  - If parents do not wish life-sustaining care in such an infant, their view should be respected.
  - If the infant appears unexpectedly vigorous or more mature, full treatment should be started.

24–25+6wk gestation

- Resuscitation would be expected.
- A senior paediatrician/neonatologist should be present.
- Chest compressions and resuscitation drugs are generally not recommended as the outcome after full resuscitation is poor (check local unit policy).
- If resuscitation is withheld on a delivery ward, the infant should be kept warm and comfortable, as well as offered to parents to cuddle. (For management after death, see ❍ Perinatal death, pp. 180–1.)

Management after birth

Clinical progress after initial resuscitation and further discussion with the parents will dictate whether it is appropriate to continue or withdraw life-sustaining treatment. *When doctors and parents, or parents themselves, cannot agree as to the best or most appropriate management, it is almost always best to continue as the situation will become clearer with time and agreement is usually then reached.*

Outcome following prematurity

Risk of complications and associated morbidity/mortality lessen as gestation advances. Infants at >32wk gestation who are well in the first 24h are at low risk of adverse outcome. The EPICure1 and 2 studies give the best guide to UK outcomes for infants born at <26wk gestation (see Table 4.1). Preterm survival is continuing to trend upwards.

Table 4.1 Likely outcomes in the UK for infants born at <26wk gestation

	Weeks of gestation		
Survival to discharge (%)	22–23	24	25
1995	19	35	54
2006	26	47	67
Statistically significant increase?	No	Yes +	Yes ++
Overall survival of live births free of disability at age 6y (EPICure 1)	<0.5	9	20

EPICure1 survivors with disability

Categorized as: one-third severe, one-third moderate, one-third mild.

Typical disabilities
- *CNS:* cerebral palsy (CP), most commonly spastic (diplegia > quadriplegia > hemiplegia); hearing loss; epilepsy.
- *Cognition:* impaired; behavioural disorders, e.g. attention-deficit/hyperactivity disorder (ADHD)].
- *Eyes:* squint (strabismus), blindness.

Local outcomes

Knowledge of your unit's outcome is important. However, numbers will be small, and national figures should be used. Many things influence outcome, e.g. singleton infant with spontaneous birth at 25wk gestation after an otherwise uncomplicated pregnancy in a mother given 48h of steroids has a better prognosis than a triplet born suddenly at 26wk in a mother with severe chorioamnionitis.

Basic obstetrics

The aim of obstetrics is to:
- *Monitor* and promote fetal and maternal well-being during pregnancy and labour.
- *Identify and manage* high-risk pregnancies or complications.

In the UK, most women choose in-hospital delivery, although planned home deliveries are increasing. Depending on local provision, women may also choose a birthing centre, a community midwifery unit, or a midwife-led unit attached to an obstetric centre.

High-risk deliveries
- All deliveries in a consultant-led obstetric unit.
- Clear protocols should be in place for transferring of women from outlying centres if problems arise during labour.

Antenatal care of low-risk pregnancy

In the UK, care is usually shared amongst the GP, community midwife, and obstetrician:
- *First antenatal ('booking') visit:* usually at 10–12wk gestation when significant risk factors should be identified.
- *Fetal US:* performed to determine gestational age.
- *Assess* every few weeks to monitor:
  - General: health, Hb, BP, urine glucose, and albumin.
  - Fetus: growth, movements, HR, and lie (liquor volume).
- Routine *prenatal screening*.
- *Maternal testing* is offered for:
  - Blood: group and antibodies (iso-immune haemolytic disease).
  - Serology: syphilis, rubella, hepatitis B, HIV.
  - Urine: protein, glucose, and bacteria.
- *17–18wk:* offer screen for chromosomal disorders and structural anomalies. Controversy on what is cost-effective, but includes:
  - α-fetoprotein (AFP); human chorionic gonadotrophin (hCG); oestriol (combined with above two tests = 'triple test'); triple test plus inhibin ('quadruple test'); quadruple test plus pregnancy-associated protein-A (PrAP-A).
  - US for nuchal thickness; detailed fetal US looking for abnormalities is usually done at 18wk.
- *Chorionic villus biopsy* (>10wk gestation) or *amniocentesis* (usually at 15–16wk) is offered for chromosomal, enzymatic, or gene probe analysis, if screening tests show high risk of serious problems. Both tests carry risk of miscarriage (71%, slightly higher with chorionic villus biopsy). Also perform if:
  - Maternal age >35y.
  - Previous abnormal baby.
  - Family history +ve.

Induction of labour

Indicated when delivery is safer—for mother or baby—than to remain *in utero*. Use prostaglandin (oral or vaginal) or amniotomy.

Normal labour

Occurs >37wk and should result in delivery within 24h of starting:
- *First-stage*: from the onset of labour to full cervical dilatation. Once cervix is 3cm dilated, should then continue at least 1cm/h.
- *Second-stage*: time from fully dilated cervix to birth. Normal duration is 45–120min in a primiparous woman; 15–45min if multiparous. Active pushing during this stage should not usually be >60–90min.
- *Third-stage*: time from birth to placental delivery.

Intrapartum fetal assessment

Intrapartum fetal heart monitoring detects signs of fetal compromise. In low-risk labour, intermittent auscultation (by Doppler US or Pinard stethoscope) should be undertaken for 1min after contractions, at least every 15min in the first stage, and every 5min in the second stage.
- *Continuous electronic fetal monitoring*: cardiotocogram (CTG) should be undertaken in high-risk pregnancies and when:
  - Abnormal fetal HR detected.
  - Meconium staining of liquor or bleeding in labour.
  - Maternal pyrexia.
  - Oxytocin use.
  - Maternal request.
- *Fetal blood sampling*: indicated if fetal distress suspected.

Mode of delivery

Majority of term infants are born by normal vaginal delivery.
- *Caesarean section* (CS) indications include:
  - Maternal: ill health, previous CS, pregnancy-induced hypertension, maternal HIV or HSV.
  - Pregnancy: multiple, acute fetal distress, fetal malpresentation (including breech), placenta praevia.
  - Labour: failed induction, failure to progress.
  - Fetus: ongoing fetal compromise (e.g. severe IUGR), umbilical cord prolapsed, APH.
- *Instrumental delivery* (forceps or vacuum extraction) may be indicated if:
  - Prolonged second stage.
  - Malpresentation: breech delivery or occipital–posterior.
  - Fetal distress.

Obstetric problems

It is desirable for a paediatrician to attend a birth in the following categories or with the following problems:
- *Fetus:* fetal distress (including meconium-stained liquor), serious fetal abnormality, significant iso-immune haemolytic disease, severe IUGR, preterm delivery <34wk gestation.
- *CS:* emergency or elective under GA.
- *Vaginal delivery:* breech, rotational forceps.
- *Mother:* maternal insulin-dependent diabetes mellitus (IDDM).

Small for gestational age

(See → Small for gestational age, pp. 90–1.) Perform serial detailed US (including Doppler fetal umbilical and cerebral artery blood flow measurement) to determine:
- *Fetal growth rate* and whether *growth reduction* is symmetrical or asymmetrical:
  - Symmetrical SGA is usually fetal in origin.
  - Asymmetrical SGA suggests placental dysfunction.
- *Fetal health.*

There is ↑ risk of fetal hypoxia or death, requiring close antenatal and intrapartum monitoring. Early delivery may be needed. Abnormal Doppler artery measurements (e.g. absent or reversed end-diastolic flow) indicate an especially high fetal risk.

Large for gestational age

(See → Large for gestational age, p. 92.) Glucose tolerance test should be performed to detect maternal diabetes. Because of ↑ risk of obstetric complications, a senior obstetrician should supervise timing and mode of delivery, and labour. Specialist input (diabetologist) should also be sought.

Multiple pregnancy

Risks increase as fetus number increases. If ≥3, selective feticide may be indicated to improve outcome for survivors. There is a risk of:
- Preterm delivery, perinatal mortality.
- Malformations, polyhydramnios.
- Malpresentation, pregnancy-induced hypertension, APH.

Oligohydramnios

Liquor volume <500mL. Causes:
- Placental insufficiency.
- Preterm prolonged rupture of membranes (PPROM).
- Fetal urinary tract obstruction or renal disease (e.g. Potter's syndrome) (see → Classification of antenatal USS abnormalities, p. 328; → Miscellaneous congenital malformations, Table 24.2, p. 890).

Risks
- Pulmonary hypoplasia/dry lung syndrome.
- Contractures/developmental dysplasia of the hip (DDH).

Polyhydramnios

Liquor volume >2000mL. Causes:
- 50% secondary to fetal disease (e.g. upper GI tract obstruction).
- 30% idiopathic.
- 20% maternal diabetes mellitus.

Risks
- Preterm labour.
- Malpresentation.
- Umbilical cord prolapse.
- APH.

Amniotic fluid reduction and indometacin may be beneficial.

Prolonged pregnancy

Longer than 42wk gestation.
- ↑ perinatal mortality and morbidity (risk of: perinatal hypoxia due to placental insufficiency; obstructed labour due to larger fetus; meconium aspiration; and reduced skull moulding).
- Induction of labour is usually advised after 41wk.

Antepartum haemorrhage

Uterine–placental bleeding after 24wk gestation. Observations or immediate delivery, depending on severity and gestation. Associations:
- ↑ perinatal mortality and morbidity; preterm delivery.

Major causes:
- Placenta praevia, vasa praevia, placental abruption.

Umbilical cord prolapse

An obstetric emergency due to high risk of cord compression and perinatal asphyxia. Requires urgent delivery, usually by CS.

Preterm prelabour rupture of the membranes

- In 80%, preterm labour rapidly follows.
- In remaining 20%, there is significant risk of infection and, if PPROM occurs before 20wk, neonatal pulmonary hypoplasia.
- *Treatment:* give mother corticosteroids. Consider antibiotics. Tocolysis is contraindicated.

Preterm labour

(See ⊃ General management, pp. 94–5; ⊃ Birth at the limit of viability, pp. 96–7.)

Failure to progress

Neonatal and maternal morbidity increase with progressive delay.
- *Cause:* passage obstruction (malpresentation, cephalopelvic disproportion, abnormal pelvic and cervical anatomy) or uterine dysfunction.
- *Treatment:* artificial rupture of membranes (ARM), analgesia, and synthetic oxytocin to hasten delivery. CS may be necessary.

Disturbing/abnormal fetal HR patterns

May signify hypoxia. Fetal acidosis results if hypoxia prolonged or repeated.

Signs
- Loss of variability in baseline fetal HR (<5 beats/min).
- Late decelerations (in HR): lowest fetal HR is >30s after peak uterine contraction.
- Repetitive severe, variable decelerations.
- Prolonged fetal deceleration (2–9min below established baseline).
- Prolonged fetal bradycardia (<100/min).
- Persistent fetal tachycardia (>170/min).

Tests
- Fetal blood gas sampling (pH ≤7.24 = 'borderline', repeat ≤30min; ≤7.2 = 'abnormal'—consultant obstetrician and delivery).
- Postnatal umbilical artery and vein blood gases are used to determine the actual level and nature of acidaemia.

Malpresentation

Breech is the commonest form of malpresentation (3% at term). Types include: extended (hips flexed and knees extended), flexed (hips and knees flexed), and footling (feet are presenting part). Management:
- *External cephalic version:* may be successful in turning baby between 34 and 36wk.
- *Vaginal breech delivery:* associated with ↑ perinatal mortality and morbidity; CS is recommended.

Other malpresentations associated with ↑ risk of obstructed labour and CS (obligatory for brow or transverse presentation).

Shoulder dystocia

Inability to deliver shoulders after head has been delivered. Cord compression leads to rapid fetal asphyxia.
- *Treatment:* urgent delivery—experienced obstetrician, McRobert's manoeuvre (flexion + abduction of maternal hips, thighs on abdomen), suprapubic pressure, posterior fetal arm extraction ± episiotomy.
- *Risks:* perinatal asphyxia, humerus and clavicle fracture, Erb's palsy.

Maternal disorders causing neonatal disease

Any maternal disease can adversely affect fetal/neonatal health. Certain maternal illnesses (e.g. CHD) raise the risk of inheritance in newborns:
- Spontaneous abortion and fetal death.
- IUGR and/or preterm delivery.

Maternal drug ingestion

Maternal medications or substance abuse can affect the newborn:
- Maternal anticonvulsants (see ➔ Miscellaneous congenital malformations, Table 24.2, p. 890).
- Tobacco; alcohol abuse and fetal alcohol syndrome (see ➔ Miscellaneous congenital malformations, Table 24.2, p. 890).
- Neonatal abstinence syndrome (see ➔ Neonatal abstinence syndrome, p. 168).

Hypertensive diseases

Pregnancy-induced hypertension, e.g. pre-eclampsia, eclampsia, haemolytic anaemia, elevated liver enzymes, low platelet count (HELLP) syndrome, is associated with fetal loss, preterm delivery, IUGR, neonatal leucopenia, and thrombocytopenia. Maternal drug treatment (e.g. β-blockers) causes neonatal hypoglycaemia and hypotension.

Systemic lupus erythematosus

Associated with:
- ↑ risk of spontaneous abortion.
- IUGR and preterm delivery.
- Neonatal lupus syndrome (rare; associated with anti-Ro and anti-La antibodies): complete heart block, haemolytic anaemia, leucopenia, thrombocytopenia, and discoid erythematous skin rash.

Antiphospholipid syndrome

Maternal antiphospholipid antibodies (e.g. lupus anticoagulant or anticardiolipin antibodies) are associated with spontaneous abortion, IUGR, fetal death, and need for preterm delivery.

Thyroid disease

(See ➔ Neonatal thyrotoxicosis, p. 414.) In 10% of women with Graves's disease, thyroid-stimulating hormone (TSH) receptor-stimulating antibodies cross the placenta, causing neonatal thyrotoxicosis. Fetus affected by high maternal serum immunoglobulin G (IgG) or by mother's treatment in pregnancy. Cord blood: TSH, free T4 (fT4), TSH receptor antibody (TRAB); repeat day 5 if abnormal.

Myasthenia gravis

In 10%, transplacental passage of IgG antibodies to motor end-plate acetylcholine (ACh) receptors causes transient neonatal myasthenia gravis.

Diabetes mellitus

(See ➔ Infant of a mother with diabetes mellitus, p. 93.)

Maternal infection

(See ➔ Prevention of neonatal infection, pp. 166–7.)

Birth trauma

Risk factors

LGA, cephalic–pelvic disproportion, malpresentation, precipitate delivery, instrumental delivery, shoulder dystocia, prematurity.

Head

- *Caput succedaneum:* oedema of the presenting scalp. Can be particularly large following ventouse delivery (chignon). Rapidly resolves.
- *Cephalohaematoma:* common fluctuant swelling(s) due to subperiostial bleed(s). Most often occurs over parietal bones. Swelling limited by suture lines. Resolves over weeks.
- *Subaponeurotic haematoma:* rare; bleeding not confined by skull periosteum, so can be large and life-threatening. Presents as fluctuant scalp swelling, not limited by suture lines.

Skin

- *Traumatic cyanosis:* bruising and petechiae of presenting part.
- *Lacerations:* caused by forceps, ventouse cap, scalp electrodes, scalp pH sampling, or scalpel wounds during CS. Close with Steri-Strips® or suture if required.

Nerve palsies

- *Brachial plexus:* commonest is Erb's palsy (C5–C6 nerve routes). May result from difficult assisted delivery (e.g. shoulder dystocia); the arm is flaccid, with a pronated forearm and a flexed wrist (waiter's tip position). Complete recovery occurs within 6wk in two-thirds of cases. X-ray clavicle to exclude fractures. Refer to physiotherapy (PT) for assessment and follow-up.
- *Facial nerve palsy:* follows pressure on face from either maternal ischial spine or forceps. Presents as facial asymmetry that is worse on crying (affected side shows lack of eye closure and lower facial movement; mouth is drawn to normal side). Majority recover in 1–2wk. May require eye care with methylcellulose and specialist referral.

Fractures

- *Clavicle:* commonest.
- *Long bone fractures:* usually lower avulsion fractures of the femoral or tibial epiphyses, or mid-shaft fractures of the femur or humerus. Infant presents as unsettled, with affected limb pseudo-paralysis or obvious deformity or swelling. Confirm by X-ray.
- *Skull fracture:* associated with forceps delivery and usually no treatment needed unless depressed; if so, neurosurgical referral required.
- *Treatment:* analgesia; often no need for surgical options; immobilize limb (arm inside baby-grow); usually heals and remodels in weeks.

Soft tissue trauma

- *Sternocleidomastoid tumour:* overstretching of muscle leads to haematoma. Subsequent contraction of muscle results in non-tender 'tumour' and torticollis (head turns away from affected muscle). PT almost always curative. Possible indication of malposition *in utero*— consider ↑ risk of DDH (see ➲ Developmental dysplasia of the hip, p. 681).
- *Fat necrosis:* tender, red subcutaneous swelling caused by pressure over bony prominences, e.g. forceps. It usually resolves spontaneously. May be extensive with risk of ↑ Ca^{2+}, and so there is a need to monitor serum level.

Non-specifically ill neonate

Early recognition of serious neonatal illness is an important skill. The nurse or parent may say that the infant is just 'not right'. Listen, examine the baby carefully, and act if in any doubt! Any serious disease can present non-specifically.

Major causes

- *Infection:* e.g. group B *Streptococcus* (GBS), septicaemia, meningitis (see ➲ Neonatal infection, pp. 162–3).
- *Hypothermia* (may be sign of infection).
- *Metabolic:* e.g. hypoglycaemia (see ➲ Hypoglycaemia, pp. 112–13); IEM (see ➲ Inborn errors of metabolism, p. 169).
- *Cardiac:* e.g. CHD, arrhythmias (see ➲ Congenital heart disease, p. 48; ➲ Congenital heart disease, p. 197; ➲ Dysrhythmias, p. 49).
- *GI:* e.g. NEC (see ➲ Necrotizing enterocolitis, pp. 160–1).
- *CNS:* e.g. intracranial haemorrhage, seizures (see ➲ Neonatal seizures, pp. 114–15; ➲ Cerebral haemorrhage and ischaemia, pp. 158–9).

Presentation

- *Skin:* pallor, mottling, peripheral cyanosis, cool peripheries, CRT >2s, rash, jaundice.
- *Temperature:* ↑ or ↓.
- *CNS:* lethargy, weak or unusual cry, generalized hypotonia, irritability, jittery, seizures.
- *Respiratory:* apnoea, expiratory grunting, flaring nostrils, tachypnoea (>60 breaths/min), intercostal or subcostal recession, tracheal tug.
- *CVS:* tachycardia (>160/min), weak or absent pulses (bradycardia <80/min or hypotension are late/pre-terminal signs).
- *GI:* vomiting, distended abdomen (ileus), diarrhoea, bloody stools; abdominal tenderness; bilious vomit or aspirate.
- *Metabolic:* ↑ or ↓ blood glucose.

Management of non-specifically ill neonate

Quickly assess ABC. Secure the airway; give O₂ if required, and provide ETT intubation and MV if needed; then:

- Transfer to neonatal unit as soon as safe to do so (get a nurse/midwife to accompany you on the move).
- Obtain vascular access [IV/umbilical vein (UV)/IO], and give bolus NS 10–20mL/kg if circulatory compromise. Repeat if necessary.
- Monitor breathing, SpO₂, HR, BP (consider arterial access), and temperature.
- Measure BP, blood glucose, U&E, FBC, and ABG. Consider clotting studies and CRP. ETT and MV early if respiratory failure.
- Full septic screen: blood culture; CXR/AXR; LP (only postpone if baby very unstable) for CSF, MC&S, protein, and glucose; stool culture and virology; urine [suprapubic or midstream urine (MSU) if antibiotics can be delayed].
- Consider cranial ultrasound scan (USS) if preterm/at risk.

Start broad-spectrum antibiotics (consult local protocols):

- IV benzylpenicillin and an aminoglycoside (e.g. gentamicin), unless possible *Listeria* infection, in which case substitute ampicillin for benzylpenicillin.
- If >48h old, and particularly if indwelling lines were present before illness, consider flucloxacillin, or vancomycin, and gentamicin.
- If meningitis, ensure broad-spectrum cover and good CSF penetration, e.g. cefotaxime. Treat for 14–21 days if meningitis present.
- If all cultures are –ve and index of suspicion of sepsis is low, antibiotics can be stopped after 48h. If not, treat for 5–7 days, changing antibiotics according to sensitivities of significant identified pathogens. If any doubt, consult microbiologist.

Other specific treatment, as appropriate, e.g. correct hypoglycaemia, inotropic support if persistently hypotensive, blood transfusion if significant haemorrhage, clotting factors to correct DIC.

Neonatal jaundice

(See also ➲ Jaundice, pp. 282–3.) Jaundice is common (60% term, 80% pre-term in first week) and usually unconjugated. Significant jaundice may indicate underlying disease. High serum unconjugated free bilirubin may cause kernicterus (deafness, athetoid CP, seizures).

Physiological jaundice

Common and appears after 24h, peaks around day 3–4, and usually resolves by day 14. It is due to immaturity of hepatic bilirubin conjugation, but poor feeding (particularly in breastfed infants) can contribute. Jaundice progresses in a cephalic–caudal direction.

- *Measure bilirubin* (transcutaneous or serum): in jaundiced babies. Action required when serum bilirubin (SBR) is above age/gestation cut-offs or rapidly rising (see Fig. 4.2).
- *Causes of elevated SBR:* exaggerated physiological jaundice (e.g. preterm, bruising), sepsis, haemolytic disorders, hepatic disease.

Treatment of elevated SBR

- Stop bilirubin rising to level that may cause kernicterus (see ➲ Bilirubin encephalopathy, p. 177).
- Treat any underlying cause, e.g. sepsis.
- Start 'blue light' phototherapy (converts bilirubin to water-soluble form that can then be excreted in urine).
- See chart for phototherapy (see Fig. 4.2). Risk factors: family history, exclusive breastfeeding, rhesus (Rh) or blood group incompatibility.
- Measure SBR frequently (4- to 24-hourly depending on circumstances) and stop when falls below treatment level.
- Ensure adequate hydration.
- Cover eyes (phototherapy side effects: decrease/increase temperature, eye damage, diarrhoea, dehydration, rash, separation from mother).
- Exchange transfusion ± intravenous immunoglobulin (IVIG) if very high SBR (e.g. >450 micromoles/L in term infant at 48h) or rapid rise (>8.5 micromoles/L/h).

In the UK, the National Institute for Health and Care Excellence (NICE) has produced guidance on investigation and management of newborn jaundice (see Fig. 4.2)—the full guideline includes gestation-specific treatment thresholds and charts (available at: ℘ http://guidance.nice.org.uk/CG98).

Jaundice in the first 24h

Assume it is pathological. Start phototherapy. Check SBR, FBC, direct Coombs' test (DCT), and blood group. Consider septic screen/TORCH.

- *Causes:* haemolysis (e.g. Rh disease), red cell enzyme defects (e.g. G6PD deficiency), red cell membrane defects (congenital spherocytosis, elliptocytosis), sepsis, severe bruising.

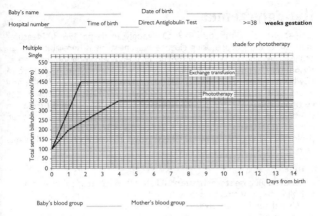

Baby's name _____   Date of birth _____

Hospital number _____ Time of birth _____ Direct Antiglobulin Test _____   >=38   **weeks gestation**

Baby's blood group _____   Mother's blood group _____

Fig. 4.2 Bilirubin thresholds for phototherapy and exchange transfusion in infant with hyperbilirubinaemia.

Reproduced from *Neonatal Jaundice*. National Collaborating Centre for Women's and Children's Health, May 2010, with permission of Royal College of Obstetricians and Gynaecologists.

Prolonged jaundice (>14 days, term infant; >21 days, preterm)

Investigate conjugated bilirubin—if conjugated hyperbilirubinaemia, more investigation needed. Ask about pale stools/dark urine.
- *Causes:* breastfeeding (benign, self-limiting, and usually resolves by 12wk), enclosed bleeding (e.g. cephalohaematoma), prematurity, haemolysis, sepsis, hypothyroidism, conjugated jaundice, hepatic enzyme disorders (e.g. Crigler–Najjar syndrome, Lucy–Driscoll disease).
- *Initial investigations:* look for pale stools and/or dark urine, total and conjugated bilirubin, FBC, blood group determination (mother and baby) and direct antiglobulin test, urine MC&S (local policy varies), metabolic screening (including congenital hypothyroidism); review and check thyroid function tests (TFTs).
- *Treatment:* depends on cause. Rarely phototherapy is beneficial (e.g. Crigler–Najjar syndrome).

Conjugated jaundice (conjugated SBR >25 micromoles/L)

Stools may be clay-coloured in obstructive jaundice.
- *Causes:* sepsis, total parenteral nutrition (TPN), biliary tract obstruction (e.g. biliary atresia, choledochal cyst), viral hepatitis; TORCH infections, α1-antitrypsin deficiency, CF, inspissated bile syndrome after haemolytic disease, galactosaemia, other IEM, idiopathic giant cell hepatitis.
- *Initial investigations:* (see ➲ Prolonged jaundice, p. 111). Further investigations: radiology, enzyme testing, viral serology, liver biopsy, histology. Investigate for biliary atresia with urgent US, as timeline for severe liver complications is a few weeks.
- *Treatment:* depends on cause.

Hypoglycaemia

(See ➜ Hypoglycaemia, pp. 78–9; ➜ Hypoglycaemia, pp. 496–8.) Measurement of blood glucose using glucose reagent strips is unreliable. Use an analyser or laboratory measurement. In the newborn period, defined as <2.6mmol/L, but new guidance suggests <2.0mmol/L in healthy term newborns (check local policy). Blood glucose drops naturally in the few hours after birth, before normalizing—newborns have the ability to use ketones/lactate for energy. All infants should be encouraged to feed in the first hour, if well. Those at risk of hypoglycaemia: infant of diabetic mother (IDM), weight <2500g or < 3rd centile, <37/40 gestation, maternal β-blockers, and birth asphyxia. Check blood glucose urgently in all infants who are unwell, lethargic, or jittery.

Causes

- Reduced glucose store: preterm, IUGR, LBW, IEM (e.g. galactosaemia).
- ↑ glucose consumption: sepsis, hypothermia, perinatal hypoxia, polycythaemia, haemolytic disease, seizures.
- Hyperinsulinism: maternal diabetes mellitus, BWS, pancreatic islet cell hyperplasia, transient.
- Miscellaneous: maternal β-blockers, malfunctioning IV infusion (IVI).
- Rare: fetal alcohol syndrome, pituitary insufficiency, adrenal insufficiency.

Presentation

Commonly asymptomatic. Jitteriness, apnoea, poor feeding, drowsiness, seizures, irritability, hypotonia, macrosomia (if hyperinsulinism).

Investigations

- *Measure blood glucose* before the second feed in asymptomatic high-risk infants. Apart from regular blood glucose measurements, further investigation is not usually required if cause evident (e.g. IDM).
- *Suspicious patterns of hypoglycaemia meriting investigation include:*
  - Recurrent hypoglycaemia in term infant despite functioning IVI of dextrose 10%.
  - Severe (<1mmol/L) and/or recurrent (>1) hypoglycaemia.
  - Symptomatic hypoglycaemia.
  - High glucose infusion rate (>8mg/kg/min) (see ➜ Therapy, p. 82; ➜ Box 3.16, p. 82; ➜ Investigation, p. 79).
  - Hypoglycaemia and prolonged jaundice (panhypopituitarism) or Na⁺ abnormalities (adrenal problems).
  - Hypoglycaemia with genital or midline abnormalities.
- First-line tests (taken when hypoglycaemic) (see ➜ Metabolic investigations, p. 496).

Treatment of hypoglycaemia

Symptomatic or severe hypoglycaemia (glucose <1.0mmol/L):
- IV bolus 2.5mL/kg of dextrose 10%.
- Follow with 10% dextrose IVI (4–6mg/kg/min).

Asymptomatic (glucose <2.0mmol/L or 2.0–2.6mmol/L, twice):
- Enterally fed infants:
  - Review feed chart (frequency/volume, etc.).
  - Dextrogel® 0.4mL/kg PO, followed by a feed if glucose ≥1.0–1.9mmol/L, can be used.
  - If reluctant to feed—consider NGT.
  - If not tolerating milk—consider IV.
  - Give early milk feed (consider larger volume).
  - Monitor with pre-feed blood glucose levels.
- Infants on IV fluids:
  - Check IV line is working.
  - If glucose <1.0mmol/L—give bolus, then increase infusion rate/concentration.
  - If glucose >1.0mmol/L—increase infusion rate/concentration.

Resistant hypoglycaemia (GIR >8mg/kg/min):
- Seek specialist advice, as hyperinsulinism likely.
- Increase background glucose infusion concentration (central IV access needed).
- Glucagon 0.5mg IM can be given in emergency—rebound ↑ insulin secretion will occur.
- Specialist treatment options include:
  - Diazoxide (give chlorothiazide to counteract fluid retention).
  - Somatostatin (octreotide).
  - Nifedipine.
  - Surgery (subtotal pancreatectomy).
- Enteral feeding promotes normality. Aim to wean off IV as soon as able.
- High concentrations of dextrose (>12.5%) require central IV access.
- Monitor plasma Na$^+$ if on IV fluids.

Prevention of hypoglycaemia in at-risk infants

Adequate feed soon after birth (<1h) and then at least 3-hourly. Monitor blood glucose levels (pre-feed), keep warm, and support feeding.

Prognosis

Profound/prolonged hypoglycaemia can cause neurological damage—exact level/duration after which this may occur is unclear.

Neonatal seizures

(See also ➲ Epilepsy syndromes: neonatal, p. 370.) Incidence ~2–4/1000 live births. Usually occurs 12–48h after delivery. Can be generalized or focal, and tonic, clonic, or myoclonic. Many 'seizures' have clinical–electrical dissociation, i.e. clinical seizures not associated with electrical seizure activity and vice versa. Also, subtle seizures (lip-smacking, limb-cycling, eye deviation, apnoea, etc.) are difficult to identify and differentiate from benign conditions that mimic seizures:

- Startle or Moro reflexes.
- Normal 'jittery' movements (fine, fast limb movements that are abated by holding affected limb).
- Sleep myoclonus: during rapid eye movement (REM) sleep.

Causes

With better neuroimaging, fewer infants are being categorized as 'benign'/ 'idiopathic' seizures. Neonatal stroke is increasingly recognized.

Brain injury
- Hypoxic–ischaemic encephalopathy (HIE).
- Intracranial haemorrhage.
- Cerebral infarction (ischaemic or haemorrhagic), stroke.
- Cerebral oedema.
- Birth trauma.

CNS infection
- Meningitis (e.g. GBS, coliforms).
- Encephalitis [e.g. herpes simplex virus (HSV), CMV].
- Cerebral malformation.

Metabolic and IEM
- Hypoglycaemia.
- Hypo- or hypernatraemia.
- Hypocalcaemia, hypomagnesaemia.
- Pyridoxine-dependent seizures.
- Non-ketotic hyperglycinaemia.
- Neonatal withdrawal from maternal medication or substance abuse.
- Kernicterus (see ➲ Bilirubin encephalopathy, p. 177).

Rare syndromes
- Benign familial neonatal seizures [autosomal dominant (AD)].
- Early myoclonic encephalopathy.

Initial investigation and management

- Review the family history, pregnancy, and delivery.
- Complete a full examination.
- Evaluate for infection, U&E, Ca²⁺, Mg²⁺, glucose, and ABG.
- If available, start signal-processed EEG with devices such as *cerebral function analysis monitoring* (CFAM).

Treatment of seizures with antiseizure medication

- *Immediate:* give O_2, maintain airway, insert IV access, check glucose, treat underlying cause. When to start ASMs is controversial because risks and benefits of treatment have not been properly evaluated; usual indication of >3 seizures/h or single seizure lasting >3–5min, particularly with cardiorespiratory compromise.
- *First-line ASM:* IV phenobarbital (10–20mg/kg bolus; give further 10–15mg if seizures persist after 30min; maintenance 5mg/day).
- *Second-line ASM:* IV clonazepam, IV midazolam, or IV phenytoin.
- *Intractable seizures:* consider trial of parenteral pyridoxine (50mg). Depending on cause, probably safe to stop ASMs after a few days of no seizures, but many clinicians prefer to wait several months before ceasing.

Further investigation

If appropriate, further investigation may include:
- Imaging: e.g. brain MRI ± spectroscopy ± MRA.
- Blood/urine: toxicology screening, serum ammonia, urine organic acids, serum amino acids, karyotype, and TORCH screening.

Prognosis

Prognosis varies according to the cause of seizures.
Generally good for:
- Idiopathic seizures.
- Sleep myoclonus.
- Hypocalcaemia.
- Benign familial neonatal seizures.

Significant risk of adverse neurodevelopmental outcome after:
- Meningitis.
- HIE.
- Hypoglycaemia.
- Cerebral infarction.
- Hypo- or hypernatraemia.
- Cerebral malformations.
- Kernicterus and some IEM.

The floppy infant

(See ⊃ Neuromuscular disorders, pp. 384–7; ⊃ Congenital myasthenia gravis, p. 388; ⊃ Myotonic dystrophy, p. 390; ⊃ Congenital myopathies, p. 391.) The causes are divided as:
- *Central:* involving the CNS (so-called 'floppy strong').
- *Peripheral:* involving lower motor neurons, neuromuscular junction (NMJ), or primary muscle disease ('floppy weak').

Range of clinical features

- *Common to both 'central' and 'peripheral' diseases:* generalized hypotonia, 'frog leg' posture, respiratory failure, obstetric problems (e.g. polyhydramnios due to impaired swallowing, breech presentation), HIE.
- *Central conditions:* encephalopathy, dysmorphism, reasonable muscle strength, ↑ or normal tendon reflexes.
- *Peripheral causes:* normal conscious level, muscle signs (weakness, myotonia, fasciculations, or fatiguing), ↓ or normal tendon reflexes, little facial expression, micrognathia, high-arched palate, ptosis, undescended testes, limb contracture/deformities (severe in arthrogryposis multiplex congenita), and hip dislocation.

Management

- *Exclude severe systemic illness:* eg treat sepsis promptly.
- *Treat respiratory failure:* O₂ or MV as required.
- *Elicit history:* e.g. maternal myotonic dystrophy and antenatal features such as movements and polyhydramnios.
- *Examine* for above clinical features to help distinguish cause; examine both parents for possible disease (e.g. maternal myasthenia gravis or myotonic dystrophy, possibly undiagnosed!).
- *'Central' causes:* consider—blood glucose, U&E, Ca²⁺, Mg²⁺, septic screen, ESR/CRP, TFTs, karyotype, IEM screen; imaging with cranial US, CT/MRI; EEG; maternal drug screen; genetics opinion if dysmorphic.
- *'Peripheral' cause:* most tests are available in tertiary centres, but consider: serum CPK; cytogenetics (e.g. myotonic dystrophy); echocardiogram (storage diseases); muscle US; electromyography (EMG) and nerve conduction studies; muscle or sural nerve biopsy; edrophonium 20mcg/kg test dose, then followed 30s later (if no adverse reaction) with 80mcg/kg IV (causes dramatic improvement in some forms of myasthenia gravis).
- *Spinal cord damage (rare):* consider in the infant who has flaccid paralysis from birth. Associated with rotational forceps delivery. Immobilize neck. Seek specialist advice. MRI.
- Referral to paediatric neurologist.

Box 4.1 Causes

'Floppy strong' or 'central' involving CNS
- Prematurity.
- HIE.
- Hypoglycaemia.
- Sepsis.
- Electrolyte disturbance.
- Drug-related.
- IEM.
- Hypothyroidism (see ➔ Congenital hypothyroidism, p. 410).
- Chromosomal disorders (e.g. trisomy 21).
- CNS malformations.
- Benign congenital hypotonia.
- Underlying syndrome [e.g. Prader–Willi syndrome (PWS)].
- Cervical spinal cord trauma (birth injury).

'Floppy weak' or 'peripheral' involving lower neurology, NMJ, or primary muscle disease
- SMA, particularly type 1 (previously known as Werdnig–Hoffman disease).
- Myasthenia gravis (transient or congenital).
- Congenital myotonic dystrophy (AD inheritance from mother).
- Congenital muscular dystrophies.
- Congenital myopathies.
- Metabolic myopathies.
- Peripheral neuropathies.
- Spinal cord injury.

Prognosis

Causation-dependent (see Box 4.1) and very variable, given the advent of new gene and biological therapies for some previously fatal conditions.

Hydrops fetalis

Characterized by abnormal fluid accumulation in skin and body compartments, which results from rate of interstitial fluid production exceeding absorption. The incidence is ~1/2500 to 1/4000 births, and it results in severe illness. *In utero*, US of the fetus shows:
- Gross generalized oedema.
- Ascites.
- Pleural ± pericardial effusions.

Causes

Box 4.2 summarizes the causes of hydrops which broadly is due to underlying disease, singularly or in combination, that results in: ↑ capillary hydrostatic pressure, ↓ colloid osmotic pressure, lymphatic obstruction, and capillary leaking.

Box 4.2 Causes of hydrops fetalis

Immune
- Haemolytic disease of the newborn: alloimmune, Rh, Kell, other.

Non-immune
- Cardiac: structure—Ebstein's anomaly, *in utero* closure of ductus arteriosus, hypoplastic left or right heart; arrhythmia—SVT, atrial flutter; cardiomyopathies—TORCH or other viral infection.
- Genetic: Turner's, chromosomal trisomies (21, 13, 18, etc.).
- Fetal anaemia: twin-to-twin transfusion, α-thalassaemia, fetal-to-maternal haemorrhage.
- Infection: TORCH, parvovirus B19.
- Malformation: congenital cystic adenomatoid malformation (CCAM), bowel atresia.
- AVM.
- Lymphatic (cystic hygroma).
- Idiopathic.

Associated complications
- Intrauterine/perinatal death.
- Obstetric complications, e.g. shoulder dystocia.
- Preterm labour.
- Pulmonary hypoplasia (pleural effusions).
- Perinatal asphyxia.

Management

Disorders treatable antenatally
- Intrauterine blood transfusion (IUT) for haemolytic disease or parvovirus infection.
- Anti-arrhythmia drugs to treat fetal SVT.
- Laser ablation of fetal vessels (twin–twin transfusion syndrome).

Birth planning
Before birth, organize expert help.
- If anaemia likely, have available fresh CMV –ve, O –ve blood, irradiated (if previous IUT), cross-matched blood against the mother.
- Prepare for full resuscitation, MV, UVC insertion, paracentesis (ascites), or pleural effusion drainage.

Neonatal management
- Resuscitation:
  - ETT intubation, MV.
  - Paracentesis, thoracentesis.
  - Blood transfusion or partial exchange transfusion.
- Supportive management:
  - Cardiac support—vasopressors, inotropes.
  - Respiratory support—MV.
  - Chest tube placement, drainage of ascites.
  - Fluid and electrolyte management.
  - Treat anaemia: blood transfusion or partial exchange.
  - Transfusion.
  - Treatment of infections.
- Octreotide to treat chylothorax and ascites.

Prognosis

For fetuses or infants with non-immune hydrops, survival rates are variable, in the range of 50%. Neurodevelopmental outcome depends on cause.
- *Higher survival* in infants with SVT, chylothorax, and parvovirus infections. Survival rates with immune hydrops is >80%.
- *Lower rate of survival* in those with chromosomal abnormalities.

Routine care of the newborn

Routine measurements *within 1h of birth* include *weight* (term, mean ~3.5kg) and *occipitofrontal head circumference* (OFC) (mean ~35cm).

Usually babies are not weighed again until day 3–5 and then on alternate days while they remain in hospital. It is normal to lose weight after birth because of water loss, but weight loss should not exceed 10% of birth-weight. Birthweight should generally be regained by day 7. Subsequent mean growth is 20–30g/day until age 6mth.

Vitamin K (phytomenadione)

To prevent haemorrhagic disease of the newborn, vitamin K1 is routinely given within 48h of birth.
• *Dose*: 1mg IM (preferred) in term infants, or 2mg PO on days 1 and 7, and if breastfeeding, also on day 28.

Cord care

Immediately after birth, clamp the cord with a purpose-made device. Keep the umbilicus clean and dry. The cord usually detaches after 7–10 days. If umbilical granulomas develop:
• Keep the area clean from faecal soiling.
• Use warm boiled water and soap, and allow the area to dry with air.
• Consider chemical cautery (silver nitrate stick).

Thermal care

Birth should occur in a warm room—dry baby with a warm towel; then immediately wrap or place skin-to-skin on mother's front, and then cover baby with a warm towel and a hat.

Bathing

Not until day 2 or 3. Use tepid water. Genitalia should be cleaned superficially only. Do not retract the foreskin; it is attached to the glans.

Biochemical screening

(See also ⊃ Congenital hypothyroidism, p. 410; ⊃ Newborn screening, p. 511.) In the UK, all infants undergo the newborn blood spot (heel prick, four drops) test using a special card between day 3 and day 10 ('Guthrie' test). Some regional variation exists, although nine rare, but serious, conditions are screened (see Box 4.3). +ve tests require follow-up and more detailed testing.

Newborn hearing screening

(See also ⊃ Hearing assessment, pp. 854–5; ⊃ Secondary prevention, pp. 896–7.) All infants in the UK will have their hearing screened [otoacoustic emission (OAE)] within the first 4wk of life. Automatic auditory brainstem response (AABR) testing is carried out if any uncertainty in OAE response.

Box 4.3 Biochemical newborn screening in the UK (UK incidence by births)

(See also ◑ Newborn screening, p. 511; ◑ Congenital hypothyroidism, p. 410).

- Sickle-cell disease (SCD) (1/2000).
- CF (1/2500); ↑ immune-reactive trypsin.
- Congenital hypothyroidism (1/3000); ↑ TSH.
- Six inherited metabolic diseases [1/10 000 babies born with PKU or medium-chain acyl-CoA dehydrogenase deficiency (MCAD); other metabolic conditions are rarer, occurring in 1/100 000–150 000 babies]:
  - PKU; ↑ phenylalanine.
  - MCAD.
  - Maple syrup urine disease.
  - Isovaleric acidaemia.
  - Glutaric aciduria type 1.
  - Homocystinuria (pyridoxine-unresponsive).

Milk feeding

The methods for milk feeding include:
- Breastfeeding
- Bottle.
- Tube feeding (if too ill/immature to suck).
- Naso-/orogastic tube (NGT/OGT).
- Silastic nasojejunal tube (NJT) used in severe gastro-oesophageal reflux (GOR), aspiration, or recurrent apnoeas.
- Gastrostomy (if required long-term, older children).

Breastfeeding

Breastfeeding is a learnt skill for both mother and baby. Establishing feeding can take time, and it is vital that good support is available (use breastfeeding advisors or midwives with appropriate training).

Advantages
- ↓ maternal post-partum haemorrhage.
- Mild maternal contraceptive effect.
- ↑ bonding.
- ↓ maternal breast cancer risk.
- Cheap.
- ↓ infant mortality (less relevant in developed world).
- ↓ GI and respiratory infection rates.
- ↓ later autoimmune disease incidence [e.g. type 1 diabetes mellitus (T1DM), atopic diseases].
- Reported increase in later intelligence quotient (IQ).

Problems
- Cracked/sore nipples.
- Maternal anxiety (breastfed babies can gain weight slower than their bottle-fed counterparts—give reassurance and support).
- Small risk of hypernatraemic dehydration if low milk intake (suspect if weight loss >10% birthweight).

Contraindications
- +ve maternal HIV status (in developed countries).
- Certain maternal medications (e.g. amiodarone).
- Maternal herpes zoster over breast.
- Infantile galactosaemia or phenylketonuria (PKU).
- Primary lactose intolerance (very rare).

Expressed breast milk (EBM)

Usually mother's own breast milk, but some units have donor breast milk banks which can be of value in extreme preterm infants. EBM is usually used to establish feeding in preterm infants but is also useful when top-up feeds are required, if mother and baby are separated for any reason, or if there are other maternal problems (e.g. cracked/sore nipples or breast engorgement). Once expressed, EBM can be refrigerated and used within 24–48h, or frozen and used for up to 3mth.

Formula milk

Normal volume required is 150mL/kg/day. See Box 4.4 for different types of formula milk available.
- *Advantages:* paternal involvement, milk intake determined.
- *Problems:* constipation, oral thrush.

Box 4.4 Types of formula milk available

- *Cow's milk formula* (standard milk): extensively modified (e.g. to decrease solute load and increase iron and vitamins). Formula used from birth is predominantly whey protein, while 'follow-on' milks (for 'hungrier' infants >6mth) are predominantly casein-based.
- *Soya milk:* previously recommended for cow's milk protein allergy or lactose intolerance, but now not recommended because of high phyto-oestrogens and availability of alternatives.
- *Hydrolysed cow's milk formula* (e.g. Nutramigen®): contains short peptides. Indicated for prophylaxis or treatment of cow's or soya milk protein allergy.
- *Elemental formulas* (e.g. Neocate®): cow's milk protein is fully hydrolysed to amino acids. Use in severe milk protein allergy or malabsorption.
- *Other specialized formula milks* for conditions such as: preterm/LBW infants, GOR (thickened with cornstarch), IEM, lactose intolerance (lactose-free milk), poor growth (high-energy formulas), and malabsorption (e.g. Pregestimil®).

Trophic feeding (gut-priming)

Trophic feeding is the practice of feeding small volumes of milk (0.5–1mL/kg/h of EBM) to enhance gut structure and function in infants too ill or immature to tolerate substantial amounts of milk feeds. The evidence suggests that in the preterm infant, it improves GI motility and function, as well as achieving clinical outcomes (i.e. ↑ weight gain, ↑ head growth, ↓ risk of infection, and later improved milk tolerance).

Routine neonatal examination

Each baby must be examined at least once in the first week, usually on day 1 after birth.

Purpose

- Maternal reassurance.
- Health education: explaining common variations.
- Detecting asymptomatic problems, e.g. CHD, DDH.
- Screening for rare, but serious, conditions.

Order of examination

- *Attending midwife:* ask if there are any concerns or problems.
- *Mother:* check patient notes for relevant details of the maternal medical history, family history, antenatal and obstetric history, and social history. Ask about feeding and whether baby has passed meconium/urine.
- *Baby:* when baby is *quiet* (if needed, use calming techniques like pacifiers, sucking a clean finger, examination after a feed), note:
  - General posture and movements.
  - Skin colour.
  - Listen to the heart and lungs.
  - Examine the eyes for size and strabismus (see ⊃ Vision screening in the UK, p. 967).
  - Use an ophthalmoscope to examine the eyes for bilateral red reflexes to exclude cataract or retinoblastoma (see ⊃ Anterior segment examination, p. 968; ⊃ Retinoblastoma, p. 597; ⊃ Cataract, p. 978).

The rest of the examination should proceed as described in Box 4.5.

Box 4.5 Rest of routine neonatal examination

The baby should be completely undressed. Examination proceeds as follows, in head-to-toe order (be systematic and learn your style!):

- *Cranium:* measure maximum OFC (normal 33–37cm at term); assess skull shape, fontanelle positions, tension, and size (anterior may be up to 4cm × 4cm, posterior 1cm).
- *Face:* assess any dysmorphism, nose, and chin size. Inspect mouth. Visualize and palpate palate for possible clefts.
- *Ears:* assess position, size, shape, and external meatus patency.
- *Neck:* inspect and assess movements; palpate clavicles.
- *Chest:* assess shape, symmetry, nipple position, RR (normal 40–60/min), pattern, and effort. Palpate precordium and apex heartbeat.
- *Abdomen:* inspect shape and umbilical stump. Check for inguinal hernias. Palpate for masses, liver (normally palpable up to 2cm below costal margin), spleen (normally palpable up to 1cm), kidneys (normally palpable), and bladder.
- *Genitalia:*
  - Girls—inspect (NB: the clitoris and labia are normally large).
  - Boys—assess size, shape, and position of urinary meatus; palpate for descended testes (NB: retractile testes are normal).
- *Femoral pulses:* palpate (absence or weakness may indicate aortic arch abnormalities).
- *Anus:* assess position and patency.
- *Spine:* any deformity (e.g. sacral naevi, dimple, pit, hair, patch, lipoma, or pigmentation may indicate underlying abnormality).
- *Limbs:* assess symmetry, shape, passive and active movements, and digit number and shape. Assess palmar creases. Examine hips for DDH (see ⊃ Developmental dysplasia of the hip, p. 681).
- *CNS:* in addition to evaluation of above, assess tone during handling by pulling baby to sitting position (hold wrists) and ventral suspension (baby should hold head almost horizontally); check Moro reflex (is it symmetrical?) (see ⊃ Primitive reflexes, p. 726).
- *Urine and meconium:* check they were passed in first 24h.

Normal variations and minor abnormalities

Skin

- *Vernix:* normal 'cheesy' white substance on skin at birth.
- *Peripheral cyanosis:* normal in first few days after birth.
- *Post-mature skin:* dry peeling and prone to cracking; common in post-mature babies, but topical emollients are often beneficial.

Head

- *Skull moulding:* overriding skull bones with palpable ridges are part of moulding and are harmless. Resolves within 2–3 days.
- *Pre-auricular* pits, skin tags, or accessory auricles. Usually isolated but can be associated with hearing loss or other abnormalities. Test hearing and consider surgical referral for cosmetic reasons.
- *Caput succedaneum*, chignon, and cephalohaematoma (see ⊃ Head, p. 106).

Eyes

- *Blocked lacrimal duct:* leads to recurrent sticky eye. Responds to regular eye toilet until ducts open. This problem may persist for months, but only consider surgery if >12mth. If purulent, then secondary bacterial conjunctivitis is likely (swab for MC&S, including for *Chlamydia*). Treat with antibiotic eye drops (see also ⊃ Neonatal conjunctivitis, p. 976).
- *Subconjunctival haemorrhage:* associated with precipitate deliveries or cord around the neck. Harmless and resolves within a few weeks.

Mouth

- *Epstein's pearls:* self-resolving white inclusion cysts on palate/gums.
- *Tongue-tie:* shortened tongue frenulum (see ⊃ Ankyloglossia (tongue-tie), p. 844).
- *Ranula:* self-resolving bluish mouth floor swelling (mucus retention cyst).
- *Oral candidiasis (thrush):* mucosal white flecks and erythema. Treat with oral antifungal, e.g. nystatin suspension 1mL 6-hourly.

Heart

(See ⊃ Heart murmurs, p. 192.) Murmurs are detected in 1–2% of all newborns, but only ~1 in 12 will have CHD. Compare pre- (right arm) and post-ductal (foot) SpO_2 and evaluate with other findings: cyanosis, signs of heart failure, and peripheral pulses. Consider ECG and four-limb BP. Obtain echocardiography in concerning infants.

Innocent heart murmur is likely if:

- Grade 1–2/6 systolic murmur, not harsh, loudest at left sternal edge, no radiation.
- Remaining cardiovascular examination is normal.
- If murmur persists in an otherwise well infant, in whom no echocardiography has been performed, arrange a repeat examination in a few days to weeks and consider referral for cardiac assessment.

Umbilicus

(See also ➲ Umbilical anomalies, p. 836.)

- *Umbilical hernia:* protuberant swelling involving the umbilicus. Rarely strangulates. Almost all spontaneously resolve within 1y.
- *Single umbilical artery:* usually isolated and of no significance; can be associated with several syndromes and IUGR.

Genitalia

- *Undescended testes:* differentiate from retractile testes (i.e. can be 'persuaded' into scrotum). If still undescended at 1y, refer to surgeon (see ➲ Undescended testes, p. 840). Bilateral undescended (non-retractile) testes in newborns require investigation for ambiguous genitalia.
- *Hydrocele:* common and most resolve by 1y. If persists, refer to a surgeon (see ➲ Hydroceles, p. 830).
- *Vaginal mucoid or bloody discharge:* due to maternal oestrogen withdrawal. Almost always spontaneously resolves.
- *Vaginal/hymenal skin tags:* spontaneously shrink (see ➲ Labial adhesions, p. 844).
- *Inguinal hernias:* can be present from birth (see ➲ Inguinal hernias, p. 830). Refer to a surgeon (NB: there is relatively high likelihood of strangulation/ incarceration).

Limbs

- *Single palmar crease:* found in 72% of normal babies. May be associated with chromosomal abnormalities (e.g. trisomy 21).
- *Polydactyly:* can be isolated or associated with other abnormalities. Refer to a surgeon.
- *Syndactyly:* commonest between the second and third toes. Often familial. If toes only are affected, no treatment required.
- *Postural deformities:* common, especially after oligohydramnios or malpresentation (e.g. breech). Positional talipes is usually equinovarus or calcaneovalgus. If affected joint can easily be massaged back to normal neutral position, deformity will rapidly resolve. If fixed (structural), refer to orthopaedic surgeon/PT. These children are also at ↑ risk of DDH (see ➲ Developmental dysplasia of the hip, p. 681).

Miscellaneous

- *Jaundice* (see ➲ Neonatal jaundice pp. 110–11).
- *Sacral coccygeal pits:* require no action if within natal cleft and base can be seen. Higher pits require spinal imaging.
- *Breast swelling:* may lactate, and almost always due to maternal hormones. Spontaneously resolves over weeks; if not, then refer for endocrinology investigation.

Newborn fluid and electrolyte balance

Normal

The newborn baby is largely water (~75% term, ~85% at 26/40). The extra-cellular compartment is large (65% of body weight at 26/40, compared to 40% by term and 20% in adult), and after birth, there is rapid loss of extra-cellular fluid. In regard to postnatal water homeostasis:

- *Pulmonary vascular resistance:* postnatal decrease, increases blood flow to left atrium, thereby inducing ↑ release of atrial natriuretic peptide (which results in the sequence of ↑ glomerular filtration rate (GFR), ↓ Na$^+$ reabsorption, and ↓ activity of the renin–angiotensin–aldosterone system).
- *Urine output:* a physiological increase at ~12–24h after birth.
- *Na$^+$/K$^+$ ATPase activity:* low at birth, but increases steadily. Na$^+$/K$^+$ ATPase is involved in renal tubular Na$^+$ reabsorption, which creates a gradient for glucose and amino acid reabsorption.

Preterm and sick babies

There is an immaturity in the system described above, hence:

- Tendency for urine Na$^+$ loss over first weeks as ↑ GFR exceeds ability to resorb Na$^+$.
- Variable ability to excrete Na$^+$ load, but excellent ability to deal with water load (modulated by ADH osmo- and baroreceptors).
- High transepidermal water loss (TEWL) with evaporation from skin in <28/40. Reduce TEWL by nursing in incubator at 80% humidity.
- Respiratory water losses (MV or spontaneously breathing) can be countered with warm, humidified ventilatory gases.

Sick infants (e.g. RDS) will also have delayed diuresis, and so giving additional Na$^+$ will further delay diuresis and may worsen their outcome. Furthermore, attempts to induce diuresis with furosemide is unlikely to be helpful.

Postnatal weight loss

Weight loss after birth is normal, and up to 10% is lost in well term infants over the first week of life—greater in preterm/VLBW. Weigh all babies on day 3 (some suggest day 5). Be concerned if there is:

- Failure to lose weight may suggest fluid retention/overload.
- If >10% weight loss:
  - Infant requires assessment of feeding; usually breastfed infants with unrecognized poor feeding; infant may even require admission for NG feeds or IV fluids.
  - Support mother with breast-expressing/top-up feeds.
  - Check U&E if weight loss >12%; rising Na$^+$ suggests dehydration in term and preterm infants and there is a risk of hypernatraemic dehydration.

Specific electrolyte disturbances

(See also ➲ Fluid and electrolytes in dehydration, pp. 71–72; ➲ Other fluid and electrolyte abnormalities, pp. 72–4.)

Hyponatraemia
Na⁺ <130mmol/L.
- *Causes:*
  - Water overload (commonest in first week).
  - Maternal fluid overload.
  - Iatrogenic.
  - Sick infant (e.g. birth asphyxia, sepsis).
  - Excess renal loss (common 'late' cause in preterm infants).
  - GI loss (e.g. diarrhoea, NG aspirates, high-output stoma).
  - Drainage of ascites/CSF.
  - Other (e.g. hypoadrenalism of any cause, Bartter syndrome, Fanconi syndrome).
- *Symptoms:* irritability, apnoeas, seizures.
- *Treatment:* depends on cause (e.g. fluid restriction or Na⁺ supplementation), and be aware that too rapid correction can cause brain injury.

Hypernatraemia
Risk of seizures if Na⁺ >150mmol/L.
- *Causes:*
  - Water depletion (usual).
  - Excess Na⁺ input (unusual because water is usually retained too).
  - High risk: extreme preterm infants in first week of life (excess water losses, TEWL), breastfed infants with poor intake (see ➲ Breastfeeding, p. 122).
- *Treatment:* increase fluid intake; enteral feeding or IV fluids (caution with rapid correction).

Hypokalaemia
K⁺ <2.5mmol/L.
- *Causes:*
  - Excess losses (e.g. diarrhoea, vomiting, NG aspirate, stoma, renal/diuretics).
  - Inadequate intake (failure to recognize daily requirement, TPN).
- *Treatment:* correct with supplementation IV or enteral; be cautious with enteral if there is any GI disturbance; *extreme caution* with IVI because of risk of arrhythmia.

Hyperkalaemia
K⁺ >7.5 OR >6.5mmol/L with ECG changes.
- *Causes:*
  - Failure of K⁺ excretion (e.g. renal failure).
- *Treatments:* myocardial stabilization with calcium gluconate; K⁺ elimination with calcium resonium (polystyrene sulfonate) or dialysis; K⁺ redistribution with salbutamol or insulin/dextrose.

Respiratory distress syndrome

RDS is a lung disease caused by surfactant deficiency. It is largely seen in preterm infants, being less common after 32wk gestation.

Causes

Surfactant deficiency causes alveolar collapse, ↑ work of breathing, and hypoxia (due to intrapulmonary shunt). ↑ risk of RDS is associated with CS delivery, hypothermia, perinatal hypoxia, meconium aspiration, congenital pneumonia, maternal diabetes mellitus, and past family history.

Presentation

Cyanosis, tachypnoea, chest in-drawing, and grunting within 4h of birth. If untreated, the disease worsens over 48–72h and then (depending on severity) resolves over 5–7 days.

Investigations

- CXR (see Figs 4.3–4.6): bilateral and diffuse 'ground-glass' appearance (generalized atelectasis), air bronchograms, reduced lung volume (see Fig. 4.3).
- SpO$_2$ monitoring and blood gases.

Management

- Good delivery room resuscitation: this care may involve ETT intubation and administration of surfactant (extremely preterm) or nasal CPAP/ high flow.
- Respiratory support will depend on the severity: may need O$_2$, nasal CPAP/high flow (see ➲ Neonatal respiratory support, pp. 140–1), or MV (see ➲ Conventional positive pressure ventilation, pp. 142–3).
- Surfactant (Curosurf® or Survanta®): requires ETT intubation and MV and should be considered in all extremely preterm (<27/40) infants and when FiO$_2$ >0.3–0.4.
  - Give first dose as bolus down ETT.
  - Less invasive administration using a surfactant delivery tube is now being used in a few centres with research into efficacy.
  - Give second dose if FiO$_2$ remains high (>0.3).
  - Further doses are sometimes required.
- Antibiotics (e.g. penicillin and gentamicin): until congenital pneumonia has been excluded, as it can mimic or coexist with RDS.
- Nutrition: use IV fluids until the baby is stable. Then start gastric tube feeds with minimal volumes and slowly increase as tolerated. If unstable, start TPN.

Prognosis

The majority of infants have good recovery. Mortality is 5–10% and depends on severity and gestation. BPD may develop (~15% and inversely proportional to gestational age).

Prevention
- Corticosteroids (betamethasone/dexamethasone, two doses, 12-hourly) given to mother 1–7 days before birth decrease the incidence and mortality by 40%. Maximum benefit 24h after first dose and lasts 7 days.
- Treat coexisting morbidities that inhibit surfactant production developing, e.g. hypothermia, acidosis, infection.

Acute respiratory diseases

All of the diseases presented below have signs of respiratory distress (see
➲ Respiratory distress syndrome, pp. 130–1). Cerebral hypoxia, CHD,
and metabolic acidosis can induce respiratory distress (suspect if CXR is
normal).

Transient tachypnoea of the newborn (TTN)

Caused by delayed clearance/absorption of lung fluid after birth. Presents
within 4h of birth. Common after elective CS.

- CXR: shows streaky perihilar changes and fluid in lung horizontal
  fissures.
- Treatment: supplemental O_2. Consider nasal CPAP/high flow and
  antibiotics.
- Prognosis: spontaneously resolves within 24h.

Congenital pneumonia

Caused by aspiration of infected amniotic fluid and presents on the
first day. Associated with prolonged rupture of membranes (PROM),
chorioamnionitis, and fetal hypoxia. Infection usually GBS, *Escherichia coli*,
other Gram –ve bacteria, *Listeria*, or *Chlamydia*.

- CXR: patchy shadowing and consolidation.
- Treatment: respiratory support, antibiotics (benzylpenicillin, or ampicillin
  if *Listeria*, and gentamicin—consult local antibiotic protocols) after septic
  screen, and chest physiotherapy.
- Prognosis: depends on severity and associated sepsis or presence of
  persistent pulmonary hypertension of the newborn (PPHN).

Meconium aspiration syndrome

Five per cent of term infants with meconium-stained liquor develop MAS
(1–5/1000 live births). Hypoxia results in gasping and meconium passage *in
utero*, a combination that leads to aspiration. Meconium aspiration inhibits
surfactant, obstructs the respiratory tract, and induces pneumonitis. Soon
after birth, these infants develop respiratory distress, pulmonary air leaks,
and PPHN.

- Prevention: if liquor is meconium-stained, expedite the delivery to
  prevent further hypoxia and gasping. If baby is apnoeic at birth, visualize
  the larynx and suck out any meconium from the larynx/trachea.
  Tracheal suction is *not* recommended in vigorous infants.
- CXR: generalized pulmonary over-inflation, with patchy collapse/
  consolidation ± air leaks.
- Treatment: supplemental FiO_2; intermittent positive pressure ventilation
  (IPPV) or high-frequency oscillatory ventilation (HFOV) if MV required;
  surfactant; antibiotics (since *Listeria* can cause antenatal meconium
  passage); treat PPHN (see ➲ Persistent pulmonary hypertension of the
  newborn, p. 148); and consider ECMO if severe.
- Prognosis: mortality <5%. Survivors do well, but there is a risk of
  asthma and, if ECMO is needed, neurological sequelae.

Air leaks: pulmonary and abdomen

Commonly secondary to respiratory disease (e.g. RDS, MAS) or MV.

Pneumothorax

Spontaneous pneumothorax seen in 72% of term infants (↑ in prematurity and respiratory disease). Majority small and asymptomatic, and resolve spontaneously; when large, presents with respiratory distress. Tension pneumothorax is life-threatening (signs: respiratory distress, cyanosis, mediastinal shift away from affected side, poor movement and air entry on affected side, affected side transilluminates).

- CXR: shows ipsilateral translucency, lack of peripheral lung markings, and collapsed lung (see Fig. 4.4).
- Treatment: none if asymptomatic. Give O_2 as required. If severe symptoms or worsening, insert chest drain (see ➔ Needle thoracentesis and chest drain, pp. 24–5). In emergency, perform needle aspiration before chest drain.
- Prognosis: excellent in term infants. Mortality doubled in infants with RDS. Also risk of periventricular haemorrhage in preterms.

Pulmonary interstitial emphysema (PIE)

Lung parenchymal air leak with small airways/alveoli collapse. Follows IPPV, particularly in severe RDS or MAS. Signs: respiratory distress; chest hyperinflated with poor air entry, and coarse crackles.

- CXR: hyperinflation; 'honeycomb' pattern of cystic lucencies/bullae, generalized or local (see Fig. 4.5).
- Treatment: high FiO_2; try low peak/positive inspiratory pressure (PIP), low PEEP, and fast rate on IPPV; HFOV may be superior. Unilateral PIE: place infant affected side down. Refractory cases: consider selective ETT intubation to ventilate healthier lung.
- Prognosis: mortality 25–50%. There is ↑ risk of BPD.

Air leak to the mediastinum, pericardium, or peritoneum

Important consequences of pneumothorax/PIE or IPPV. Pericardial air can lead to life-threatening tamponade (quiet heart sounds, hypotension, bradycardia, cyanosis) and must be recognized and treated.

- CXR: mediastinal air shows lucency around the heart extending superiorly and 'sail sign' (thymus lifted and splayed); pericardial air gives sharp borders around a small heart.
- AXR: confirms peritoneal air often originating from the chest, which could impair ventilation.
- Treatment: none needed for mediastinal air; pericardial air needs urgent needle drainage inserted (see ➔ Pericardiocentesis, p. 27); drain peritoneal air if symptomatic.
- Prognosis: symptomatic pneumopericardium has high mortality.

Massive pulmonary haemorrhage

Occurs in 1/1000 live births. Usually due to haemorrhagic pulmonary oedema in VLBW infants. Small bleeds are associated with tracheal trauma from ETT or suction. It is associated with: PDA, heart failure, PIE, hydrops fetalis, perinatal hypoxia, sepsis, coagulopathy, fluid overload, and surfactant therapy.

Signs
- Rapid systemic collapse.
- Profuse bloodstained fluid welling up from upper airway.
- Respiratory crackles on auscultation.
- Imaging: CXR 'white-out'; consider echocardiography for PDA.

Treatment
- Increase FiO_2; optimize MV pressures, suction ETT frequently.
- Correct hypovolaemia and coagulation; consider blood transfusion.
- Consider surfactant.
- Treat known associations/comorbidities.

Milk aspiration

Term infants can may aspirate a feed. The usual causes are:
- Swallowing incoordination (e.g. preterm, neurological disease).
- Upper airway or oesophageal disorders [e.g. tracheo-oesophageal fistula (TOF), GOR].

Presentation
Sudden choking or respiratory distress during/after a feed, often with excessive milk in the mouth, or aspiration pneumonia. CXR is normal or shows patchy collapse/consolidation in the upper lobes.

Treatment
If well, observe only. If unwell, respiratory support and broad-spectrum antibiotics are needed. Investigate the cause, and use gastric or nasojejunal tube feeding. Period of IV fluids or feeding may be necessary.

Apnoea

Apnoea can result from any severe illness and may need supportive MV. Investigate and correct the primary cause.

Apnoea of prematurity

Episodes of apnoea in a baby who is well between episodes (common in <34wk gestation). Exclude other diagnoses (see ➋ Respiratory failure, pp. 38–9; ➋ Non-specifically ill neonate, p. 108).

Treatment
Tactile stimulation, blood transfusion, continuous gastric tube feeds, caffeine or theophylline, nasal CPAP/high flow or IPPV.

Prognosis
Short-lived apnoeas appear to be harmless and should resolve by 34wk gestation.

Neonatal X-rays

(See Figs. 4.3–4.8.)

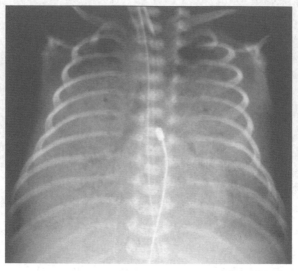

Fig. 4.3 Respiratory distress syndrome. Bilateral diffuse 'ground-glass' appearance (due to generalized atelectasis), airway bronchograms, and reduced lung volume.

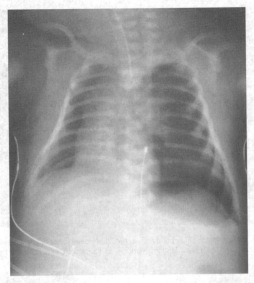

Fig. 4.4 Left tension pneumothorax. Left chest is hyperlucent and hyperinflated, with left lung collapse (absence of peripheral lung markings). The mediastinum is shifted to the right.

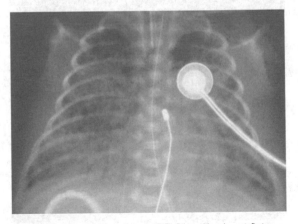

Fig. 4.5 Pulmonary interstitial emphysema (PIE). Bilateral lung hyperinflation (hyperlucent with downward displacement of the diaphragm), with multiple radiolucent cystic areas. PIE may be unilateral. Isolated large bullae may appear. Cardiac compression may occur.

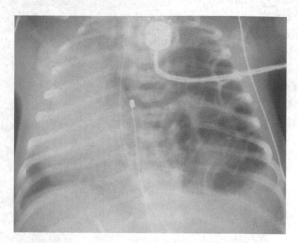

Fig. 4.6 Congenital diaphragmatic hernia. Air-filled bowel loops fill the left hemithorax, with absence of left lung markings and a mediastinal shift to the right.

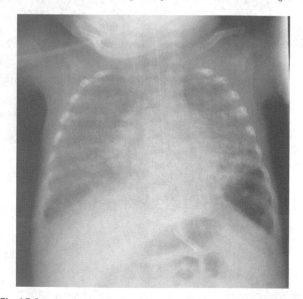

Fig. 4.7 Bronchopulmonary dysplasia. Hyperexpanded chest with diffuse patchy collapse and fibrosis interspersed by radiolucent cystic areas, and an area of emphysema in the left lower lung.

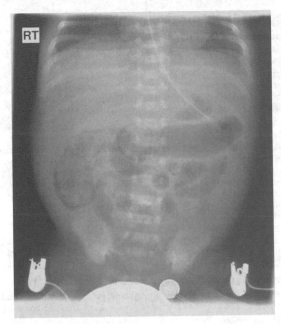

Fig. 4.8 Necrotizing enterocolitis (NEC). Dilated loops of thick-walled bowel and pathognomonic appearance of gas in the gut wall (pneumatosis intestinalis) evident in the left lower abdomen (gut seen side on) and centre (gut seen end on—'halo sign'). Gas in the portal venous system may also be seen and indicates severe disease (not present on this X-ray).

Neonatal respiratory support

Supplemental O_2 (FiO_2 >0.21, room air)

All infants given supplemental O_2 must have SpO_2 monitoring. If significant hypoxia, consider an arterial line to directly monitor PaO_2.
- Term infants: SpO_2 >95% on air—usually ≥97%.
- Preterm infants (≤32/40, ≤1500g): 'correct' SpO_2 range is 90–95%, as suggested by Neonatal Oxygenation Prospective Meta-analysis (NeOProM) collaboration; avoid 'swings' in SpO_2 and FiO_2.

Supplemental O_2 is given via:
- Head box (concentration easily monitored).
- Nasal cannula (<2L/min): cannot monitor effective FiO_2—depends on gas flow rate, FiO_2, and tidal volume; ineffectively humidified.
- Nasal high flow (nHF): humidified, heated, and blended O_2/air at flow rate of >2L/min via nasal cannula. Flow in the upper/lower airways is more laminar, which leads to PEEP generation versus airway CO_2 washout. Tight face mask and strap are not needed, so babies are comfortable and less prone to nasal trauma. nHF is used for:
  - Primary treatment for RDS.
  - Treatment and/or prevention of apnoea of prematurity.
  - As NIV: support in extremely preterm and preterm infants; for infants with parenchymal lung disease.

Continuous positive airway pressure

Prevents airway collapse and low lung volume, maintains functional residual capacity (FRC) above closing volume, and reduces work of breathing. It is used:
- For respiratory support in RDS, particularly for preterm infants.
- For post-extubation.
- In upper airway obstruction.

Method
Nasal mask or binasal prongs, rarely face mask or via ETT:
- Usual pressure is 5–6cmH_2O. Probable safe upper level is 8cmH_2O, but risk of pulmonary air leaks as pressure increases.
- Some equipment can deliver bi-level CPAP with or without synchronization to spontaneous breaths.

Complications
- Pulmonary air leaks (e.g. pneumothorax), particularly if treating RDS in an infant who has not received surfactant.
- Nasal trauma.
- Baby upset, leading to hypoxia.
- ↑ airway resistance and work of breathing.
- Upper GI distension or perforation: insert gastric tube on free drainage to reduce risk, so rarely seen with modern equipment.

Positive pressure ventilation
- IPPV (see ➔ Conventional positive pressure ventilation, pp. 142–3).
- HFOV (see ➔ High-frequency oscillatory ventilation, pp. 144–5).

Synchronized ventilation

The nomenclature is confusing but includes the following:

- Synchronized intermittent positive pressure ventilation (SIPPV), assist control, patient-triggered ventilation (PTV): every spontaneous patient breath can trigger time-limited +ve pressure inflation.
- Synchronized intermittent mandatory ventilation (SIMV): rate of triggered breaths is preset; any other spontaneous patient breaths are unassisted—in the case of apnoea, the set rate is given.
- Pressure support: all spontaneous breaths are supported by +ve pressure for as long as inspiratory flow continues above a defined threshold. Can be combined with other modes.

Studies in newborns show no advantage of SIPPV or SIMV, compared with conventional IPPV for RDS. These modes may be useful during weaning from support or if there is patient–ventilator dyssynchrony. Smaller infants may be unable to trigger breaths (older ventilators). Autocycling can cause over-ventilation in PTV.

Extracorporeal life support (ECLS)

ECLS is mechanical support that functions as the lungs ± heart. ECMO provides a 'window' during which the lungs have a period of 'rest and recovery' (i.e. they are not being exposed to injurious MV). In the UK, a small number of specialist centres provide ECLS/ECMO for infants with severe respiratory disease (e.g. MAS, PPHN). Early transfer to a centre is important for the best likelihood of optimal outcomes in these critically ill infants. The criteria for eligibility include severe, but reversible, cardiac or respiratory disease and oxygenation index (OI) persistently >30–40 where:

$$OI = [(mean\ airway\ pressure \times FiO_2)/PaO_2\ (kPa)] \times 100$$
NB: FiO_2 is a decimal, e.g. 30% O_2 = 0.30.

Contraindications
- Weight <1.8kg.
- Gestation <34wk.
- Severe congenital malformation.
- Intracranial haemorrhage or poor CNS prognosis (e.g. severe IIIC).
- Coagulopathy.

Outcome
Survival rate is high for reversible lung pathologies. Up to 10% of ECMO survivors suffer major long-term problems related to the support or the underlying disease. At the time of ECMO, major complications include CNS haemorrhage, ischaemia, or thromboembolism, as well as pathology in the GI tract and kidneys.

Conventional positive pressure ventilation

IPPV via ETT with continuous flow of heated and humidified gas allows the non-paralysed baby to breathe spontaneously. The ventilator is time-cycled, pressure-limited, (TCPL), and the user sets the PIP, inspiratory time (Ti), and ventilator rate. The tidal volume (V_T) is determined by lung compliance. Some ventilators can adjust PIP within a set range to deliver a set V_T (volume guarantee). Some ventilators can terminate inspiration when a set volume is reached or when inspiratory flow is declining below a threshold. Whichever method you use, you must be familiar with the ventilator's operation and limitations.

Indications

- Worsening respiratory failure (e.g. RDS).
- Impending or actual respiratory arrest from any cause.
- Recurrent apnoeas.
- Massive pulmonary haemorrhage.
- Severe cardiac failure.
- PPHN.
- Severe congenital lung malformation (e.g. diaphragmatic hernia).
- Severe HIE.
- Anaesthesia.

Ventilation parameters

- PIP.
- PEEP.
- Ti and expiratory (TE) time (often expressed as I:E ratio).
- Inspired O_2 % or FiO_2.
- Gas flow (L/min) through ventilator circuit (may not be adjustable).

Monitoring ventilation

Review and adjust ventilation settings soon after commencing (see Box 4.6 for care principles), followed by ABG monitoring to adjust ventilation as appropriate. Acceptable limits depend on the clinical situation. As a guide in preterm infants, the targets are: pH 7.2–7.35, $PaCO_2$ 5–8kPa, PaO_2 6–10kPa, SpO_2 90–95%, and expired V_T ~5mL/kg.

- *PaO_2 too low:* increase FiO_2 or increase mean airway pressure (by either increasing PIP or PEEP; or decreasing TE, which will increase rate as Ti is constant). Do the opposite if PaO_2 is too high.
- *$PaCO_2$ too high:* increase alveolar ventilation (i.e. minute volume)—increase PIP, or decrease PEEP, or increase rate. Do the opposite if $PaCO_2$ is too low.

Box 4.6 Care principles in assisted ventilation in newborns

- *ETT:* use correct size and secure appropriately.
- *Elective intubation:* use sedation with opiate (e.g. morphine or fentanyl) and muscle relaxant (e.g. suxamethonium) ONLY if staff experienced in airway management are present for the procedure.
- *Minimal handling:* reduces episodes of deterioration.
- *Sedation/analgesia:* no evidence for routine morphine infusion in ventilated preterms, but needed in older infants, unless obtunded.
- *Prolonged neuromuscular relaxation (e.g. vecuronium):*
  - Consider in specific circumstances (e.g. severe MAS).
  - Give sedation/analgesia to paralysed infants (as paralysis is distressing), e.g. morphine infusion.
- *Feeding:* once stable, ventilation is not a contraindication to careful gastric feeding. Very ill babies may not tolerate feeding, and gastric distension can cause diaphragmatic splinting.
- *Humidify and warm inspired gas.*
- *Minimal routine suctioning.*
- *Continued monitoring:*
  - HR, BP, RR, VT.
  - SpO$_2$, transcutaneous O$_2$ pressure (TcO$_2$), EtCO$_2$.
  - Intermittent blood gas analysis (capillary or arterial).

Acute deterioration during ventilation

Remember 'DOPE': Displaced ETT, Obstructed ETT, Pneumothorax, Equipment failure. May present as systemic collapse, fall in PaO$_2$, or ↑ PaCO$_2$. Non-respiratory disease may also be contributory, e.g. intraventricular haemorrhage (IVH), gut perforation.

Slow deterioration during ventilation

Slow deterioration in overall condition with ↑ PaCO$_2$ ± ↓ PaO$_2$. Consider worsening respiratory disease, partial ETT obstruction, airway circuit leak, or non-respiratory disease.

Ventilation weaning

As the infant's condition improves, aim to wean supportive ventilation:
- FiO$_2$: wean to lowest needed to maintain adequate PaO$_2$ (decreases risk of retinopathy).
- PIP: as lung compliance improves, wean to maintain appropriate expired V$_T$ (decreases risk of pulmonary air leak) in 2cmH$_2$O steps until 12–14cmH$_2$O (monitor blood gases). Then wean rate by five or ten increments until 10–20 breaths/min. Following extubation, it is often helpful in preterm infants to start nasal CPAP 5cmH$_2$O or nHF (see ➋ Neonatal respiratory support, pp. 140–1). Extubation without CPAP/nHF may be appropriate after short-term ventilation.

High-frequency oscillatory ventilation

A continuous +ve distending pressure (mean airway pressure, P_{aw}) is applied, and around P_{aw} is an amplitude (or Zp) in oscillated pressure. (At high frequency, there is an attenuation in Zp down the airway, such that the alveolus 'sees' 10% of the pressure amplitude in the upper airway.) Zp is produced by a diaphragm or an interrupter device in what is essentially a CPAP circuit. HFOV has an efficacy equivalent to IPPV in the primary treatment of RDS. Since the alveolus does not see swings in pressure delivery (compared to conventional ventilation which works by applying PIP and PEEP), it has the potential to reduce baro-/volume trauma. HFOV may be indicated for:
- Rescue treatment when IPPV has failed.
- Pulmonary air leaks (see ➔ Air leaks: pulmonary and abdomen, p. 133).
- MAS (see ➔ Meconium aspiration syndrome, p. 132).
- PPHN (see ➔ Persistent pulmonary hypertension of the newborn, pp. 148–9).
- Pulmonary hypoplasia.
- Congenital diaphragmatic hernia (CDH) (see Fig. 4.6). (see ➔ Congenital diaphragmatic hernia, p. 814)

Ventilation parameters
- P_{aw}.
- FiO_2.
- Airway pressure difference around P_{aw} (Zp; 'wobble').
- Oscillation frequency per second (Hz).
- Circuit gas flow.

Oxygenation (PaO$_2$) is dependent on both P_{aw} and FiO_2. As P_{aw} increases, PaO_2 will improve as FRC increases. At some point in the pressure–volume relationship, there is *hysteresis* and further P_{aw} increase will decrease PaO_2. This point is recognized either by a fall in PaO_2 with an increase in P_{aw} and/or by the appearance of 'overdistension' on CXR.

CO_2 removal (PaCO$_2$) depends on alveolar ventilation and so on both the Hz and Zp. Unlike IPPV, ventilator constraints make V_T inversely proportional to the Hz. It is normal for V_T generated be less than that physiologically required, yet adequate ventilation occurs—this apparent paradox is explained by complicated air flow physics of HFOV that augment CO_2 diffusion and *pendelluft*. Once the Hz is set, CO_2 removal is ↑ by increasing P_{aw}, and vice versa.

Commencing ventilation

The appropriate settings when using HFOV as the initial form of MV in an infant are:
- HFOV: P_{aw} 8cmH$_2$O; Zp 20cmH$_2$O; Hz 10Hz.
- FiO_2: 0.5 (i.e. 50%).

If transferring from IPPV:
- HFOV: set initial P_{aw} 2cmH$_2$O higher than P_{aw} used in IPPV; Zp 20cmH$_2$O and titrate; 10Hz.
- FiO_2: same as used on IPPV.

Monitoring ventilation

Once ventilated, observe the infant's chest expansion and oscillation, and alter settings as required.

- CXR: perform after 1h to assess chest expansion, with optimal at eight posterior ribs visible above the diaphragm until the baby is stable.
- Monitoring: same as for IPPV (see ➔ Monitoring ventilation, p. 142). Be aware that rapid over-ventilation can occur with high CO_2 elimination and hypocapnia. Anticipate and monitor closely ABG/transcutaneous readings.
  - If PaO_2 is too low: increase either FiO_2 or P_{aw} by 1–2cmH$_2$O every 30–60min (avoid chest overexpansion), and vice versa.
  - If CO_2 is too high: increase Zp by 2cmH$_2$O increments, and vice versa.
  - Optimal CO_2 elimination occurs at 10Hz, and hence the frequency does not usually need to be changed.

Weaning ventilation

As clinical status improves:

- Decrease FiO_2 to 0.5 and then decrease P_{aw} by 2cmH$_2$O steps until 6–7cmH$_2$O is tolerated.
- Also progressively decrease Zp to the minimum required to maintain normal $PaCO_2$.

Some babies will tolerate weaning to what is essentially CPAP, while others, below a certain P_{aw}, do better if changed to slow-rate IPPV.

Bronchopulmonary dysplasia

(See also ➔ Chronic lung disease of prematurity, pp. 246–7.) BPD is a form of chronic lung disease (CLD) that affects infants born preterm. Over the last decade, advances in neonatal care, including the increasing use of antenatal steroids and early surfactant therapy, have modified a change in the underlying pathology in many cases.

• *'Old' BPD* was a disease of scarring and repair, and was associated with long periods of MV, often with high PIP and high FiO_2.
• *'New' BPD* is a condition of impaired alveolar development, with less destruction and scarring. Mechanical, oxidative, and inflammatory factors contribute to lung injury. The CXRs are less dramatic (see Fig. 4.7), but impairment in lung function continue through childhood and is associated with other disorders.

Definition

The definition of BPD has evolved with time; the most commonly used is 'O_2 requirement at 36/40 corrected gestational age (CGA)'. This definition does not have any grading of severity and encompasses a wide spectrum of disease.

> ### US National Institute of Child Health and Human Development; National Heart Lung and Blood Institute (2001 definitions)
> • *Mild:* need for supplemental O_2 at 28 days, but not at 36/40 CGA.
> • *Moderate:* need for supplemental O_2 <30% at 28 days and 36/40 CGA.
> • *Severe:* MV or requiring O_2 >30% at ≥36/40 CGA.
>
> *'Walsh' test (2003)*
> • Test at 36 ± 1/40 CGA. Aim to maintain SpO_2 >88%.
> • BPD if need ≥30% O_2 to maintain SpO_2 >88% (or MV).
> • If <30% O_2, then FiO_2 is gradually ↓ to air. BPD is defined as inability to maintain SpO_2 >88% for 1h.

Incidence and risk factors

Incidence is dependent on the definition used. Wide variations between centres, with a range of 4–58% (mean 23%) of at-risk babies. BPD is more likely with:
• Gestational immaturity.
• LBW.
• ♂.
• Caucasian heritage.
• IUGR.
• Family history of asthma.
• History of chorioamnionitis.

Prevention of BPD

No evidence of effect
- Surfactant and antenatal steroids (effect may be offset by ↑ survival?).
- Closure of PDA.
- Diuretics.
- Inhaled steroids.
- Inhaled nitric oxide.
- HFOV, compared to IPPV.
- Treating *Ureaplasma urealyticum* (more research needed).

May be of benefit in certain infants
- Systemic corticosteroids ☌ (↑ risk of CP).
- nCPAP/nHF versus ETT intubation.

Evidence of effect
- Caffeine citrate for apnoea of prematurity in infants <1250g.
- Vitamin A supplementation for infants <1000g.

Treatment of established BPD

- ☌ No therapies are known to improve outcome in BPD. However:
- O₂ is the most commonly used treatment, and the suggested dose is that needed for SpO₂ 90–95% (see NeOProM collaboration).
- Other treatments are: diuretics, corticosteroids, sildenafil, and optimizing nutrition.
- Immunization for at-risk infants with monoclonal respiratory syncytial virus (RSV) antibody is recommended by the UK Department of Health, ☌ which requires monthly injections in the RSV season.

Outcome

↑ survival of preterm infants has led to an increase in the number surviving with BPD. Mortality has improved (previously 10–20% would die from cor pulmonale or respiratory infection). Other problems include:
- ↑ risk of CP.
- Poorer cognitive functioning and academic performance.
- High risk of re-hospitalization with respiratory illness.
- Poorer lung function.
- Respiratory problems seem to lessen as children get older, perhaps reflecting the lung's continued growth and development.

Circulatory adaptation at birth

Fetal circulation

Oxygenated placental blood (PaO_2 75kPa) returns to the fetus via the umbilical vein. Blood bypasses the liver via the ductus venosus and flows into the IVC and then the right atrium. This blood is then channelled to the left atrium and so to the left ventricle (via the foramen ovale). Oxygenated blood is then pumped to the cerebral and coronary vessels. The right ventricle mostly receives deoxygenated blood from the superior vena cava (SVC). About 15% is pumped to the lungs and the rest is diverted, via the ductus arteriosus, to the descending aorta so that it can go to the placenta via the umbilical arteries.

Postnatal circulation

At birth, inhaled air with O_2 leads to pulmonary arterial vasodilatation, leading to ↓ pulmonary vascular resistance (PVR) and ↑ pulmonary blood flow. At the same time, systemic vascular resistance increases due to loss of the low-resistance placental circulation. The ductus arteriosus constricts as PaO_2 increases. The foramen ovale closes as pulmonary venous return to the left atrium increases and right atrial pressure decreases. Although initially rapid, these changes consolidate over 2–3wk.

Persistent pulmonary hypertension of the newborn

Failure of PVR to fall after birth causes ↓ pulmonary blood flow; incidence 1/1000–1500 live births.

Causes

Rarely primary/idiopathic due to disease of pulmonary vasculature. More commonly, it is secondary to severe illness.

Presentation

- Hypoxia disproportionate to any difficulty with CO_2 elimination.
- Discrepancy between pre- and post-ductal SpO_2 >10%.
- Mild breathlessness (as $PaCO_2$, not PaO_2, is the main physiological determinant of RR), acidosis, hypotension.
- Loud single second heart sound.
- Echocardiography shows ↑ pulmonary arterial pressure, large right-to-left shunt at level of foramen ovale and ductus arteriosus. Echocardiography also needed to rule out cyanotic or duct-dependent CHD.

Management
- Treat cause and use minimal handling.
- Give O_2 (it acts as a pulmonary vasodilator).
- Optimize BP, pH (aim high-normal), Hb, U&E, and blood glucose.
- Ventilate (aim for high PaO_2 and normal $PaCO_2$). HFOV may be helpful.
- Inhaled nitric oxide (results in selective pulmonary vasodilatation): dose 20ppm for 6h initially, and monitor for toxic levels of nitrogen dioxide (NO_2) and methaemoglobin.
- Inotropes may be used to boost BP above that of the raised pulmonary pressure, and so reduce right-to-left shunt. Aiming for mean BP of >60mmHg may be needed.
- ECMO if severe.

Prognosis
- 10–30% mortality.
- Risk of neurodevelopmental impairment in survivors.

Patent ductus arteriosus

(See also ➲ Persistent ductus arteriosus, p. 200.) PDA is failure of the ductus arteriosus to close after birth. The ductus is normally functionally closed by day 1–3 after birth in term infants. Common in preterms (>50% if VLBW).

Presentation

- Small: asymptomatic.
- Large: poor growth, feeding difficulty, respiratory difficulty, systolic/continuous 'machinery' murmur at the upper left sternal edge radiating to back, heart failure.
- CXR: cardiomegaly, pulmonary plethora.
- Echocardiography: confirms PDA and degree of shunt.

Complications

- Poor growth.
- Heart failure, pulmonary haemorrhage, and ↑ risk of BPD.

Management

💣 There is uncertainty about treatment of PDA in preterm infants and what the optimal is. There is wide variation in practice and here is a reasonable approach:

> If *asymptomatic*, observe because most close spontaneously.
> If *symptomatic AND preterm*, consider the following:

- Restrict fluids, e.g. 100–120mL/kg/day.
- Optimize blood oxygenation, e.g. blood transfusion if anaemic.
- Treat heart failure, e.g. furosemide 1mg/kg 12-hourly PO or IV.
- Consider pharmacological closure with indometacin or ibuprofen. If duct fails to close, a repeat course may be given. Side effects:
  - ↓ renal blood flow: oliguria, fluid retention ± hyponatraemia.
  - ↓ cerebral blood flow.
  - GI complications (bleeding, ulceration).
  - Bleeding (↓ platelet function).
  - Displaced protein binding of bilirubin. Indometacin is contraindicated in severe jaundice, NEC, thrombocytopenia, and renal failure. Pharmacological closure is contraindicated when there is duct-dependent pulmonary blood flow (e.g. some forms of CHD).
- Surgery if medical management fails to control symptoms or if there is heart failure, MV dependence, or prolonged failure to close.

Prognosis

Generally good, but infants given treatment often have comorbidities that also affect prognosis, including severe BPD. Surgery has a risk of death. In term infants, PDA is less likely to close or respond to medical treatment.

CNS malformations

Overall incidence ~4–5/10 000 births (falling over the last 50y).

Neural tube defects

Failure of primary neural tube closure during fourth week of gestation.

Prevalence is decreasing because of prenatal diagnosis (detected by ↑ AFP and antenatal US) leading to termination, and maternal periconceptual folate therapy.

Anencephaly

Lethal condition comprising absence of skull bones, forebrain, and upper brainstem.

Encephalocele

Midline skull defect with brain tissue herniation. The lesion is covered with skin and requires surgical excision and closure. Associated brain abnormality usually leads to poor neurodevelopment.

Spina bifida

Several types, all secondary to failure of midline fusion of dorsal vertebral bodies. All forms require specialist advice and treatment.

- *Spina bifida occulta:* no herniation of neural tissue. Often overlying dermal sinus, dimple, lipoma, or hairy naevus is present (perform spinal US or MRI). Associated with diastematomyelia or cord tethering.
- *Meningocele:* herniation of meninges and fluid only, with skin covering. Requires surgical closure. Excellent prognosis.
- *Myelomeningocele:* herniation of spinal neural tissue, which may be covered by meninges/skin or be open. Adjacent spinal cord is always abnormal. Usually thoraco-lumbar, lumbar, or lumbo-sacral.
  - Problems include: flaccid paralysis below the lesion, urinary and faecal incontinence, urinary tract dilatation, hydrocephalus, bulbar paresis secondary to Chiari malformation, and vertebral anomalies (e.g. kyphosis).
  - Treatment: surgical closure and hydrocephalus drainage.
  - Prognosis: related to severity of other problems. Prognosis worst if lesion very large or high. Palliative care may be appropriate.

Congenital hydrocephalus

Excessive head growth caused by CSF accumulation (see also ⊃ Hydrocephalus, p. 380) and confirmed by head US and cranial MRI:

- *Causes:* congenital (aqueduct stenosis, Dandy–Walker malformation, CMV infection, cerebral tumour); acquired (IVH, subarachnoid haemorrhage, CNS meningitis).
- *Features:* OFC above the 97th centile, with wide cranial sutures and bulging fontanelle, 'sun-setting' sign of eyes.
- *Treatment:* surgical insertion of ventriculo-peritoneal shunt.

Dandy–Walker malformation

Cerebellar vermis hypoplasia associated with:
• Hydrocephalus.
• Posterior fossa CSF collection ('cyst') expanding into fourth ventricle.

This malformation is also associated with a variety of syndromes: fetal alcohol and trisomy 13 and 18. Prognosis depends on associated syndromes, abnormalities, and underlying conditions.

Agenesis of the corpus callosum

Non-specific feature of numerous conditions and is associated with a wide variety of conditions. It may be total or partial, or an incidental finding. Prognosis depends on associated syndromes, abnormalities, and underlying conditions.

Hydrancephalus

Absence of cerebral hemispheres, with cavity filled with CSF. The brainstem and midbrain are usually spared.
• *Cause:* severe (vascular) cerebral insult leading to extensive cortical necrosis.
• *Prognosis:* usually lethal. Survivors have severe neurodevelopmental impairment.

Microcephaly

(See also ➜ Microcephaly, p. 379.) OFC progressively falls away and below 3rd centile. The primary defect is reduction in brain size.
• *Causes:* intrauterine infection (including the recent outbreak of Zika), chromosomal defects, various syndromes, maternal drug/alcohol abuse, brain injury. (See ➜ Zika, p. 645.)
• *Prognosis:* generally poor neurodevelopmental outcome.

Holoprosencephaly

Severe developmental defect of the forebrain. There is a single central cerebral ventricular cavity, with varying degrees of development and separation of the hemispheres. Midline facial defects are common. May be isolated or associated with chromosomal defects, particularly trisomy 13. Poor prognosis.

Neuronal migration defects

Includes lissencephaly (smooth brain), pachygyria (very few gyri), polymicrogyria (numerous underdeveloped gyri), schizencephaly (deep cerebral cleft), and neuronal heterotopia (foci of neurons in abnormal locations within the brain). All are associated with poor neurodevelopmental outcome and seizures, but eventual outcome is dependent on severity of malformation.

Hypoxic–ischaemic encephalopathy

HIE is a clinical syndrome of brain injury secondary to a hypoxic–ischaemic insult. In developed countries, incidence of 2–5/1000 live births (moderate to severe incidence is 1–2/1000 live births).

Causes

- ↓ umbilical blood flow (e.g. cord prolapse).
- ↓ placental gas exchange (e.g. placental abruption).
- ↓ maternal placental perfusion.
- Maternal hypoxia from whatever cause.
- Inadequate postnatal cardiopulmonary circulation.

Presentation

Varies depending on severity of cerebral hypoxia. An infant may have a range of symptoms and signs affecting: LOC, muscle tone, posture, tendon reflexes, suck, HR, and CNS homeostasis. Before concluding that an infant may have HIE secondary to an intrapartum hypoxic–ischaemic event, assess for evidence of an intrapartum problem, e.g. CTG abnormality, sentinel event such as abruption or cord prolapse. There should be respiratory depression at birth and a need for resuscitation, including IPPV (Apgar score at 5min <5). There should be moderate to severe acidosis soon after birth (pH <7.0, base excess worse than −12mmol/L). The baby should develop HIE within 24h of birth, with other causes of encephalopathy excluded.

Management

- Resuscitate at birth; insert IV ± arterial lines.
- *Avoid hyperthermia.*
- Assess CNS and neurology:
  - Eligibility for therapeutic hypothermia (TH) (see Box 4.7).
  - Start cerebral function (EEG analysis) monitoring (CFAM).
  - Assess for features of dysmorphism and birth trauma.
  - Exclude other encephalopathies (e.g. meningitis, metabolic disturbances, maternal drugs, CNS malformation, haemorrhage).
- Expect and manage multiorgan failure (e.g. cardiac or renal).
- Monitor and maintain homeostasis (e.g. U&E, Ca^{2+}, Mg^{2+}, blood glucose, Hb, ABG, coagulation). Support BP.
- Mild fluid restriction initially (e.g. 40mL/kg/day with 10% dextrose) as there may be oliguria. Omit milk feeds for 1–2 days if HIE severe, and then introduce feeds slowly.
- Treat seizures if prolonged or recurrent. (see ➔ Neonatal seizures, pp. 114–15.)

Therapeutic hypothermia

TH is standard for term infants with moderate/severe HIE (see Box 4.7). Cooling achieved with temperature-controlled mattress/wrap, and target 33–34°C by 6h of insult. TH for 72h, then gradual re-warming.

Box 4.7 Criteria for therapeutic hypothermia

A. *Infants >36/40 and >1800g and <6h old with one of:*
- Apgar ≤5 or continued need for resuscitation at 10min.
- Acidosis: cord pH (or any blood gas in first hour) <7.0 or base excess ≤ −16mmol/L.

B. *Moderate or severe encephalopathy with altered LOC (lethargy/stupor/coma) and one of:*
- Hypotonia.
- Abnormal reflexes (e.g. Moro, suck, gag, pupillary, oculovestibular).
- Clinical seizures.
  If criteria A and B are both met, then assess for criterion C using CFAM:

C. *At least 30min of CFAM recording which shows either abnormal background activity or seizures (clinical or electrical).*
  If CFAM is unavailable and criteria A and B are met, cooling can be started after senior doctor discussion (e.g. before/during transfer).

CFAM

Single- or two-channel machines available (two-channel = left and right hemispheres). Displays 'raw' EEG and a compressed 'amplitude-integrated' (aEEG) recording. Pattern of EEG is used for classification of background activity (see Figs. 4.9–4.12). Normal CFAM (aEEG) recording in term infants:
- Lower margin ≤5 microvolts (when awake), upper margin ≥10 microvolts.
- Evidence of sleep–wake cycling, no seizures.

Prognosis

Without cooling, the risk of later disability or death by Sarnat grade is:
- *Grade I* [mild: hyperalert, normal muscle tone, mild distal flexion, overactive tendon reflexes, weak suck, strong Moro, generalized sympathetic (S) dysfunction, tachycardia, absent seizures]: <2%.
- *Grade II* [moderate: lethargic, mild hypertonia, strong distal flexion, overactive tendon reflexes, weak/absent suck, weak/incomplete Moro, generalized parasympathetic (P) dysfunction, bradycardia, common focal/multifocal seizures]: 24%.
- *Grade III* (severe: coma, flaccid, intermittent decerebration, ↓ or absent reflexes, absent suck, absent Moro, both P and S dysfunction, variable HR, absent/difficult-to-control seizures): 78%.

Disabilities
Likely to include spastic quadriplegia, dyskinetic CP, severely reduced IQ, cortical blindness, hearing loss, and epilepsy.

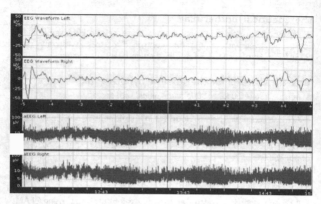

Fig. 4.9 Normal CFAM trace. Note sleep–wake cycling (narrowing and widening of trace).

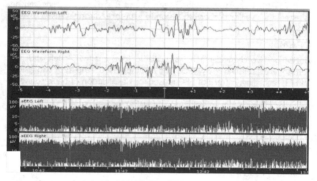

Fig. 4.10 Moderately abnormal CFAM trace. Note the widened aEEG trace (baseline <5) and suppressed raw EEG with periodic high-voltage complexes.

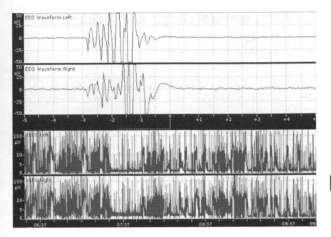

Fig. 4.11 Severely abnormal CFAM trace—burst suppression. Note the very low baseline voltage (<5) with high-voltage discharges (as seen on raw trace below), giving a spiked pattern to the aEEG.

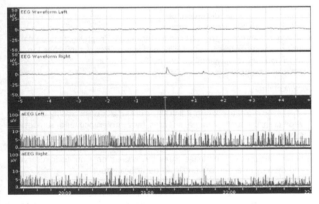

Fig. 4.12 Severely abnormal CFAM trace—continuous low voltage. Note that there is almost no electrical activity.

Cerebral haemorrhage and ischaemia

Periventricular haemorrhage and intraventricular haemorrhage

Periventricular haemorrhage (PVH) and IVH are rare at >32wk gestation. Haemorrhage starts in the vascular germinal matrix (subependymal). Bleeding may extend and dilate the lateral ventricles in IVH; also, haemorrhagic periventricular infarction secondary to impaired cerebral venous drainage by IVH.

- *Incidence:* 10–15% of infants born <32wk. Risk increases with being more premature.
- *Causes:* related to rapid alteration in cerebral blood flow, e.g. severe RDS, pneumothorax, hypotension, hypoxia, high/low $PaCO_2$.
- *Presentation:* most occur within 72h of birth. Seldom occur before birth unless there is alloimmune thrombocytopenia. Up to 50% are asymptomatic. Larger bleeds may present as sudden catastrophic systemic collapse, bulging fontanelle, neurological dysfunction (e.g. seizures or paucity/abnormal movements), anaemia, and jaundice.
- *Diagnosis:* confirmed using cranial US. At-risk groups or preterm infants <32wk should be screened by cranial US (at day 1, 1wk, and 1mth, or after sudden deterioration; local policies for screening schedules will vary). Several grading systems exist, but it is better to describe the location and extent of haemorrhage as one of:
  - subependymal only; or
  - IVH ± ventricular dilatation; or
  - IVH ± parenchymal involvement.
- *Prevention:* antenatal steroids reduce incidence. Prophylactic neonatal indometacin treatment reduces incidence but does not improve long-term neurodevelopmental outcome.
- *Treatment:* supportive.

Complications

- *Post-haemorrhagic ventricular dilatation (PHVD):* secondary to obstruction of CSF flow or absorption. Clinical features include: increasing OFC, wide cranial sutures, apnoea, seizures, feed intolerance, and 'sun-setting' eyes. Diagnosis confirmed and monitored by measuring ventricular index on cranial US; 50% resolve spontaneously. Progressive, symptomatic PHVD requires CSF drainage either by serial LP or ventricular reservoir, and then by insertion of ventriculo-peritoneal shunt.
- *Haemorrhagic periventricular infarction:* occurs in 15%. Blood in the lateral ventricles impairs adjacent venous drainage, which results in adjacent cerebral infarction. Cranial US: cystic parenchymal area(s) adjacent to, and communicating with, lateral ventricle (porencephalic cyst).

Prognosis

Subependymal or uncomplicated IVH does not affect neurodevelopment. CP is common if either PHVD present and treatment is required (50%) or there is parenchymal extension (80%).

Term intracranial haemorrhage

- *Subdural:* ↑ risk with difficult extraction.
- *Subgaleal:* potential massive blood loss with systemic collapse. Boggy swelling all over scalp, not limited by sutures.
- *Subarachnoid:* asymptomatic or may present with seizures/irritability.
- *Parenchymal or intraventricular:* usually haemorrhagic infarction—seizures possible.
- *Cephalohaematoma:* subperiosteal bleed, limited by suture lines, may take weeks to resolve, and may partially calcify.

Periventricular leucomalacia (PVL)

PVL is usually associated with extreme prematurity. Severe HIE can lead to cortical neuronal necrosis, basal ganglia injury, focal cerebral infarct, or subcortical leucomalacia. There are periventricular white matter lesions (i.e. ↑ US echogenicity or cysts), which may not be apparent for several weeks after birth.

- *Cause:* poor cerebral perfusion or ischaemia, inflammation.
- *Risk factors:* extreme prematurity, hypotension, severe illness, hypocarbia.
- *Diagnosis:* periventricular echodensities/cysts on cranial US.
- *Prognosis:* higher risk of CP (especially spastic diplegia), particularly if there is cyst formation.

Cerebral infarction (perinatal stroke)

A perinatal stroke is a vascular event around the time of delivery.
- *Incidence:* 1/1600 to 1/5000 births.
- *Presentation:* depends on timing and nature of event and includes focal seizures, encephalopathy, apnoea, poor feeding, and asymmetrical reflexes/movement/tone. A stroke may be associated with maternal/neonatal coagulation disorders (e.g. factor V Leiden, protein C or S deficiency).
- *Management:* supportive, cover infection, correct any metabolic (e.g. hypoglycaemia) or haematological (e.g. polycythaemia) abnormalities. Start CFAM and treat seizures.
- *Investigations:* FBC, coagulation screen, U&E, Ca^{2+}, Mg^{2+}, LFTs, glucose. Others include MRI and EEG.
- *Prognosis:* depends on site and nature of lesion. ~50% of affected children will carry some neurological impairment into childhood.

Necrotizing enterocolitis

Incidence

The commonest neonatal surgical emergency. Incidence 1–3/1000 live births (5–10% in VLBW infants). Incidence is reduced 6-fold in preterm infants fed on breast milk. Typically, a sporadic condition affecting preterm infants (~90% of cases), but can be epidemic or occur in term infants in situations such as significant hypoxic event or systemic collapse leading to gut ischaemia. The disease may just involve an isolated area of the gut or be extensive. The distal terminal ileum and proximal colon are most frequently affected. Multiorgan failure is associated with diffuse disease.

Cause

Multifactorial. Severe intestinal necrosis is the end-result of an exaggerated immune response within the immature bowel, leading to inflammation and tissue injury. NEC rarely occurs before milk feeding commences, but timing of the first feed does not appear to be relevant. Predisposing factors include:
- Prematurity.
- IUGR (causes chronic bowel ischaemia).
- Hypoxia.
- Polycythaemia.
- Exchange transfusion.
- Hyperosmolar milk feeds.

Presentation

Commonest in the second week after birth.

Early
- Non-specific illness.
- Vomiting/bilious aspirate from gastric tube.
- Poor feed toleration (increasing gastric aspirates).
- Abdominal distension.

Late
- Additional abdominal tenderness.
- Stool: blood, mucus, or tissue in stools.
- Systemic: shock, DIC, multiorgan failure.
- Abdomen: bowel perforation—signs of intestinal perforation are free peritoneal gas or gas outlining of falciform ligament ('football' sign). AXR shows intestinal distension (see Fig. 4.8), pneumatosis intestinalis, and hepatic portal venous gas.

Management

- *Prophylaxis:* antenatal steroids and breast milk are protective. Evidence for prevention by administration of probiotic bacteria.
- *Investigations:* FBC, U&E, creatinine, coagulation screen, albumin, ABG, blood culture, AXR, group and cross-match.
- *General care:* 'Bell staging' (see Table 4.2) may be useful in grading severity. Start by *stopping milk feeds* for 10–14 days ●※. Insert gastric tube on free drainage.
- *IV antibiotics:* for 10–14 days (e.g. benzylpenicillin, gentamicin, and metronidazole).
- *Systemic support:* e.g. IPPV, correct BP and DIC, PN.
- *Surgical opinion:* surgery used for GI perforation, deterioration despite above medical treatment (necrotic bowel likely), GI obstruction secondary to stricture formation (late). If localized disease, surgical resection of involved bowel with primary repair. If more extensive, 2-stage repair with bowel resection(s) and enterostomy, followed later by intestinal re-anastomosis.

Prognosis

Overall mortality is ~22%. ↑ mortality is associated with:
- VLBW.
- Extensive intestine involvement.
- Multiorgan failure.
- Intrahepatic portal gas.

Extensive bowel resection may result in short bowel syndrome (see ➔ Short bowel syndrome, p. 299). Excellent prognosis is seen in those who respond to medical treatment, but subsequent stricture may develop.

Table 4.2 Bell staging of NEC

Stage I (suspected NEC)	Predisposed infant; systematic manifestations (temperature instability, lethargy, apnoea, bradycardia); GI manifestations (feed intolerance, vomiting—may be bilious, occult blood in vomit or stool, mild abdominal distension); AXR with bowel distension only
Stage II (definite NEC)	As above plus mild/moderate acidosis and/or thrombocytopenia; persistent occult or gross GI bleeding, marked abdominal distension; AXR shows distension and bowel wall thickening, and intramural gas (portal vein or a fixed bowel loop)
Stage III (advanced NEC)	As above plus shock, severe acidosis, electrolyte abnormalities, thrombocytopenia, DIC; marked GI bleeding; AXR may show pneumoperitoneum

Neonatal infection

Neonatal infection can be acquired transplacentally (congenital; see ➔ Transplacental (congenital infection), p. 164) by ascent from the vagina, during birth (intrapartum infection), or postnatally from the environment or contact with others. Infections are categorized as early-onset (first 48h of age) versus late-onset sepsis (>48h). Preterm infants are at greater risk for both types of infections.

Risk factors

- PROM >18h, especially if preterm.
- Signs of maternal infection (e.g. maternal fever, chorioamnionitis, UTI).
- Vaginal carriage or previous infant with GBS.
- Preterm labour; fetal distress.
- Skin and mucosal breaks.
- Risk factors for late-onset sepsis.
- Central lines and catheters.
- Congenital malformations (e.g. spina bifida).
- Severe illness, malnutrition, or immunodeficiency.

Early-onset neonatal infection

Incidence 2–5/1000 live births. Infection caused by organisms acquired from the mother, usually GBS, *E. coli*, or *Listeria*. Other possibilities include herpesvirus, *Haemophilus influenzae*, anaerobes, *Candida*, and *Chlamydia trachomatis*.

Presentation (symptomatic)

Includes temperature instability, lethargy, poor feeding, respiratory distress, collapse, DIC, and osteomyelitis or septic arthritis.

Initial investigations

Including blood culture, CSF (glucose, protein, MC&S), FBC, and CXR. The diagnostic value of CRP in early neonatal sepsis is unclear ⬤. Failure to respond to antibiotics within 24h should prompt further investigation.

Treatment

- Supportive (may require IPPV, volume expansion, and inotropes).
- Broad-spectrum antibiotics (e.g. penicillin and gentamicin; consider ampicillin/amoxicillin if *Listeria* is a possibility).
- If meningitis is confirmed or strongly suspected, then treatment with cefotaxime (± ampicillin/amoxicillin).
- Length of antibiotic course and choice of antibiotics will depend on local sensitivities/policy, as well as on age/gestation of baby.
  - If infant has remained well and initial index of suspicion was low, then consider stopping antibiotics if culture results are −ve (~48h), and observe.
  - In CSF +ve meningitis, treat for 14–21 days (or greater). A repeat LP demonstrating resolution at the proposed end of treatment may be of value in deciding the length of course.

In the UK, there is national guidance on when to investigate and commence treatment for early-onset neonatal infection.[1]

Prognosis
Up to 15% mortality (up to 30% if VLBW).

Late-onset neonatal infection

Incidence 4–5/1000 live births. Infection is caused by environmental organisms such as coagulase –ve staphylococci, *Staphylococcus aureus, E. coli*, and other Gram –ve bacilli, *Candida* species, and GBS.

Investigation
FBC, blood culture; urinalysis (clean catch) and urine culture; CSF MC&S, glucose, and protein.

Treatment
• Give IV antibiotics:
  • Broad-spectrum, e.g. flucloxacillin and gentamicin.
  • Consider cefotaxime if meningitis is likely.
  • Use vancomycin if coagulase –ve *Staphylococcus* sepsis likely, (e.g. preterm infant with indwelling CVC).
• Decisions on removing/continuing to use any CVL should be made by a senior doctor.
• Fungal sepsis is relatively uncommon in the UK (1% of VLBW infants). However, it should be considered in any infant who fails to respond to standard therapy or has additional risk factors.

Transplacental (congenital infection)

Causes
- 'TORCH' infections.
- Other viruses: herpes zoster, parvovirus B19, syphilis, enterovirus, HIV, hepatitis B, and zika.
- Rarely bacterial (e.g. GBS, *Listeria monocytogenes, Neisseria gonorrhoeae*).

Presentation
- TORCH infection: SGA, jaundice, hepatitis, hepatosplenomegaly, purpura, chorioretinitis, micro-ophthalmos, cerebral calcification, micro-/macrocephaly, hydrocephalus.
- Rubella and CMV: also cause deafness, cataracts, CHD, and osteitis (rubella only).
- Parvovirus B19: rubella-like rash, aplastic anaemia ± hydrops.
- Herpes zoster: cutaneous scarring, limb defects, multiple structural defects.
- Congenital syphilis: SGA, jaundice, hepatomegaly, rash, rhinitis, bleeding mucous membranes, osteochondritis, meningitis.
- Bacterial infections presenting with non-specific or multiorgan failure. Gonorrhoea causes purulent conjunctivitis (ophthalmia). Listeriosis causes preterm labour and meconium-stained liquor.

Investigation
Consider:
- *Blood:* blood culture; pathogen-specific IgM and IgG (paired for herpes zoster, *Toxoplasma*); Venereal Disease Research Laboratory (VDRL) test.
- *Maternal-specific serology.*
- *Other cultures:* urine CMV culture; throat swab viral culture; CSF culture and latex particle agglutination (GBS); stool viral culture; skin vesicle viral culture and electron microscopy (EM).

Treatment
Most congenital infections have no specific treatment. General treatment is supportive and involves careful follow-up to identify sequelae (e.g. deafness and CMV). Consider specific therapies:
- *Toxoplasma*: spiramycin (4–6wk 100mg/kg/day) alternating with pyrimethamine (3wk 1mg/kg/day) plus sulfadiazine (1y 50–100mg/kg/day).
- Syphilis: benzylpenicillin 14 days 30mg/kg 12-hourly IV.
- Symptomatic CMV: IV ganciclovir, then PO valganciclovir 💣.

Prognosis
Variable and depends on disease severity.

Prevention of neonatal infection

General measures

- Good handwashing with antiseptic solutions and use of gloves.
- Avoidance of overcrowding.
- Low nurse-to-patient ratio.
- Nurse cohorting.
- Patient isolation and barrier nursing.
- Minimal handling.
- Rational antibiotic use.
- Minimize indwelling vascular access.

Group B streptococcal disease

The incidence of early-onset GBS disease in term infants without antenatal risk factors in the UK is 0.2 cases/1000 births. The best approach to minimize early-onset sepsis due to GBS infection is uncertain because there have not been trials that permit the overall risks and benefits of intrapartum antibiotic prophylaxis (IAP) to be judged. IAP reduces the number of newborns with +ve blood cultures, but with a very low disease incidence and a very high rate of maternal GBS colonization (around 25%), a very large number of women must be treated to prevent one case if bacteriological screening programmes are implemented. Routine bacteriological screening of pregnant women is not presently recommended in the UK. Current practice follows a risk factor-based approach. UK NICE guidance (2012) exists.[1] The Royal College of Obstetrics and Gynaecology recommends that intrapartum IV penicillin (or clindamycin) should be offered to women with:

- *Mother:* previous baby with neonatal GBS disease; GBS carriage detected on low vaginal swab culture or GBS bacteriuria.
- *Perinatal:* intrapartum fever >38°C; preterm (<37/40); PROM >18h.

Management

Not much evidence, but any ill newborn infant should have cultures taken and be treated with broad-spectrum antibiotics that are effective against GBS and other common neonatal pathogens. Well infants exposed to the above risk factors should be evaluated and observed. Because >90% of cases of early-onset GBS disease present in the first 12–24h after birth, infants who are well after this time are not at ↑ risk of disease, in comparison with infants without risk factors. There is no need to send investigations on infants who are not ill. If there are multiple risk factors, or a previous child has been affected by GBS sepsis, many would consider blood culture and starting appropriate antibiotics.

Hepatitis B

Usually contracted at birth. Routine antenatal screening detects maternal carrier state [i.e. hepatitis B surface antigen (HBsAg) +ve]. Transmission risk ~10% if the mother is a low-risk carrier (i.e. anti-HBe +ve). To reduce vertical transmission, give hepatitis B vaccine to infant within 24h of birth. Also give specific hepatitis B immunoglobulin 200IU IM if mother is a high-risk carrier (i.e. mother HBeAg +ve, or anti-HBe –ve, or antibody/antigen status unknown), since the untreated transmission risk is 90%. In both groups, subsequent hepatitis B vaccine is required at 1, 2, and 12mth (UK schedule).

Human immunodeficiency virus

(See → Human immunodeficiency virus, pp. 648–9.)Vertical transmission rate 15–25%. Risk markedly reduced by:
- Maternal antiretroviral drug therapy to minimize viral load during third trimester and labour, and then postnatal treatment of baby for 6wk.
- Elective lower-segment Caesarean section (LSCS).
- Avoidance of breastfeeding (in developed world).

Infants are usually asymptomatic at birth and require testing at 3 and 6mth. Infection is very unlikely if all of the following tests are –ve at 6mth and baby is well:
- HIV viral PCR.
- P24 antigen.
- Specific immunoglobulin A (IgA).

Herpes simplex

Eighty-five per cent of neonatal HSV is contracted at birth from active maternal genital lesions. Elective CS reduces transmission if mother has active genital herpes. Treat infant with prophylactic IV aciclovir if born by vaginal delivery and there is primary maternal herpes (transmission risk of 50%, compared with 3% in secondary herpes). To prevent infection from carers with cold sores, the lesions should be covered with a mask and the sores treated with topical aciclovir.

Herpes zoster

Perinatal infection can cause severe disseminated disease, with high mortality (30%), if:
- Maternal rash occurs in the period between 7 days antenatally and 7 days postnatally.
- LBW infant (<1mth old) has contact with varicella and whose mother is non-immune (i.e. check maternal antibody status if unsure).

Prevention
PO aciclovir and specific zoster immunoglobulin (ZIG) 100mg IM given soon after delivery.

Neonatal abstinence syndrome

A cluster of symptoms caused by withdrawal from a dependency-inducing substance. In the UK, this is commonly related to methadone (± heroin) or benzodiazepines. However, withdrawal is documented with cocaine, amphetamine, selective serotonin reuptake inhibitors (SSRIs) (e.g. fluoxetine), alcohol, caffeine, and nicotine.

Presentation

- *Timing depends on substance:* heroin and SSRIs often present soon after birth, methadone within 24h, and benzodiazepines later.
- *CNS symptoms:* irritability, sleepiness, hyperactivity, tremors, seizures.
- *Non-CNS symptoms:* poor/disorganized feeding, vomiting, diarrhoea (can cause severe nappy rash), sneezing, tachycardia, sweating, respiratory depression, fever (be cautious—sepsis may coexist or present with similar symptoms).

Management

Observe 'at-risk' infants for signs of withdrawal for several days after birth. Several scoring systems exist for quantifying withdrawal.

- *General and supportive measures:* swaddling, minimal handling, dark and quiet environment, frequent low-volume feeding.
- *Drug treatment:* a pragmatic approach to starting low-dose PO morphine would be to start if significantly symptomatic (e.g. sleeping <1h after feeds, continuous high-pitched cry, unable to feed). Once stable, wean morphine slowly over several days.
- *Apnoea monitor:* start if preterm or requires large doses of morphine.
- *Seizures:* control with phenobarbital (also drug of choice to treat barbiturate withdrawal).
- *Other points* to consider are:
  - Does baby need urine screen (remember this will effectively drug-test the mother)?
  - Ensure social services are aware as child protection and family support must be considered.
  - Consider infection with HIV or hepatitis B or C infection.
  - Mother can breastfeed unless she is taking high doses of methadone (>20mg/day), amphetamines, or cocaine, or is HIV +ve.

Prognosis

It is difficult to establish whether adverse outcomes are related to drug exposure from the literature. There is an ↑ risk of:

- Prematurity, IUGR, SIDS.
- Congenital HIV, hepatitis B/C infections.
- Social problems.
- Neurodevelopmental impairment.

Inborn errors of metabolism

(See also ➔ Unexplained metabolic acidosis, p. 75; ➔ Inborn errors of metabolism, p. 82; ➔ Chapter 12.) The common presentations of IEM are as follows:

- *Encephalopathy without metabolic acidosis:* e.g. pyridoxine-dependent seizures, urea cycle enzyme defects (hyperammonaemia).
- *Encephalopathy with metabolic acidosis:* e.g. organic acidurias.
- *Hepatic failure:* e.g. galactosaemia.
- *Non-immune hydrops:* can be haematological (e.g. β-thalassaemia) or due to lysosomal storage disorder (e.g. Gaucher disease).
- *Significant dysmorphism:* these can be divided into lysosomal disorders (e.g. mucopolysaccharidosis), peroxisomal disorders (e.g. Zellweger syndrome), mitochondrial disorders, biosynthetic defects (e.g. albinism), and receptor defects (e.g. pseudo-hypoparathyroidism).
- *Other:* non-specific illness (see ➔ Non-specifically ill neonate, p. 108), severe hypotonia, resistant hypoglycaemia, cataracts, odours, cardiomyopathy, severe diarrhoea.

Investigations

- *Initial:* blood for U&E, SBR, gas analysis, glucose, Ca^{2+}, Hb, ammonia, and AG (normal range 12–16mmol/L). Urine for ketones and reducing substances.
- *'Metabolic screen':* for amino acid and organic acid analysis, take and save blood in heparinized (1–2mL) and EDTA (3–5mL) tubes and save urine (5–10mL) in sterile container with no preservatives.
- *Subsequent investigation:* after discussion with expert.
- *If child dies before diagnosis:* seek permission to take:
  - Further blood for storage (clotted and heparinized).
  - Skin biopsy placed in sterile saline.
  - Liver and muscle biopsy.
  - Send immediately to pathology laboratory for preservation.

Acute management

Supportive
- Stop all protein intake, including milk, and start 10% dextrose IVI.
- Correct electrolyte/acid–base imbalance.
- Broad-spectrum antibiotics in case crisis was precipitated by infection.

Specific treatments
After expert advice.

Prognosis
Depends on disease.

Retinopathy of prematurity

(See also → Retinopathy of prematurity, p. 982.)

ROP is a leading cause of preventable blindness. Infants born <32/40 and those weighing <1500g at birth are at greatest risk. The incidence is decreasing and recent data suggest that ~90% of infants born weighing >1000g will have no ROP. However, this number drops to only 38% for those <750g at birth. The cause is multifactorial. *In utero*, retinal vasculature develops in a relatively hypoxic environment, with vessels stimulated to grow towards the most hypoxic regions. This development is disrupted with preterm delivery. ROP is associated with retinal arterial hyperoxic vasoconstriction and retinal ischaemia during retinal development before 32wk gestation. It is therefore essential to monitor and prevent hyperoxia in infants requiring supplemental O_2. Minimizing variability in oxygenation may also be important.

Classification

ROP is a proliferative retinopathy classified according to internationally accepted guidelines (see Box 4.8).[2]

Screening criteria

- ≤27/40: first screen at 30–31/40 CGA.
- 27–32/40: first screen at day 28–35 of life.
- Screen 2-weekly thereafter, unless any of the following, which needs 1-weekly screening:
  - Any stage 3 disease.
  - Any plus/pre-plus disease.
  - Vessels ending in zone 1 or posterior zone 2.

Screening is performed by indirect ophthalmoscopy after pharmacological pupil dilatation or increasingly by wide-field digital retinal imaging. Screening continues until vascularization has progressed into zone 3 (usually >36/40).

Treatment

Diode laser treatment within 72h (48h if aggressive disease) of meeting any of the treatment criteria (see Box 4.8). Babies should be ventilated, adequately sedated, and given a muscle relaxant. Atropine should be available. Side effects of treatment include:

- Need for re-ventilation.
- Bradycardia.
- Apnoea.
- Ocular haemorrhage.
- Eyelid trauma.
- Laser burns.

Infants should be re-examined 5–7 days following treatment, and if no regression, re-treatment should be performed at 10–14 days after initial therapy. Steroid eye drops may be useful in decreasing post-operative swelling. Direct injections of monoclonal antibodies against vascular endothelial growth factor (VEGF) are showing promise as an alternative.

Prognosis

Almost all cases can be treated effectively, so blindness is a rare outcome. There may be reduced visual fields in severe cases. Refractive errors are common.

Box 4.8 Classification of ROP[2]

Severity
- Stage 1: demarcation line visible.
- Stage 2: ridge evident.
- Stage 3: ridge with extraretinal fibrovascular proliferation.
- Stage 4: subtotal retinal detachment (4A, extrafoveal; 4B involves fovea).
- Stage 5: total retinal detachment.

Location
- Zone 1 extends a radius of 30° from the optic disc.
- Zone 2 extends from the nasal retina periphery in a circle around the anatomical equator.
- Zone 3 involves the anterior residual crescent of the temporal retina.

Extent: recorded as clock hours in each eye in the appropriate zone.

'Plus' (+) disease: indicates aggressive disease and is used when there is engorgement and tortuosity of posterior pole retinal vessels, iris rigidity or vessel engorgement, or vitreous haze.

Treatment criteria
- Zone 1, any stage if 'plus' disease present.
- Zone 1, stage 3 (no 'plus').
- Zone 2, stage 3 with 'plus' disease.
- Seriously consider if zone 2, stage 2 with 'plus'.

Metabolic bone disease

Also known as osteopenia of prematurity, the incidence is 32–90% in pre-term infants (mostly ELBW).

Cause

Chronic substrate deficiency—usually PO_4^{3-}, rarely Ca^{2+} or vitamin D. Risk is ↑ if:
- Prolonged PN.
- Breastfed (low in PO_4^{3-}).
- Chronic diuretic treatment.

Presentation

Bone mineral biochemical derangement; must measure serum Ca^{2+}, PO_4^{3-}, and alkaline phosphatase (ALP) weekly in infants <33wk gestation.
- ↓ linear growth.
- Rib or distal long bone fractures.

Investigations

- Biochemistry: PO_4^{3-} <1.2mmol/L; Ca^{2+} >2.7mmol/L; ALP >500–1000IU/L (local policies vary for cut-offs).
- Bone X-ray: osteoporosis, features of rickets, fractures.
- Urine Ca^{2+}:PO_4^{3-} ratio >1 after 3wk of age (high renal PO_4^{3-} reabsorption).

Treatment

- Oral PO_4^{3-} 1mmol/kg/day supplement if milk-fed.
- Increase TPN Ca^{2+} and PO_4^{3-} (consult pharmacist).

Prevention

In infants <2kg or <33wk gestation:
- Supplement breast milk with oral PO_4^{3-} 1mmol/kg/day (not required if fed preterm formula as it contains added PO_4^{3-}).
- Oral vitamin D 400IU/day.
- Ensure TPN contains Ca^{2+} 2mmol/kg/day and PO_4^{3-} 2.5mmol/kg/day (organic phosphate solution avoids mineral precipitation).
- Passive exercise 10min/day appears beneficial.

Prognosis

Stature is reduced at age 18mth. Bone mineralization and fracture risk appear to be normal by 2y.

Orofacial clefts

(See also ➔ Cleft lip and palate, p. 808.)

Orofacial clefts are due to failure of fusion of maxillary and pre-maxillary processes. They may be unilateral or bilateral and result in cleft lip and/or cleft palate. The incidence is ~1/1000 live births.

Causes

Multifactorial and includes genetic and environmental factors; 66% of clefts are isolated. Majority have no obvious cause.

- *Enviromental factors:* maternal folic acid deficiency; maternal exposure to alcohol, tobacco, steroids, anticonvulsants, and retinoic acid.
- *Syndromic (~30%):* e.g. Pierre–Robin syndrome (large midline posterior cleft palate, mandible hypoplasia, prone to upper airway obstruction due to a posteriorly displaced tongue).

Treatment

- *Refer to specialist:* 'cleft lip and palate' multidisciplinary team (MDT).
- *Possible upper airway obstruction:* a recognized complication of large cleft palate (e.g. Pierre–Robin syndrome). If it occurs or is likely:
  - Nurse prone.
  - Nasopharyngeal airway may be helpful.
  - Monitor SpO_2—low or worsening SpO_2 is an ominous sign and should be taken very seriously.
  - ETT intubation: may be difficult and requires specialist (ENT) support.
- *Feeding problems:* common and need specialist nursing input; special feed devices and prosthetic plate (obdurator) may all be required if cleft palate is too large to allow adequate suck.
- *Risk of infection:* be aware of ↑ risk from aspiration pneumonia, and later secretory otitis media with conductive hearing loss. Treat as appropriate.
- *Surgical repair:* lip repair is usually at 3mth; palate at 6–12mth.
- *Later speech defects and dental problems:* can occur and require speech therapy and dental input, respectively.

Prognosis

Repair of unilateral complete or incomplete lesions usually produces a good result. As well as those complications described above, later problems may include:

- Hindered parental bonding.
- Psychological morbidity.

Neonatal haematology

Anaemia

(See also ➲ Chapter 14.)

Causes

Antenatal

- Alloimmune haemolytic disease, e.g. rhesus disease.
- Twin-to-twin transfusion syndrome.
- Parvovirus B19 infection.
- APH.
- Red cell defects or aplasia.

Postnatal

- Nutritional deficiency, chronic illness.
- Anaemia of prematurity occurs 6–12wk after preterm delivery and is caused by:
  - Repeated and frequent blood sampling.
  - Shorter HbF red cell half-life.
  - ↓ erythropoietin.
  - Fast growth rate.

Presentation

- Pallor and tachycardia, ↑ O_2 requirement or apnoea.
- Poor feeding 🔊, growth failure 🔊.

Treatment

- *Iron:* start supplement at 4wk for 12mth if <35wk gestation.
- *Blood:* research needed to establish transfusion thresholds for preterm infants. So transfuse, if indicated, with volume (mL) = desired rise in Hb (g/dL) × weight (kg) × [4 (packed cells) or 6 (whole blood)]. Or give 20mL/kg over 4h of CMV –ve and irradiated blood (check local policy). The UK National Health Service Blood & Transplant (NHSBT) has guidelines and an app (see ➲ Further reading, p. 182).
- *Erythropoietin:* useful, but not cost-effective for routine use and may increase risk of ROP. Use is limited to infants from Jehovah's Witness families.

Polycythaemia

(See also ➲ Polycythaemia, pp. 560–1.) Arterial or venous PCV >65%. Commoner if placental insufficiency, maternal diabetes mellitus, Down's syndrome, or after twin-to-twin transfusion. Risk of complications due to thrombosis and/or microvascular sludging.

Treatment

- *Symptomatic* (lethargy, seizures, respiratory distress, poor feeding, thrombocytopenia, stroke, renal failure, NEC): dilutional exchange transfusion with 20–30mL/kg of NS over 30–60min.
- *Asymptomatic:* consider dilutional exchange transfusion if PCV >70% to prevent complications—discuss with expert neonatologist.

Thrombocytopenia

(See also ➔ Thrombocytopenia, p. 576.) Common neonatal causes include:
- Sepsis, including congenital infection, DIC, and NEC.
- IUGR.
- Maternal idiopathic thrombocytopenic purpura (ITP) due to passive transfer of autoimmune IgG antiplatelet antibodies.
- Neonatal alloimmune thrombocytopenia (NAIT) from transplacental maternal-specific IgG antiplatelet antibodies sensitized to differing fetal human platelet antigen (HPA). In 85%, antibody to HPA1.
- Placental dysfunction.
- Pre-eclampsia.

Presentation
- Petechiae.
- Thrombocytopenia.
- Intracranial haemorrhage (10–20%), particularly with NAIT.

Treatment
Platelet transfusion 10–15mL/kg if platelet count is <50 × 10^9/L and active bleeding, or <30 × 10^9/L plus additional haemorrhagic risk factor, or <20 × 10^9/L in a well baby.

NAIT-specific treatment
- *Antenatal:* fetal platelet transfusion. Maternal IVIG.
- *Postnatal:* observe if platelets >40 × 10^9/L. If platelets less or infant symptomatic, give platelet transfusion (HPA1 −ve if relevant) and consider corticosteroids, IVIG, or even exchange transfusion (liaise with blood transfusion/haematology).

Coagulation disorders

(See also ➔ Chapter 14.)
The commonest neonatal cause is DIC. Rarely, there is a specific coagulation defect (e.g. haemophilia or haemorrhagic disease of the newborn).

Haemorrhagic disease of the newborn
- Bleeding due to deficient vitamin K-dependent factors from:
  - Poor transplacental supply.
  - Lack of enteric bacteria.
  - Maternal anticonvulsants.
  - Low vitamin K levels in breast milk.
- *Typical presentation:* is at 2–7 days with bruising and spontaneous bleeding from umbilicus, GI tract, or intracranial.
- *Investigation:* shows ↑ prothrombin time (PT) and partial thromboplastin time (PTT), with normal platelet count.
- *Prevention:* vitamin K1 at birth (see ➔ Vitamin K (phytomenadione), p. 120).
- *Treatment:* immediate IV vitamin K1 1mg and FFP 10mL/kg.

Rh disease (rhesus haemolytic disease)

Haemorrhage of fetal blood of differing Rh group into maternal circulation leads to maternal anti-D IgG production (usually fetus RhD +ve, mother RhD –ve). Transplacental antibody leads to fetal haemolysis. Asymptomatic or mild in first affected pregnancy; severity increases with subsequent pregnancies. Maternal blood group and Rh antibody status checked in early pregnancy. High or rising titre needs further fetal investigation (e.g. serial anti-Rh titres, US, blood sampling). The risk of disease is predicted by maternal anti-Rh titre:

- Unlikely when maternal anti-Rh titre <4U/mL.
- 10% when titre is 10–100U/mL.
- 70% when fetal Hb <7g/dL or titre >100U/mL.

Iso-immunization may occur with other blood group incompatibilities (e.g. ABO—usually baby A or B and mother O), other Rh groups (e.g. c, C, e, E), Kell, Kidd, and Duffy. Clinical presentation is usually milder than with RhD (particularly ABO).

Presentation

- *Antenatal:* fetal anaemia, hydrops fetalis.
- *Postnatal:* hydrops fetalis, early jaundice, kernicterus (see ➔ Bilirubin encephalopathy, p. 177), skin 'blueberry muffin' lesions, hepatosplenomegaly, coagulopathy, low platelets, leucopenia.
  Late: anaemia, inspissated bile syndrome.

Investigations

- *Maternal blood:* group (usually RhD –ve), ↑ anti-Rh titre.
- *Cord/neonatal blood:* ↓ Hb, ↑ reticulocytes, low platelets, DCT +ve, group (usually RhD +ve), ↑ SBR.
- *After diagnosis:* monitor SBR 4-hourly (until rate of rise known), blood glucose, and rate of Hb fall. Check coagulation screen.

Treatment

(See also ➔ Hydrops fetalis, pp. 118–19.)

- Close antenatal supervision ± intrauterine blood transfusion.
- After birth: cord SBR and Hb, start high-risk infants on intensive phototherapy and await results. If SBR >100 micromoles/L, prepare infant for exchange transfusion and consider IVIG (see ➔ Neonatal jaundice, pp. 110–11; ➔ Intravenous immunoglobulin, p. 580).
- Supportive treatment as required (e.g. correct coagulopathy).
- If treatment required, PO folic acid 250mcg/kg/day for 6mth.
- Check Hb every 1–2wk to detect anaemia for up to 12wk. Transfuse if symptomatic or Hb <7g/dL.
- Audiology screening if exchange transfusion required.
- Prophylaxis: Rh anti-D IgG given to RhD –ve mothers after birth of Rh +ve fetus or possible feto-maternal haemorrhage.

Prognosis

Mortality <20%, even if hydropic. Risk of late-onset anaemia.

Bilirubin encephalopathy (kernicterus)

A clinical syndrome resulting from the development of excessive neurotoxic unconjugated bilirubin levels. Toxic levels lead to selective damage of the cerebellum, basal ganglia, and brainstem auditory pathways. It may occur in the healthy neonate if serum bilirubin is >360 micromoles/L, but usually only occurs at significantly higher serum levels (>430 micromoles/L after 48h of life), unless:

- Infant is <24h old.
- Infant is preterm.
- Infant is severely ill (any cause).
- Infant is acidotic.
- Caused by iso-immunization haemolytic disease.
- Reduced albumin binding caused by drugs or hypoalbuminaemia.

Presentation

- Lethargy progressing to hypertonia, then hypotonia.
- Poor feeding.
- Fever.
- High-pitched cry.
- Opisthotonos.
- Seizures and coma.
- Main differential diagnosis is meningoencephalitis/sepsis. Neonatal tetany may also present with opisthotonos.

Treatment

- Supportive (likely to require full intensive care).
- Urgent reduction of SBR by intensive phototherapy and exchange transfusion.
- Give IVIG.
- Treat underlying cause.

Prognosis

Majority survive, but there is a high risk of athetoid CP, deafness, and low IQ.

Neonatal dermatology

(See also ➔ Congenital naevi (birthmarks), p. 802.) Neonatal skin is covered with vernix at birth and is poorly keratinized. There is reduced resistance to bacterial infection, ↑ water loss, and ↑ absorption of drugs (all more pronounced with prematurity).

The following benign conditions resolve without treatment, often within a few weeks of birth:

- *Milia:* <2mm yellowish-white spots, usually on the face, secondary to blocked sebaceous/sweat glands.
- *Erythema toxicum (erythema neonatorum):* discrete erythematous, macular–papular lesions, often with a white centre, mostly over the knees, elbows, trunk, and face. Common in post-mature infants.
- *Harlequin colour change:* marked erythema or pallor in different halves, or quadrants, of the body. Secondary to vasomotor immaturity.
- *Cutis marmorata (livedo reticularis):* marble-like colour change in well baby, secondary to vasomotor immaturity.
- *Sucking blisters:* common on hand, wrist, or upper lip.
- *Superficial capillary haemangioma (salmon patches, stork marks):* erythematous vascular marks on eyelids, face midline, and posterior scalp, particularly the nape of the neck (tends to persist at latter site).
- *Mongolian blue spots:* bluish-black macules, most often in lumbar–sacral region, common in non-Caucasians. May last several years.

Nappy rash

(See ➔ Napkin dermatitis, p. 786.) Usually a contact dermatitis from ammonia released by bacterial breakdown of urine.

Treatment includes:
- *Frequent nappy changes.*
- *Barrier cream:* e.g. zinc and castor oil cream; expose to air.
- *Suspect secondary Candida infection:* if worse in flexures or satellite lesions present. Treat with topical antifungal, e.g. nystatin ointment 6-hourly (if severe, may need PO antifungal simultaneously).

Infantile seborrhoeic eczema

Very common. Usually appears after a few weeks. Erythema and scaling rash affects face, neck, behind ears, axillae, scalp (cradle cap), upper trunk, napkin area, and flexures. Majority spontaneously resolve within weeks. Minority will go on to develop atopic eczema, particularly if there is a family history.

Treatment
- Avoid detergents (i.e. soap) and use topical emollients.
- Mild topical steroid/antifungal preparation (e.g. 1% hydrocortisone cream).

Perinatal death

Causes

- Extreme prematurity (40%).
- Congenital abnormalities (30%).
- RDS.
- Sepsis.
- Perinatal asphyxia.
- Pulmonary hypoplasia.
- Miscellaneous.

After death

- Take photographs and mementos (e.g. footprints) according to parents' wishes.
- Inform all relevant professionals [e.g. general practitioner (GP), obstetrician].
- Refer to coroner (Procurator Fiscal in Scotland) if necessary. UK criteria are:
  - Cause of death unknown.
  - No medical practitioner attended illness, leading to death.
  - Intraoperative death or prior to recovering from anaesthetic.
  - Suspicious circumstances.
- Explain and offer post-mortem to parents. Possible benefits include:
  - Determines cause of death.
  - Identifies unknown comorbidities.
  - Determines degree of normality.
  - Audits clinical care.
  - Research and medical education.
- Unexpected/unexplained death. As soon as possible, consider (with consent!):
  - Blood for culture—save serum for possible later testing (IEM).
  - Throat, eye, and ear surface swabs for bacterial and viral culture.
  - Suprapubic aspiration (SPA) of urine to be saved (IEM).
  - Axilla skin biopsy for fibroblast culture (send in sterile NS).
- Additional blood: U&E, CRP, LFTs (consult local protocol).
- Organ donation is an area that may develop, given recent changes to neonatal determination of death by neurological criteria in the UK.
- If able, issue death certificate to parent/guardian who is then responsible for registering the death. In the UK, there is a specific certificate required for a neonatal death (i.e. <28 days old).
- Offer follow-up appointment with senior doctor at 4–6wk to discuss issues surrounding death, post-mortem findings, and bereavement.

Withholding or withdrawal of life support

(See also ➲ Withholding or redirecting treatment in children, pp. 960–1.)
Up to 70% of deaths on UK NICUs follow withholding or elective with-
drawal of life-sustaining treatment. The Royal College of Paediatrics and
Child Health (RCPCH) states that there are five situations when with-
holding or withdrawal of life-sustaining treatment may be appropriate.
Three are relevant to newborns and are summarized here:

* 'No chance': life-sustaining treatment simply delays death without
  significant alleviation of suffering.
* 'No purpose': although the baby may be able to survive with treatment,
  the degree of physical or mental impairment will be so great that there
  is no quality of life.
* 'An unbearable situation': treatment is more than can be borne by the
  baby and/or family when the illness is progressive and irreversible.

The other two situations relating to 'brain death' and 'permanent vegetative
state' previously were not diagnosed in newborns in the UK, although this
is changing. Withholding or withdrawing life-sustaining treatment must be
discussed with the parents. Almost always a joint decision can be made in
the child's best interests. Time, rather than court proceedings, is the best
approach, the latter being best reserved for extreme situations.

Procedure for withdrawal of life-supporting treatment

Remember, withdrawal of life-sustaining treatment does not equal
withdrawing care:

* If possible, allow parents and family to say their goodbyes, spend time
  alone with the baby, and conduct appropriate religious services.
* Parents may wish to be present at the time of withdrawal. Offer options
  of being present or holding the child in a private quiet room during
  withdrawal or afterwards.
* Stop all non-palliative infusions and remove all peripheral vascular lines
  and gastric tubes. Clamp central lines and chest drains.
* Switch off all alarms/monitors.
* If on IPPV, disconnect and remove ETT.
* Dress or swaddle the infant and then allow parents to cuddle the infant.
* Give parents/family space and privacy.
* After death, carry out relevant tasks (see ➲ After death, p. 180).

References

1. National Institute for Health and Care Excellence. (2012). *Neonatal infection (early onset): antibiotics for prevention and treatment*. Clinical guideline [CG149]. Available at: ℘ https://www.nice.org.uk/guidance/cg149.
2. Royal College of Ophthalmologists, Royal College of Paediatrics and Child Health Medicine. (2008). *Guideline for the screening and treatment of retinopathy of prematurity*. Available at: ℘ https://www.rcophth.ac.uk/wp-content/uploads/2014/12/2008-SCI-021-Guidelines-Retinopathy-of-Prematurity.pdf.

Further reading

Blood Components (NHS Blood & Transplant) Smartphone App. A useful application for blood transfusion thresholds.

NeoMate Smartphone App. A useful application for fast calculations relevant for intubation, central lines, and resuscitation drugs; includes HIE cooling criteria.

Hawkins KC, Scales A, Murphy P, Madden S, Brierley J. Current status of paediatric and neonatal organ donation in the UK. *Arch Dis Child* 2018; **103**: 210–15.

Marlow N, Wolke D, Bracewell MA, et al. Neurologic and developmental disability at six years of age after extremely preterm birth. *N Engl J Med* 2005; **352**: 71–2.

National Institute for Health and Care Excellence. (2010). *Jaundice in newborn babies under 28 days*. Clinical guideline [CG98]. Available at: ℘ http://guidance.nice.org.uk/CG98.

Public Health England. (2013). *Green Book: Immunisation against infectious disease*. (holds guidance for neonates and pregnant mothers) Available at: ℘ https://www.gov.uk/government/collections/immunisation-against-infectious-disease-the-green-book.

Royal College of Obstetrics and Gynaecology. (2003). *Prevention of early-onset neonatal group B streptococcal disease*. Green-top Guideline No. 36. Available at: ℘ https://www.rcog.org.uk/en/guidelines-research-services/guidelines/gtg36/.

Cardiology

Common presentations

The majority of children with cardiovascular disease will present with one or more of the following clinical problems:

- Cyanosis (see ● Cyanosis, p. 190).
- Heart failure (see ● Heart failure, pp. 190–1).
- Heart murmur (see ● Heart murmurs, p. 192).
- Chest pain (see ● Chest pain, p. 194).
- Syncope (see ● Syncope, p. 195).
- Palpitations (see ● Palpitations, p. 196).

History

Like all history and examination in paediatrics, the question needs to match the age of the child and the possible pathologies being considered. While asking about palpitations is relevant to a teenager, a history of sweating during feeding may be telling in an infant. However, many signs and symptoms of cardiac disease in paediatrics overlap with other organ dysfunction (e.g. respiratory, neurology, etc.) and differentiating the cause may need further investigation. Specific signs and symptoms are considered in more detail later in the chapter.

Points that can relate to a cardiac pathology

- Increasing fatigue, breathlessness, FTT, recurrent chest infections.
- Collapse/syncope associated with exercise, exertion, water/swimming, loud noise.
- Chest pain or palpitations associated with symptoms of pallor, breathlessness, or feeling faint.
- Previous cardiac surgery.
- History of unoperated CHD.
- Known cardiomyopathy.
- Known arrhythmia.
- Recent illnesses such as streptococcal sore throat or viral illness.
- First-degree relative with a connective tissue disorder [e.g. Marfan's syndrome (MFS)].
- Details of antenatal scans and obstetric history (e.g. cardiac abnormalities detected), maternal factors that increase the risk of CHD disease (e.g. illness, medication).
- Family history of CHD in first-degree relatives.
- Family history of arrhythmia (e.g. long QT), cardiomyopathy, or sudden unexplained death in the young.

Examination

On examination, key findings to elicit are:
- Presence of dysmorphism and signs suggesting an underlying genetic syndrome.
- Presence of central cyanosis; tachypnoea, breathless, sweating.
- Fingers clubbing, splinter haemorrhages, Janeway lesions.
- Perfusion: skin, level of alertness, passing urine?
- Pulses: palpable brachial and femoral pulses, volume of pulses, and whether they feel equal.
- Chest: thrills and murmurs; crackles audible on auscultation.
- HR, rhythm, and JVP in an older child.
- Hepatomegaly, tissue oedema.

Genetic and metabolic disorders with cardiac features

(See ➲ Genetic disorders with cardiac features, pp. 876–7; ➲ Systems—cardiac, p. 508).

Electrocardiogram

Salient aspects when reading paediatric ECG

- ECG lead positions are the same as in adults. By the age of puberty, the ECG should resemble that of an adult. Sometimes V5 and V6 are placed on the right side of the chest because of space, and they should be labelled as V5R and V6R, respectively, to avoid confusion (they will appear as a mirror image of what would be expected if placed on the left side of the chest).
- Check ECG is calibrated appropriately: voltage, 1mV/cm (i.e. ten small squares) and speed 25mm/s (i.e. one small square = 0.04s).
- A systematic approach to ECG evaluation includes:
    1. *Rate:* is HR appropriate for age?
    2. *Rhythm:* Is the patient in sinus rhythm (P wave before each QRS complex and upright P waves in leads I and aVF)?
    3. *Is P wave morphology normal?* Tall P waves >3mm height [right atrial hypertrophy (RAH)]; broad P waves >3mm length and 'bifid' [left atrial hypertrophy (LAH)]; broad + tall + 'bifid' (bi-atrial hypertrophy)
    4. *Are Q waves present?* Q waves should be narrow (0.02s), <5mm deep in left chest leads and aVF, but allowed up to 8mm in lead III in young children (<3y); Q waves usually absent in right chest leads and, if present, may indicate right ventricular hypertrophy (RVH).
    5. *What is the QRS axis?*
        a. Right axis deviation (RAD) in neonates is normal because of right ventricular (RV) dominance—resolves by 3mth to 0° to +90°.
        b. Superior axis is abnormal until proven otherwise [atrioventricular septal defect (AVSD) is a common association].
    6. *Look for pre-excitation* (WPW syndrome): slurred upstroke of QRS ('delta wave') and short PR interval—predisposes to SVT.
    7. *Are T-waves inverted?* T-wave inversion is normal in leads V1–V3 until puberty; however, T-wave should be upright in V1 in first week of life).
    8. *QTc interval:* calculate it yourself as the machine is often inaccurate. Should be 0.35–0.45s. Bazett's formula used to correct for HR is QTc = QT interval/√(preceding R–R interval).

Normal development of ECG

(See Table 5.1.)

Table 5.1 Normal range in ECG findings by age

	PR interval	QRS axis	R-waves	T-waves
Newborn	<3mm (0.12s)	RAD (< +180°)	Dominant tall R-waves; right chest leads (<10mm)	+ve V1 on day 1 of life, then −ve by day 3
1wk to 1mth	<3mm (0.12s)	RAD	Dominant in right chest leads still	−ve V1 and usually V2 (up to V3)
1–6mth	<3mm (0.12s)	Usually < +90°, but up to +125° is normal	Dominant in V1 still. Narrow RSR′, with normal amplitude (<10mm) in V1 normal	−ve V1 and usually V2 (up to V3)
6mth to 3y	<3mm (0.12s) in <1y; <4mm (0.16s) in child	Between 0 and < +90°	Dominant in V6	−ve V1 and usually V2 (up to V3)
3–8y	<4mm (0.16s)	Between 0 and +90°	Dominant in V6 (dominant S in V1)	−ve V1 (allowed in V2 up to V3)
8–16y	<5mm (0.2s)	Between 0 and < +90°	Dominant in V6 (dominant S in V1)	May all be +ve now, but −ve T-waves in V1–V3 are still acceptable
Adults	<5mm (0.2s) in adult	Between 0 and < +90°	Dominant in V6 (dominant S in V1)	+ve V2–V6 (can be +ve in V1 also)

Table 5.2 ECG and CXR findings in paediatric cardiology

Diagnosis	ECG findings	CXR findings
Small VSD	Normal	Normal
Myocarditis	Ischaemia, e.g. inverted T-waves, ST depression/elevation	Cardiomegaly, plethoric lung fields
VSD, ASD secundum, AVSD partial, PDA	RVH + LVH + RAD + RBBB Prolonged PR, superior axis normal or LVH	Mild cardiomegaly + ↑ pulmonary markings
HLHS, HOCM	Normal/LVH	Cardiomegaly
AS	LVH	Enlarged left ventricle
ToF	RAD, RVH	Small boot-shaped heart + oligaemic lung fields
TGA	Normal	Narrow mediastinum, heart 'egg on side' + ↑ pulmonary vascular markings
CoA	RVH (neonate); LVH	Rib-notching
PS	Normal or RVH	PA post-stenotic dilatation

AS, aortic stenosis; ASD, atrial septal defect; AVSD, atrioventricular septal defect; CoA, coarctation of the aorta; HLHS, hypoplastic left heart syndrome; HOCM, hypertrophic obstructive cardiomyopathy; LAD, left axis deviation; LVH, left ventricular hypertrophy; PA, pulmonary artery; PDA, patent ductus arteriosus; RAD, right axis deviation; RBBB, right bundle branch block; RVH, right ventricular hypertrophy; TGA, transposition of the great arteries; ToF, tetralogy of Fallot; VSD, ventricular septal defect.

Abnormal childhood ECG

(See Table 5.2.)

Criteria for right ventricular hypertrophy

The more +ve criteria present, the more likely RVH is present:
1. RAD more than expected for patient's age (see Tables 5.2 and 5.3).
2. ↑ voltage and dominant rightward R waves in chest leads for patient's age.
3. Upright T-wave V1 in patients >3 days of life and <6y.
4. Q wave in V1.
5. T-wave axis in the 0° to −90° (+ve in lead I, −ve in aVF) can indicate RV strain pattern.

Criteria for left ventricular hypertrophy (LVH)

The more +ve criteria present, the more likely LVH is present:
1. Left axis deviation (LAD) for patient's age (see Tables 5.2 and 5.3).
2. ↑ voltage and dominant leftward forces in chest leads for patient's age.
3. Q wave V5 and V6 ≥5mm, coupled with tall symmetrical T-waves in same leads.
4. T-wave inversion leads I and aVF.

Criteria for combined ventricular hypertrophy (CVH)

Equiphasic and large QRS complexes in two or more limb leads and in mid-precordial leads (V2–V5):
1. +ve voltage criteria for RVH and LVH (in the absence of bundle branch block or pre-excitation).
2. Voltage criteria +ve for RVH or LVH; relatively large voltages for the other ventricle.

Cyanosis

A *centrally cyanosed* child will have a blue tongue due to hypoxia, which may be due to a cyanotic heart lesion or any other cause of hypoxia. *Peripheral cyanosis* is due to poor peripheral perfusion and will occur when there is central cyanosis, but also if peripheral perfusion is affected by other mechanisms (e.g. cold environment, fever, etc.). In dark-skinned children, a tip to spotting central cyanosis is to ask the child to stick out their tongue and compare the colour to that of the carer's tongue—the difference is usually marked.

Heart failure

Heart failure may be manifested by symptoms of poor tissue perfusion alone, which are usually non-specific (e.g. fatigue, poor exercise tolerance, confusion), and/or by more telling symptoms of congestion of circulation (e.g. dyspnoea, hepatomegaly). Peripheral oedema is uncommon in young children. The underlying pathophysiological mechanisms that compromise cardiac stroke volume and output—so that the heart is unable to meet the demands of the body—include:
* ↑ afterload (pressure work), e.g. CoA.
* ↑ preload (volume work), e.g. ventricular septal defect (VSD).
* Myocardial abnormalities (deficient intracellular contractility), e.g. cardiomyopathy.
* Tachyarrhythmias (poorly coordinated and ineffective contractility), e.g. SVT.

Causes of heart failure
* *Large left-to-right shunt:* e.g. large VSD (not in first few days of life).
* *Left-sided obstructive lesions:* CoA, hypoplastic left side of the heart (within first few days of life).
* *Cardiomyopathy:* hypertrophic, dilated, restrictive.
* *Myocarditis:* viral, rheumatic fever.
* *Endocarditis:* usually bacterial.
* *Myocardial ischaemia:* anomalous left coronary artery, KD.
* *Tachyarrhythmias:* SVT.
* *Acute hypertension.*
* *High-output:* severe anaemia, thyrotoxicosis, AVMs.

Clinical features
The clinical features of heart failure depend on the degree of cardiac reserve and whether there is congestive or single-chamber failure. In addition, there may be compensatory mechanisms of sympathetic nervous stimulation, evidenced by:
* Sweating.
* Breathlessness, tachypnoea, coughing, lung crepitations.
* Poor feeding (infant), poor weight gain, and FTT.
* Hepatomegaly.
* Cardiomegaly.
* Tachycardia or 'gallop' heart rhythm.

NB: unlike adults, there are usually few clinical signs of congestive cardiac failure. Only children with chronic heart failure or adolescents may have 'adult' signs such as peripheral oedema, orthopnoea, paroxysmal nocturnal dyspnoea, and elevated JVP.

Investigations

These are directed at finding a cause and quantifying function.
- SpO_2: compare pre-ductal (right arm) with post-ductal (either foot).
- CXR:
  - Cardiac enlargement?
  - Lungs—oligaemia/oedema?
- Echocardiography: congenital heart defects and function.
- ABG: reduced PaO_2 and metabolic acidosis.
- ECG: rarely diagnostic, but may assist in establishing aetiology.
- Serum electrolytes: hyponatraemia due to water retention.

Management

The underlying cause of heart failure must be treated because measures that relieve symptoms (e.g. diuretics) will only give temporary relief. Specific interventions usually include surgical repair, but this is limited to dedicated paediatric cardiology centres of expertise, and general measures may be employed while awaiting more definitive treatment.

General measures

- Supplemental O_2: give if acute hypoxia (caution in left-to-right shunt because pulmonary vasodilation may increase left-to-right shunting).
- Diet: sufficient caloric intake to enable growth (NB: ↑ metabolic demands in cardiac failure).
- Diuretics: reduce volume load.
- ACE inhibitors: reduce afterload.
- Respiratory support: reduces preload and volume load, and MV assists left ventricular function.
- Inotropic support: if acute cardiac decompensation is detected.

Heart murmurs

Heart murmurs should be characterized in terms of type, location, radiation, and quality of sound. Murmurs are classified as follows:
- *Systolic:* pansystolic; ejection systolic.
- *Diastolic:* early diastolic; mid-diastolic.

The location where a murmur is best heard and radiates to may give a clue to the underlying cause.
- *Loudest above the nipple line*—usually *ejection systolic*:
  - Aortic stenosis (AS), radiates to neck.
  - Pulmonary stenosis (PS), radiates to back.
  - Atrial septal defect (ASD), radiates to back.
  - PDA, radiates to back.
  - CoA, radiates to back.
- *Loudest below the nipple line*—usually *pansystolic*:
  - VSD, may radiate to axilla.
  - Mitral regurgitation (MR), may radiate to axilla.
- Diastolic murmurs—usually due to:
  - Aortic regurgitation (AR).
  - Pulmonary regurgitation (PR).
  - Mitral stenosis (MS).
  - Tricuspid stenosis (TS).

Innocent heart murmurs

These are the commonest cause of a heart murmur in children. They arise due to the rapid flow and turbulence of blood through structurally normal great vessels and across normal heart valves. These are non-pathological and do not signify the presence of any underlying cardiac abnormality.

Characteristics of innocent heart murmur
- Systolic in timing. *Never* diastolic.
- Short-duration/low-intensity sound.
- Intensifies with ↑ cardiac output (e.g. exercise/fever).
- May change in intensity with change in posture and head position.
- No associated cardiac thrill or heave.
- No radiation.
- Asymptomatic patient.

Types of innocent heart murmur
Venous hum (uncommon)
- 'Machinery'-quality sound. Heard on both sides of the sternum.
- Due to blood flow in great veins.

Flow murmur
- Short systolic murmur. Mid-left sternal edge.
- Often heard during acute illness with fever, disappears when fever resolves.

Musical (Still's) murmur
- Systolic murmur. Lower left sternal edge. Often loudest on lying supine.

Clinical features

Table 5.3 summarizes likely diagnoses, given the clinical characteristics of the murmur.

Table 5.3 Likely diagnoses based on clinical features of murmur

Location of murmur	Diagnoses	Additional features
Continuous machinery murmur		
Left clavicular	PDA	Acyanotic, bounding pulse, wide pulse pressure
Long systolic murmur		
Lower left sternal edge (pansystolic)	VSD	Acyanotic, may also have a parasternal thrill
Apex	MR	Acyanotic, rheumatic fever
Mid-left sternal edge	Tetralogy of Fallot	Cyanotic, single S2 (PS murmur loudest later)
Ejection systolic murmur		
Upper left sternal edge	ASD secundum	Acyanotic, fixed split S2
	AVSD partial	Acyanotic, fixed split S2 + apical pansystolic murmur
Upper left sternal edge ± thrill	PS	Acyanotic
Upper left sternal edge	CoA	Acyanotic, weak or absent femoral pulses (if neonate), *hypertensive* in right arm (if older)
Upper right sternal edge	AS	Acyanotic, carotid thrill, delayed soft S2, radiation to the neck

Chest pain

Fewer than 4% of cases of chest pain in children are cardiac in origin.

History

The key to differentiating cardiac from non-cardiac causes of chest pain is a detailed history of the pain and establishing risk factors (e.g. past history and family history) for cardiovascular disease. The commonest causes of chest pain in children are:
- Costochondritis.
- Musculoskeletal strain or trauma of the chest wall.
- Respiratory causes (via cough or pleuritic pain).
- Less common: oesophagitis, psychogenic, haematological (e.g. SCD).

Presentation

Cardiac chest pain will present with typical dull or heavy-pressure central chest pain; may radiate to arms or neck.
- *Associated features:* physical exertion, sweating, breathlessness, dizziness, syncope, palpitations. If pericarditis, there may be a history of sharp central chest pain relieved by leaning forward.
- *Cardiac causes of chest pain include:*
  - Ischaemia: severe AS, PS, hypertrophic obstructive cardiomyopathy (HOCM); coronary abnormality, congenital or acquired (e.g. KD), aortic dissection (e.g. MFS).
  - Arrhythmia.
  - Inflammatory: pericarditis, myocarditis.
  - Drugs: cocaine.

Investigations

- *CXR:* may be helpful to rule out cardiomegaly or respiratory causes, depending on the clinical features present.
- *12-lead ECG:* useful to look for ischaemic changes and predisposition to arrhythmia, if the history sounds cardiac.
- *Cardiac enzymes:* only indicated if there is a typical cardiac sounding history or ischaemic/inflammatory ECG changes.

Cardiac chest pain is unlikely if:
- Non-exertional.
- Description of pain is not suggestive.
- The family history is –ve for hereditary heart disease: long QT syndrome or other channelopathies; cardiomyopathy; unexplained sudden death, especially in young people.
- Cardiovascular examination is unremarkable.
- Other features are found on examination, suggesting non-cardiac causes, e.g. costochondral tenderness.
- Normal 12-lead ECG.

Syncope

Syncope definition

Transient loss of consciousness and muscle tone due to inadequate cerebral perfusion. *Pre-syncope* refers to feeling one is about to pass out with a brief loss of postural tone, while remaining conscious.

Prevalence

Up to 15% of young people aged 8–18y have a syncopal event.

Causes

Cardiac (rare)
- Severe left or right outflow tract obstructions: AS, PS, HOCM.
- Acute aortic valve incompetence/dissection: e.g. MFS.
- Arrhythmias.
- Poor cardiac contractility: cardiomyopathies, myocarditis, any cause of ischaemia.

Non-cardiac (common)
- Autonomic: orthostatic, vasovagal, micturation, breath-holding, reflex-anoxic. Syncope usually <1min in duration.
- Neurological/psychogenic, e.g. seizure; hyperventilation.
- Metabolic, e.g. hypoglycaemia.

Diagnosis

Key is a good history.
- Does this sound cardiac or non-cardiac?
- Predisposing lifestyle factors: adequacy of oral fluid intake in the day, skipping meals.
- What happened before, during, and after the event.
- Activity at the time of event.
- Loss of consciousness and for how long; recovery time to be back to normal.
- Associated symptoms.
- Recurrence of event.
- Red flags in child's past history and family, i.e. long QT syndrome or other channelopathies; cardiomyopathy; unexplained sudden death, especially in young people.

Refer to cardiology

- Syncope associated with exertion/exercise, water/swimming, and loud noises (long QT association).
- +ve family history.
- >1min loss of consciousness.
- Abnormal cardiac examination or ECG.

Palpitations

Definition

Subjective, unpleasant awareness of feeling one's own heart beating. It may be fast, irregular, slow, and painful. (See also ➲ Cardiac arrhythmias, pp. 220–1.)

History

A good history is essential as the nature of palpitations may suggest the cause. If possible, ask the child to 'tap out' the rhythm of their symptoms on a desk. History may suggest:

- Isolated 'jumps' or 'skips', suggesting premature/ectopic beats.
- Sudden start/stop of rapid heartbeat or pounding in the chest suggests SVT. May appear sweaty, pale, or breathless during event.
- Gradual onset and cessation suggest sinus tachycardia.
- Slow HR may suggest sinus dysfunction or AV node dysfunction.
- If related to exercise, with no other symptoms, and gradually gets better at rest, it is more difficult to differentiate normal exercise sinus tachycardia from exercise-induced arrhythmias.
- Are there symptoms of syncope or pre-syncope, or breathlessness?
- Related to posture, e.g. orthostatic.
- Stimulants: caffeine in foods/drinks, recreational drugs, medication.
- Known cardiac history.
- Other predisposing factors: hyperthyroidism, drugs affecting electrolytes such as diuretics.
- Are there any red flags in the personal or family history?

Causes

- *Cardiac:* arrhythmias (due to ischaemia, cardiomyopathy, some CHD, post-cardiac surgery, stimulants, electrolyte imbalance).
- *Non-cardiac:* sinus tachycardia (anxiety, emotion, hyperthyroidism, catecholamine excess, electrolyte imbalance, stimulant drugs/ medications, pain, fever, exercise), with no other red flag features.

Investigations

- *12-lead ECG:* look for sinus rhythm, sinus tachycardia, heart block, arrhythmia and/or pre-disposition to arrhythmia (e.g. pre-excitation WPW syndrome or long QT).
- *Ambulatory ECG:* Holter recording (for common events), event recorder (events occurring up to every 30 days), or implantable device recorder (for rare events).

Management

- If ECG normal or just sinus tachycardia during an episode of palpitations, the cause is not arrhythmia.
- If arrhythmia is recorded, use specific management. If possible arrhythmia, stop precipitating medications or stimulant in drinks/food.
- Treat any underlying identifiable trigger, e.g. electrolyte imbalance.

Congenital heart disease

Definition
Failure of normal cardiac development or persistence of the fetal circulation after birth.

Incidence
- 8/1000 live births.
- 10–15% are complex lesions with >1 abnormality.
- 10–15% of CHD patients also have a non-cardiac abnormality.

Causes
Unknown in the most cases, but commonly associated with:
- Chromosomal defects: e.g. Down's syndrome, Turner's syndrome.
- Gene defects: e.g. 22q deletion, Noonan's syndrome (NS).
- Congenital infections: e.g. rubella.
- Teratogenic drugs: e.g. phenytoin, warfarin, alcohol.

Classification
The diagnosis of a specific lesion is made after clinical examination, CXR, ECG, and echocardiography. Can be classified into *acyanotic* or *cyanotic* types, depending on whether the predominant presentation is with or without central cyanosis. The latter is caused by deoxygenated blood mixing with systemic oxygenated blood, owing to either mixing or right-to-left shunting.

Acyanotic ('pink') CHD: left-to-right shunts or outflow tract obstructions
- ASD (see ➔ Atrial septal defect, p. 198).
- VSD (see ➔ Ventricular septal defect, p. 199).
- AVSD (see ➔ Complete atrioventricular septal defect, p. 199).
- PDA (see ➔ Persistent ductus arteriosus, p. 200).
- AS (see ➔ Aortic stenosis, p. 200).
- PS (see ➔ Pulmonary stenosis, p. 202).
- CoA (see ➔ Coarctation of the aorta, p. 202).
- Dextrocardia (see ➔ Dextrocardia, p. 203).

Cyanotic ('blue') CHD: right-to-left shunts and common mixing lesions
- ToF (see ➔ Tetralogy of Fallot, pp. 204–5).
- Transposition of the great arteries (TGA) (see ➔ Transposition of the great arteries, p. 206).
- Tricuspid atresia (TA) (see ➔ Tricuspid atresia, p. 206).
- Ebstein's anomaly (see ➔ Ebstein's anomaly, p. 207).
- Pulmonary atresia (see ➔ Pulmonary atresia, p. 207).
- Hypoplastic left heart syndrome (HLHS) (see ➔ Hypoplastic left heart syndrome, p. 207).
- Total anomalous pulmonary drainage (TAPVD) (see ➔ Total anomalous pulmonary venous connection, p. 208).
- Truncus arteriosus (see ➔ Truncus arteriosus, p. 208).

Atrial septal defect

ASD may be subtyped as ostium secundum or partial AVSD (ostium primum).

Ostium secundum defect

This defect is in the region of the foramen ovale. The AV valves are normal. The defect is usually isolated, found incidentally, and three times commoner in girls.

- *Clinical features:* most children are asymptomatic. ASDs may rarely result in heart failure, and murmur is usually audible as an ejection systolic murmur at upper left sternal edge. Fixed splitting of second heart sound may be detected.
- *Prognosis:* ostium secundum defects are well tolerated, and symptoms and complications usually only present in third decade or later.
- *Treatment:* ASD closure is required and advised for all patients, even if asymptomatic. Usually, closure is achieved by inserting an occlusion device at cardiac catheterization or by open heart surgery. Intervention should be performed in early childhood, before school entry. NB: in the first year of life, differentiation of ASD from a patent foramen ovale (PFO) may be technically challenging, so usually monitored without intervention until preschool age.

Partial atrioventricular septal defect

This is the more serious ASD, affecting the endocardial cushion tissue that gives rise to the mitral and tricuspid valves. It is located in the lower atrial septum and is associated with a 'common' AV valve (instead of separate tricuspid and mitral valves). These abnormalities result in a left-to-right shunt with valve incompetence.

- *Clinical features:* most children with small defects are asymptomatic. Those with larger defects are predisposed to recurrent chest infections and heart failure, with ejection systolic murmur at upper left sternal edge and fixed split second heart sound.
- *Prognosis:* depends on the degree of left-to-right shunt, pulmonary hypertension, and severity of MR. Without surgical repair, congestive cardiac failure may develop in infancy/early childhood.
- *Management:* definitive treatment with surgical closure of the defect is indicated preschool.

Ventricular septal defect

VSDs account for 25% of all CHDs (2/1000 live births). They may occur in isolation or as part of complex malformations. The clinical features depend on the size and location of the defect.

Subtypes
- Large/small VSD.
- Perimembranous.
- Muscular.
- Multiple/small defects.

Clinical features
- Asymptomatic (typical/early).
- Heart failure (breathlessness—after first few days of life as pulmonary pressures drop).
- Recurrent chest infections.
- Endocarditis (late).

Examination
Pansystolic murmur—lower left sternal edge; parasternal thrill sometimes.

Prognosis
The majority of defects will close spontaneously.

Management
- *Medical:* treat heart failure if present.
- *Surgery:* indicated if severe heart failure or pulmonary hypertension. This is performed at 3–6mth of age, before pulmonary hypertension causes pulmonary vascular disease and cyanosis due to reversal of flow to right-to-left shunting (Eisenmenger syndrome).

Complete atrioventricular septal defect

Complete AVSD is often found in conjunction with Down's syndrome. There is a large defect often from the middle of the atrial septum down to the middle of the ventricular septum. In addition, there is no separate mitral and tricuspid valves, but there is a common AV valve of five leaflets guarding the AV junction.

Clinical features
- May be pink or cyanosed, depending on degree of mixing.
- Breathless with signs of heart failure if mostly left-to-right shunting.
- Most patients with Down's syndrome are screened for CHD with an echocardiogram.
- An ECG will show a superior axis.

Treatment
- *Medical:* treat heart failure if present.
- *Surgery:* performed at 3mth of age, before pulmonary hypertension causes pulmonary vascular disease (Eisenmenger syndrome).

Persistent ductus arteriosus

(See → Patent ductus arteriosus, p. 150.) PDA is common and seen in 1–2/ 1000 live births. Sometimes it follows on from a preterm delivery. It is defined as a duct still being present 1mth after the date that the child should have been born.

Clinical features

Low diastolic pressure due to blood flow back to the pulmonary artery; may be in heart failure (breathlessness) due to left-to-right shunting.

Examination

- Wide pulse pressure or bounding peripheral pulses and precordium.
- Continuous or machinery murmur in the left infraclavicular area.

Prognosis

- The majority of defects will close spontaneously.

Management

- *Medical:* diuretics to treat failure. In symptomatic neonates, indometacin or ibuprofen.
- *Cardiac catheter:* device closure usually at 1y.
- *Surgical:* ligation (rarely).

Aortic stenosis

Congenital AS accounts for ~5% of all CHDs and is the commonest cause of left ventricular outflow obstruction. It is due to thickening of the aortic valves, although subvalvular (subaortic) stenosis is an important form of obstruction. Congenital AS is commoner in boys (3:1). A supravalvular form is also recognized, which may be sporadic or familial; supravalvular AS is associated with Williams syndrome (WS).

Clinical features

Features depend on severity of AS and age at presentation. Ejection systolic murmur is loudest at the right upper sternal edge, classically radiating to the neck, and thrill often palpable in the suprasternal notch/over carotid arteries:
- *Mild AS:* usually asymptomatic; found on routine examination.
- *Severe neonatal AS:* present with heart failure and collapse.
- *Severe AS in older child:* syncope and chest pain on exertion.

Management

- Surgical or balloon dilatation is indicated if symptomatic or if a high resting pressure gradient of >64mmHg is present.
- Avoidance of competitive sports recommended if severe.

Prognosis

Good in the majority with mild or moderate AS. In severe AS, sudden death may occur. Eventually, aortic valve replacement will be required (e.g. Ross procedure).

Pulmonary stenosis

This is a common form of CHD due to the following:
- Isolated thickened deformed pulmonary valves (usually).
- Isolated infundibular stenosis; supravalvular PS.
- Branch pulmonary artery stenosis.

Clinical features

Pulmonary valve stenosis is seen in NS:
- Asymptomatic (mild to moderate stenosis).
- Poor exercise tolerance (severe stenosis).
- RV failure/cyanosis (critical stenosis).
- Ejection systolic murmur at upper left sternal edge radiating to back.

Prognosis

Mild to moderate PS is compatible with normal activities. Monitor because worsening obstruction and significant pressure gradients may develop, which predispose to heart failure when very severe.

Treatment

When severe, needs transvenous balloon dilatation.

Coarctation of the aorta

CoA occurs anywhere in the aorta, but majority (98%) are distal to the left subclavian artery at the level of the ductus arteriosus. Neonates (commonest) become symptomatic at 48h at duct closure. Older children—elevated BP in proximal (above) arteries, with extensive collaterals. CoA is commoner in boys (2:1), but it is common in Turner's syndrome. An abnormal bicuspid aortic valve is often present.

Clinical features

- Heart failure and collapse may occur in neonates.
- Disparity in pulse volume, with weak or absent femoral pulses.
- Mild defects may present later with hypertension (right arm) and rib notching on CXR.

Prognosis

Outside the neonatal period, mortality from untreated hypertension is high and usually occurs aged 20–40y. Complications include premature coronary artery disease (CAD), congestive cardiac failure, hypertensive encephalopathy, and intracranial haemorrhage.

Treatment

- Neonates require resuscitation, commencement of prostaglandin E (PGE) infusion to maintain ductal patency, and early surgery.
- Older children or adolescents require stent insertion at cardiac catheter or surgical resection.

Dextrocardia

Abnormal position of the heart, with location of the left atrium on the right side, and vice versa (i.e. situs inversus), is classified according to the position of the left atrium, the main bronchi, and the abdominal organs. Inversion of viscera (abdominal situs inversus) is always associated with atrial inversion. No malformations of heart structures are found when dextrocardia and abdominal situs inversus (i.e. mirror-image dextrocardia) are present in combination. Major malformations of heart structures are usually found in either of the following:
- Dextrocardia + normal position of abdominal organs.
- Normal position of heart (laevocardia) + abdominal situs inversus.

Characteristic heart malformations include: PS, TA, TGA, anomalous pulmonary venous drainage, AVSD, and single ventricle.

Tetralogy of Fallot

The commonest form of cyanotic CHD, characterized by four cardinal anatomical cardiac anomalies:

- Large VSD.
- Overriding aorta.
- RV outflow obstruction (infundibular and valvular PS).
- RVH.

Systemic venous return to the right side of the heart is normal. In the presence of PS, however, blood is shunted right-to-left across the VSD into the aorta, and SpO_2 desaturation and cyanosis result. The severity of cyanosis depends on the degree of RV outflow obstruction, and when moderate, a balanced shunt across the VSD occurs and cyanosis may be mild or absent.

Clinical features

ToF presents in early infancy with the following:

- *Cyanosis:* usually not present at birth, but increasing from a few weeks' age and leading to clubbing of fingers.
- *Paroxysmal hypercyanotic spells (infancy):* spontaneous/unpredictable onset, tachypnoea, restlessness, and increasing cyanosis, then becoming white and floppy. Potentially dangerous. Duration ranges from a few minutes to hours; severe episodes result in syncope and occasionally in convulsions/hemiparesis.

Treatment

- Severe ToF: worsening cyanosis in early neonatal period requires IV PGE and surgery [e.g. modified Blalock–Taussig (BT) shunt] to maintain pulmonary blood flow and oxygenation.
- Definitive surgery to repair the underlying heart defects is carried out from 4mth of age onwards.
- *Management of hypercyanotic spells:* see Box 5.1.

Prognosis

Untreated, the combination of right-to-left shunt, chronic cyanosis, and polycythaemia predisposes to:

- Cerebral thrombosis and ischaemia.
- Brain abscess.
- Bacterial endocarditis.
- Congestive cardiac failure.

Patients are often asymptomatic after surgical corrections. Long-term follow-up (up to 30y) suggests that improved quality of life is maintained and most have unrestricted lives. Some will require pulmonary valve replacement in teenage years. Cardiac conduction defects, including complete heart block, are seen post-operatively and require treatment.

Box 5.1 Tetralogy of Fallot ('cyanotic spell')

Patients may have attacks of paroxysmal hyperpnoea and ↑ cyanosis that occur spontaneously or after early morning feeds, prolonged crying, or defecation.

Emergency treatment
- Place the patient in the knee to chest position.
- Administer high-flow O_2.
- Insert IV line and administer NS bolus and morphine sulfate.
- Prolonged attacks need $NaHCO_3$, phenylephrine, and propranolol.
- Refer to cardiac centre.

Transposition of the great arteries

The great arteries are transposed—the aorta arises from the right ventricle, and the pulmonary artery from the left ventricle. Consequently, systemic venous blood passing through the right side of heart returns directly to the systemic circulation. Pulmonary venous blood returning to the left side of the heart is returned directly to the pulmonary circulation. This condition is not compatible with life, unless there is adequate mixing of blood from both circulations via an ASD or PDA.

Clinical features

Infants usually present in the first few hours or days with worsening duct-dependent cyanosis. Hypoxia is usually severe, but heart failure is not a dominant feature. This is a medical emergency, and early diagnosis and intervention are required to avoid severe hypoxia.

Treatment

- Commence PGE infusion for ductal patency and to allow mixing of circulations.
- Maintain body temperature, as hypothermia will worsen the metabolic acidosis of hypoxaemia.
- Prompt correction of acidosis and hypoglycaemia.
- Balloon atrial septostomy is usually needed to allow further mixing of the circulations at the atrial level.
- Definitive arterial switch procedure is performed in the first 2wk of life.

Tricuspid atresia

In TA, there is no connection between the right atrium and the RV. Venous blood is diverted to left side via a PFO. Pulmonary blood flow is dependent on associated VSD or PDA.

Clinical features

Most patients with TA present in the first few days to early months of life with increasing cyanosis. The clinical features will vary, depending on other associated cardiac abnormalities. The ECG shows a superior axis. CXR shows massive right atrial enlargement ('wall-to-wall heart')

Treatment

In an emergency, duct patency is achieved with PGE infusion. Surgical palliation and procedures include:
- BT shunt (neonatal period).
- Pulmonary artery banding (neonatal period).
- Glenn shunt (6mth of age).
- Fontan procedure (preschool).

Ebstein's anomaly

The tricuspid valve is inferiorly displaced. There is a range in severity. Essentially, the more inferiorly displaced the valve is, the smaller the RV chamber becomes, and therefore, its capacity to function as a pumping chamber diminishes, compromising the forward blood flow to the lungs. In the worse form, the lesion behaves like a TA.

Pulmonary atresia

In pulmonary atresia, the pulmonary valve is not patent and will either be a closed membrane or be replaced by a segment of blind-ending muscle tissue. Deoxygenated blood cannot exit the right ventricle to reach the lungs and therefore is shunted right-to-left across an atrial communication and a VSD if present. In order for blood to reach the lungs and pick up O_2, ductal patency is essential for survival.

Clinical features

- Cyanosis, acidosis, collapse in early neonatal period.

Management

- Resuscitation.
- PGE infusion to maintain ductal patency.
- If a membranous atresia, perforation using cardiac catheter.
- Emergency BT shunt or stenting of duct to secure pulmonary blood flow.
- May require single ventricle palliation (see ➲ Surgical palliation procedures, p. 209) depending on size and function of the right ventricle: often underdeveloped.

Hypoplastic left heart syndrome

HLHS is a group of disorders associated with underdevelopment of left-sided heart structures. The LV is small and non-functional, and the RV maintains both pulmonary and systemic circulations. The latter is achieved by pulmonary venous blood passing through an ASD or PFO, or retrograde flow via a PDA.

Clinical features

- Early onset (days): central cyanosis and heart failure, leading to collapse and death within the first few days of life.
- Most infants will appear sick (greyish-blue colour) with poor peripheral perfusion and weak peripheral pulses.

Treatment

- Medical management aimed at maintaining patency of the ductus is necessary to support systemic blood flow.
- Surgery is either palliative (2–3 stages: initial Norwood operation or hybrid procedure, followed later by Fontan operations) or definitive (heart transplantation).

Total anomalous pulmonary venous connection

Pulmonary veins connect and drain to the systemic venous circulation (not the left atrium). Therefore, all blood returning to the heart (systemic and pulmonary) returns to the right atrium, and an obligatory PFO or ASD is necessary for survival in order for pink blood to reach the left side of the heart. The pulmonary veins may join the systemic venous side through either above the heart (supracardiac) via the SVC, inside the heart via the coronary sinus (intracardiac), or below the heart (infracardiac) via the IVC.

Clinical features
• First few days of life with varying degrees of obstruction, cyanosis, and congestive cardiac failure.
• Presentation will depend on the degree of obstruction to the pulmonary venous return.

Treatment
• Often a surgical emergency: anastomosis of the common pulmonary channel to the left atrium, with closure of ASD, and interruption of connections to the systemic venous circuit are required.
• Maintaining ductal patency with prostaglandin is usually not helpful for this condition.

Truncus arteriosus

There is a common arterial trunk overriding a large VSD. Therefore, pink and blue blood from both ventricles mixes at the VSD and is ejected through the common trunk. The pulmonary arteries arise from the common trunk and the trunk then continues as the aorta. The child will be cyanosed. This is a precarious lesion based on the balance of pulmonary and systemic blood flow from a single vessel. Needs surgical correction.

Surgical palliation procedures

Blalock–Taussig shunt

Systemic arterial-to-pulmonary artery shunt. Used to secure a temporary blood supply to the pulmonary circulation. Often a prosthetic ('modified') shunt usually connecting either the innominate artery or the right subclavian artery to the right pulmonary artery. Eventually the child will outgrow the prosthetic shunt, and so a Hemi-Fontan/Glenn procedure will be needed later. Sometimes the subclavian artery is anastomosed directly to the pulmonary artery ('classic' BT shunt) and the radial pulse in the corresponding arm will be absent.

Norwood procedure

In HLHS, a 'neo-aorta' is created by fusing together the main pulmonary artery (MPA) to the atretic ascending aorta. To do this, the MPA has to be disconnected from the branch pulmonary arteries. In order to secure pulmonary blood flow, a BT shunt is placed (see ➔ Blalock–Taussig shunt, p. 209). The right ventricle acts as the systemic ventricle, pumping mixed oxygenated and venous blood to the body via the neo-aorta.

Hemi-Fontan/Glenn procedure

Used for single ventricle lesions, the single ventricle acts as the systemic pumping chamber and pulmonary blood flow is secured by anastomosing the SVC directly into one of the pulmonary arteries. Therefore, blood flow to the pulmonary circulation is passive. This procedure may be done following an earlier temporary BT shunt or a hybrid (stenting of PDA) procedure.

Fontan procedure

Used following the Hemi-Fontan procedure described above, completion of creating a passive systemic venous return to the pulmonary circulation, also known as total caval pulmonary circulation (TCPC), is achieved by anastomosing the IVC directly into the pulmonary arteries. The Norwood and Hemi-Fontan procedures, and then completion of the Fontan procedure is often the standard three-operation palliation pathway for HLHS.

Looking after a child with a complex palliation procedure

This procedure is often a source of anxiety for those not used to seeing such patients. A few basic principles are listed below. Always inform the child's named cardiology team if they get admitted to hospital and ask for their specialist advice, including whether to continue their regular medications.

BT shunt

- Ensure you can hear the murmur of the BT shunt.
- If you cannot hear it and they are more hypoxic than expected, then this is an emergency.
- Record the SpO_2 and ensure the values fall in the expected range that is normal for that child.

Cyanotic CHD

- Ensure adequate hydration (as they are often polycythaemic and prone to sluggish blood flow if dehydrated).
- Usually will be prescribed a blood-thinning agent, such as aspirin, especially if they have a BT shunt.

Record a 12-lead ECG

- Check they are in sinus rhythm and for any new signs of ischaemia.
- Compare with previous ECGs—is there a change? ECGs often appear abnormal after previous heart surgery and assessing if there is a new abnormality is difficult without seeing old ECGs.

Check SpO_2

- Assess if the patient is in the expected range.
- SpO_2 that is too low needs investigating.
- SpO_2 consistently above what is normal is abnormal too (e.g. excessive pulmonary flow via BT shunt) and needs cardiologist review.

Check BP

- Indicative of dropping cardiac output.

Check an ABG with [lactate]

- Indicative of cardiac failure.

Acquired heart disease in childhood

Acquired heart disease is uncommon in childhood but carries the risk of significant morbidity and mortality.

The acquired heart conditions include:
- KD (see ◗ Kawasaki disease, pp. 630–1).
- Infective bacterial endocarditis (see ◗ Infective bacterial endocarditis, pp. 212–13).
- Rheumatic fever (see ◗ Rheumatic fever, pp. 214–15).
- Pericarditis (see ◗ Pericarditis, pp. 216–17).
- Myocarditis (see ◗ Myocarditis, p. 218).

Kawasaki disease

This is the leading cause of acquired heart disease in children in the developed world. This disease carries a significant risk of coronary artery aneurysm (see ◗ Kawasaki disease, pp. 630–1).

Infective bacterial endocarditis

There are both acute and subacute forms of infection of the endocardium. Children at risk are those with turbulent blood flow through the heart or where prosthetic material has been inserted following surgery, e.g. PDA or VSD, CoA, previous rheumatic fever. The commonest pathogens associated with infective bacterial endocarditis are:

- *Streptococcus viridans (50% cases)*: often after dental procedures.
- *Staphylococcus aureus*: often related to central venous catheters.
- *Group D Streptococcus (Enterococcus)*: often after lower GI surgery.

An organism is not found in up to 10% of cases.

Clinical features

In the early stage, symptoms are mild. Prolonged fever persisting over several months may be the only feature. Alternatively, rapid onset of high intermittent fever can occur. Non-specific symptoms include:

- Myalgia and arthralgia.
- Headache, weight loss, and night sweats.

Examination

This may be variable, but classic signs include:

- Pallor/anaemia.
- Nail bed—splinter haemorrhages.
- Tender nodules—fingers/toes (Osler's nodes).
- Erythematous palms/soles of feet (Janeway lesions).
- Finger clubbing (late).
- Necrotic skin lesions.
- Splenomegaly.
- Haematuria (microscopic).
- Retinal infarcts (Roth's spots).
- Heart murmurs (change in character with time).

Diagnosis

A high index of suspicion is required. Blood tests include FBC [raised white cell count WCC)], ESR, CRP, and repeated blood cultures (typically three blood cultures from different sites over 3–4h). Echocardiography is needed to look for valve 'vegetations'.

Prophylaxis

This is no longer routinely advised.

Treatment

- *Antibiotic therapy:* should be started as soon as possible (preferably after repeated cultures have been taken). Delays may result in progressive endocardial damage and deterioration in cardiac function. High-dose IV antibiotics (e.g. penicillin/vancomycin) are required for a minimum of 6wk.
- *Bed rest:* is recommended and heart failure should be treated.
- *Surgery:* to remove infected prosthetic material and may be needed for removal of vegetations and repair of affected valves.

Prognosis

Even with antibiotic treatment, mortality may be as high as 20% and complications (50–60%) include heart failure. Systemic emboli from left-sided vegetations may result in brain abscess and stroke.

Rheumatic fever

This is an important cause of heart disease worldwide, but rarely seen in developed countries. Acute rheumatic fever develops in response to infection with group A β-haemolytic *Streptococcus*. It is seen in children aged 5–15y, and the incidence is highest in those from socially and economically disadvantaged areas.

Clinical features

There is a latent period of 2–6wk between onset of symptoms and previous streptococcal infection (e.g. pharyngitis). The grouping together of clinical features makes the diagnosis more likely (Jones criteria). These are categorized into major or minor (see Box 5.2).

> **Box 5.2 Jones criteria**
>
> *Major features*
> - *Pancarditis (50%):* endocarditis/myocarditis/pericarditis.
> - *Polyarthritis (80%):*
>   - *Flitting*—<1wk.
>   - *Migratory*—to other joints over 1–2mth.
>   - *Joints*—knees/ankles/wrists.
> - *Erythema marginatum (<5%):*
>   - Early/trunk and limbs.
>   - Pink border/fading centre.
> - *Subcutaneous nodules* (rare): pea-size/hard/extensor surfaces.
> - *Sydenham's chorea (10%)* (see ➲ Chorea, p. 400):
>   - *Late feature*—2–6mth post-infection.
>   - *Involuntary movements*—choreoathetoid.
> - *Emotional lability.*
>
> *Minor features*
> - Fever.
> - Arthralgia.
> - *Abnormal ECG:* prolonged PR interval.
> - Elevated ESR/CRP.
> - *Evidence of streptococcal infection*, e.g. raised ASOT.
> - History of previous rheumatic fever.

Diagnosis of acute rheumatic fever

- Two major features; *or*
- One major + two minor features; *and*
- Evidence of group A streptococcal (GAS) infection.

Management

In the acute phase, treatment will include:
- Bed rest.
- Anti-inflammatory drugs (e.g. aspirin).
- Corticosteroids (2–3wk).
- Diuretics/ACE inhibitors if in heart failure.
- Antibiotics (e.g. phenoxymethylpenicillin for 10 days).

Long-term therapy is aimed at prevention of further attacks of acute rheumatic fever and the development of chronic rheumatic heart disease. Antibiotic prophylaxis (daily PO penicillin, or monthly IM benzylpenicillin) is recommended.

Chronic rheumatic heart disease

Recurrent bouts of acute rheumatic fever with associated carditis result in scarring and fibrosis of the heart valves (most commonly mitral valve) and may result in incompetent valves requiring replacement.

216 CHAPTER 5 **Cardiology**

Pericarditis

Inflammation of the pericardium may be primary or a manifestation of more generalized illness. The principal causes of pericardial inflammation are:
- *Infections:*
  - Viral, e.g. Coxsackie B, Epstein–Barr virus (EBV).
  - Bacterial, e.g. *Streptococcus, Mycoplasma*.
  - Tuberculosis (TB).
  - Fungal, e.g. histoplasmosis.
  - Parasitic, e.g. toxoplasmosis.
- *Rheumatological:*
  - Rheumatoid arthritis (RA).
  - Rheumatic fever.
  - Systemic lupus erythematosus (SLE).
  - Sarcoidoisis.
- *Metabolic:*
  - Hyperuricaemia.
  - Hypothyroidism.
- *Malignancy.*
- *Radiotherapy.*

Clinical features

The features depend on the extent of involvement of the pericardium. The predominant symptom is precordial pain that is typically sharp, exacerbated by lying down, and relieved by sitting or leaning forward. The pain is often referred to the left shoulder. Other symptoms include cough, dyspnoea, and fever. The accumulation of sufficient fluid to cause cardiac tamponade and heart failure is rare, but an emergency.

Examination

Specific diagnostic findings will relate to the amount of fluid within the pericardial sac, including pulsus paradoxus, pericardial rub, and quiet/distant heart sounds.

Investigations

Investigations directed at confirming the diagnosis include:
- Echocardiogram.
- ECG (typical low-voltage QRS complexes).

Other investigations should be directed at identifying the underlying cause of the pericarditis and will include: pericardiocentesis, bacterial/viral culture, and biochemical analysis; and blood serology for viral studies, anti-streptolysin O titre (ASOT), and connective tissue disease.

Management

Treatment is directed both at the underlying cause (e.g. antibiotics) and symptoms:
- *Analgesia* for pain relief.
- *Anti-inflammatory* drugs to reduce pericardial inflammation.
- *Pericardiocentesis* for pericardial effusion causing cardiac tamponade and heart failure.

Constrictive pericarditis

Previous pericardial inflammation may predispose to this condition. However, most cases of constrictive pericarditis occur in the absence of any preceding illness or generalized systemic disease. The fibrosed restrictive pericardium impairs cardiac contractility.

Clinical features
- Include evidence of heart failure, hepatomegaly, and neck vein distension.
- On auscultation, heart sounds are distant and a characteristic pericardial 'knock' is often heard.
- CXR may reveal calcification of the pericardium.

Treatment
Requires pericardiectomy.

Myocarditis

Myocarditis may be due to:
- *Infections:* viral, e.g. Coxsackie B, EBV.
- KD.
- *Drugs:* doxorubicin (adriamycin).
- *Rheumatological disease:* SLE, RA, rheumatic fever, sarcoidosis.

Clinical features

Variable and will depend on the age of the patient and on the time course of underlying disease. Specific cardiovascular symptoms include progressive worsening of dyspnoea and congestive cardiac failure. Sudden onset of ventricular arrhythmia may occur.

Examination

Typical cardiovascular examination includes:
- Weak pulses.
- Tachycardia.
- Gallop heart rhythm.
- Distant heart sounds.

Diagnosis

Echocardiography shows poor ventricular function. Definitive histological diagnosis is made after percutaneous endomyocardial biopsy. CXR shows cardiomegaly; ECG shows reduced QRS complex size.

Treatment

This is directed at the underlying cause and at controlling symptoms of congestive heart failure. Arrhythmias should be treated. Cardiac transplantation is needed in patients with refractory heart failure.

Cardiomyopathy

Cardiomyopathy may be primary or secondary to systemic or metabolic disease. Primary cardiomyopathy may be classified as:
• Hypertrophic (obstructive).
• Dilated (congestive).
• Restrictive.

Hypertrophic obstructive cardiomyopathy

Massive ventricular hypertrophy, principally involving the septum. All portions of the left ventricle are affected, and the right ventricle may also be involved. There is myocardial fibrosis, resulting in stiff muscle with ↓ distensibility. Ventricular filling is ↓, but systolic pumping is maintained until late in disease. HOCM occurs at all ages and seen in other family members (dominant inheritance sometimes occurs).

Clinical features
• Most children are asymptomatic.
• Ejection systolic murmur (may be incidental finding).
• Symptoms, when present, include fatigue, dyspnoea, chest pain, and syncope on exertion (because of left outflow tract obstruction).
• Important cause of sudden unexpected death.

Prognosis
Unpredictable, especially in those without symptoms.

Treatment
Avoidance of competitive sports and strenuous activity is encouraged. Therapy is aimed at reducing the outflow obstruction:
• *Medical therapy:* β-blockers; Ca^{2+} antagonists, pacemaker.
• *Surgical therapy:* ventricular septal myotomy, transplantation.

Dilated (congestive) cardiomyopathy

This condition is rare and characterized by massive dilatation of the ventricles and cardiomegaly. Cause is unknown in most cases, but it can be post-viral or occur in IEM (see ➲ Systems–Cardiac, p. 508).

Clinical features
Insidious onset of progressive congestive cardiac failure is common. The course is usually progressive, and the prognosis poor.

Management
Mainly directed at treating heart failure and, where possible, any underlying cause. Heart transplantation if severe heart failure.

Restrictive cardiomyopathy

A rare condition characterized by poor ventricular compliance and inadequate ventricular filling. Clinical features similar to constrictive pericarditis (see ➲ Constrictive pericarditis, p. 217). It is sometimes seen in Löffler hypereosinophilic syndrome (multisystem disorder of the skin, lungs, nervous system, and liver) and results in endocardial fibrosis of the AV valves and ventricles. Prognosis is poor and heart transplantation is often required.

Cardiac arrhythmias

(See ➔ Dysrhythmias, p. 49; ➔ Palpitations, p. 196.) Sinus arrhythmia is normal in children and adolescents. Other arrhythmias are rare in childhood and may be transient or permanent. Congenital arrhythmias may occur in structurally normal or abnormal hearts. They may be secondary to myocardial disease (e.g. rheumatic fever, myocarditis) or follow exposure to toxins, drugs, or surgery to the heart. Children with suspected arrhythmia require a detailed history and examination. The arrhythmia should be identified and characterized by ECG. Underlying CHD should be excluded by echocardiography.

Supraventricular tachycardia

The commonest abnormal arrhythmia in childhood. Re-entry within the AV node is the commonest mechanism of SVT.

Clinical features

Sudden onset (and cessation) lasting from seconds to hours; HR 240–300 beats/min. SVT is well tolerated in older children, but heart failure may occur in the young infant. Often precipitated by febrile illness.

Treatment

• *Medical:* adenosine (emergency), β-blocking medication (flecainide, amiodarone under specialist guidance).
• *Interventional:* electrophysiology, intracardiac ablation at teen age.

Wolff–Parkinson–White syndrome

Pre-excitation syndrome predisposing to SVT. Due to abnormal re-entry circuit of the AV node and an accessory conduction pathway connecting the atrium to the ventricle on the right or left lateral cardiac border or within the ventricular septum. It may be associated with Ebstein's anomaly, post-surgical repair, and cardiomyopathy. ECG shows short PR interval and delta wave (slow upstroke of QRS complex).

Ventricular tachycardia long QT syndrome (LQTS)

LQTS may be associated with sudden loss of consciousness during exercise, stress, or emotion, usually in late childhood. If unrecognized, sudden death from VT may occur. Inheritance is AD, but there are several phenotypes. Prolongation of the QT interval on ECG is associated with many drugs, electrolyte disorders, and head injury. LQTS is a channelopathy caused by specific gene mutations with gain or loss of function. There is a range of effects from long QT, short QT, and Brugada syndromes and cardiomyopathy. Anyone with a family history of sudden unexplained death or syncope on exertion must be assessed for these.

Congenital complete heart block

Rare. Mothers of affected children are usually +ve for serum anti-Ro or anti-La antibodies and have an underlying connective tissue disorder.

Clinical features
- Significant bradycardia.
- Fetal hydrops and intrauterine death.
- *Neonate*: heart failure.
- *Childhood*: asymptomatic, syncope.

Management
Isoprenaline as temporizing measure if symptomatic or profound bradycardia in neonatal period; endocardial/epicardial pacemaker.

Further reading

Useful resources and websites for patients and clinicians

British Heart Foundation. Congenital heart disease and arrhythmia. Available at: ℘ http://www.bhf.org.uk/heart-health/children-and-young-people.

European Society of Cardiology (ESC). Clinical practice guidelines. Available at: ℘ http://www.escardio.org/Guidelines/Clinical-Practice-Guidelines.

Great Ormond Street Hospital for Children. *Conditions treated by the Paediatric Cardiology department*. Available at: ℘ http://www.gosh.nhs.uk/medical-information/clinical-specialties/cardiology-information-parents-and-visitors/conditions-we-treat.

Syncope Trust and Reflex anoxic Seizures (STARS). Available at: ℘ http://www.stars.org.uk.

Paediatric ECG tables

Park MK, Guntheroth WG. *How to Read Pediatric ECGs*, fourth edition. Mosby Elsevier, Philadelphia, PA; 2006.

Park MK. *Park's The Pediatric Cardiology Handbook*, fifth edition. Elsevier Saunders, Philadelphia, PA; 2015.

Respiratory medicine

Respiratory assessment

The respiratory system is the most commonly affected body system in acute paediatric disease, with presentations across the whole spectrum of health care—from primary care to hospital admissions to paediatric intensive care units (PICUs). A respiratory system-focused history and examination for paediatric patients are outlined below.

History

- *General information:* growth and general body proportions, weight loss, immunizations.
- Age of onset of symptoms or problem.
- Description of respiratory sounds in lay terminology from parents.
- Any video (e.g. mobile phone) footage of the child when symptomatic?
- Have there been any triggers to this illness, e.g. dust or cold air?
- What makes the problem worse? Exercise (e.g. asthma), sleep (e.g. adenotonsillar hypertrophy and snoring)?
- What makes the problem better, e.g. bronchodilators in asthma?
- *Other symptoms:* haemoptysis, cough, sputum production, choking, GOR, apnoea, coryza, chest/abdominal pain.
- *Past respiratory history:*
  - Neonatal: any intubations (risk of subglottic stenosis), how premature, how long on IPPV (risk of chronic lung disease), any previous surgery?
  - Postnatal: any hospital admissions, any PICU admissions, any previous respiratory investigations?

Examination

- *General:* growth parameters, clubbing, lymphadenopathy, temperature, LOC, colour, SpO_2, HR.
- *RR* (know the normal ranges; see ⊅ Table 3.1): the single best indicator of respiratory illness.
- *Effort of breathing:* recession (subcostal/intercostal/sternal), tracheal tug, grunting, nasal flare, head bobbing.
- *Effect of breathing:* SpO_2 (± ABG or venous blood pCO_2), presence of cyanosis, Harrison's sulcus.
- *Pattern of breathing:* e.g. episodic, periodic, apnoea; duration of expiration.
- *Nose and speech:* allergic crease across the bridge of the nose and nasal discharge (e.g. allergic rhinitis); hyponasal speech (e.g. palate and nasal problems); nasal or mouth breather.
- *Facial appearance:* size of midface, lower jaw, tongue (e.g. craniofacial syndrome).
- *Tonsillar hypertrophy.*
- *Cough:* paroxysms, barking, high-pitched?
- *Breathing cycle:* inspiratory stridor indicates airway obstruction above the thoracic inlet; expiratory prolongation or wheeze indicates intrathoracic airway obstruction.

- *Breath sounds:* presence of crepitations (coarse or fine), wheeze (high-pitched, bronchiolar constriction), rhonchi (low-pitched, larger airway obstruction), bronchial breathing (loud expiratory sounds associated with pneumonia).
- *Chest appearance:* hyperexpansion, Harrison's sulcus (in chronic obstructive airway disease).
- Chest expansion (usually reduced on pathological side), percussion note (high in hyperinflation, 'stony dull' in effusion), vocal fremitus (reduced over effusions).

Respiratory investigations

Chest X-ray

CXR is often the first-line investigation in respiratory disease. A structured approach will help avoid missing subtle pathology without overestimating normal variants. A suggested structure follows:

- Check *identity of patient* is confirmed on the CXR.
- Check *orientation of the film* and whether it was taken AP (antero-posterior) or PA (postero-anterior); the radiographer will indicate this on the film.
- Check *level of penetration*: intervertebral spaces should be clearly seen, and spinous processes of the vertebrae just visible—this is particularly important when you want to review changes on a series of films.
- Check *alignment*: look for asymmetry of rib shape, clavicular heads, and/or anterior ribs, indicating the film is rotated.
- Check *lung expansion* (an expiratory film makes further interpretation very unreliable): how many ribs can be counted (usually 8–9 posterior ribs)? Are the hemi-diaphragms in the usual position (right slightly higher than left)? Is the horizontal fissure visible and correctly placed?
- Check *airways*: position of trachea, any FB?
- Check *bones*: adequate mineralization, any fractures?
- Check *cardiac silhouette*: is there any blurring of the margins (suggesting adjacent lung may be consolidated)? Is the shape abnormal (suggesting cardiac defect)? Is the size normal (cardiothoracic ratio usually no more than 60%)?
- Check *hilar regions* for lymphadenopathy.
- Check *lung fields*: are lung markings present throughout (rule out pneumothorax)? Are the costophrenic angles clear (rule out effusion)? Is there asymmetry of any lung fields (radio-opaque suggests fluid or solid tissue replacing normally aerated lung tissue)?

Lung function testing

Spirometry can be achieved in very compliant 5y olds, but measurements are more likely to be successful in ≥7y olds. Many modern spirometers use incentive games to encourage children to use good technique. Measurements include:

- FEV_1 (forced expiratory volume in 1s): reduced in obstructive airway disease.
- FVC (forced vital capacity): reduced in restrictive lung disease (e.g. bronchiectasis).
- FEV_1/FVC (forced expiratory volume in 1s as a fraction of forced vital capacity): values <70% of predicted suggest obstructive airway disease. Use upper and lower limits of normal parameters for age (available on most spirometers if body weight and height are known).
- *Exercise testing*.

- *Bronchodilator responsiveness* (i.e. reversibility): improvement of FEV_1 by >12% after administering a bronchodilator is a +ve result.
- *Peak expiratory flow rate* (PEFR): easily obtained from a peak flow meter. While limited in comparison to spirometry, it does offer the advantage of being cheap and portable and it can be used at home.

Exhaled nitric oxide (eNO)

The eNO test is largely used to help identify inflammatory airway disease (e.g. asthma). High levels [over 35 parts per billion (ppb)] are indicative of ongoing inflammation and support escalation of anti-inflammatory treatment (e.g. inhaled corticosteroids).

Sweat test

The sweat test is used in the diagnosis of CF. Sweating is induced in an area of the forearm using pilocarpine iontophoresis, and a capillary tube is used to collect the sweat. A minimum of 15 microlitres (and preferably >30 microlitres) of sweat should be collected. In CF, abnormal function of the Cl^- channel (also present in sweat glands) results in higher concentrations of Cl^- in sweat:

- *Suspicious:* >40mmol/L (>30mmol/L in newborn screened babies).
- *Diagnostic:* >60mmol/L.

Other respiratory investigations

Chest computerized tomography
Useful for assessing abnormalities in airways, as well as abnormalities in parenchymal tissue density, and requires cooperation (or GA) to achieve quality images on inspiration and expiration.

Flexible bronchoscopy
Used to assess directly the airway from nose to distal bronchus; used to:
- Visualize airway anatomy (e.g. identify bronchomalacia, vascular rings causing compression, etc.).
- Obtain broncho-alveolar lavage (BAL) for MC&S.
- Microscopy of BAL samples for fat-laden macrophages (suggest GOR) and eosinophils (suggest inflammatory airway disease).

Common presentation: wheeze

Wheeze is the typically high-pitched sound produced by flow through a partially obstructed small airway.

Clinical characteristics

- Associated with prolongation of the expiratory phase of the breathing cycle, as airway diameter contracts further during expiration, leading to trapped air (dynamic hyperinflation).
- Typically, high-pitched sound—the pitch can help indicate the size of airway obstructed (cf. lower-pitched wheeze—also called rhonchi—associated with larger airways).
- Typically polyphonic (e.g. in asthma), but monophonic wheeze may indicate single airway obstruction (e.g. FB) versus multiple airways.
- Associated crepitations may occur when significant airway oedema is present (commoner in infants with bronchiolitis).

Differential diagnosis

Intrinsic change causing lower airway obstruction
- Asthma.
- Bronchiolitis.
- Bronchitis and bronchiectasis.
- CF or primary ciliary dyskinesia (PCD).
- Airway haemangioma/polyps.
- Bronchomalacia.

Extrinsic lower airway compression
- *Lung parenchyma:* e.g. pneumonia, pulmonary oedema, bronchogenic cyst.
- *Vascular:* e.g. enlarged left atrium compressing left main stem bronchus, pulmonary artery vascular ring.
- *Lymphatic:* e.g. enlarged hilar lymph nodes.
- *Chest deformity:* e.g. scoliosis.

Intraluminal lower airway obstruction
- Aspiration of food or milk from GOR.
- FB inhalation.
- Mucus, pus, blood.

Common presentation: stridor

Stridor is a high-pitched inspiratory sound indicating either dynamic or fixed extrathoracic airway obstruction (i.e. above the thoracic inlet/upper trachea). *Stertor* is a lower-pitched inspiratory sound associated exclusively with the nasopharynx (e.g. snoring). When it arises acutely and is associated with respiratory distress, stridor requires immediate attention.

Differential diagnosis

Nose and nasopharynx

- Congenital obstruction, e.g. choanal atresia (rare) (see ➔ Congenital abnormalities: upper airway, pp. 808–9).
- Inflammation: e.g. rhinitis and sinusitis (common).

Mouth, oropharynx, and hypopharynx

- *Congenital obstruction*: e.g. macroglossia and glossoptosis (rare).
- *Inflammation*: e.g. tonsillar hypertrophy (common).
- *Masses*: e.g. cystic hygroma or other malformation (rare).

Larynx

- *Congenital obstruction*: e.g. laryngomalacia (common); laryngeal web or cleft, vocal cord paralysis (rare).
- *Inflammation*: e.g. GOR (rare).
- *Infection*: e.g. croup (common), acute epiglottitis (very rare post-immunization).
- *Masses*: e.g. haemangiomas, abscess (rare).
- *Acquired obstruction*: e.g. subglottic stenosis (common), FB inhalation (rare, but must not be missed).

Trachea

- *Congenital obstruction*: e.g. tracheomalacia, TOF (rare).
- *Infection*: e.g. bacterial tracheitis (rare).

There are specific treatments for many of these conditions. In persistent, non-medical causes of stridor, airway surgery may be required after endoscopy.

Common presentation: cough

Cough is a protective response for removing secretions and particulate matter from the airway. Like fever, it often generates much anxiety in parents but is not a danger per se. It is the cause of cough that must be identified and treated if needed. For these reasons, cough suppressants are *not recommended* in paediatric practice.

Differential diagnosis—acute cough

Upper airway disease
- *Common cold*: e.g. rhinovirus, coronavirus.
- *Other infections*: e.g. sinusitis, tonsillitis, laryngitis, croup, viral (influenza and parainfluenza), bacterial (e.g. GAS).
- *Allergic rhinitis* and post-nasal drip of secretions, especially when supine at night.
- *Vocal cord dysfunction*.

Lower airway disease
- Asthma.
- *Infection*: e.g. bronchiolitis.

Lung parenchymal disease
- *Infection*: e.g. viral and bacterial pneumonia, empyema.
- *Atypical pneumonia*: e.g. *Mycoplasma pneumoniae* infection.

Differential diagnosis—chronic cough

A chronic cough is one that has persisted for >8wk. Possible causes are as follows.

Long-standing upper airway disease
- *Infection*: e.g. chronic sinusitis.
- *Inflammation*: e.g. persistent GOR.

Long-standing lower airway disease
- *Congenital abnormalities*: e.g. TOF, cleft larynx, pulmonary artery sling.
- *Infection*: e.g. post-bronchiolitis symptoms, persistent bacterial bronchitis.
- *FB*.
- *Bronchiectasis*: e.g. damage to the airway from chronic infection and TB, or immunodeficiency.
- *CF and PCD*.

Lung parenchymal disease
- *Infection*: e.g. atypical pneumonia and empyema.

Central causes
- Psychogenic cough.
- Tourette disease: with a tic involving throat clearing or cough.

Asthma

Asthma is a disease of chronic airway inflammation, bronchial hyperreactivity, and reversible airway obstruction. It affects 10% of the population and can develop at any age, but typically half of paediatric cases present aged <10y. There is often a family history of asthma or atopic disease. Different phenotypes of asthma exist, based on triggers, with allergic triggers (e.g. pollen) being more responsive to medication than infectious triggers (e.g. viral).

Diagnosis

No single 'asthma test' is diagnostic and smaller children rarely cooperate with formal lung function testing. A combination of factors must be evaluated to give a clinician-led diagnosis.

History

- Recurrent episodic symptoms of wheeze, chest tightness, cough, and breathlessness.
- Identify triggers: e.g. viral URTI, allergen exposure, exercise.
- Cough after exercise or sometimes in the night, disturbing sleep.
- Look for daily or seasonal variation in symptoms.
- History of atopy: food allergy, eczema, allergic rhinitis.
- Family history of atopy (in siblings or parents).
- Note cough in isolation is rarely an indication of asthma.

Examination

Common findings include:
- Barrel-shaped chest.
- Hyperinflation leading to hyperresonance on percussion.
- Wheeze and prolonged expiratory phase of respiration.

CXR

Rarely useful, unless to rule out other pathology, but in asthma:
- Hyperinflation: flattened hemi-diaphragms, ↑ anterior rib spacing.
- Peribronchial cuffing.
- Rarely air leak (e.g. pneumothorax/pneumomediastinum).

Spirometry

- PEFR: +ve if >20% below level predicted for height.
- FEV_1/FVC: +ve if <70% of lower limit of normal for age.
- Concave, scooped shape in expiratory flow–volume curve.
- Bronchodilator response to β-agonist (i.e. 12% ↑ in FEV_1 or PEFR).
- Fractional eNO (FeNO): +ve if >35ppb at ages 4–16y.

Other investigations

- Validated symptoms questionnaire, e.g. Asthma Control Test.
- Tests for aero-allergens [either blood IgE or skin prick tests (SPTs)]: grass, tree pollens, cat/dog/horse/hamster, moulds (see ➔ Asthma, p. 533; ➔ Allergy test, pp. 514–15).
- Blood eosinophil count.

Aids when diagnosis is uncertain or of intermediate probability

For example, some, but not all, are typical of asthma:

- Perform spirometry with bronchodilator reversibility as above.
- Monitor PEFR variability for 2–4wk (20% variability over 3 days is suggestive of diagnosis).
- Commence inhaled corticosteroids (e.g. 8wk trial) and repeat lung function tests thereafter.
- If spirometry normal, consider IgE tests for allergens and measurement of FeNO to identify eosinophilic inflammation. FeNO >35ppb is a +ve test.
- Alternatively, consider watchful waiting if child is asymptomatic.

Unlikely asthma or low probability

For example, when there are symptoms reported, but no typical features of asthma:

- Normal or obstructive spirometry, FeNO <34ppb and –ve peak flow variability.
- Consider alternative diagnosis.

Management

The main medications used as maintenance therapy for asthma are bron-chodilators, which give short-term relief of symptoms, and prophylactic therapy to reduce chronic inflammation and bronchial hyperreactivity. Deaths in asthma are frequently associated with undertreatment.

Education

- *Asthma action plan:* all children (and their carers) should have a written plan detailing medication and what to do if an exacerbation.
- *Correct inhaler technique.*
- *Trigger avoidance.*
- *Smoking avoidance.*

Bronchodilators

- *Short-acting β2-agonists:* salbutamol, terbutaline.
- *Long-acting β2-agonists:* salmeterol, formoterol.
- *Short-acting anticholinergic:* ipratropium bromide.

Chronic treatment of inflammation and hyperreactivity

- *Inhaled corticosteroids:* beclometasone, ciclesonide, fluticasone. Categories: very low dose, low dose, or medium dose.
- *PO steroids:* prednisolone.
- *Leukotriene inhibitors:* montelukast.
- *Methylxanthines:* theophylline.
- *Combination inhalers:* containing inhaled steroids and long-acting β2-agonists, e.g. fluticasone with salmeterol (Seretide®).
- *Maintenance and reliever therapy (MART) regimen:* a form of combined inhaled steroids and a fast long-acting β2-agonist, e.g. budesonide with formoterol (Symbicort®) used when symptomatic.

Preschool wheeze

Preschool recurrent wheeze presents a particular challenge:
- Many of these children do not go on to develop asthma in later childhood.
- Evidence base for use of asthma medications is much weaker in this cohort.
- Lack of objective respiratory function testing leaves them open to greater inter-clinician interpretation of signs and symptoms.

Preschool wheeze—according to clinical presentation—can be classified as either:
- Episodic viral wheeze (EVW, commonest), *or*
- Multi-trigger wheeze (MTV, resembles asthma).

Risk factors for preschool wheeze include exposure to tobacco smoke, prematurity, intrauterine growth retardation (IUGR), exposure to viruses and bacteria, and allergens.

Management strategy
- Carer tobacco avoidance.
- Trial of bronchodilator.
- Consider PO corticosteroids during a severe episode requiring hospitalization.
- Consider trial of low-dose inhaled corticosteroids for 8wk, with aim to review and stop.
- If symptoms do not resolve within 8wk of therapy, consider alternative diagnosis, e.g. airway anatomical defect, protracted bacterial bronchitis, etc.
- Consider trial of leukotriene inhibitor for 8wk, with aim to review and stop.
- If symptoms recur within 4wk of stopping, repeat 8wk trial.

Adolescent asthma

Characteristics
- Age 10–19y, as defined by the WHO.
- Compliance is often poor, as is inhaler technique.
- Major depression, panic attacks, and anxiety disorders are common comorbidities.

Management strategy
- Tobacco avoidance.
- Consider Quality of Life Questionnaire, a screening questionnaire for anxiety or depression.
- Transition to adult services should start well before transfer to adult services (usually at age 16–18y).

Side effects of chronic asthma treatment

(See also ➔ Asthma: long-term management, p. 236.)

Steroids
When long-term PO steroids or high-dose inhaled steroids are used, special attention will need to be given to unwanted effects, including:
- *Impaired growth:* can affect growth in height, so suspect if poor height velocity with no other identified reason.
- *Adrenal suppression.*
- *Oral candidiasis.*
- *Altered bone metabolism.*

Theophylline
Now less commonly used in children, but blood level monitoring is recommended to avoid side effects, including:
- Vomiting.
- Sleep disturbance or ↑ sleeping.
- Headaches.
- Poor concentration and deterioration of performance at school.
- Arrhythmias.

Asthma: long-term management

(For acute management of asthma, see ⊃ Status asthmaticus, pp. 42–3.)

Long-term therapy

Having reviewed the history and categorized your patient in terms of clinical pattern and severity, use a logical, stepwise approach to escalating therapy (see Box 6.1).

Box 6.1 The stepwise approach to drugs

Before altering a treatment, ensure that treatment is being taken in an effective manner. The use of numbered steps is avoided in recent national/international guidelines but given below to assist the novice in asthma management.

Step 1
- Short-acting β2-bronchodilator as required, *AND*
- Inhaled corticosteroid at very low dose (e.g. Clenil Modulite® 100mcg bd or fluticasone 50mcg bd).
- Oral leukotriene inhibitor may be used as alternative in under 5y olds.

Step 2
- Continue very low-dose corticosteroid, *AND*
- Add long-acting bronchodilator for over 5y olds as combination inhaler to aid compliance (e.g. Seretide® 50mcg bd) or leukotriene inhibitor for under 5y olds.

Step 3
- If no benefit from long-acting bronchodilator, then discontinue.
- Increase to low-dose inhaled steroid (e.g. Clenil Modulite® 200mcg bd).
- Consider adding leukotriene inhibitor if not already done so.
- Consider move to a MART regimen (e.g. Symbicort® 100/6 two puffs bd and if symptoms occur).

Step 4
- Increase steroid to medium-dose inhaled steroid (e.g. Clenil Modulite® 400mcg bd or fluticasone 250mcg bd).
- Consider addition of slow-release theophylline.

Step 5
- Add regular low-dose PO corticosteroid.
- Consider alternative diagnoses.
- Consider anti-IgE antibody therapy (omalizumab).
- Refer to specialist centre.

Take consideration of the following

Monitoring
- After starting or adjusting medication for asthma, review in 4–8wk for response. Adjust asthma action plan with any changes.
- Always aim for the lowest dose of inhaled corticosteroid to obtain control of symptoms.
- Consider reducing maintenance therapies when asthma symptoms controlled for at least 3mth.
- Review inhaler technique at each consultation or acute presentation.

Allergen avoidance
- Removal of feather bedding.
- Wrapping of mattress in plastic.
- Cleaning of carpets and furniture.
- No pets in the house if the child is allergic to them.

Passive smoking
- No smoking in the house or car.
- Parents/carers must be strongly encouraged to stop smoking completely.

Education
Patients and parents encouraged to learn more about the condition and how it is best treated. For example:
- Which medication to use and when.
- Best inhaler technique.
- What to do if asthma is getting worse.
- Share asthma action plan with all carers, including nursery and school.
- Not to smoke.
- To gargle with water after steroid inhaler use to avoid oral thrush.

Uncontrolled asthma
When asthma is poorly controlled, consider the following:
- Lack of adherence.
- Suboptimal inhaler technique.
- Alternative diagnosis, e.g. dysfunctional breathing, bronchiectasis.
- Psychological factors.

Asthma: drug delivery devices

There are a number of drug delivery devices available for use in children. Choice of device may be determined by the choice of drug:

- *Nebulizer:* use in emergency treatment at all ages for delivery of bronchodilator with 6–8L/min O_2 flow. Air-delivered nebulizers for use in home/community are not recommended.
- *Large- or small-volume spacer with MDI:* use in infancy to any age (face mask for under 3y and mouthpiece for older children). This device uses a plastic chamber with a valve at one end and a place where an MDI can be inserted at the other end. The spacer allows aerosol particles from the inhaler to be slowed and inhaled on each breath. It reduces depositing in the mouth and optimizes drug delivery to bronchioles.
- *Propellant MDI (PMDI):* these are the preferred method of delivery, with a spacer for bronchodilators and inhaled corticosteroids for small children.
- *Breath-activated inhaler:* a PMDI inhaler that activates delivery on detection of inspiratory air flow from patient. Limited to use in older children/adolescents; particularly consider if poor compliance with use of spacer device (e.g. Qvar Easi-Breathe®)
- *Dry powder device:* terbutaline sulfate (*Bricanyl Turbohaler*®), salbutamol (*Ventolin Accuhaler*®). Use also limited to older children with good inhaler technique.

Inhaler technique

In the clinic, you will need to make sure that your patient is getting and taking the medication prescribed. In all children, you will need to see that they have the appropriate technique and device for their age.

Child >3y

Look for 5-breath tidal volume breathing technique.
- *Stand* to allow full use of the diaphragm.
- *Shake MDI.*
- *Place MDI into spacer.*
- *Place device in mouth.*
- *Firm seal with mouth around mouthpiece.*
- *Breathe in and out tidally:* when good rhythm, activate device (only once).
- *Continue breathing five times.*
- *If second dose is needed:* then shake MDI and repeat as above.

Infant

Note that if the infant is crying, less drug will be inhaled. Make sure that the person giving the medication:
- Tilts the spacer, so that the valve is open (in small-volume device, you do not need to tip as the valve is low-resistance).
- Lets the infant take at least *five breaths from each dose* actuated.

Cystic fibrosis

CF is an AR genetic disorder leading to a defect in the CF transmembrane receptor (CFTR) protein, which results in defective ion transport in exocrine glands. In the lung, abnormal Na^+ and Cl^- ion transport causes thickening of respiratory mucus. The lung is therefore prone to inadequate mucociliary clearance, chronic bacterial infection, and lung injury. There are also similar effects in other organs that lead to pancreatic insufficiency, liver disease, and, in the ♂, infertility. There are over 1500 mutations in the *CFTR* gene; the commonest is ΔF508 deletion. Carriage rate is highest in Caucasian ethnic groups (1/2500).

Diagnosis

Screening
Since 2007, in the UK, all newborn babies are screened for CF, looking for abnormally raised immunoreactive trypsinogen (IRT) and 29 *CFTR* gene mutations from blood-spot analysis, as part of the national newborn screening programme.

History

Give particular attention to:
- Cough and wheeze.
- Shortness of breath (SOB).
- Sputum production.
- Haemoptysis.
- Stool type (e.g. fatty, oily, pale) and frequency.
- Weight loss or poor weight gain.

About 10–20% of CF patients present in the neonatal period with meconium ileus. However, most children with CF present with:
- Malabsorption.
- FTT.
- Recurrent chest infection.

Examination

Full assessment of:
- Respiratory system.
- Liver and GI system.
- Growth and development.

Investigations

- Sweat test showing ↑ Cl^- levels (>60mmol/L).
- *CXR:* hyperinflation, ↑ AP diameter, bronchial dilatation, cysts, linear shadows, and infiltrates.
- *Lung function:* obstructive pattern with ↓ FVC and ↑ lung volumes.

Cystic fibrosis: problems

Lifelong therapy and supervision are required in CF. There is a variety of problems that can be expected at different ages.

Infancy

- Meconium ileus.
- Neonatal jaundice (prolonged).
- Hypoproteinaemia and oedema.

Childhood

- Recurrent lower respiratory tract infections (LRTIs).
- Bronchiectasis (occasionally).
- Poor appetite.
- Rectal prolapse.
- Nasal polyps.
- Sinusitis (rare to have symptoms).

Adolescence

- Bronchiectasis.
- Diabetes mellitus.
- Cirrhosis and portal hypertension.
- Distal intestinal obstruction.
- Pneumothorax.
- Haemoptysis.
- Allergic bronchopulmonary aspergillosis.
- ♂ infertility.
- Arthropathy.
- Psychological problems.

Cystic fibrosis: management (1)

Management of the child with CF requires close cooperation between local hospitals and regional centres. Patients and their families gain much from expert clinics and from other patients and their families. Effective management requires an MDT approach, which should include:

• A paediatric pulmonologist.
• A physiotherapist.
• A dietician.
• A nurse liaison or practitioner in CF.
• A primary care team.
• A teacher.
• A psychologist.

All patients with CF should have a thorough annual multisystem review (see Table 6.1).

Table 6.1 Annual multisystem review of a CF patient

Blood tests
- *Haematology:* FBC, clotting (APTT, PTT).
- *Biochemistry:* creatinine, urea, Na$^+$, K$^+$, Cl$^-$, HCO$_3^-$ (Mg^{2+}, Ca^{2+} if on IV colistin), iron studies, vitamin A, D, and E levels.
- *Liver function:* ALP, ALT, bilirubin, albumin, protein.
- *Glucose control:* random glucose, HbA1c, oral glucose tolerance test (OGTT) (>10y). (See also ➲ Cystic fibrosis-related diabetes, p. 486.)
- *Immunology:* IgE, IgG, radioallergosorbent test (RAST) to *Aspergillus*, *Pseudomonas* precipitins.

Radiology
- *X-rays:* CXR.
- *US:* liver and bowel.
- *Dual-energy X-ray absorptiometry (DEXA) scan:* consider in children >10y or those on increasing doses of steroids or who have increasing fractures.

Lung function
- *Measurements:* FEV$_1$, FVC, PEFR, residual volume (RV), total lung capacity (TLC).
- *Oximetry:* testing SpO$_2$.

Bacteriology
- *Sputum/cough swab:* cultures, including *Burkholderia cepacia*, acid-fast bacilli.

Morbidity
- *Hospital:* number of admissions and days in hospital.
- *Chest:* number of courses of IV antibiotics.

Reviews
- *Auxology:* plot height and weight on sex-appropriate growth chart.
- *Medications:* requirements (dose).
- *PT:* technique, education, equipment, exercise review.
- *Nutrition:* education, enzymes, supplements.
- *Social:* family support, genetics, housing, school, statement of special needs.
- *Psychology:* patient and family support by clinical psychologist.
- *CF specialist nurse:* equipment review.

Cystic fibrosis: management (2)

Pulmonary care

Physiotherapy

All children with CF should have PT at least twice a day. Parents and older children are taught how to do some of the following:

- Chest percussion.
- Postural drainage.
- Self-percussion.
- Deep breathing exercises.
- Use of flutter or Acapella® device.

Antimicrobial therapy

Most experts recommend antibiotic therapy:

- PO during periods when well: against *Staphylococcus aureus* and *Haemophilus influenzae*.
- IV for acute exacerbations: initially courses of antibiotics can be administered via an indwelling long-line that should last a number of weeks if needed. As infections become more frequent, a permanent form of IV access (such as an indwelling Portacath) will help.
- Nebulized for those chronically infected with *Pseudomonas aeruginosa*.

Other therapies

- Annual: influenza immunization.
- Bronchodilators for those with reversible airway obstruction.
- *Mucolytics:* dornase alfa or inhaled hypertonic (7%) saline used before PT.
- PO azithromycin (long-term anti-inflammatory effect).

Gastrointestinal management

Distal intestinal obstruction (meconium ileus equivalent)

- *Lactulose:* 10–20mL bd.
- *PO acetylcysteine solution:* 100mg tds.
- *Gastrografin®:* PO dose can be used as a single treatment dose. Fluid intake should be encouraged for 3h after administration.

Nutrition

- *Pancreatic insufficiency:* pancreatic enzyme replacement therapy. Commonly used Creon® to be taken with all meals, snacks, and drinks.
- *High-calorie diet:* children with CF require 120–150% of normal energy intake.
- *Salt supplements:* salt depletion is a risk in CF patients during the first year of life and in the summer months in older patients.
- Fat-soluble vitamin supplements.
- *Multivitamins:* Dalivit® drops 1mL/day or multivitamin tablets.
- Vitamin E.
- *Vitamin K:* if there is evidence of liver disease (hepatosplenomegaly or abnormal clotting).

Primary ciliary dyskinesia

PCD is a genetic disorder leading to recurrent infections of the upper and lower respiratory tract due to impaired mucociliary clearance.

Diagnosis

History

- Usually symptoms emerge during infancy.
- SOB, signs of respiratory distress (mild to severe).
- History of persisting wet cough outside neonatal period.
- Recurrent episodes of pneumonia, rhinitis, otitis media, and sinusitis.
- Episode of bronchiectasis.
- Family history of PCD.
- ♂ infertility and low fertility in ♀.

Examination

If suspicious of PCD, look for the following:
- Signs of pneumonia, otitis media, and sinusitis.
- Signs of situs inversus (50% of patients).

Investigations

- CXR.
- CT chest.
- Nasal eNO level (for children over 5y old) used to screen patients with suspicion of PCD.
- Spirometry.
- Transmission electron microscopy (TEM) of ciliary ultrastructure obtained via nasal or bronchial brush biopsy.
- Ciliary beat frequency (CBF) and ciliary beat pattern (CBP) assessment via brush biopsy of epithelium.
- Genetics.
- Semen analysis in post-pubertal ♂.

Treatment

Multidisciplinary approach

- *Respiratory:* individual-based, but similar to management of patients with CF, including respiratory PT.
- *Surgery:* lobectomy of isolated areas of bronchiectasis.
- *ENT:* as per management of rhinosinusitis. Tympanoplasty and endoscopic sinus surgery occasionally performed.
- *Hearing:* hearing aids may be required for conductive hearing loss.
- *Vaccinations:* influenza and pneumococcal vaccines recommended.

Complications

- Conductive hearing loss.
- Impaired fertility.

Chronic lung disease of prematurity

(See also ➲ Bronchopulmonary dysplasia, pp. 146–7.) As the quality and outcome of neonatal intensive care for premature babies have improved, more and more infants with CLD are being seen. There are a variety of lung conditions that affect premature babies and necessitate MV and put babies at risk of developing CLD. These include:

- RDS (premature infants).
- Neonatal pneumonia.
- Meconium aspiration.
- Diaphragmatic hernia.
- Pulmonary hypoplasia.
- Alveolar capillary membrane dysplasia.
- Interstitial lung disease.
- Surfactant protein deficiency.

On follow-up in the paediatric clinic, you may see O_2 dependency due to any of these conditions. CLD in this context is defined as abnormal CXR and use of supplementary O_2 beyond 28 days.

Management

A multisystem and MDT approach is needed. This should include home and community liaison—the neonatal unit nurse specialist and health visitor are particularly helpful.

Nutritional support and therapy

- *Weight gain and growth:* these should be monitored, and if there is a problem with inadequate intake, consult a dietician for advice.
- *Gastrostomy:* procedure sometimes required to enable full feeding.
- *GOR:* the 'flat' position of the diaphragm, lung hyperinflation, and tachypnoea promote the development of vomiting and GOR. The lungs need to be protected and adequate feeding needs to be ensured. Initially try medical therapy such as acid suppressants. If these measures fail, fundoplication and gastrostomy feeds are required.
- *Vitamins:* appropriate vitamin supplements are used until the child is thriving well (i.e. vitamin compound drops, folic acid, iron).

Antimicrobial strategy

- *Vaccination:* all immunizations should be up-to-date. Patients should be offered the annual influenza vaccine. They may be eligible to receive the RSV vaccine (check your local guidance).
- *Antibiotics:* viral or bacterial illness may result in significant deterioration in CLD and be hard to differentiate clinically. Take sputum, throat swab, and nasopharyngeal aspirate for viral and bacterial cultures. Have a low threshold for starting antibiotics.

Obstructive airway disease

Wheeze is a common symptom in infants with CLD. Asthma treatments are often used in these children to relieve any bronchoconstrictive element.

O_2 therapy
The aim of supervision of these patients is to withdraw O_2 in a safe and timely manner. The target SpO_2 in patients on nasal cannula O_2 (NC-O_2) is ≥92%. Withdrawal is appropriate when the infant is clinically well, and gaining weight, and has an SpO_2 that is consistently ≥92%, with NC-O_2 requirement ≤0.1L/min. Children can be weaned from continuous low-flow O_2 to night-time and naps only or remain on continuous O_2 throughout 24h until the child has no requirement at all. Weaning can be directed by regular SpO_2 sleep studies. O_2 equipment should be left in the home for at least 3mth after the child has stopped using it. If this is in winter, it is usually left until the end of winter.

Congenital respiratory tract disorders

The following congenital abnormalities of the upper and lower airway are discussed in Chapters 4 and 22.

Congenital abnormalities of the upper airway

- Choanal atresia (see ➔ Choanal atresia, p. 808).
- Laryngeal atresia.
- Cleft lip and palate (see ➔ Orofacial cleft, p. 173).
- Pierre–Robin sequence (see ➔ Pierre–Robin sequence, p. 809).
- TOF (see ➔ Congenital abnormalities: tracheo-oesophageal, pp. 810–11).

Congenital abnormalities of the lower airway

- CCAM (see ➔ Congenital pulmonary airway malformations (CPAM), p. 812).
- Sequestration (see ➔ Sequestration, p. 812).
- Congenital lobar emphysema (see ➔ Congenital lobar emphysema, p. 812).
- CDH (see ➔ Congenital diaphragmatic hernia, p. 814; ➔ Figure 4.6).
- Hiatus hernia (see ➔ Hiatus hernia (HIH), p. 814).

Sleep apnoea

Obstructive sleep apnoea (OSA) presents as snoring associated with periods of ineffective breathing of >2 breaths (e.g. breathing at 20/min, this would be 6s). The commonest causes of OSA are upper airway obstruction (UAO) due to adenotonsillar hypertrophy or obesity.

Central apnoeas are rare and defined by pauses in breathing of >20s in an otherwise well child. They are usually associated with a significant CNS disorder (acute injury or long-standing neurodisability). Very rarely caused by central hypoventilation syndrome.

OSA syndrome (OSAS) may be due to tonsillar/adenoidal hypertrophy, obesity, macroglossia, or micrognathia. OSAS can cause metabolic, cardiac, and neurocognitive disorders in children if left untreated.

Diagnosis

History
- Snoring and sleep disturbance.
- Daytime sleepiness or inattention.
- Enuresis.
- Only ~15% of snoring children have significant airway obstruction.

Examination
Findings commonly found on physical examination include:
- Symptoms of UAO and OSAS are more likely to be due to adenoidal hypertrophy, rather than just tonsillar hypertrophy.
- Middle ear infection and chronic effusion: these are features associated with adenoidal hypertrophy.
- Mouth breathing: leading to dry mouth and cracked lips.
- FTT and behavioural problems.

Investigations
A thorough history and examination should identify children who need further treatment. However, consider the following useful tests:
- *Sleep study:* this could include just overnight SpO_2, but to diagnose impaired gas exchange, transcutaneous CO_2 measurement is necessary as well. In cases of diagnostic difficulty, more extensive polysomnography may be needed, mainly to differentiate OSA from central sleep apnoea.
- *CXR and ECG:* to look for secondary right heart cardiac consequences of UAO (e.g. RVH).

Treatment

Medical
CPAP for a select group because of often poor adherence. Weight loss is recommended for all obese patients.

Surgery
- Adenotonsillectomy: when evidence of airway obstruction.
- Uvulopalatopharyngoplasty.
- Tracheostomy: very rare.

Allergic rhinitis

(See also ➲ Allergic rhinitis, pp. 534–5.)

Up to 20% of the population have symptoms of allergic rhinitis, which include nasal congestion, itching, sneezing, and discharge.

Diagnosis

History

Identify symptoms and history of atopy and environmental exposures:
- Tree pollens tend to be present in early spring (March to May), and grass later (May to July).
- House dust mite is perennial and ever present.
- Environmental exposures such as parental smoking, pets, dust mite-favoured stuffed toys, carpet, bedding, etc.

Examination
- Look for clinical signs of nasal crease and nasal inflammation.

Treatment
- Allergen avoidance and medication, e.g. PO antihistamines, nasal corticosteroid sprays.
- Allergic trigger for both rhinitis and asthma: be particularly aggressive in avoidance. Consider adding montelukast to treat both nose and lower airways, in addition to other medications.

Upper airway infections

(See also ➔ Table 16.3.)

Ear, sinus, nose, and throat infections account for 80% of respiratory infections. The diagnosis 'URTI' may mean any of the following:

- *Common cold (coryza):* commonly due to rhinoviruses, coronaviruses, and RSV (the latter more often causes acute bronchiolitis).
- *Pharyngitis and/or tonsillitis:* pharyngitis is usually due to viral infection with adenovirus, enterovirus, and rhinovirus. Tonsillitis associated with purulent exudates may be due to group A β-haemolytic *Streptococcus* or EBV.
- *Ear infection (acute otitis media):* common pathogens include viruses, Pneumococcus, group A β-haemolytic *Streptococcus*, *H. influenzae*, and *Moraxella catarrhalis*.
- *Sinusitis:* presents with facial pain and/or fever—it may occur with viral or bacterial infection but is rare in the preschool child.

Clinical findings

Although most commonly caused by viral infections, consider a bacterial cause if atypical presentation or systemically unwell:

- *Ears:* acute otitis media presents with fever, pain, and bright red, bulging tympanic membrane (otoscopy loss of normal light reflex).
- *Pharynx:* acute tonsillitis diagnosed if purulent exudates on red, inflamed tonsils ('mildly erythematous' tonsils with fever is not diagnostic). Look for associated reactive cervical lymphadenopathy.

Treatment

Symptom relief

- *Fever:* use paracetamol or ibuprofen.
- *Earache:* use paracetamol or ibuprofen.

Antibiotics

Virus infection causes the majority of URTIs and antibiotics *should not* be prescribed. However, if bacterial pharyngitis or tonsillitis suspected due to group A β-haemolytic *Streptococcus*, take a throat swab for bacterial and/or viral culture.

- *Tonsillitis and pharyngitis:* avoid amoxicillin because it may cause maculopapular rash in EBV infection. Use phenoxymethylpenicillin, or erythromycin in allergic patients, for 10 days.
- *Acute otitis media:* co-amoxiclav will cover the common bacterial causes of otitis media and be effective against β-lactamase-producing *H. influenzae* and *M. catarrhalis*.

Laryngeal and tracheal inflammation

There are a number of laryngeal and tracheal causes of inflammation and airway obstruction. In the acute setting, you will be concerned with three common conditions.

- *Viral laryngotracheobronchitis (croup):* mucosal inflammation affecting anywhere from the nose to the lower airways that is commonly due to parainfluenza and other respiratory viruses in children aged 6mth to 6y.
- *Spasmodic or recurrent croup:* barking cough and hyperreactive upper airways, with no apparent lower respiratory tract symptoms.
- *Acute epiglottitis:* life-threatening swelling of the epiglottis and septicaemia due to *H. influenzae* type B (HiB) infection—most commonly in children aged 1–6y. This is now very rare since routine HiB immunization.

Diagnosis

History
(See Table 6.2.)

Examination
Do not examine the throat until full assessment is complete. Take a careful assessment of severity, including:
- Degree of stridor and associated signs of respiratory distress.
- RR.
- HR and signs of sepsis.
- LOC (drowsiness), tiredness, and exhaustion.
- SpO_2.

Table 6.2 Differentiating between viral croup and acute epiglottitis

	Croup	Epiglottitis
Time course	Days	Hours
Prodrome	Coryza	None
Cough	Barking	Slight if any
Feeding	Can drink	No
Mouth	Closed	Drooling saliva
Toxic	No	Yes
Fever	<38.5°C	>38.5°C
Stridor	Rasping	Soft
Voice	Hoarse	Weak or silent

Treatment

Priority
The main priority is airway protection. Avoid startling the child and try to keep the child, their family, and staff calm. Alert the emergency otolaryngologist and anaesthetist to the possibility of a need for emergency airway support.

Viral croup

Children with mild illness can be managed at home, but advise parents that if there is intercostal recession and stridor at rest, then they will need to attend hospital. Infants <12mth need closer monitoring. Treatments include the following:

- *Steroids:* PO dexamethasone (0.15mg/kg 12-hourly) or nebulized budesonide (2mg stat dose) reduces the severity and duration of croup. They also reduce the need for ETT intubation.
- *Nebulized adrenaline (epinephrine):* can provide transient relief of symptoms. The effects of nebulized adrenaline last 2–3h; therefore, if it is administered, the child should be observed closely for returning symptoms. Repeated doses may be necessary.

In cases that require ETT intubation, steroids should be given, and if there is evidence of secondary bacterial infection or bacterial tracheitis, antibiotics should be added.

Acute epiglottitis

The child with acute epiglottitis will need to be managed in PICU after ETT intubation. Once this procedure has been completed, take blood cultures and start IV antibiotics.

- *Second- or third-generation cephalosporin* (e.g. cefuroxime, ceftriaxone, or cefotaxime) IV for 7–10 days.
- *Rifampicin prophylaxis* to close contacts.

Bronchial disease

Acute infection of the bronchi can occur in children and often overlaps with bronchiolitis or virus-induced wheeze.

Pertussis (whooping cough)

Bordetella pertussis infection typically induces three stages of illness:

- *Catarrhal (1–2wk):* mild symptoms with fever, cough, and coryza.
- *Paroxysmal (2–6wk):* severe paroxysmal cough, followed by inspiratory whoop and vomiting.
- *Convalescent (2–4wk):* lessening symptoms that may take a whole month to resolve.

A whooping cough-like syndrome may also be caused by *Bordetella parapertussis*, *M. pneumoniae*, *Chlamydia*, or adenovirus.

History

There may be a typical history. In young infants, however, whoop is often absent, and apnoea is a commoner finding. In older children, and parents, there may be a history of persistent and irritating cough.

Examination and investigations

- *Eyes:* subconjunctival haemorrhages are common.
- *CXR:* rarely pertussis pneumonia occurs (high mortality rate).
- *Blood count:* significant lymphocytosis with low/normal neutrophil count is typical.
- *Pernasal swab:* culture of *B. pertussis*.

Management

- *Infants:* admission for those with a history of apnoea, cyanosis, or significant paroxysms. ARDS, seizures, and encephalopathy are rare.
- *Isolation:* patients should be isolated for 5 days after starting treatment with antibiotics.
- *Antibiotics:* erythromycin for 14 days (or clarithromycin for 7 days) to reduce infectivity, but this may have minimal effect on the cough.
- *Immunization of contacts:* recommended for children <7y and pregnant contacts (see public health advice).
- *Prophylactic antibiotics:* should be given to close contacts.

Persistent bacterial bronchitis (PBB)

Common cause of chronic cough, especially in the under 5y olds. Defined as persisting infection of the conducting airways.

History

Based on clinical criteria, the diagnosis is based on:
- Chronic, wet-sounding cough daily for >4wk.
- Absence of systemic symptoms and signs, e.g. weight loss, clubbing, chest wall deformity.
- Cough resolves after 2wk of antibiotics.
- Child looks well, with normal growth velocity.
- No evidence of an alternative diagnosis on initial investigations.

Causes

Typical organisms that cause PBB include:
- Streptococcal pneumonia.
- *M. catarrhalis*.
- *H. influenzae*.

Investigations
- BAL helpful but is not always feasible.

Treatment

Prolonged course of antibiotics (e.g. co-amoxiclav) for a minimum of 2wk, extended for further 2–4wk if good clinical response.

Bronchiolitis

Bronchiolitis, most commonly due to RSV, infects almost all children by the age of 2y. There is an ↑ risk of severe infection in infants with CHD, CLD of prematurity, immunodeficiency, and other lung disease. RSV invades the nasopharyngeal epithelium and spreads to the lower airways where it causes ↑ mucus production, desquamation, and then bronchiolar obstruction through airway oedema and mucus plugging. The net effect is varying degrees of pulmonary hyperinflation and atelectasis. Other causes include infection with:

- Viruses: parainfluenza, influenza, adenovirus, rhinovirus, metapneumovirus.
- *Chlamydia*.
- *M. pneumoniae*.

Diagnosis

History

In winter months, infants typically present with coryza, then cough and worsening breathlessness. Other features in the history include:

- Wheeze; episodes of apnoea (especially infants <1mth of age).
- Feeding difficulty.

Rarely, other presenting histories in babies include:

- Sudden-onset apnoea and near-miss sudden infant death syndrome (SIDS).
- Encephalopathy with seizures due to hyponatraemia.

Atypical findings should raise suspicion of alternative diagnosis, e.g.:

- High-grade/persistent fever: consider bacterial pneumonia (particularly onset of fever after several days of illness).
- Associated lactic acidosis, hepatomegaly, persistent tachycardia: suggest possible decompensation of underlying cardiac disease.

Examination and investigations

Examination findings are characterized by bilateral wheeze and/or crepitations with associated signs of respiratory distress. Additional common findings include:

- Cyanosis, chest hyperinflation.
- Prolonged expiratory phase, respiratory pauses or apnoea.

Key investigations include:

- SpO_2.
- *CXR:* only if other diagnoses are suspected (e.g. cardiac disease, secondary bacterial pneumonia). In bronchiolitis, expect CXR signs of hyperinflation, atelectasis, and consolidation.
- *ABG:* CO_2 retention is often a late sign of respiratory failure.
- *Nasopharyngeal aspirate or throat swab:* useful if diagnostic doubt and for cohorting admissions. Viral respiratory panels may detect RSV, influenza A and B, rhinovirus, coronavirus, human metapneumovirus, and adenovirus.

Hospital treatment

Treatment of RSV bronchiolitis is mainly supportive and includes:
- O_2 to achieve SpO_2 >92%.
- If significant respiratory distress, limit enteral feeding volumes to 2mL/kg/h (or two-thirds maintenance rates; NB: risk of SIADH) and use an NGT to reduce energy expenditure during feeding.
- *Bronchodilators for wheeze:* there is no evidence for bronchodilators being effective in acute bronchiolitis.
- *Mucolytic therapy:* while an attractive therapeutic option, evidence base for hypertonic saline (e.g. 4mL of 3% saline nebulized 6-hourly) is limited. *Dornase alfa* is expensive but may be used in life-threatening cases (usually in PICU).
- *Non-invasive therapy:* CPAP and humidified high-flow nasal cannula (HHFNC) therapy show reduction in need for ETT and MV, but limited effects on hospital length of stay.
- MV for infants showing recurrent apnoea or clinical signs of respiratory failure ('tiring').
- Antiviral therapy with oseltamivir indicated for influenza-confirmed cases, most effective if started within 48h of disease onset.

Prophylaxis

Palivizumab is a monoclonal antibody to RSV and can be used as prophylaxis. Preterm babies and O_2-dependent infants at risk of RSV infection can receive a monthly IM injection (for 5mth starting in October), according to local protocols.

Follow-up

Recurrent cough, wheeze, and tachypnoea may occur after RSV infection. These may require treatment and are best assessed in the outpatient clinic. A significant minority of patients go on to develop asthma, and associated atopic conditions should raise clinical suspicion and a trial of asthma medication.

Pneumonia

Pneumonia is an infection of the lower respiratory tract and lung parenchyma that leads to consolidation.

- Viruses alone account for approximately half of all community-acquired pneumonia (CAP) cases in childhood. Similar viral agents to bronchiolitis can also cause pneumonia.
- *Influenza* pneumonia can be life-threatening. Treatment is supportive and similar to other forms of pneumonia (see ⊃ Pneumonia: treatment, p. 260). Vulnerable children require annual immunization.

Common bacterial causes, by age, are:

- *Neonates:* GBS, *Escherichia coli, Klebsiella, S. aureus.*
- *Infants:* Streptococcus pneumoniae, Chlamydia.
- *School age:* S. pneumoniae, S. aureus, GAS, B. pertussis, M. pneumoniae.

Certain groups of children are at risk of pneumonia, e.g. those with:

- Long-standing neurodisability (especially if significant scoliosis).
- CLD.
- Immunodeficiency.
- CF.
- SCD.

Diagnosis

History

Common symptoms include:

- Temperature ≥38°C.
- SOB.
- Cough, with sputum production in older children (>7y).
- Abdominal pain.
- Pleuritic chest pain.

Examination

Check for the following:

- *RR:* fever and tachypnoea may be the *only* features.
- *Associated signs of respiratory distress:* recession, grunting, etc.
- *SpO₂ <92%:* indicates need for admission and O₂ therapy.
- *Nutritional/hydration status:* not common as SIADH frequently occurs and renal retention of fluid maintains hydration status.
- *Auscultation:* bronchial breathing may be hard to detect, dullness to percussion; crackles; ↓ breath sounds; reduced vocal fremitus; reduced chest expansion on affected side.

Investigations

In uncomplicated CAP, clinical assessment should be sufficient without the need for investigations. In more complicated cases, investigations that help in diagnosis include (see also Box 6.2):

- *Sputum/cough swab:* culture may be of limited value and hard to obtain (small children tend to swallow respiratory secretions).
- *Nasopharyngeal aspirate:* viral respiratory panel, especially in infants.
- *Blood:* culture should be done in all children with severe bacterial pneumonia (not necessary in CAP).

- *CXR*: not as routine, but indicated if atypical features or signs of effusion/empyema. Atypical infections (e.g. *Mycoplasma*, TB, *Pneumocystis* pneumonia) give characteristic CXR appearances.
- *Pleural fluid*: when there is a significant pleural effusion, an aspirated sample should be sent for culture and antigen testing once a drain is inserted.

Box 6.2 Investigations to consider in children with chronic or recurrent pneumonia

Step 1: initial blood tests
- *Haematology*: FBC, complement screen, ESR.
- *Immunology*: IgA, IgE (and *Aspergillus* RAST), IgG, IgM, antibody response to immunizations (tetanus and *Pneumococcus*), rheumatoid factor (RF).
- *Antibodies*: *Aspergillus* precipitins, ANA.
- *Genetics*: CF genotype.

Step 2: other tests
- Sweat test.
- *Microbiology*: sputum culture.
- *Lung function*: spirometry, lung volumes, and reversibility.
- *Radiology*: CXR, barium swallow for vascular ring, sinus radiography.

Step 3: further investigations
- *Haematology*: neutrophil and monocyte function, lymphocyte subsets, and cellular immune function.
- *Imaging*: HRCT scan of the chest.
- *pH/oesophageal impedance study*: for GOR.
- *Videofluoroscopy*: for silent aspiration.
- *Nasal ciliary biopsy*: microscopy and function (unnecessary if there is normal nasal eNO) to rule out PCD.
- *Bronchoscopy*: visualization of dynamic airway function, as well as sputum analysis for culture, fat-laden macrophages (aspiration), eosinophil counts (inflammatory airway disease).

Pneumonia: treatment

(See also ➲ Table 16.3.) Oral antibiotics are safe and effective in the treatment of CAP. IV antibiotics are used in children who cannot tolerate oral antibiotics or in those with severe symptoms. The specific choice of antibiotic is based on the following:

• Age of the child.
• Host factors.
• Severity of illness.
• Information about cultures if known.
• CXR findings if known.

Antibiotic therapy for pneumonia

Under 5y

S. pneumoniae is the most likely pathogen. The causes of atypical pneumonia are M. pneumoniae and Chlamydia trachomatis.

• *First-line treatment:* amoxicillin.
• *Alternatives:* co-amoxiclav or cefaclor for typical pneumonia; erythromycin, clarithromycin, or azithromycin for atypical pneumonia.

Over 5y

M. pneumoniae is commoner in this age group.

• *First-line treatment:* amoxicillin is effective against the majority of pathogens, but consider macrolide antibiotics if Mycoplasma or Chlamydia is suspected.
• *Alternatives:* if S. aureus is suspected, consider using a macrolide or a combination of flucloxacillin with amoxicillin.

Severe pneumonia

• *Antibiotics:* co-amoxiclav, cefotaxime, or cefuroxime IV.
• *Antivirals:* oseltamivir if suspicion of influenza.

Supportive therapies

Consider whether any of the following are needed:

• *Antipyretics:* for fever.
• *IV fluids:* consider if dehydrated or not drinking, but restrict fluid volumes (e.g. two-thirds of maintenance rates because of risk of SIADH).
• *Supplemental O_2:* use NC-O_2 or face mask, so that SpO_2 is >92%.
• *Chest drain:* for fluid or pus collections in the chest, as in empyema.

Physiotherapy

Chest PT is generally not beneficial in children with pneumonia and should not be performed unless unable to produce effective cough (e.g. significant neurodisability) or evidence of life-threatening mucus plugging of airways.

Pleural effusions and empyema

The presence of a small effusion, in association with pneumonia, that does not cause any respiratory distress can be managed conservatively without the need for aspirating a sample. A fluid sample, however, is needed if there is:

• A large effusion.
• Significant hypoxia/respiratory distress.
• No clear underlying diagnosis.
• Persistent fever despite antibiotic treatment.

Fluid sample

After USS of the chest and checking blood-clotting studies, a small chest drain (or pigtail drain) should be inserted into the pleural space. Samples should be sent for the following:

• *Microbiology:* bacterial culture and sensitivity, acid-fast bacilli.
• *Cytology:* presence of pus cells and microscopic assessment of aberrant cell types. Cytology for lymphoma may give false −ve results in up to 10% of cases.

Diagnosis of empyema

The diagnosis of empyema can be based on the presence of:

• *Fluid:* pH <7.2, glucose <3.3mmol/L, protein >3g/L, pus cells.
• *USS:* loculation or fibrin strands seen.

Fluid drainage

After inserting a small-bore drain or pigtail catheter, fluid should be allowed to drain into standard commercially available systems (e.g. underwater seal system). The drain can be removed if draining <50mL in 24h.

Urokinase for empyema

In empyema, as opposed to simple pleural effusion, instillation of urokinase via the chest drain is recommended:

• *Dose example:* 40 000U urokinase in 40mL (10 000U in 10mL if <1y), given 12-hourly for 3 days.
• *Method:* instil via the chest drain and then clamp the drain and encourage the patient to move and roll around over the next 4h.
• *Suction:* use a low-pressure suction device (e.g. Robert's pump) to maintain suction of 20cmH$_2$O between doses.
• *LA:* bupivacaine around the drain site may control pleural pain. Consult the pain control team.

Surgical referral

If the effusion or empyema fails to resolve over a period of 7 days, get a surgical opinion. Chest CT scan may help identify loculated areas or abscess formation. A definitive surgical procedure or large-bore drain and manual disruption of loculation may be needed.

Pulmonary tuberculosis

(See also ⊃ Tuberculosis: presentation and diagnosis, pp. 639–40.)
Worldwide, TB of the lung remains a significant cause of childhood mortality. TB should always be considered in children from endemic areas, as well as those at risk of immunodeficiency or taking immunosuppressive agents. Once diagnosed, TB is a notifiable disease and contact tracing is required, so that those exposed to the patient undergo tuberculin testing and CXR screening. Bacille Calmette–Guérin (BCG) vaccination appears to be protective against miliary spread, but evidence for prevention of pulmonary disease is weak and in many countries, it is no longer routinely administered to low-risk infants.

Mycobacterium tuberculosis is spread from person to person by droplet infection. Once inhaled, some bacilli remain at the site of entry and the rest are carried to regional lymph nodes. The bacilli multiply at both sites; the primary focus, along with the regional lymph nodes, are collectively described as the primary focus. Organisms can then spread via blood and lymphatics. The pathological sequence after infection is as follows:

- *4–8wk:*
  - Febrile illness.
  - Erythema nodosum.
  - Phlyctenular conjunctivitis.
- *6–9mth:*
  - In most cases, progressive healing of primary complex.
  - Effusion: focus may rupture into pleural space.
  - Cavitation: focus may rupture into bronchus.
  - Coin lesion on CXR: focus may enlarge.
  - Regional lymph nodes: may obstruct bronchi.
  - Regional lymph nodes: may erode into bronchus or pericardial sac.
  - Miliary spread.

Drug management

NB: resistance patterns vary worldwide and consultation with local infectious disease guidelines is strongly recommended.

Active TB without CNS involvement

- *2mth:* isoniazid, rifampicin, pyrazinamide, and ethambutol added as a fourth drug.
- *Then 4mth:* isoniazid and rifampicin.

Active TB with CNS involvement

- *2mth:* isoniazid, rifampicin, ethambutol, and pyrazinamide.
- *Then 10mth:* isoniazid and rifampicin.

Other respiratory disorders

Aspiration syndromes

- *Acute aspiration* of fluid or particulate matter may occur at any age and the typical presentation is choking and coughing. In infants, some aspiration episodes go unrecognized in the acute phase. These babies may present later with consolidation that fails to improve.
- *Chronic aspiration* may present with recurrent pneumonia—different lobes at different times. Airway anomalies should be sought as an underlying cause. Swallowing abnormalities need to be excluded, e.g. videofluoroscopy by a speech and language therapist.

Interstitial lung disease

A rare group of disorders in childhood, and children (usually infants) present with progressive tachypnoea and hypoxia. The CXR shows widespread reticular shadowing, but a high-resolution CT (HRCT) scan is needed for diagnosis. Treatment should be undertaken in specialist centres, as these children require lung biopsy and may need long-term steroids or chloroquine. Supplemental O_2 therapy is common.

Lymphoid interstitial pneumonitis (LIP)

LIP has the appearance of fibrosing alveolitis, but it is a pulmonary feature of HIV infection that responds to steroids.

Immunodeficiency

(See also ➲ Immunodeficiency disorders, p. 646.) Recurrent infection of the lower airways is common in immunodeficiencies such as:
- IgG subclass deficiency.
- Defective cell-mediated immunity: viral or fungal infection.

Dysfunctional breathing

Defined as presence of an altered breathing pattern leading to intermittent or chronic respiratory symptoms. Examples include:
- Vocal cord dysfunction.
- Hyperventilation.
- Habit cough.
- Sighing dyspnoea.

Take a detailed history, focusing on time of onset and recovery of symptoms. Examination and investigations (e.g. spirometry) are typically normal, with no reversibility to therapies such as bronchodilators.

Treatment options include:
- Reassurance.
- PT.
- Speech therapy.
- Cognitive behavioural therapy (CBT).

Further reading

Barker N, Everard M. Getting to grips with 'dysfunctional breathing'. *Paediatr Respir Rev* 2015; **16**: 53–61.

British Thoracic Society and Scottish Intercollegiate Network Guidelines. (2016). *British guideline on the management of asthma (SIGN 153)*. Available at: https://www.clinicalguidelines.scot.nhs.uk/ggc-paediatric-guidelines/other-guidelines/british-guideline-on-the-management-of-asthma-sign-153.

National Institute for Health and Care Excellence. (2016). *Tuberculosis*. NICE guideline [NG33]. Available at: https://www.nice.org.uk/guidance/ng33.

National Institute for Health and Care Excellence. (2017). *Asthma: diagnosis, monitoring and chronic asthma management*. NICE guideline [NG80]. Available at: https://www.nice.org.uk/guidance/ng80.

Shields MD, Bush A, Everard ML, et al. BTS guidelines: recommendations for the asssessment and management of cough in children. *Thorax* 2008; **63**(Suppl 3): iii1–15.

Gastroenterology and nutrition

Healthy eating for children

Infants

(See also ⦿ Milk feeding, pp. 122–3.)

- Breast milk is the ideal feed for almost all infants.
- Solids are not recommended until age 6mth (decrease food allergies), although often given from 4mth.
- Initial solids should be based on baby rice, fruit, and vegetables.
- Gluten is acceptable from age 6mth.
- Following introduction of solids, infants should experience and progress through a wide variety of tastes and appropriate textures.
- Finger foods should be introduced from around age 7mth.
- Continue complementary breast or formula feeds until age 1y.
- Normal full-fat cow's milk may then be introduced as main drink.
- Avoid addition of salt and sugar to food.
- Low-fat products are not suitable for infants.
- Supplemental vitamins A, C, and D are recommended until age 5y.

Age 1–5y

A well-balanced diet in early childhood is important to establish a lifetime pattern of healthy eating. By age 5y:

- Avoid excessive sugars.
- Decrease fat to 35% energy intake by avoiding excess high-fat foods, and use semi-skimmed at 2y and skimmed at age 5y.
- Include wholegrain cereals and five portions per day of fruits and vegetables to increase fibre intake.
- Moderate salt intake, e.g. not adding salt to cooking or at the table.
- Monitor weight velocity (accelerating), and avoid overweight/obesity which increases long-term risk of adverse health outcomes.
- Avoid iron deficiency anaemia: milk ≤1 pint/day; eat foods rich in iron (red meat, cereals, beans, pulses, egg yolk, dark green vegetables, and dried fruit); some fruit juice (vitamin C) at meals increases iron absorption; avoid tea at meals as it decreases iron absorption.
- Avoid excessive consumption of fruit juices or squashes which contributes to chronic non-specific diarrhoea of childhood (toddler diarrhoea) and contributes to feeding problems and the risk of obesity.

Older children

Schoolchildren should eat a wide variety of foods. Nutritional guidelines for school meals are set out by UK local authorities and healthy eating is in the UK national curriculum. A healthy diet includes:

- At least one starchy food at each mealtime, e.g. wholemeal bread, potatoes, pasta, and rice.
- Five portions per day of fruits and vegetables.
- Two servings of meat or alternatives each day.
- 2–3 portions a day of skimmed milk, low-fat yoghurt, fromage frais, or cheese (1 portion = 1 yoghurt, 1/3 pint milk, 30g cheese).
- Only small and occasional amounts of sugar and fats.

Vomiting

A common symptom in childhood. Three clinical scenarios are recognized (see Box 7.1):

- *Acute:* discrete episode of moderate to high intensity. Commonest and usually associated with an acute illness.
- *Chronic:* low-grade daily pattern, frequently with chronic illness.
- *Cyclic:* severe, discrete episodes associated with pallor, lethargy ± abdominal pain. The child is well between episodes; often a family history of migraine or vomiting.

Causes

- *Acute:* GI infection, non-GI infection (e.g. UTI), GI obstruction (congenital or acquired, e.g. malrotation, pyloric stenosis), adverse food reaction, poisoning, raised ICP, endocrine/metabolic disease (e.g. DKA). If vomiting is bile-stained, then consider surgical causes.
- *Chronic (usually GI):* peptic ulcer disease, GOR, chronic infection, gastritis, gastroparesis, food allergy, psychogenic, bulimia, pregnancy.
- *Cyclic (usually non-GI cause):* idiopathic, CNS disease, abdominal migraine/cyclical vomiting syndrome, endocrine (e.g. Addison's disease), metabolic (e.g. acute intermittent porphyria), intermittent GI obstruction, fabricated induced illness.

Management

- *Full history:* e.g. early morning vomiting with CNS tumour, or family members with similar illness.
- *Full examination:* including ENT, growth; assess for dehydration.

Treatment

- *Supportive treatment as needed:* e.g. PO or IV fluids.
- *Treat cause:* e.g. pyloromyotomy for hypertrophic pyloric stenosis.
- *Pharmacological:* antihistamines, phenothiazines (side effects: extrapyramidal reactions), prokinetic drugs (e.g. domperidone), 5-HT$_3$ antagonists (e.g. ondansetron) for post-operative or chemotherapy-induced vomiting. Serotonin antagonists (e.g. pizotifen) are useful as prophylaxis of migraine/cyclic vomiting syndrome.

Complications

Dehydration, plasma electrolyte disturbance (e.g. ↓ K$^+$, ↓ Cl$^-$, alkalosis with pyloric stenosis), acute or chronic GI bleeding (e.g. Mallory–Weiss tear), oesophageal stricture, Barrett's metaplasia, pulmonary aspiration, faltering growth, iron deficiency anaemia.

Psychogenic vomiting

- *Causes:* anxiety, manipulative behaviour, disordered family dynamics. A family history of vomiting is common.
- *Management:* exclude organic disease. Explanation and reassurance. Refer to child psychologist.

Box 7.1 Investigation for vomiting

Acute (if severe)
- FBC.
- U&E, glucose.
- Creatinine.
- Stool for culture and virology.
- Consider AXR.
- Test feed and/or abdominal US for pyloric stenosis if suspected.
- Surgical opinion if vomiting bile-stained.
- Surgical opinion if obstruction suspected.
- Consider systemic disease.

Chronic
- FBC.
- ESR/CRP.
- U&E, glucose.
- LFTs.
- *H. pylori* testing.
- Coeliac antibody screen.
- Urinalysis.
  If indicated:
- Abdominal US.
- Small bowel imaging (barium, MRI).
- Sinus X-rays.
- Brain imaging (CNS tumour).
- Urine pregnancy testing in teenage girls.
- Upper GI endoscopy.

Cyclic
As for chronic vomiting, plus the consider the following:
- Serum amylase.
- Serum lipase.
- Serum ammonia.

Acute diarrhoea

- Normal stool frequency and consistency vary, e.g. breastfed infants can pass up to 10–12 stools per day, while primary schoolchildren can pass stool anything from three times a day to once every 3 days.
- Diarrhoea is a change in consistency and frequency of stools, with enough loss of fluid and electrolytes to cause illness.
- Diarrhoea kills 3 million children per year worldwide.

Causes

- Infective gastroenteritis. Commonest cause (see ➲ Gastrointestinal infection, pp. 306–7).
- Non-enteric infections, e.g. respiratory tract.
- Food hypersensitivity reactions (see ➲ Food allergy, p. 284).
- Drugs, e.g. antibiotics.
- Henoch–Schönlein purpura (HSP) (see ➲ Henoch– Schönlein purpura, pp. 698–9).
- Intussusception (<4y) (see ➲ Intussusception, p. 822).
- HUS (see ➲ Haemolytic uraemic syndrome, pp. 354–5).
- Pseudomembranous enterocolitis.

Presentation

- Fever ± vomiting (infectious gastroenteritis).
- Diarrhoea ± bloody stools (colitis—infectious or non-infectious).
- Dehydration and ↓ consciousness.

Management

- Assess hydration and vital signs, pallor (blood loss), abdominal tenderness, and signs of associated illness (e.g. petechial rash in HSP).
- *Mild/moderate dehydration:*
  - No tests necessary.
  - Replace fluid and electrolyte losses with oral glucose–electrolyte-based rehydration fluid.
- *Severe/shock dehydration:*
  - U&E, creatinine, FBC, ABG, stool MC&S/virology, tests for specific disease (e.g. USS in suspected intussuseption).
  - IV fluid and electrolyte replacement (see ➲ Fluid and electrolytes in dehydration, pp. 71–72; ➲ Other fluid and electrolyte abnormalities, pp. 72–4).
- Anti-motility drug treatment is not recommended; it can be harmful, particularly in acute infection/inflammation.
- Cause is more commonly viral than bacterial. Antibiotics are not given unless the cause is proven, e.g. *Yersinia* or *Campylobacter* infection, parasitic infection, NEC, or bacteraemia/systemic infection.
- Pseudomembranous colitis (*Clostridium difficile*) requires specific treatment with metronidazole or PO vancomycin.
- Other treatments are disease-specific: some diarrhoeal processes require removal of the offending agent such as in lactose intolerance, coeliac disease, or allergic gastroenteritis. Others may require bowel rest or surgery, e.g. NEC or intussusception.

- Once rehydrated, resume normal diet. Replace ongoing losses. Continue breastfeeding. There is no evidence that prolonged starvation is beneficial in infective gastroenteritis.
- Prevent cross-infection with strict handwashing and barrier nursing. In the less developed world, breastfeeding, provision of clean water, and adequate sanitation are also important to reduce risk of infection.

Investigations

(See Box 7.1.)

Prognosis

The majority of cases, particularly if caused by infective gastroenteritis, make a complete recovery with appropriate treatment.

Other diarrhoea

Chronic diarrhoea

Defined as diarrhoea persisting for >14 days. Many of the diseases that cause acute diarrhoea can lead on to chronic diarrhoea. The pathophysiology may involve:

- Reduced GI absorptive capacity, e.g. coeliac disease.
- Osmotic diarrhoea, e.g. lactase deficiency.
- Inflammatory, e.g. UC.
- Secretory diarrhoea (rare), e.g. vasoactive intestinal peptide (VIP)-producing tumour.

Causes

Age 0–24mth

- Malabsorption (see ➲ Malabsorption, p. 302), e.g. post-infective gastroenteritis syndrome, lactose intolerance, CF, coeliac disease.
- Food hypersensitivity, (see ➲ Cow's milk protein allergy, p. 522).
- Chronic non-specific diarrhoea (toddler diarrhoea); child is usually thriving (see ➲ Chronic non-specific diarrhoea (toddler diarrhoea), p. 273).
- Excessive fluid intake, particularly fruit juices (fructose intolerance).
- Protracted infectious gastroenteritis.
- Immunodeficiencies, including HIV.
- Hirschsprung's disease (see ➲ Hirschsprung's disease, p. 832).
- Rarer causes (intractable diarrhoea) include congenital mucosal transport defects and autoimmune enteropathy.
- Tumours (secretory diarrhoea).
- Fabricated induced illness.

Older children

- Inflammatory bowel disease (IBD).
- Constipation (spurious, overflow diarrhoea).
- Irritable bowel syndrome (IBS)—diarrhoea predominant.
- Malabsorption—see above.
- Chronic infections, including giardiasis, bacterial overgrowth, and pseudomembranous colitis.
- Laxative abuse.
- Excessive fluid intake, particularly fruit juices (fructose intolerance).
- Fabricated induced illness.

History

Nature and frequency of stool, presence of undigested food, relationship to diet changes (e.g. weaning) or travel, stool blood or mucus, weight loss.

Examination

Features of poor nutritional status or other illness, e.g. peri-anal disease in IBD or finger clubbing in CF.

Investigations to consider

- *Stool:* inspection; microscopy for bacteria or parasites, leucocytes, fat globules (pancreatic diseases), fatty acid crystals (diffuse mucosal defects); culture; pH (<5.5 = carbohydrate malabsorption); reducing substances (>0.5% = carbohydrate malabsorption); faecal occult blood (colitis); electrolytes (↑ Na+ and K+ = secretory diarrhoea; ↑ Cl– = congenital chloridorrhoea); faecal elastase (reduced in pancreatic insufficiency); faecal calprotectin (elevated in IBD).
- *Blood:* U&E; FBC (↓ Hb = haematinic deficiency or blood loss; ↑ eosinophil = food hypersensitivity or parasites); ↑ CRP/ESR (inflammatory); ABG; RAST (food allergy); hormone level [vanillylmandelic acid (VMA), catecholamines, VIP for secretory tumours].
- *Radiology:* AXR, USS, small bowel imaging (barium, MRI).
- *Other:* hydrogen breath test (lactose malabsorption or bacterial overgrowth); GI endoscopy biopsy (e.g. upper for coeliac disease, upper and lower for suspected IBD); sweat test/genetic testing (CF); rectal biopsy (Hirschsprung's disease).

Treatment

- Treat underlying cause.
- Nutritional intervention if deficiencies are present.
- Antibiotics only if systemic illness or prolonged infection is present, e.g. *Salmonella*, *Campylobacter*, giardiasis, or amoebiasis.
- Rarely, other drugs useful, e.g. loperamide or colestyramine.

Chronic non-specific diarrhoea (toddler diarrhoea)

- Occurs from 6mth to 5y.
- Colicky intestinal pain, ↑ flatus, abdominal distension, loose stools with undigested food ('peas and carrots' stools).
- Child is otherwise well and thriving.
- Examination and investigations are normal.

Treatment

Reassurance; dietary (normalize fibre intake; avoid excess fruit juice and sugary drink intake); loperamide occasionally may be necessary.

Encopresis

- Voluntary defecation in unacceptable places, including the child's pants in older children.
- No organic abnormality is present; it is a symptom of an emotional disorder.
- Constipation is often a factor with overflow diarrhoea.
- It is three times commoner in boys.
- Once organic disease or spurious diarrhoea secondary to constipation with loading are excluded (see ➜ Constipation, pp. 274–5), consider behavioural problems and referral to a child and adolescent psychiatrist.

Constipation

(See also ➋ Constipation and soiling, pp. 906–7.) Defined as infrequent passage of stool associated with pain and difficulty, or delay in defecation.

- Constipation is common in childhood.
- 95% of infants pass one stool/day.
- 95% of schoolchildren pass three stools/wk.
- ~5% of schoolchildren suffer constipation, usually functional.
- Presentation can be with overflow soiling.
- Organic cause more likely if: delayed passage of meconium beyond 24h of age, onset in infancy, severe, and associated with faltering growth or abnormal physical signs (include per anal examination).

Causes

Idiopathic (commonest)

Commonest due to a combination of:

- Low-fibre diet.
- Lack of mobility and exercise.
- Poor colonic motility (55% have a +ve family history).

Gastrointestinal

- Hirschsprung's disease.
- Peri-anal disease (infection—streptococcal, fissure, stenosis, ectopic, hypertonic sphincter).
- Partial intestinal obstruction.
- Food hypersensitivity.
- Coeliac disease.

Non-gastrointestinal

- Hypothyroidism.
- Hypercalcaemia.
- Neurological disease, e.g. spinal cord disease.
- Chronic dehydration, e.g. diabetes insipidus (DI).
- Drugs, e.g. opiates and anticholinergics.
- Sexual abuse.

Presentation

- ↓ growth.
- Poor dietary intake.
- Straining and/or infrequent stools.
- Involuntary soiling or spurious diarrhoea (liquid faeces passes around solid impaction).
- *Abdomen:* pain and distension; flatulence; palpable abdominal or rectal faecal masses, usually indentible.
- *Anus:* pain on defecation; fresh rectal bleeding (anal fissure).
- *Rectal examination:* usually unnecessary unless child fails to respond to initiation of simple treatment, except in infancy when anal stenosis should be considered; abnormal anal tone.

Investigations

Usually unnecessary. If an organic cause is suspected, consider:

- *Blood*: FBC, coeliac antibody screen, TFTs, serum Ca^{2+}, RAST.
- *Imaging*: AXR, spinal imaging (neurological cause).
- *Bowel*: transit studies (older child) and anal manometry.
- *Rectal biopsy*: for Hirschsprung's disease.

Management

(See Box 7.2.)

Box 7.2 Treat in a stepwise manner

- Treat any underlying organic cause.
- Dietary: increase PO fluid and fibre intake; natural laxatives, e.g. fruit juice.
- Behavioural measures: toilet footrests; regular 5min toilet time after meals; star charts and rewards for child passing stool; reassure parents and encourage them not to show concern to the child.
  The aim of medication is to disimpact stool and then to maintain:
- Emphasize the need for consistency and adherence.
- Poor adherence and failure to evacuate faecal masses preclude improvement.
- Treat for at least 3mth. Do not wean therapy too soon.
- Regular PO faecal softeners, e.g. macrogols (Movicol®), lactulose, or sodium docusate, will aid disimpaction.
- Maintenance treatment should continue once disimpaction is achieved.
- PO stimulant laxatives, e.g. senna, bisacodyl, sodium picosulfate, may be required.
- Consider treatment of any anal fissure with topical anaesthetic (2% lidocaine ointment) to reduce pain and remove voluntary inhibition to defecate.
- Consider Picolax® (sodium picosulfate plus magnesium citrate) or high-volume polyethylene glycol (PEG) electrolyte solution bowel clean-out (may require NG administration for rapid infusion) in severe cases.
- Enemas, e.g. Micralax® or phosphate enemas, only if no response to intensive treatment with above.
- Hospital admission may be required for the most severe cases.

Prognosis

The majority of children can be 'cured' by a sympathetic paediatrician with complete evacuation of any stool masses, maintaining soft stools, and defecation training. Many children need long-term therapy. Do not underestimate the misery of this condition on child and family.

Faltering growth (failure to thrive)

Faltering growth, also known as failure to thrive (FTT), is when there is failure to grow at the expected rate (i.e. growth 'falls away' from standardized weight or height centile). Weight is the most sensitive indicator in infants and young children, while height is better in the older child. Under stress, OFC growth is more preserved than linear growth, which, in turn, is more than weight gain.

- In infancy, birthweight reflects the intrauterine environment. It is a poor guide to the child's correct 'genetic potential' and weight may naturally fall until the correct centile 'level' is attained (catch-down growth). The infant would then be expected to track that centile.
- In a well and happy child, consider constitutional small stature (normal growth velocity in a healthy child of small stature parents).

Causes

The majority of cases of FTT are caused by not enough food being offered or taken. In developing countries, poverty is the main cause. In the UK, causes include socio-economic difficulties, emotional deprivation, unskilled feeding, or a particular belief system regarding appropriate nutrition.

Organic causes

- ↓ appetite, e.g. psychological or secondary to chronic illness.
- Inability to ingest, e.g. GI, structural, or neurological problems.
- Excessive food loss, e.g. severe vomiting [GOR disease (GORD), pyloric stenosis, dysmotility], diabetes mellitus (urine).
- Malabsorption (see ⊃ Malabsorption, p. 302).
- ↑ energy requirements, e.g. CHD, CF, malignancy, sepsis.
- Impaired utilization, e.g. various syndromes, IEM, endocrinopathies.

Causes may overlap (e.g. in CF, there is simultaneous anorexia, malabsorption, and ↑ energy requirements, exacerbated by chronic infection).

Management

- *Detailed history:* including age of onset of FTT and timing of weaning. Consider a paediatric dietetic assessment.
- *Full examination:* including accurate measurement of growth.
- *If organic disease possible:* basic investigations should include:
  - FBC, ESR/CRP, U&E, creatinine, total protein and albumin, Ca^{2+}, PO_4^{3-}, LFTs.
  - Immunoglobulins.
  - Coeliac antibody screen.
  - Urinalysis, including MC&S.
- *Further investigations:* are indicated if there are suggestive symptoms or the faltering growth is severe, and include:
  - Blood: IEM screen, karyotype, serum lead (pica).
  - Sweat test.

- Oesophageal pH monitoring, upper endoscopy and small intestinal biopsy, faecal occult blood.
- Imaging: CXR, bone age, skeletal survey [non-accidental injury (NAI)], abdominal US, head CT/MRI.
- ECG.
- *If non-organic disease is likely:* seek dietary advice, preferably from a paediatric dietician; involve the health visitor/primary care:
  - *If FTT resolves in the next few weeks:* give +ve reinforcement and supervise subsequent growth as an outpatient.
  - *If FTT persists:* admit to hospital for basic investigations and observe the response to supervised adequate dietary input. Adequate growth in hospital suggests a non-organic cause; explore and support family dynamics.
  - *Should FTT occur again at home:* after improvement in hospital, and then refer to social services for family assessment and appropriate intervention.
  - *If FTT continues in hospital:* despite adequate dietary input, occult organic disease is most likely and requires extensive investigation as above.
- Provide dietetic input, whatever the cause, to support nutritional correction and education.
- Identify and correct associated comorbidities, e.g. developmental delay or early presentation of neurological disorder such as CP; fall-off in head growth is suggestive.

Prognosis

The prognosis depends on the severity of FTT. It is good if mild. Severe FTT, whatever the cause, may be associated with later neurodevelopmental and behavioural problems.

Recurrent abdominal pain

- Defined as >2 discrete episodes in a 3mth period interfering with school and/or usual activities.
- *Incidence:* 10–15% in school-age children.

Causes

No organic cause is found in 90%. Organic factors include: constipation, IBS—constipation or diarrhoea predominant, poor diet, food intolerance (lactose or fructose), peptic ulcer (*Helicobacter pylori*), coeliac disease, abdominal migraine (cyclic vomiting syndrome), gall bladder disease, renal colic, dysmenorrhoea, UTI, and physical or sexual abuse.

Presentation

Non-organic disease

This form occurs in a thriving, generally well child, with short episodes of peri-umbilical pain, good appetite, no other GI symptoms, no family history of migraine or coeliac disease, and normal examination. Coexisting symptoms such as headache, joint symptoms, and fatigue can occur and this is referred to as recurrent abdominal pain syndrome.

Organic cause

Likely if presentation is different to above or child <2y.
- *'Red flag' symptoms* include weight loss, diarrhoea, blood PR, joint symptoms, skin rashes, family history of IBD, or coeliac disease.

Management

History

Episodes of pain, severity—exacerbating and relieving factors, how pain is dealt with.
- *Red flags:* associated symptoms—constipation, poor diet, anxiety, school absence. Family history, including anxiety/emotional disorders.

Full examination

Investigations
- If *non-organic disease is likely:* no or very little investigation is needed, e.g. FBC, ESR/CRP, U&E, LFTs, coeliac antibody screen, urine MC&S, faecal MC&S (if there is a recent history of foreign travel). Stool faecal calprotectin if IBD suspected.
- If *organic disease is likely:* investigate as above, plus consider US, small bowel imaging, upper and lower GI endoscopy, hydrogen breath test (lactose intolerance), and ^{13}C breath test (*H. pylori*).

Treatment

Non-organic disease

- Confident reassurance; education that condition is common and pain is genuine (just like headaches); personal support; avoidance of associated stressful events (e.g. bullying); acknowledge symptom, while at same time down-play pain; minimize secondary gains from abdominal pain, e.g. school avoidance; ↑ dietary fibre intake may be beneficial; formal psychotherapy in complex and resistant cases. Multidisciplinary support and engagement of the family are essential.
- *Organic disease:* treat the underlying cause.

Prognosis

~25% of children with functional recurrent abdominal pain continue to have pain or headaches in adulthood. Functional sequelae are common.

Abdominal migraine

Abdominal pain is associated with pallor, headaches, anorexia, nausea ± vomiting. The condition overlaps with periodic syndrome and cyclic vomiting syndrome. Usually, a strong family history of migraine.

Treatment

- *Dietary:* avoid citrus fruits, chocolate, caffeine-containing drinks (e.g. cola), Marmite™, and solid cheeses.
- *Pharmacological:* pizotifen, sumatriptan, gabapentin, or amitriptyline may be helpful.

Gastrointestinal haemorrhage

This condition is relatively rare in childhood. Upper GI tract bleeding may present as haematemesis (vomiting of frank blood or 'coffee grounds') or melaena (black, tarry, foul-smelling stools). Haematochezia (bright or dark red blood PR) indicates lower GI tract bleeding. Beware of spurious haemorrhage, e.g. black stools after bismuth/iron ingestion, red vomit after beetroot, urate crystals in nappies, or normal pseudomenstruation in newborns. Use Dipstix test or laboratory testing to confirm blood if you are unsure.

Causes

Neonates
- Swallowed maternal blood, i.e. not GI haemorrhage.
- Dietary protein intolerance.
- Coagulopathy.
- Stress ulcers.
- Gastritis, vascular.
- Malformations.
- Duplication cyst.
- NEC.
- Infectious colitis, including pseudomembranous colitis.
- Inflammatory colitis.

Infants
Most of the above, plus:
- Oesophagitis.
- Swallowed blood from upper airway, e.g. epistaxis.
- Intussusception (see ➔ Intussusception, p. 822).
- Meckel's diverticulum (often presents as a massive painless rectal bleed) (see ➔ Meckel's diverticulum, p. 827).
- Anal fissure.

Older children
Most of the above, plus:
- Mallory–Weiss tear.
- Peptic ulcer disease.
- Oesophageal varices.
- Non-steroidal anti-inflammatory drugs (NSAIDs).
- Intestinal polyps.
- IBD (see ➔ Inflammatory bowel disease, pp. 300–1).
- GI infection, e.g. dysentery.
- HSP (see ➔ Henoch–Schönlein purpura, pp. 698–9).
- HUS (see ➔ Haemolytic uraemic syndrome, pp. 354–5).

Management

(See Box 7.3.)

- *Detailed history:* e.g. is there associated abdominal pain?
- *Examination:* specifically, vital signs; skin (pallor, abnormal blood vessels); ENT examination (e.g. epistaxis); organomegaly (e.g. splenomegaly); abdominal tenderness; anal inspection (e.g. fissure or fistula); rectal examination. Examine vomit or stool to confirm nature of bleed.
- *Supportive treatment:* fluids, blood product transfusion, airway protection with NGT or ETT intubation as necessary.
- *Drug treatment:* proton pump inhibitors (PPIs); somatostatin or vasopressin reduces splanchnic blood flow, and thereby upper GI bleeding secondary to portal hypertension.
- *Therapeutic endoscopy:* In severe bleeds (e.g. electrocautery), bleeding vessel ligation, paravariceal injection, balloon tamponade.
- *Treat underlying cause:* e.g. surgery for Meckel's diverticulum.

Box 7.3 Investigations for GI haemorrhage

Guided by findings from examination and history, these may include:

- FBC.
- U&E.
- Coagulation studies.
- LFTs.
- ESR/CRP.
- Apt test in newborns (confirms swallowed maternal blood by distinguishing adult from fetal Hb).
- Stool MC&S.
- Stool *C. difficile* toxin assay (pseudomembranous colitis).
- Formal ENT examination.
- Abdominal USS (e.g. intussusception or portal hypertension).
- Upper GI barium meal.
- Nuclear medicine scan (Meckel's diverticulum).
- Labelled RBC scan (occult bleeding).
- CXR (in case haemoptysis is true cause).
- Endoscopy (oesophagogastroduodenoscopy if melaena or haematemesis; flexible sigmoidoscopy or colonoscopy if haematochezia).
- Laparoscopy.

Jaundice

(See also ➔ Neonatal jaundice, pp. 110–11.) Jaundice occurs when serum bilirubin >25–30mmol/L. It is rare outside the neonatal period. First determine the SBR and conjugated (direct) fraction. Unconjugated bilirubin is rarely due to liver disease. Conjugated bilirubin (>20% of total or >20mmol/L) suggests liver disease and needs further assessment and investigation.

Unconjugated jaundice

Due to excess bilirubin production, impaired liver uptake, or conjugation.

Causes
- Physiological/breast milk jaundice.
- Haemolysis (spherocytosis, G6PD deficiency, sickle-cell anaemia, thalassaemia, HUS).
- Defective bilirubin conjugation (Gilbert syndrome, Crigler–Najjar syndrome).

Intrahepatic cholestasis

Jaundice is due to hepatocyte damage ± cholestasis. There is unconjugated ± conjugated hyperbilirubinaemia.

Causes
Infectious
- Viral hepatitis, including chronic hepatitis.
- Bacterial hepatitis [leptospirosis (Weil's disease), septicaemia, *Mycoplasma*, liver abscess].
- *Toxoplasma gondii.*

Toxic
- Drugs or poisons, e.g. paracetamol overdose, sodium valproate, anti-TB drugs, cytotoxic drugs.
- Fungi (*Amanita phalloides*).

Metabolic
- Galactosaemia, hereditary fructose intolerance, hypothyroidism.
- Tyrosinaemia type 1; Wilson's disease; α1-antitrypsin deficiency.
- Peroxisomal disorders, e.g. Zellweger syndrome.
- Dubin–Johnson syndrome, rotor syndrome.

Biliary hypoplasia
- Non-syndromic.
- Syndromic, e.g. Alagille syndrome.

Cardiovascular
- Budd–Chiari syndrome.
- Right heart failure.

Autoimmune
- Autoimmune hepatitis.

Cholestatic (obstructive) jaundice

Conjugated hyperbilirubinaemia is due to bile tract obstruction.

Causes
- Biliary atresia.
- Choledochal cyst.
- Caroli's disease.
- Cholelithiasis (may be secondary to chronic haemolysis).
- Cholecystitis.
- CF.
- Primary sclerosing cholangitis (commonly associated with IBD).
- Obstructive tumours or cysts.

Management of jaundice

- *Full history:* e.g. medications, family history, overseas travel, past blood transfusions, jaundice contacts, pale stools, or dark urine (cholestasis).
- *Examination:* vital signs, conscious level (hepatic coma), hepatic stigmata (= chronic liver disease), pallor (haemolysis), hepatomegaly, splenomegaly, ascites, peripheral oedema.

Investigations
Depending on which of the above pattern presents, these may include:
- Blood/serum: FBC, blood film, reticulocyte count, coagulation studies; U&E, SBR (total and conjugated), LFTs, albumin, total protein, TFTs, vitamins A, D, and E.
- Viral serology (hepatitis A, B, and C; EBV; CMV), blood culture, *Leptospira* and *Toxoplasma* antibody titres.
- IEM screen, ammonia, copper studies (serum copper ↑, ↓, or normal; serum caeruloplasmin ↓ in Wilson's disease), blood glucose, α1-antitrypsin level, galactose-1-uridyl-phosphatase level.
- Immunoglobulins, ANA, smooth muscle and liver/kidney antibodies (autoimmune hepatitis).
- Abdominal US, abdominal CT/MRI, biliary scintigraphy, e.g. hepato-iminodiacetic acid (HIDA) scan.
- Liver biopsy.

Treatment
- Remove or treat underlying cause.
- Correct blood glucose if it is low.
- Correct any clotting abnormalities.
- Phototherapy may be helpful only if jaundice has a significant unconjugated component, e.g. Crigler–Najjar syndrome.
- Conjugated hyperbilirubinaemia in early infancy should prompt thought of biliary atresia (surgery <12wk improves outcome).
- Treat any associated anaemia if due to haemolysis.
- Treat liver failure as appropriate.

Adverse reactions to food

Food allergy

(See also ➔ Chapter 13.) Defined as an abnormal immunological response to food (incidence is 6–8% in children aged <3y).

- Immediate allergic reactions involve production of food-specific IgE antibodies (type 1-mediated hypersensitivity).
- 70% of cases have a family history of atopy.
- Allergy becomes less common as age increases.
- The commonest food allergens are cow's milk proteins, eggs, peanuts, wheat, soya, fish, shellfish, and tree nuts.

Presentation—depends on whether immediate or delayed onset

- Vomiting.
- Urticaria.
- Erythematous rash, particularly perioral.
- Wheeze, circulatory disturbance.
- Anaphylaxis.
- Eczema.
- Asthma.
- Diarrhoea ± blood/mucus.
- Faltering growth (FTT).
- Abdominal pain.
- Dysphagia, GOR symptoms.

Non-allergic symptoms: food intolerance

Intolerance involves adverse reactions to food that are mediated by non-immunological reactions. This is generally thought to be commoner than food allergy. Presentation can be similar. Fructose intolerance is very common due to usage of high-fructose corn syrup in prepared foods and beverages. Other food intolerances may be due to:

- GI enzyme deficiency, e.g. lactose intolerance (see ➔ Lactose intolerance, p. 286), congenital sucrase–isomaltase deficiency.
- Pharmacological reactions to agents contained in food, e.g. caffeine, histamine, tyramine, tartrazine, acetylsalicylic acid.
- Reactions to food toxins or microbes, e.g. haemagglutinins in soy or mycotoxin present in mould-contaminated cereals.

Management of suspected food allergy or intolerance

(See Box 7.4 for clinical approach.)

Treatment
- *Dietary treatment:* exclusion of offending food(s) from diet, e.g. milk-free, soya-free, egg-free diet.
  - Involve a paediatric dietician in the diagnosis and management.
  - Extensively hydrolysed or amino acid-based milks can be used.
  - Consider dietary exclusion in mother if breastfeeding.
- *Drug treatment:* regular therapy may have a role, e.g. oral sodium cromoglicate, antihistamines, and corticosteroids.
- IM adrenaline is used for anaphylactic reactions, particularly if IgE-mediated and respiratory or systemic signs.
- After 6–12mth of being symptom-free on exclusion diet, consider food challenge if there is a food allergy. If the previous reaction was severe, this should only be done in hospital.

Prophylaxis
Unclear. In newborns with a first-degree relative with food allergy, exclusive breastfeeding to age 1y reduces the risk of allergy. Alternatively, a hydrolysed milk formula can be used. After weaning (delayed till 6mth), temporary avoidance of at-risk foods may reduce risk.

Box 7.4 Approach to adverse food reaction

History
Including diet history and examination. A food diary may be helpful.

Investigations
RAST or ELISA to detect specific food IgE antibodies; serum ↑ total IgE or eosinophils; favourable response to dietary elimination of suspected food protein and then recurrence after challenge; allergen SPT or patch skin testing. If the diagnosis is still in doubt, consider a double-blind controlled food antigen challenge. Upper and lower GI endoscopy (eosinophilic/non-specific inflammatory infiltrate) in children with predominantly gut symptoms.

In severe cases when allergen(s) cannot be identified, start a full elimination diet in which only a few hypoallergenic foods are given for 1–2wk, e.g. lamb, rice, water, pears, followed by a gradual re-introduction of increasingly allergenic foods until a food reaction(s) is detected.

Prognosis of food allergy or intolerance
Prognosis depends on cause. Most infant-onset food-allergy resolves by 2y, except peanut allergy that tends to persist. Allergies in older children are more likely to become chronic.

Lactose intolerance

- Most commonly due to post-viral gastroenteritis lactase deficiency, e.g. rotavirus. Most cases are transient and short-lasting (<4–6wk).
- In older healthy children and adults, lactase levels commonly decline, with subsequent variable tolerance (especially in certain populations, e.g. South East Asian and Afro-Caribbean).
- Rare causes include congenital lactase deficiency (primary). Infants present with severe diarrhoea after lactose exposure (present in high quantities in breast milk).
- *Presentation:* diarrhoea, excessive flatus, colic, peri-anal excoriation, stool pH <5.
- *Treatment:* lactose-free formula milk (soya milk not recommended in children under 6mth).

Cow's milk protein allergy

(See ⊃ Cow's milk protein allergy, p. 522).
- Commonest food allergy in infancy.
- Symptoms depend on where the allergic inflammation is:
  - *Upper GI tract*—vomiting, feeding aversion, pain.
  - *Small intestine*—diarrhoea, abdominal pain, protein-losing enteropathy, FTT.
  - *Large intestine*—diarrhoea, colitis with blood and mucus in stools, rarely chronic constipation.
- Limited use for RAST or SPT in infancy.
- May occur in breastfed infants; the reaction is to cow's milk protein secreted into breast milk following maternal ingestion. Usually presents as allergic colitis in an otherwise healthy, happy infant.
- In infants, first treat by limiting cow's milk protein intake (and soy protein):
  - In exclusively breastfed infants, this is achieved by a maternal exclusion diet to these proteins.
  - In formula-fed infants, feed with a hydrolysed protein formula (short peptides).
  - If symptoms severe or unresponsive to hydrolysed formula, then an elemental (amino acid) formula may be required.
- Anti-inflammatory medications are very rarely needed.
- Avoid using goat's or sheep's milk as a cow's milk substitute, as 25% will also develop allergy to these milks (cross-reactivity). Similar cross-reactivity also often occurs with soya milk. Use of soya milk is not recommended under age 6mth.
- After weaning, introduce a cow's milk protein-free diet (supplement with PO Ca^{2+} if required).
- Consider a cow's milk protein challenge after 6–12mth.

Nutritional disorders

Malnutrition is a common cause of child death and morbidity. There is a wide spectrum of nutritional disorders, varying from protein–energy malnutrition (PEM) to micronutrient nutritional deficiencies to overweight/obesity (see Table 7.1). In non-industrialized nations, malnutrition and associated infection are leading causes of child death.

Causes of nutritional impairment

- Diets low in protein, energy, or specific nutrients.
- Strict fad or vegetarian diets.
- Diseases causing malabsorption (e.g. coeliac disease, CF, CD), severe GORD, immunodeficiency, chronic infection.
- Eating disorders, e.g. anorexia nervosa (see ➲ Chapter 19).

Assessment of nutritional status

Refer to a paediatric dietician and consider the following:
- Assessment of food intake—consider food diary in chronic cases.
- Accurately plot serial heights and weights (falling across 2nd centile lines or < 3rd centile may indicate nutritional impairment).
- Plot body mass index (BMI) [BMI = weight (kg)/height (m)^2].
- Recent weight loss (≥10% over 3mth is suggestive of impaired nutritional status).
- Percentage weight for height [= (actual weight/expected weight for height centile) × 100]; a value of ≤90% may indicate impairment.
- Mid-arm circumference divided by OFC (malnutrition if <0.31).

Protein–energy malnutrition

Kwashiorkor and marasmus occur together. Because of oedema, mid-upper arm circumference is a better guide to malnutrition than weight.
Kwashiorkor is severe deficiency of protein/essential amino acids.
- *Clinical features:* growth retardation, diarrhoea, apathy, anorexia, oedema, skin/hair depigmentation, abdominal distension with fatty liver.
- *Investigations:* ↓ serum albumin; normo- and microcytic anaemia; ↓ Ca^{2+}, Mg^{2+}, and PO_4^{3-}; and ↓ glucose.

Marasmus is due to severe energy (calories) deficiency.
- *Clinical features:* height is relatively preserved, compared to weight; wasted appearance; muscle atrophy; listless; diarrhoea; constipation.
- *Investigations:* ↓ serum albumin, Hb, U&E, Ca^{2+}, Mg^{2+}, PO_4^{3-}, and glucose; stool MC&S for intestinal ova, cysts, and parasites.

Treatment

- Correct dehydration and electrolyte imbalance (IV if required).
- Treat underlying infection and/or parasitic infections.
- Treat concurrent/causative disease.
- Treat specific nutritional deficiencies.
- Orally refeed slowly—watch out for refeeding syndrome (see ➲ Method, p. 291).

Table 7.1 Specific nutritional deficiencies

Name	Causes	Presentation	Treatment
Iron	Low dietary intake, chronic blood loss (e.g. intestinal parasites or malaria), prematurity	Common ~10% in children in the UK). Microcytic hypochromic anaemia, developmental delay, angular stomatitis, koilonychia, serum ferritin <7mg/L, serum iron <5mcmol/L, total iron-binding capacity >90mmol/L	PO 4–6mg/kg iron daily
Vitamin A	Fat malabsorption states, e.g. CF; deficient indigenous diet	↑ morbidity and mortality from infections, follicular hyperkeratosis, xerophthalmia, night blindness. Plasma retinol <0.7mmol/L	PO vitamin A supplementation
Vitamin D	Common. Dietary deficiency, low ultraviolet light, fat malabsorption, hepatic or renal failure	Rickets (limb X-rays: distal bony cupping and fraying), ↓ serum Ca²⁺ and PO₄³⁻, ↑ ALP, plasma 25-hydroxy colecalciferol <25nmol/L	PO 40–125mcg/day vitamin D; Ca²⁺ and PO₄³⁻ supplements
Vitamin K	Congenital, fat malabsorption states, small bowel bacterial overgrowth	Bleeding, including haemorrhagic disease of the newborn	IV 1mg vitamin K₁
Vitamin B₁	Dietary deficiency (particularly when polished rice staple diet)	Beriberi (muscle weakness, oedema, heart failure), Wernicke's encephalopathy; red cell thiamine pyrophosphate <150nmol/L	PO 5mg vitamin B₁ daily
Vitamin B₁₂	Vegan diets, distal small bowel disease (e.g. CD), pernicious anaemia	Macrocytic megaloblastic anaemia, peripheral neuropathy, motor weakness. Vitamin B₁₂ level <75pmol/L, Schilling test of B₁₂ absorption	IM vitamin B₁₂ 1mg every 1–3mth
Vitamin C	Lack of fresh fruits and vegetables	Scurvy: petechiae, ecchymosis, bleeding gums, painful subperiosteal bleeding of legs, motor weakness. Plasma vitamin C level <6–11 micromols/L	PO vitamin C 25mg qds for 4 days, then bd
Vitamin E	Prematurity, fat malabsorption	Haemolytic anaemia, neurological symptoms, visual impairment. Serum vitamin E level <5mg/L	PO 75–100mg vitamin E daily
Folic acid	Small bowel disease, malignancy, drugs (anticonvulsants, cytotoxics)	Macrocytic megaloblastic anaemia, thrombocytopenia, irritability, FTT, red cell folate <160ng/mL	PO 0.5–1mg folic acid daily
Zinc	Prematurity, dietary insufficiency, intestinal disease or chronic diarrhoea, acrodermatitis enteropathica (inborn error of zinc absorption)	Peri-orofacial and anal dermatitis, diarrhoea, alopecia, FTT, neurological dysfunction. Serum zinc <11 micromoles/L	Infants: PO 1mg/kg/day Children: 1–5y, 5mg/ day; >10y, 10mg/day
Iodine	Dietary deficiency, endemic in some regions	Hypothyroidism and delayed development. Low urine iodine:creatinine ratio	PO 100–300mcg/day iodine and PO levothyroxine replacement

Nutritional support

Nutritional support can be enteral (EN) or parenteral (PN). EN, when possible, is preferred as it is cheaper, technically less demanding, more physiological, and associated with fewer complications.

* Paediatric dietician to assess nutritional status and requirements.
* Beware of 'refeeding syndrome'—potentially fatal cardiorespiratory failure induced by electrolyte disturbance (PO_4^{3-}, Mg^{2+}) following nutritional therapy in severe malnutrition.

Indications

* Severely ill patients, e.g. extreme preterm infants, ill preterm infants.
* Nutritional supplementation is required, e.g. FTT, CF.
* Swallowing difficulty, e.g. severe CP.
* Metabolic diseases, e.g. PKU.
* GI disease, e.g. malabsorption, failure, short bowel syndrome.
* Other primary disease state, e.g. chronic renal failure (CRF).

Oral supplementation

Includes high-energy milks, mineral/vitamin supplementation.

Specialized foods

Huge range of specialized milk and feeds exist for many conditions (elemental/polymeric diets for CD, hypoallergenic milk for milk protein allergy/intolerance, high calorie-dense milks for children with chronic medical conditions).

Enteral tube feeding

* Can be orogastric, NG, nasojejunal, and gastrostomy (including gastro-jejunal).
* Liquid feeds are given as boluses or continuously, e.g. overnight.
* *Indications:* swallowing problems (e.g. severe CP, prematurity), cardiorespiratory compromise, GORD, anorexia, generalized debilitation, e.g. trauma.
* *Feeds:* standard polymeric diets (e.g. ready-to-feed nutritionally complete whole protein products), elemental diets and semi-elemental diets requiring little/no digestion, or specific formulations.
* Gastrostomy reduces orofacial complications/discomfort, but complications include: gastric leakage, localized skin infection or inflammation, and GI perforation/trauma/haemorrhage.

Trophic feeding

* *Synonyms:* minimal enteral feeding, gut priming.
* *Indications:* during PN in newborn infants, particularly if preterm.
* *Rationale:* prolongation of enteral starvation leads to loss of normal GI structure and function despite PN-induced anabolic body state. Small milk volumes appear to prevent this. Also promotes GI development in newborn infants.
* Typically, 0.5–1mL/kg/h milk is fed within 2–3 days of birth.
* *Evidence of beneficial effects (in newborns) includes:* less sepsis, fewer days of PN, improved growth, and improved gut function.

Parenteral nutrition

IV PN may be supplemental or for TPN. Parents can be trained to give long-term PN at home.

Indications

- Preterm infants.
- Post-operative, e.g. abdominal or cardiothoracic.
- After severe trauma or burns.
- Acute pancreatitis.
- Oral feeds are contraindicated, e.g. NEC.
- Intestinal failure, e.g. short bowel syndrome, congenital enteropathy.
- Protracted vomiting or diarrhoea.
- GI obstruction, e.g. chronic intestinal pseudo-obstruction.
- Oncology patients, e.g. severe mucositis, GVHD.

Administration

- An MDT comprising a clinician with an interest in PN, a pharmacist, a paediatric dietician, and a nutrition nurse specialist should be involved in supervising PN.
- Follow unit/hospital dietetic/pharmacy guidelines for individual needs.
- Allowance should be made of body weight (you may need to estimate a working weight, e.g. if oedematous or gross ascites), recent weight trends, clinical condition, fluid and nutritional requirements, and additional infused fluids.

Method

Once requirements are calculated, sterile pharmacy-prepared solutions are given via central (preferable) or peripheral venous lines. Rapid commencement of PN may risk 'refeeding syndrome' in chronically undernourished patients. When significant malnutrition exists, measure and correct electrolyte abnormalities before commencing PN, and introduce slowly. PN is usually supplied and administered as two components:

- *Lipid component:* contains fat (triglyceride emulsion, e.g. Intralipid® 20%) and fat-soluble vitamins. Usually infused over 20h.
- *Aqueous component:* contains carbohydrate (glucose solution), protein (crystalline L-amino acid solution), electrolytes, water-soluble vitamins, minerals, trace elements (zinc, copper, manganese, selenium ± iron). Usually infused over 24h.

Monitoring

Serious, unexpected biochemical disturbances occur rarely as a result of PN. An appropriate monitoring regimen is suggested in Table 10.2.

Weaning PN

PN should be weaned slowly, so that hypoglycaemia is avoided. This also allows GI mucosal recovery as enteral feeding is ↑. When weaning is protracted, PN can be administered over shortened periods. A paediatric dietician should assess the contribution of both enteral and parenteral feeds to ensure nutritional adequacy.

Complications/problems

- *Electrolyte/metabolic disturbances:* e.g. glucose ↑ or ↓.
- *Sepsis:* usually *Staphylococcus epidermidis, Staphylococcus aureus, Candida, Pseudomonas, E. coli.*
- *Central line:* occlusion, breakage, displacement.
- *Vascular:* thrombophlebitis, thromboembolism, extravasation injuries.
- *Cardiac tamponade:* avoid by placing CVL tip proximal to right atrium.
- *From amino acids:* PN-associated liver disease, including, steatosis, cholestasis, or rarely cirrhosis or portal hypertension.
- *From lipids:* platelet dysfunction, hyperlipidaemia, fatty liver, pulmonary hypertension.
- *Metabolic bone disease:* due to insufficient Ca^{2+} and PO_4^{3-}.
- *Demanding:* in time expertise, cost, etc.

Table 7.2 Guidelines for monitoring stable patients during short-term PN

Measurements	Pre-PN	During First week	Second week	Third and subsequent weeks
Weight	✓	Daily	Daily	Daily
FBC	–	–	× 1	× 1
Creatinine, urea, Na$^+$, K$^+$	✓	× 2	× 2	× 2
Ca^{2+}	✓	× 1	× 1	× 2
Mg^{2+}	✓	× 1	× 1	Monthly
PO$_4^{3-}$	✓	× 2	× 1	× 2
ALP, ALT, bilirubin, albumin	✓	× 1	× 1	× 2
Glucose	✓	Daily blood glucose	Urine dipstick daily	Urine dipstick daily
Copper, zinc, selenium, fat-soluble vitamins	–	–	–	Monthly
Triglycerides	✓	× 1	× 1	× 1

The unwell/malnourished infant/child is likely to need more frequent monitoring tailored to the specific needs of the individual.

Oesophageal disorders

(See also ➔ Congenital abnormalities: tracheo-oesophageal, pp. 810–11.)

Gastro-oesophageal reflux (GORD)

GOR occurs when there is inappropriate effortless passage of gastric contents into the oesophagus. It is very common in infancy. GORD is when reflux is repeated and severe enough to cause harm.

GOR is associated with slow gastric emptying, liquid diet (milk), horizontal posture, and low resting lower oesophageal sphincter (LOS) pressure.

Other causes in infancy and older children include: LOS dysfunction (e.g. hiatus hernia), ↑ gastric pressure (e.g. delayed gastric emptying), external gastric pressure, gastric hypersecretion (e.g. acid), food allergy, and CNS disorders (e.g. CP).

Presentation of GORD

- *GI*: regurgitation, non-specific irritability, rumination, oesophagitis (heartburn, difficult feeding with crying, painful swallowing, haematemesis), faltering growth (calorie deficiency due to profuse reflux of ingested calories, irritability with feeds).
- *Respiratory*: apnoea, hoarseness, cough, stridor, lower respiratory tract disease (aspiration pneumonia, asthma, CLD).
- *Neurobehavioural symptoms*: e.g. Sandifer's syndrome (extension and lateral turning of head, dystonic postures).
- *Complications*:
  - Faltering growth.
  - Anaemia (chronic blood loss).
  - Lower respiratory tract disease.
  - Oesophageal stricture (dysphagia).
  - Barrett's oesophagus (premalignant intestinal metaplasia).

Management of GORD

- *History*: e.g. effortless regurgitation, relationship to feeds.
- *Examination*: including growth, possible anaemia, respiratory.
- *Investigations*: appropriate when diagnosis is uncertain, there is a poor response to treatment, or complications occur. May include: upper GI endoscopy, oesophageal biopsy, 24h oesophageal pH/impedance probe, barium swallow with fluoroscopy, radioisotope 'milk' scan (aspiration), oesophageal manometry (oesophageal dysmotility), and CXR (associated respiratory disease).

Treatment

Treatment is carried out in a stepwise fashion.

- *Positioning*: nurse infants on head-up slope of 30° ± prone.
- *Dietary*: thickened milk feeds (infants); small frequent meals; avoid food before sleep; avoid fatty foods, citrus juices, caffeine, carbonated drinks, and 'alcohol and smoking'.

- *Drugs:* gastric acid-reducing drugs, e.g. ranitidine or omeprazole (if oesophagitis); Gaviscon® (contains antacids and an alginate that forms a viscous surface layer to reduce reflux); prokinetic drugs, e.g. domperidone; mucosal protectors, e.g. sucralfate; corticosteroids (allergic oesophagitis).
- *Surgery:* usually Nissen's fundoplication is performed when medical treatment has failed.
  - Indications for surgery are: failed intense medical treatment, oesophageal stricture, Barrett's oesophagus, and severe oesophagitis.
  - Complications of surgery include: 'gas bloating' syndrome, dysphagia, profuse retching, and 'dumping' syndrome.

Prognosis
Vast majority of infants outgrow symptoms by 1y. In older children, 50% develop a chronic, relapsing course.

Oesophageal foreign body

(See also ◆ Ingested foreign bodies, p. 818.) This usually occurs in toddlers or older children with neurological or psychiatric conditions. If the object reaches the stomach, 90% will pass spontaneously. Confirm position with AP and lateral CXR. Remove endoscopically if:
- Dysphagia or drooling persists.
- Object is still in the oesophagus for >12h.
- Object is sharp (risk of perforation).
- Object is hazardous, e.g. mercuric oxide disc batteries.

Upper oesophageal dysfunction

This disorder is usually due to diffuse CNS dysfunction.
- *Presentation:* choking, cough, drooling, dysphagia, nasal regurgitation.
- *Diagnosis:* barium swallow with videofluoroscopy or oesophageal manometry.
- *Treatment:* treat primary underlying disorder. Rarely, cricopharyngeal myotomy is helpful.

Achalasia

This rare idiopathic condition of obstruction is due to failure of LOS relaxation.
- *Presentation:* vomiting, dysphagia with solids or liquids, FTT, aspiration.
- *Diagnosis:* barium swallow (dilated tapering of lower oesophagus) or oesophageal manometry.
- *Treatment:* endoscopic balloon dilatation, Heller's cardiomyotomy.

Benign oesophageal stricture

Causes include severe GORD, caustic ingestion, and radiotherapy.

Treatment
Treat the underlying cause, e.g. reduce gastric acid production in GORD and perform balloon endoscopic dilatation.

Pancreatitis

Acute pancreatitis

This rare disorder consists of acute pancreatic inflammation, with variable involvement of local tissues and remote organ systems.

Causes
- *Blunt abdominal trauma:* e.g. road traffic accident.
- *Viral infection:* e.g. mumps, hepatitis A, Coxsackie B.
- *Multisystem disease:* e.g. SLE, KD, HUS, IBD, hyperlipidaemia.
- *Drugs and toxins:* e.g. thiopurines, metronidazole, cytotoxic drugs.
- *Pancreatic duct obstruction:* e.g. CF, choledochal cyst, tumours.

Presentation
Abdominal pain involving the upper central abdomen, radiating to the back, chest, or lower abdomen, vomiting, fever, abdominal tenderness. Severe cases also exhibit:
- Jaundice.
- Hypotension.
- Abdominal distension.
- Cullen or Grey Turner sign (bruising of peri-umbilical area and flanks, respectively).
- Ascites.
- Pleural effusion.
- Multiorgan failure.

Investigations
- *Blood:* amylase ↑; lipase ↑; Ca^{2+} ↓; ESR/CRP ↑; deranged LFTs.
- *Radiology:* abdominal USS or CT; endoscopic retrograde cholangiopancreatography (ERCP) if structural or obstructive cause.

Treatment
Mild
- Supportive only, e.g. NGT, analgesia.
- Start short period of nil by mouth to 'rest' pancreas, with early introduction of feeds.

Severe
Treat as for mild form, plus:
- Consider admission to PICU.
- Correct hypotension.
- Treat multiorgan failure.
- Surgery if significant pancreatic necrosis, major ductal rupture (trauma), gallstones (cholecystectomy), and presence of pseudocyst.
- ERCP may be therapeutic if structural obstructive cause.

Prognosis
- Complete recovery is likely if there is minimal organ dysfunction.
- 20% mortality if there is severe disease or organ failure present, or if local complications develop (e.g. pancreatic pseudocyst).
- Most children have only a single acute episode.

Chronic pancreatitis

This very rare condition follows acute pancreatitis with continuing inflammation, destruction of pancreatic tissue, and fibrosis, leading to permanent exocrine or endocrine pancreatic failure. Causes include CF, congenital ductal anomalies, sclerosing cholangitis (IBD), hyperlipidaemia, and hypercalcaemia.

Presentation
- Repeated episodes of acute pancreatitis are separated by good health.
- Eventually, features of pancreatic exocrine failure/pancreatic endocrine failure (diabetes mellitus) can occur.

Investigations
- Abdominal US or CT scan confirms chronic pancreatitis.
- Pancreatic function tests may be useful, e.g. raised stool chymotrypsin, pancreozymin–secretin test, 72h faecal fat measurement raised.

Treatment
- Treat acute exacerbations as for acute pancreatitis.
- Give pancreatic enzyme replacement and nutritional supplementation (well-balanced diet with moderated-fat intake and fat-soluble vitamins—involve a paediatric dietician).
- Relieve any ductal obstruction by endoscopy or surgery.

Prognosis
Recovery or risk of developing long-term pancreatic exocrine and/or endocrine failure is dependent on cause and severity.

Intestinal disorders

Gastritis and peptic ulcer disease

Rare in children. It most commonly affects the duodenum.

Causes
- *H. pylori* infection (strong familial link, associated with ↑ risk of adult gastric cancer).
- Stress ulcers, e.g. post-trauma, HIE.
- Drug-related, e.g. NSAIDs.
- ↑ acid secretion [Zollinger–Ellison syndrome, multiple endocrine neoplasia (MEN) type I, hyperparathyroidism].
- CD, eosinophilic gastroenteritis; hypertrophic gastritis; autoimmune gastritis.

Presentation
- Often asymptomatic.
- Nausea ± vomiting; FTT ± anorexia.
- Chronic abdominal and epigastric pain.
- GI haemorrhage; perforation (very rare).
- Iron deficiency anaemia.

Investigations
- ^{14}C urea breath test (*H. pylori*).
- Upper GI endoscopy and biopsy (*H. pylori*).

Treatment
- Treat underlying cause, e.g. eradicate *H. pylori* with 7–10 days of PO amoxicillin (clarithromycin), metronidazole, and omeprazole (quadruple therapy).
- ↓ gastric acid, e.g. ranitidine, PPIs, H_2 antagonists; sucralfate (cytoprotective).
- Antacids, e.g. Gaviscon®.

Protein-losing enteropathy

This disorder is characterized by chronic intestinal protein loss.

Causes
- GI infection, e.g. giardiasis.
- Coeliac disease, IBD.
- Severe food hypersensitivity
- Cardiac failure
- SLE; GVHD.
- Polyposis or lymphatic obstruction.

Presentation
There is hypoalbuminaemia with diarrhoea. ↑ faecal α1-antitrypsin confirms the condition.

Treatment
Treat the underlying disease; give nutritional support and albumin infusions, as required.

Short bowel syndrome
This is due to severe intestinal disease or the surgical removal of a large portion of the small intestine. Common causes include NEC, gastroschisis (neonatal), malrotation/volvulus, and IBD. The condition manifests as malabsorption, fluid and electrolyte loss, and malnutrition.

Presentation
- Diarrhoea, steatorrhoea.
- FTT; dehydration, electrolyte loss (Na^+, K^+, Mg^{2+}, Ca^{2+}).
- Cholestasis (bile salt loss); renal stones (oxalate).
- Peptic ulcer disease (due to ↑ gastrin).
- Specific (e.g. vitamin B_{12}) ± generalized malnutritional disorders.

Treatment
- Correct fluid and electrolyte disturbance; PN.
- Specific nutritional supplements; hydrolysed protein/elemental diets.
- Gastric acid-reducing drugs, e.g. PPI or H_2 antagonists.
- Anti-diarrhoeal drugs, e.g. loperamide.
- Colestyramine (chelates bile salts).
- Parenteral somatostatin.
- PO antibiotics to reduce bacterial overgrowth.
- Surgery to reduce GI motility or small bowel transplant.

Prognosis
Prognosis is improving, with 90% 5y survival. Retention of ileo-caecal valve significantly improves prognosis.

Intestinal polyps
Most polyps are hamartomas, single, and located in the distal colon (juvenile polyps). Polyposis (multiple polyps) syndromes include:
- Peutz–Jegher's syndrome (mucocutaneous pigmentation).
- Familial adenomatous polyposis coli.
- Gardner's syndrome (GI polyps, osteomas, and soft tissue tumours).

Presentation
- Often asymptomatic.
- Haematochezia, rectal polyp prolapse, protein-losing enteropathy.
- Intussusception, mucoid diarrhoea.

Investigations
- Gastroscopy and ileo-colonoscopy, small bowel imaging.

Treatment
- Endoscopic or surgical removal.
- Periodic colonoscopy surveillance is required in polyposis syndromes because of significant risk of neoplasia.

Inflammatory bowel disease

Includes CD and UC. UK incidence is ~8/100 000/y. CD is twice as common as UC. The cause is unknown, although there is a recognized genetic disposition.

Crohn's disease

- May affect any part of GI tract, but terminal ileum and proximal colon are the commonest sites of involvement.
- Unlike UC, bowel involvement is non-continuous ('skip' lesions).

Ulcerative colitis

- Involves colon only; rectal (proctitis) is commonest or may extend continuously up to involving the entire colon (pancolitis).
- Terminal ileum may be affected by 'backwash ileitis'.

Presentation

Symptoms
- Anorexia, weight loss, lethargy, fever.
- Abdominal cramps.
- Diarrhoea ± blood/mucus, urgency, and tenesmus (proctitis).

GI signs
- Aphthous oral ulcers.
- Abdominal tenderness; abdominal distension (UC > CD), right iliac fossa (RIF) mass (CD).
- Peri-anal disease (CD), i.e. abscess, sinus, fistula, skin tags, fissure, stricture.

Non-GI signs and associations
- Fever, finger clubbing, anaemia, poor growth, delayed puberty.
- *Skin:* erythema nodosum, pyoderma gangrenosum.
- *Joints:* arthritis, ankylosing spondylitis.
- *Eyes:* iritis; conjunctivitis; episcleritis.
- Sclerosing cholangitis, renal stones.
- Nutritional deficiencies, e.g. vitamin B_{12}.

Complications
- 'Toxic' colon dilatation (UC > CD), GI perforation or strictures.
- Pseudopolyps (apparent 'polyps' resulting from inflammation).
- Massive GI haemorrhage.
- Colon carcinoma (UC, 50% risk after 10–20y disease).
- Fistula involving bowel only or bowel and skin, vagina, or bladder (CD); abscesses (CD).

Investigations

- *Blood:* FBC; ESR/CRP high; U&E; LFTs; albumin low; blood culture; serum iron low; vitamin B_{12} and folate low.

- *Serum serological markers:* ASCA (anti-*Saccharomyces cerevisiae* antibodies, better for CD); p-ANCA (perinuclear antineutrophil cytoplasmic antibody, better for UC).
- *Stool MC&S:* infectious colitis can mimic CD/UC; faecal calprotectin raised in bowel inflammation.
- *Endoscopy:* ileo-colonoscopy to determine extent and pattern of abnormal mucosa and intestinal biopsy (UC histology: crypt abscesses, mucosal inflammation only, goblet cell depletion; CD: crypt abscesses, granulomas, transmural inflammation); upper GI endoscopy (CD).
- *Radiology:* small bowel imaging—barium radiology/US/MRI (CD: mucosal 'cobblestone' appearance, ulceration, dilatation, narrowed segments, fistula, 'skip' lesions; UC: mucosal ulceration, haustration loss, colonic narrowing ± shortening).

Treatment

Supportive treatment
- If severe, e.g. bowel rest, IV hydration, PN.

Dietary treatment
Polymeric/elemental diets are useful to induce remission (CD), but the relapse rate is high. Dietary supplementation often required to minimize poor growth and correct specific nutritional deficiencies, e.g. vitamin and mineral supplements. Involve a paediatric dietician.

Drug treatment
- *Mild to moderate disease:* PO 5-aminosalicylic acid (ASA) dimers, e.g. mesalazine, may be useful to induce and maintain colonic disease remission in UC. ASA or corticosteroid enemas are effective for treating rectal disease. Dietary treatment may be useful to induce remission and so it is important to involve a paediatric dietician.
- *Moderate to severe disease:* induce remission with PO prednisolone or IV methylprednisolone 1–2mg/kg/day until condition improved (<2wk), then wean over 6–8wk.
- *Antibiotics:* e.g. ciprofloxacin or metronidazole, may also be useful.
- *Maintenance treatment or to treat resistant active disease:* immunomodifiers, e.g. azathioprine, ciclosporin, tacrolimus, methotrexate, or infliximab/adalimumab [anti-tumour necrosis factor (TNF) antibody].

Surgery
- *UC:* total colectomy/ileostomy, and later pouch creation and anal anastomosis, cure UC; 10–20% complication rate, e.g. pouchitis.
- *CD:* local surgical resection for severe localized disease, e.g. strictures, fistula, may be indicated, but there is a high re-operation rate as inflammation recurrence is universal.

Prognosis

UC and CD are marked by relapse and remission. Patients can have good quality of life. Poor prognostic factors include extensive disease, frequent disease flare-ups, and young age at diagnosis.

Malabsorption

Defined as subnormal intestinal absorption of dietary constituents with excessive faecal nutrient loss. The prognosis depends on the cause. Reduced adult height, teeth enamel defects, and osteoporosis may result from long-term malabsorption. Causes are listed in Box 7.5.

Presentation

- Diarrhoea.
- Steatorrhoea.
- Flatulence.
- FTT/weight loss.
- Muscle wasting.
- Abdominal distension.
- Peri-anal excoriation.
- Delayed puberty.
- Features of underlying illness, e.g. abdominal pain in CD.
- Signs of nutritional deficiency, e.g. ascites in hypoalbuminaemia.

Investigations

- *Initial screening tests should include:* FBC, U&E, creatinine, albumin, total protein, Ca^{2+}, PO_4^{3-}, LFTs, iron status, coeliac antibody screen, coagulation screen, and stool MC&S.

If the diagnosis still unclear:
- Upper GI endoscopy with biopsy to look for enteropathy; ileo-colonoscopy if features suggest colitis.
- Sweat test.
- Immune function tests.
- Faecal measurement of fat, elastase, calprotectin, and α1-antitrypsin.
- Exocrine pancreatic function tests.

Treatment

- Treat underlying disease, e.g. metronidazole for giardiasis, gluten-free diet for coeliac disease.
- Supplemental digestive enzymes, e.g. pancreatic enzymes in CF.
- Nutritional supplementation to correct deficiencies.
- PN if malabsorption severe or slow to recover.

Box 7.5 Causes of malabsorption

Intraluminal digestive defect

- Carbohydrate intolerance (most commonly lactose intolerance).
- PEM.
- CF.
- Shwachman–Diamond syndrome (see ◐ Schwachman–Diamond syndrome, p. 558).
- Chronic pancreatitis.
- Cholestasis.
- Pernicious anaemia.
- Specific digestive enzyme deficiency, e.g. lipase.

Mucosal abnormality

- Coeliac disease.
- Dietary protein intolerance, e.g. milk protein allergy.
- Intestinal infection or parasites, e.g. giardiasis.
- Short bowel syndrome.
- CD.
- Abetalipoproteinaemia [disorder of lipid metabolism—FTT, steatorrhoea, progressive ataxia, retinitis pigmentosa (RP), acanthocytes on FBC].
- PEM; intestinal venous or lymphatic obstruction, e.g. congestive cardiac failure, intestinal lymphangiectasia.

Miscellaneous

- Immunodeficiency syndromes, e.g. HIV.
- Drug reaction, e.g. cytotoxics, post-radiation.
- Bacterial overgrowth, e.g. pseudo-obstruction.

Coeliac disease

Coeliac disease is an enteropathy due to lifelong intolerance to gluten protein (in wheat, barley, rye, and oats by cross-contamination).
Prevalence is ~1% when populations are screened. It is associated with:
• +ve family history.
• T1DM.
• Down's syndrome.
• IgA deficiency.

Presentation

The condition may present at any age after starting solids containing gluten. The 'classic' initial features include:
• Pallor.
• Anorexia.
• FTT.
• Irritability.
• Diarrhoea.
• Pale, bulky floating stools.

Later, there is:
• Apathy.
• Ascites.
• Peripheral oedema.
• Anaemia.
• Delayed puberty.
• Arthralgia.
• Hypotonia, muscle wasting, developmental delay.
• Specific nutritional disorders.

↑ recognition and widespread practice of antibody screening of children at high risk have changed considerably the clinical spectrum of cases seen, with less classical and less severe symptoms now commoner at the time of diagnosis, e.g. presentation with iron deficiency anaemia or short stature. There are three settings in which the diagnosis of coeliac disease should be considered and screened for:
• Children with frank gut symptoms.
• Children with non-GI manifestations.
• Asymptomatic individuals with conditions associated with coeliac disease.

Coeliac crisis

Life-threatening dehydration due to diarrhoea accompanying malabsorption. Very rare, except in the less developed world.

Investigations

- Essential to be on a gluten-containing diet for diagnostic testing and to avoid gluten exclusion prior to diagnostic confirmation.
- –ve testing does not preclude getting the condition later.
- Measurement of serum tissue transglutaminase IgA antibody (TTG) is recommended for initial testing for coeliac disease. IgA sensitivity and specificity approach 100%, although false +ves are occasionally seen. Anti-endomysial IgA antibody is observer-dependent and expensive. Anti-gliadin antibody tests are less accurate and now not advised. It is important to exclude IgA deficiency as a cause of falsely –ve serology.
- Endoscopic small bowel biopsy of the third part of the duodenum shows diffuse subtotal villus atrophy, ↑ intraepithelial lymphocytes, and crypt hyperplasia. Villi normalize on a gluten-free diet.
- Most clinicians consider +ve mucosal histology and full clinical recovery on gluten-free diet ± +ve IgA antibodies sufficient for diagnosis. Antibody levels should return to normal on treatment and –ve serology is a marker of compliance.
- Avoid gluten challenge (>10g PO gluten per day for 3–4mth and re-biopsy), unless diagnosis is in doubt (e.g. initial biopsy is inadequate or not typical) or alternative diagnosis is possible (e.g. transient gluten intolerance may occur after gastroenteritis, giardiasis, or cow's milk protein intolerance).
- If TTG is >10 times normal, anti-endomysial antibody +ve, and HLA (DQ2, DQ8) confirms risk in a symptomatic case, then providing there is a good response to gluten exclusion, the diagnosis can be considered confirmed without the need for biopsy.

Treatment

- Gluten-free diet under the supervision of a paediatric dietician.
- Gluten-free foods are prescribable in the UK.
- Gluten avoidance should be lifelong if coeliac disease is confirmed.
- Nutritional supplements may be required.

Prognosis

Excellent if patient is compliant with strict, lifelong gluten-free diet. There is a possible ↑ risk of intestinal lymphoma if gluten is ingested, even in asymptomatic coeliac disease (see NICE guidance).[1]

Gastrointestinal infections

GI infections are the second commonest cause of primary care consultation after the common cold. They are the cause of over 3 million children deaths per year (mostly in lower- and middle-income countries).

Viral gastroenteritis

Transmission is by the faecal–oral route, including contaminated water. Epidemics are frequent and usually occur during winter. Breastfeeding is protective. Severity is ↑ in malnourished children.

Causes
- Rotavirus (commonest)—reduced significantly in settings where rotavirus immunization has been implemented.
- Small, round structural virus, e.g. winter vomiting disease caused by 'Norwalk agent'.
- Enteric adenovirus, astrovirus.
- CMV (in immune-comprised patients).

Presentation
- Watery diarrhoea (rarely bloody).
- Vomiting, cramping abdominal pain.
- Fever.
- Dehydration, electrolyte disturbance.
- Vomiting predominates with Norwalk virus.
- Upper respiratory tract signs common with rotavirus.

Investigations
Rarely necessary. Stool EM or immunoassay can sometimes be useful, particularly to diagnose and type an outbreak.

Treatment
Give supportive rehydration PO or with an NGT, or IV glucose and electrolyte solution if not tolerated or signs of shock. Re-introduce feeds as soon as tolerated/continue breastfeeding. Hospitalization is rarely needed (e.g. ≥10% dehydration or unable to tolerate PO fluids).

Prognosis
Symptoms last <7 days, except in enteric adenovirus infections when diarrhoea lasts >14 days. The child may develop temporary secondary lactose intolerance, particularly after rotavirus infection, which usually resolves in 4–6wk.

Prevention
Rotavirus immunization is now available and effective.

Bacterial gastroenteritis

Causes secretory and inflammatory diarrhoea. Commonest causes include:

- *Salmonella* spp.
- *Campylobacter jejuni.*
- *Shigella* spp.
- *Yersinia enterocolitica.*
- *E. coli.*
- *C. difficile.*
- *Bacillus cereus.*
- *Vibrio cholerae.*

Sources of infection include contaminated water, poor food hygiene (meat, fresh produce, chicken, eggs, previously cooked rice), and faecal–oral route.

Presentation

As for viral gastroenteritis, plus:

- Malaise, abdominal pain, tenesmus.
- Dysentery (bloody and mucous diarrhoea).
- Abdominal pain may mimic appendicitis or IBD.

Complications

- Bacteraemia, secondary infections (particularly *Salmonella, Campylobacter*), e.g. pneumonia, osteomyelitis, meningitis.
- Reiter's syndrome (*Shigella, Campylobacter*).
- HUS (*E. coli* 0157, *Shigella*).
- G-BS (*Campylobacter*).
- Reactive arthropathy (*Yersinia*).
- Haemorrhagic colitis.

Investigations

- Stool ± blood culture (some organisms need specific culture medium).
- Stool *C. difficile* toxin.
- Endoscopy if stool cultures –ve and features suggestive of IBD.

Treatment

- Rehydration, as for viral gastroenteritis.
- Antibiotics not indicated, as duration of symptoms not altered and may increase chronic carrier status, unless there is high risk of disseminated disease, presence of artificial implants (e.g. ventriculo-peritoneal shunt), severe colitis, severe systemic illness, age <6mth, enteric fever, cholera, or *E. coli* 0157. Most organisms are sensitive to ampicillin, co-trimoxazole, or third-generation cephalosporins. *Consider:*
  - Erythromycin if *Campylobacter*.
  - PO vancomycin or metronidazole if *C. difficile* (causes pseudomembranous colitis).

Intestinal parasites

Infection is usually via the faecal–oral route. Pets and livestock can be the hosts. Parasitic infection can mimic IBD (see ➜ Inflammatory bowel disease, pp. 300–1), hepatitis (see ➜ Acute hepatitis, pp. 310–11), sclerosing cholangitis, peptic ulcer disease, and coeliac disease (see ➜ Coeliac disease, pp. 304–5).

Presentation

- Fever, abdominal pain, diarrhoea, dysentery, flatulence.
- Malabsorption and FTT.
- Abdominal distension, intestinal obstruction.
- Biliary obstruction, liver disease, pancreatitis.

Investigations

- Stool MC&S for ova, cysts, parasites; staining for cryptosporidiosis.
- Stool enzyme-linked immunosorbent assay (ELISA) for giardiasis and cryptosporidiosis.
- Blood-specific serology, e.g. *Entamoeba histolytica*.
- Duodenal fluid aspiration for MC&S.
- Duodenal villus biopsy, e.g. giardiasis.

Protozoa

Giardia lamblia
- Very common.
- Swallowed cysts develop into trophozoites that attach to the small intestinal villi, causing mucosal damage.

Presentation
- Diarrhoea, flatulence, abdominal discomfort.
- Sometimes FTT.

Treatment
- Metronidazole.

Entamoeba histolytica
Symptoms are usually mild but may cause:
- Fulminating colitis (amoebic dystentery can mimic UC).
- Intestinal obstruction due to chronic localized lesion (an 'amoeboma').
- Amoebic hepatitis.
- Liver abscess (right upper quadrant pain, fever, hepatomegaly).

Treatment
- Metronidazole.

Cryptosporidium
This organism causes a mild self-limiting illness, except in immune-compromised patients where it can cause:
- Severe chronic watery diarrhoea, flatulence.
- Malaise, abdominal pain, weight loss.

Treatment
- Erythromycin, metronidazole, or spiramycin.

Nematodes

Ascaris lumbricoides

The commonest parasitic worm infection in humans, with up to 25% of the world's population infected (rare in industrialized countries). They look like earthworms and can cause Loeffler's syndrome (eosinophilic pneumonia that can mimic asthma, also caused by the parasite *Strongyloides stercoralis* and the hookworms *Ancylostoma duodenale* and *Necator americanus*). Heavy infestation can cause specific nutritional deficiencies or bowel obstruction. Infection occurs by faecal–oral transmission of eggs.

Treatment
• Mebendazole, albendazole, pyrantel pamoate.

Trichuris trichiura (whip worm)

Lives in the colon and causes diarrhoea, abdominal pain, and weight loss.

Treatment
• Mebendazole or albendazole.

Hookworms (N. americanus, A. duodenale)

Infection is by larvae penetrating the skin, e.g. bare feet. The adult worms live in the intestine, voraciously sucking blood, leading to anaemia and hypoproteinaemia.

Treatment
• Mebendazole.

Strongyloides stercoralis
• Penetrates the skin and migrates to the lungs, then coughed up and ingested into the gut.
• Causes bloating, heartburn, and malabsorption.

Treatment
• Mebendazole, albendazole, or thiabendazole.

Enterobius vermicularis (thread or pinworm)
• Very common and causes anal pruritus as ♀ emerge and lay eggs in peri-anal region.
• *Infection*: occurs by faecal–oral transmission of eggs.
• *Diagnosis*: confirmed by direct visualization of worms in peri-anal area or stool, or microscopy of Sellotape applied to the anus.

Treatment
• Mebendazole.

Cestodes (tapeworms)
• *Infection*: results from ingesting undercooked contaminated pork (*Taenia solium*), beef (*Taenia saginata*), or fish (*Diphyllobothrium latum*).
• *Diagnosis*: by microscopy of eggs or proglottides in stool.

Treatment
• Praziquantel.

Acute hepatitis

Viral causes

- *Hepatitis A (HAV)*: incubation 2–6wk, faecal–oral transmission.
- *Hepatitis B (HBV)*: incubation 6wk to 6mth. Endemic in the Far East and Africa. Infection may be transmitted from:
  - Blood products.
  - IV drug abuse, contaminated needles or syringes.
  - Sexual intercourse.
  - Close direct contact (e.g. intrafamilial, health workers).
  - Vertical (may cause fulminant hepatitis).
- *Hepatitis C (HCV)*: incubation 2wk to 6mth. Transmission is as for HBV. Usually causes a mild-severity acute illness or is asymptomatic. HCV rarely causes acute hepatitis.
- *Hepatitis E*: faecal–oral transmission, endemic in India.
- *Hepatitis D*: requires previous HBV infection.
- *Hepatitis G*: parenteral transmission.
- *Other organisms*: can cause hepatitis as part of systemic infection—EBV (common in adolescents; only 40% have hepatitis), TORCH organisms (neonatal hepatitis), HIV, CMV (immune-compromised), *Listeria*.

Other causes

- *Poisons and drugs*: e.g. paracetamol, isoniazid, halothane.
- *Metabolic disease*: e.g. Wilson's disease, tyrosinaemia type I.
- *Autoimmune hepatitis*: may present with acute hepatitis.
- *Reye syndrome*: a rare and largely historical, acute encephalopathic illness associated with aspirin therapy and microvesicular fatty infiltration of the liver.
  - *Prodrome*: nausea, vomiting, hypoglycaemia, abdominal pain; occurs 2–3 days before onset of jaundice or abnormal LFTs.

Presentation

Acute fulminant hepatic failure (encephalopathy and coagulopathy) may rarely occur. Many infections are asymptomatic, particularly HAV and HCV. There are many presentations, including:

- Fever.
- Fatigue, malaise, anorexia, nausea.
- Arthralgia.
- Right upper quadrant abdominal pain.
- Jaundice ± hepatomegaly; splenomegaly.
- Adenopathy, urticaria.

Investigations

- LFTs: raised bilirubin >20mg/L; raised AST/ALT (× 2–100).
- Low blood glucose (especially in Reye syndrome).
- Viral serology (IgM antibodies), viral PCR (HCV), EBV heterophil antibodies (Monospot or Paul–Bunnell).
- Blood culture if appropriate.
- Paracetamol level or halothane antibodies, if relevant.
- Serum immunoglobulin, complements (C3, C4), +ve autoimmune antibodies (anti-smooth muscle, anti-mitochondrial, and/or anti-liver and kidney microsomal) in autoimmune hepatitis.
- Serum copper/caeruloplasmin, 24h urinary copper (Wilson's disease).
- Urinary succinylacetone (tyrosinaemia type I).

Management

Usually none is required, except support and rest:

- Alcohol avoidance in teenagers.
- No place for antivirals unless the child is immune-compromised.
- Fulminant hepatitis requires referral to a specialist unit for PICU management and possible liver transplantation.
- *Reye syndrome:* maintain blood glucose >4mmol/L; prevent sepsis; provide intensive care support.

Prognosis

- Acute hepatitis is usually self-limiting.
- Mortality after fulminant hepatitis is ~30% if both cerebral oedema and renal failure are absent; ~70% if both are present without liver transplant.
- There is a long-term risk of:
  - Chronic hepatitis (HAV, 0%; HBV, 5–10%; HCV, ~85%).
  - Cirrhosis.
  - Hepatocellular carcinoma (HCC) (HBV and HCV).
  - Glomerulonephritis (circulating immune complexes).

Prevention

Active immunization exists for both HAV and HBV. Within 24h of infectious contact, infection may be prevented by giving pooled serum immunoglobulin for HAV and CMV, or specific HBV serum immunoglobulin for HBV.

Chronic liver disease

(See also ⊃ Systems—hepatic, pp. 506–7.)

Causes

- Chronic hepatitis (after viral hepatitis B or C).
- Non-alcoholic steatohepatitis (fatty liver disease).
- Biliary tree disease, e.g. biliary atresia.
- α1-antitrypsin deficiency.
- Autoimmune hepatitis.
- Wilson's disease (age >3y).
- CF.
- Alagille syndrome or non-syndromic paucity of bile ducts.
- Tyrosinaemia.
- Primary sclerosing cholangitis.
- Budd–Chiari syndrome.
- Toxin-induced, e.g. paracetamol, alcohol.
- PN-induced.

Presentation

- Jaundice (not always).
- GI haemorrhage (portal hypertension and variceal bleeding).
- Pruritus.
- FTT.
- Anaemia.
- Enlarged, hard liver (though liver often small in cirrhosis).
- Non-tender splenomegaly.
- Hepatic stigmata, e.g. spider naevi.
- Peripheral oedema and/or ascites.
- Nutritional disorders, e.g. rickets.
- Developmental delay or deterioration in school performance.
- Chronic encephalopathy.

Investigations

Blood tests

- LFTs [↑/normal bilirubin, ↑ AST/ALT (× 2–10), albumin <35g/L].
- FBC (low Hb if GI bleeding); low WCC and platelets (hypersplenism).
- Coagulation (PT ↑ if vitamin K deficiency).
- Low/normal blood glucose.
- U&E (low Na^+, low Ca^{2+}, ↑ PO_4^{3-}, ↑ ALP if biochemical rickets).
- Viral serology or PCR for hepatitis B and C.
- ↑ IgG, low complements (C3, C4), autoimmune antibodies.

Metabolic studies

- Sweat test (CF); α1-antitrypsin level and phenotype.
- Low serum copper and caeruloplasmin (Wilson's disease).
- ↑ 24h urinary copper (Wilson's disease).

Abdominal US/MRI
- Hepatomegaly.
- Echogenic liver.
- Splenomegaly.
- Evidence of portal hypertension
- Ascites.

Upper GI endoscopy
- Oesophageal or gastric varices.
- Portal hypertension-related gastritis.

EEG
- To confirm chronic encephalopathy if suspected.

Liver biopsy
- Histology, enzymes, EM.

Management
- Treat underlying cause and give nutritional support.
- Diet: lower protein, ↑ energy, higher-carbohydrate diet.
- Vitamin supplementation, particularly fat-soluble vitamins A, D, E, and K. Involve a paediatric dietician.

Drug therapy
- Prednisolone ± azathioprine for autoimmune hepatitis.
- Interferon-alfa ± ribavirin for chronic viral hepatitis.
- Penicillamine for Wilson's disease.
- Colestyramine may be useful to control severe pruritus.
- Vitamin K1 and FFP (10mL/kg) if significant coagulopathy or bleeding.

Oesophageal varices
- Endoscopy, i.e. sclerotherapy or surgery.

Ascites
- Fluid and Na⁺ restriction (two-thirds maintenance and 1mmol/kg/day, respectively).
- Spironolactone (1–2mg/kg 12-hourly).
- Consider IV 20% albumin (with furosemide) if ascites is resistant to above treatment.

Encephalopathy
Reduce GI ammonia absorption using PO or rectal lactulose, neomycin, or soluble fibre pectin.

Liver transplantation
(See ➔ Liver transplantation, p. 315.)

Prognosis
There is up to 50% 5y mortality without liver transplant. Poor prognostic factors are:
- Blood: bilirubin >50 micromoles/L; albumin <30g/L; PT >6s.
- Ascites, encephalopathy, malnutrition.

α1-antitrypsin deficiency

α1-antitrypsin (serum protease inhibitor) deficiency:
- Is the commonest genetic cause of liver disease in children, with AD inheritance. Prevalence is 1/2000 to 1/7000.
- Genetic variants are identified by enzyme electrophoretic mobility as medium (M), slow (S), or very slow (Z). S is associated with ~60% α1-antitrypsin level of normal; Z ~15%. Normal genotype is designated PiMM. Only PiZZ individuals are at risk of liver disease.

Presentation

- Cholestasis in infancy, may progress to liver failure.
- Cirrhosis can occur in late childhood to adult. Chronic liver disease affects 25% of patients in late adulthood.
- Pulmonary emphysema is the commonest presentation in adulthood.

Diagnosis

- Serum α1-antitrypsin level low.
- Phenotyping by enzyme isoelectric focusing.

Treatment

- Supportive treatment of liver complications.
- Strongly advise against smoking.
- Liver transplant for end-stage liver failure.

Wilson's disease

Rare AR disorder leading to toxic accumulation of copper in the liver, and subsequently the brain and eye.

Presentation

- Kayser–Fleischer rings (copper deposition in Descemet's membrane of the eye) often present (45% with hepatic presentation and 90% with neurological presentation) and pathognomonic (use slit-lamp).
- Hepatic problems usually present in childhood (hepatitis, cirrhosis, fulminant hepatic failure).
- Adolescents/young adults usually present with neurological disease.

Investigations

- Serum copper and caeruloplasmin low.
- 24h urinary copper excretion >100mcg (normal <40mcg).
- Molecular genetics—Wilson's disease gene (*ATP7B*) mutation.

Treatment

- Lifelong chelation therapy with penicillamine (reverses pre-cirrhotic liver disease, but not neurological damage).
- Liver transplantation if end-stage hepatic failure.

Liver transplantation

Indications for liver transplantation

The commonest underlying conditions leading to irreversible liver failure and transplant are:
- *Fulminant hepatic failure:* e.g. viral, toxic, Wilson's disease.
- Biliary atresia.
- *Chronic end-stage liver disease:* e.g. post-viral hepatitis with cirrhosis.
- *Liver-based metabolic conditions:* e.g. Wilson's disease, α1-antitrypsin deficiency, Crigler–Najjar syndrome, tyrosinaemia.
- *Acute liver failure following liver transplant:* e.g. primary non-function of transplant or hepatic artery thrombosis.
- Neonatal hepatitis.
- Autoimmune hepatitis.
- *Unresectable tumour confined to the liver:* e.g. hepatoblastoma.

Features requiring consideration for transplantation

- Bleeding varices due to portal hypertension.
- Failure of growth or development.
- Resistant ascites.
- Hepatic encephalopathy.
- *Poor quality of life:* e.g. pruritus, lethargy.
- Coagulopathy (PTT >2 times normal).
- *Multiorgan failure:* e.g. hepatorenal syndrome, hepatopulmonary syndrome.

Preparation for transplant

Requires multidisciplinary evaluation to include the following:
- Nutritional support.
- Development and psychological assessment of child and family.
- Education and counselling.
- Ensure vaccinations current: e.g. MMR, varicella, hepatitis A and B.
- Cardiac evaluation (ECG, echocardiogram).
- Abdominal US (patency of major hepatic blood vessels).

Post-transplant complications

- Primary non-function of the liver (<5%).
- Hepatic artery thrombosis (10–15%).
- Biliary leaks and strictures (20%).
- Acute rejection (50%).
- Chronic rejection (5–10%).
- Sepsis (main cause of death).

Prognosis

Long-term studies indicate normal psychosocial development and quality of life in survivors. Patients require lifelong immunosuppression drug therapy, e.g. ciclosporin or tacrolimus.
- 1y survival is 90%.
- 5y survival is 80%.

References

1. National Institute for Health and Care Excellence. (2015).*Coeliac disease: recognition, assessment and management*. NICE guideline [NG20]. Available at: ℜ https://www.nice.org.uk/guidance/ng20.

Nephrology

Haematuria

Blood in urine (haematuria) may be visible (macroscopic) or detected only by dipstick testing or microscopy (microscopic). Urine RBCs of ≥10 per high-power field is abnormal. Urine dipsticks are very sensitive and can be +ve at <5 RBCs per high-power field. Asymptomatic haematuria is found in up to 2% of children.

Presentation

- Episode(s) of macroscopic haematuria.
- Incidental finding of microscopic haematuria.
- Family screening and routine urinalysis.

Other causes of 'red urine'

Urine microscopy is mandatory to exclude other causes of red urine:
- Haemoglobinuria/myoglobinuria.
- Foods—colouring (e.g. beetroot).
- Drugs (e.g. rifampicin).
- Urate crystals (in young infants, usually 'pink' nappies).
- External source (e.g. menstrual blood losses).
- Fictitious—consider if no cause found.

Assessment

The history and examination will direct investigation.

History
- Haematuria at the beginning or end of the urinary stream suggests bladder or urethral cause.
- Red urine is more likely from the lower urinary tract; tea-/cola-coloured is more likely glomerular.
- Asymptomatic haematuria is commoner with familial glomerular disease or IgA nephropathy (see ⊋ Glomerular diseases, pp. 322–3).
- Symptomatic haematuria: pain suggests calculi, pelviureteric junction (PUJ) obstruction, UTI, urethritis, balanitis, vulvovaginitis.
- Symptoms of acute nephritis (see ⊋ Glomerular diseases, pp. 322–3).
- Renal tumours are very rare. Clots may be passed.

Examination
- Monitor weight and any changes.
- Check BP and any changes; check for oedema.
- Abdomen: urinary meatus and perineum, palpable masses?
- Skin: rashes?
- Joints: pain/swelling?

Investigations

All children:
- Urine:
  - Microscopy (to confirm RBCs present, and for casts—suggestive of nephritis) and culture.
  - Protein:creatinine ratio (normal <20mg/mmol).
  - Ca^{2+}:creatinine ratio (normal <0.7mmol/mmol).
- USS of urinary tract.
- If glomerular cause suspected, then blood tests:
  - U&E, creatinine, albumin.
  - FBC, clotting.
  - Complement—C3/C4, ASOT.
  - ANA and anti-double-stranded deoxyribonucleic acid (dsDNA) antibodies.
- Urinalysis of parents (hereditary causes).

Treatment
- If obvious cause (e.g. UTI), treat.
- If PUJ obstruction, urethral abnormality, calculus, or haematuria at beginning or end of urinary stream, refer to paediatric urology.
- If history and investigations suggest glomerular cause, with ↑ BP, proteinuria, and/or abnormal blood tests, refer to paediatric nephrology.
- If isolated persistent microscopic haematuria, annual follow-up to check for ↑ BP and proteinuria, with referral to paediatric nephrology, should they develop.

Proteinuria

Small amounts of protein may be found in the urine of healthy children, but are <0.15g/24h.

Detection of proteinuria

Urinalysis

Performed by dipstick testing (see Table 8.1), which is a cheap, practicable, and sensitive method that primarily detects albumin in the urine. It is less sensitive for other forms of proteinuria.

Table 8.1 Urinalysis by dipstick testing

Test result	Equivalent protein estimate (g/L)
+	0.2
++	1.0
+++	3.0
++++	≥20

Urinary protein:creatinine (Upr:Ucr) ratio

Collection of an early morning urine (EMU) specimen for measurement of Upr:Ucr ratio. Normal <20mg/mmol.

24h urinary protein excretion

This is the gold standard test and requires a 24h collection of urine to estimate urinary protein excretion.

- Normal: <30mg/24h.
- Microalbuminuria: 30–300mg/24h.
- Proteinuria: >300mg/24h.

Causes of proteinuria

Proteinuria may be due to benign or pathological causes.

Benign proteinuria

- *Transient or intermittent:* does not need investigation.
- *Fever.*
- *Exercise.*
- *Orthostatic proteinuria (postural proteinuria):* common reason for referral in older children. There is no history of significance, and a normal examination. The Upr:Ucr ratio in the first urine of the morning taken immediately on rising is normal, but levels are elevated thereafter. *A benign finding and requires no treatment.*

Pathological (persistent) proteinuria
- Glomerular diseases.
- Tubular diseases.

History and examination
- Symptoms.
- Family history.
- Growth.
- BP.
- Monitor weight and presence of oedema.

Investigations
- Urine microscopy for RBCs.
- Urine albumin-to-creatinine (Ua:Ucr) ratio or Upr:Ucr ratio.
- Urine retinol-binding protein-to-creatinine (Urbp:Ucr) ratio, or other low-molecular weight protein, when tubular disease suspected.
- Renal USS.
- U&Es, creatinine, and albumin.
- FBC.
- ASOT, C3, C4, anti-dsDNA binding, hepatitis B and C (if acute nephritis suspected).
- Check urine of parents and siblings for blood and protein.

Refer to paediatric nephrology if
- Persistent proteinuria on an EMU sample detected over a period of 6–12mth.
- If any of the above investigations are abnormal.
- Family history of proteinuria and renal disease.

Glomerular diseases

Inherited glomerular diseases

Many glomerular diseases have identified genetic causes:
- 30% of patients with steroid-resistant nephrotic syndrome have identified mutations.
- Familial haematuria:
  - Alport syndrome: nephritis, sensorineural (SN) deafness, and often eye abnormalities. Classical Alport syndrome is due to mutations in type IV collagen.
  - Thin basement membrane, once thought of as mild but may progress to chronic kidney disease (CKD), as in Alport syndrome.

Acute glomerulonephritis

- A combination of haematuria, oliguria, oedema, and hypertension, with variable proteinuria and abnormal renal function.
- The majority of cases are post-streptococcal infection, presenting 1–2wk after an URTI and sore throat.
- Any infection can be a cause.

Causes of acute glomerulonephritis (GN)

Post-infectious

Others (less common)
- C3 glomerulopathy.
- IgA nephropathy.
- SLE.
- Subacute bacterial endocarditis.
- Shunt nephritis.

Investigations
- *Urine:*
  - Urinalysis by dipstick: haematuria ± proteinuria.
  - Microscopy—casts (mostly RBC casts).
- *Throat swab:* culture.
- *Bloods:*
  - FBC.
  - U&E, creatinine, HCO_3^-, Ca^{2+}, PO_4^{3-}, albumin.
  - ASOT/anti-DNAse B.
  - Complement C3 and C4.
  - Autoantibody screen (include ANA).
- *Renal USS.*
- *CXR:* if fluid overload suspected.

Management

Most cases need admission because of fluid imbalance, worsening renal function, or hypertension. Treat life-threatening complications.

First:

- Hyperkalaemia (see ➲ Hyperkalaemia, p. 73).
- Hypertension (see ➲ Hypertension, p. 47; ➲ Hypertension management, p. 348).
- Acidosis (see ➲ Unexplained metabolic acidosis, p. 75).
- Seizures (see ➲ Status epilepticus, p. 64).
- Hypocalcaemia (see ➲ Hypocalcaemia, p. 74).

Otherwise supportive treatment:

- *Fluid balance:*
  - Weigh daily.
  - No added/restricted-salt diet.
  - If oliguric, fluid restrict to insensible losses ($400mL/m^2$) + urine output.
  - Consider furosemide 1–2mg/kg bd.
- *Hypertension:*
  - Treat fluid overload; therefore, furosemide is the usual first choice.
  - Calcium channel blocker as second choice.
  - NB: do not use ACE inhibitor (may worsen renal function).
- *Infection:*
  - A 10-day course of penicillin (does not affect natural history but limits spread of nephritogenic bacterial strains).

When to refer to paediatric nephrology unit

- Patients with life-threatening complications.
- Those with atypical features, including:
  - Worsening renal function.
  - Nephrotic state.
  - Evidence of systemic vasculitis (e.g. rash).
  - +ve ANA.
  - Persisting proteinuria at 6wk.
  - Persisting low C3 at 3mth.

Prognosis

- 95% with post-streptococcal GN recover completely.
- For other GNs, outcome depends on cause.
- Microscopic haematuria may persist for years.
- Discharge from follow-up once urinalysis, BP, and creatinine are normal.
- Ongoing proteinuria requires referral to paediatric nephrology.

Nephrotic syndrome

Nephrotic syndrome is a triad of:
- Heavy proteinuria (Upr:Ucr ratio >200mg/mmol).
- Hypoalbuminaemia (serum albumin <25g/L).
- Oedema.

Definitions

- *Congenital nephrotic syndrome:* presents during the first 3mth of life (often present before or at birth).
- *Infantile nephrotic syndrome:* presents between 3 and 12mth of age.
- *Steroid-sensitive nephrotic syndrome:*
  - *Idiopathic nephrotic syndrome:* nephrotic syndrome in the absence of other glomerular pathology mediated by systemic disease (e.g. SLE), structural glomerular changes (e.g. Alport syndrome), vasculitis, immune complex deposition (e.g. post-infectious GN).
  - *Frequently relapsing nephrotic syndrome:* two or more relapses in the first 6mth after presentation or four times within any year.
  - *Steroid-dependent nephrotic syndrome:* relapse while on steroid therapy or within 14 days of stopping.
- *Steroid-resistant nephrotic syndrome:* failure of proteinuria to resolve following at least 28 days of prednisone 60mg/m^2/day.

Clinical features

Presentation is with insidious development of oedema, initially periorbital (most noticeable in the morning on rising) and becoming generalized, with pitting oedema. Ascites, labial and scrotal swelling, and pleural effusions may develop.

Examination

- Assessment of oedema.
- Height and weight (monitor weight daily; compare with recent measurements).
- BP.
- Peripheral perfusion (core–peripheral temperature gap or CRT).

Investigations

Urine

- *Urinalysis:* proteinuria.
- *Microscopy:* haematuria/casts, which suggest causes other than minimal change disease (MCD).
- Upr:Ucr ratio (EMU specimen).

Bloods

- Serum albumin (reduced, <25g/L).
- U&E/creatinine ($\downarrow$ Na^+ and total Ca^{2+}—with normal ionized Ca^{2+}).
- C3/C4 (if $\downarrow$, suggests not MCD).
- Consider ANA, ASOT, ANCA, immunoglobulins if mixed nephritic/nephrotic picture.
- *Lipids:* total cholesterol/low-density lipoprotein (LDL)/very low-density lipoprotein (VLDL).
- Hb may be $\uparrow$ or $\downarrow$, depending on plasma volume.
- Varicella-zoster immunity status.

Management

Patients should be admitted, particularly if this is their first episode or if there are concerns regarding complications.

Treatment

- Treat hypovolaemia if present, but albumin infusion is not routine.
- Diuretics if very oedematous and no evidence of hypovolaemia (peripherally warm); furosemide/spironolactone.
- Diet (no added salt—high protein is not necessary).

Steroid therapy

- PO prednisolone 60mg/m² day for 4wk.
- Followed by 40mg/m²/alternate days for 4wk.
- Then: *stop*—slow wean is an alternative over next 4mth with slow taper, but need to consider side effects of steroids.

Steroid-resistant nephrotic syndrome

- The majority have focal segmental glomerulosclerosis (FSGS).
- A genetic cause can be found in 30%, with more genes being identified all the time.
- Because of the high risk of progression to end-stage kidney disease (ESKD), these children are followed up in a paediatric nephrology centre.

Nephrotic syndrome: complications and follow-up

Complications

Complications secondary to fluid imbalance and impaired immunity:

Infection

Predisposition to infection is due to ↓ IgG levels, and to impaired opsonization due to steroid immunosuppression. Bacterial peritonitis (especially *Streptococcus pneumoniae*) is an important complication and should be considered in any child with nephrotic syndrome who complains of abdominal pain.

Thrombosis

Nephrotic syndrome produces a hypercoagulable state and predisposition to both arterial and venous thrombus.

Hypovolaemia

Suggested by the development of oliguria and prolonged CRT (cool peripheries). Patients may complain of abdominal pain. This is a clinical diagnosis because:

- Urinary Na⁺ is not helpful in nephrotic states, as levels may be low (<10mmol/L) in both hypo- and hypervolaemia. Levels will be high when a child is on furosemide:
  - In *hypovolaemia*, levels will be low due to avid salt and water retention by the kidney.
  - In *hypervolaemia*, levels may also be low due to primary Na⁺ retention in nephrotic syndrome.
- An elevated Hb concentration is suggestive of haemoconcentration, i.e. hypovolaemia.
- Hypovolaemia should be promptly corrected with the use of 10–20mL/kg of 4.5% albumin solution or another colloid, and diuretics should be stopped or avoided.

Acute kidney injury (AKI)

Pre-renal and secondary to hypovolaemia.

Indications for renal biopsy

The majority of patients will have MCD and will respond to steroids. Biopsy is therefore reserved for those with atypical features:

- Age <12mth or >12y.
- ↑ BP.
- Macroscopic haematuria.
- Impaired renal function.
- ↓ C3/C4.
- Failure to respond after 1mth of daily steroid therapy.

Follow-up

Prognosis

- The majority of cases respond to steroids. Of these:
  - 33%—single relapse.
  - 33%—occasional relapses.
  - 33%—steroid dependence.
- These children do not develop CKD, except in the very rare cases of secondary steroid resistance.

Relapse

A relapse is defined as detection of urine dipstick ++ proteinuria for >3 days. *Frequent relapse* is defined as >2 relapses within 6mth of initial response or ≥4 relapses in any 12mth.

Management of relapses

Because of the high risk of progression to ESKD, these children are followed up in a paediatric nephrology centre. Each relapse is treated with PO steroids as above (see ◗ Nephrotic syndrome: treatment, pp. 324–25). Alternative strategies for frequent relapses include continuation of the smallest dose of prednisolone to prevent relapse ± a trial of therapy with other agents:

- Levamisole.
- Cyclophosphamide.
- Mycophenolate mofetil (MMF).
- Ciclosporin or tacrolimus.
- Anti-CD20 monoclonal antibody (rituximab).

Congenital abnormalities of the kidneys and urinary tract (CAKUT)

- Most structural urinary tract anomalies are detected during routine antenatal USS.
- Renal anomalies account for about 20% of all significant abnormalities found on detailed scans at 18–20wk gestation.
- Close liaison between obstetrician, paediatrician, and surgeon with regard to counselling the parents and follow-up is vital.
- Centres should have a postnatal management protocol, as the majority of infants will be asymptomatic.
- Low amniotic fluid volume may indicate low urine production or urinary obstruction and is associated with pulmonary hypoplasia.

Classification of antenatal USS abnormalities

Any antenatal USS abnormality will require a postnatal plan, e.g.:
- Renal tract dilatation, which may be of the renal pelvis and/or calyces (hydronephrosis) and/or ureter (hydroureteronephrosis).
- The bladder may have diverticulae, be thick-walled, and/or show poor emptying; a dilated posterior urethra may be seen [posterior urethral valves (PUVs)].
- Absent kidney(s).
- Large, small, echogenic, or cystic kidneys.

Postnatal findings

The postnatal USS of the renal tract should assess for:
- *Hydronephrosis:*
  - Unilateral: PUJ or vesicoureteric junction (VUJ) abnormality; vesicoureteric reflux (VUR).
  - Bilateral: bladder outlet obstruction, e.g. PUV, VUR.
- *Renal cysts:*
  - Multicystic dysplastic kidney (MCDK).
  - Cystic dysplasia.
  - Other non-CAKUT causes: polycystic kidney diseases (PCKDs).
- *Abnormal renal parenchyma, if echogenic:*
  - Dysplastic or cystic kidneys (any cause).
  - Congenital nephrotic syndrome (may have polyhydramnios, large placenta).

Clinical management

A ♂ infant with a thick-walled bladder or ureteric dilatation needs an urgent micturating cystourethrogram (MCUG) to exclude a PUV. Further investigations will depend on the suspected cause.

Urinary tract infection

Up to 3% of girls and 1% of boys have a symptomatic UTI. The highest incidence is in the first year of life. UTI involving the kidneys (pyelonephritis) is associated with fever and systemic upset. UTI restricted to the bladder (cystitis) leads to absent or low-grade fever. Up to half of children with UTI have structural abnormality of the urinary tract. UTI is important because if the upper tracts are involved, it may damage the growing kidney by forming a scar, predisposing to hypertension and, if bilateral, CKD.

UK NICE guidelines (available at: ℘ https://www.nice.org.uk/guidance/cg54) recommend the testing of urine in infants and children with:
- Symptoms and signs of UTI.
- Unexplained fever of ≥38°C (test urine within 24h).
- An alternative site of infection but who remain unwell (consider urine test after 24h at the latest).

Clinical features

Presentation of UTI varies:
- In the *newborn*, symptoms are non-specific; septicaemia may develop rapidly.
- The *classical symptoms* of dysuria, frequency, and loin pain become commoner with increasing age.
- The presence of loin pain, systemic upset, and fever are suggestive of *pyelonephritis*.
- Dysuria without a fever is often due to vulvitis in *girls* or urethritis or balanitis in *boys*, or to cystitis without upper tract involvement.

Examination

- Height and weight: plot on growth chart.
- BP.
- Abdomen, including genitalia.
- Spine and lower limbs if neuropathic bladder suspected.

UTI: urine collection and diagnosis

UK NICE recommended techniques for the child in nappies include:
• A 'clean-catch' sample into a waiting sterile pot when the nappy is removed; this is easier in boys.
• Absorbent urine collection pads, e.g. Newcastle sterile urine collection packs, in the nappy (not cotton wool, gauze, sanitary towels).
• Catheter sample or SPA using USS guidance when non-invasive methods are not possible.
• *Bag samples are not recommended* because of false +ve rate of 85%. However, this method can be used as a screening test. A –ve result confidently excludes a diagnosis of UTI.

In the older child
• Midstream sample. Careful cleaning and collection needed; contamination with WBCs and bacteria occurs from under the foreskin (boys) or from urine reflux into the vagina during voiding (girls).

Diagnosis
• Any growth on culture of SPA or catheter sample.
• >10^5 organisms/mL of a pure growth.
• It is important to distinguish between upper and lower tract UTI:
    • *Pyelonephritis:* bacteriuria loin pain/tenderness, systemic involvement, and fever >38°C.
    • *Cystitis:* bacteriuria, dysuria, frequency, enuresis, but no systemic features.
    • *Asymptomatic bacteriuria:* rarely of significance.

Bacterial and host factors predisposing to infection

The infecting organism
• Bowel flora enter the urinary tract via the urethra, except in the newborn, which is more often haematogenous.
• Commonest organisms: *Escherichia coli, Proteus*, and *Pseudomonas* spp.
• Virulence of *E. coli* depends on cell wall appendages (P-fimbriae), which allow attachment to the ureter and ascent to the kidney.
• Infecting organisms other than *E. coli* are more likely to be associated with structural abnormalities of the urinary tract.

Incomplete bladder emptying
The most important cause of UTI and may be due to:
• Infrequent voiding, resulting in bladder enlargement.
• Vulvitis or urethritis/balanitis.
• Hurried micturition.
• Obstruction by a loaded rectum from constipation.
• Neuropathic bladder.
• VUR.

Vesicoureteric reflux

VUR varies from reflux into the lower end of an undilated ureter during micturition to the severest form with reflux during bladder filling and voiding, with a dilated ureter, renal pelvis, and clubbed calyces.

* *Primary VUR*, a developmental anomaly of VUJ, by definition not associated with bladder pathology (~1% of young children).
* *Secondary VUR* may be due to neuropathic bladder or urethral obstruction or occur temporarily after a UTI.
* *VUR with associated ureteric dilatation* is important because:
  * Refluxed urine returning to the bladder from the ureters after voiding results in incomplete bladder emptying.
  * ↑ work placed upon the bladder may result in bladder dysfunction and decompensation over time.
  * The kidneys may become infected (pyelonephritis), particularly if there is intrarenal reflux, resulting in renal scarring.
  * Renal scarring may lead to high BP (variously estimated at up to 10%) or to CKD if bilateral.
  * Bladder voiding pressure is transmitted directly to the renal papillae; this may contribute to renal damage if there is an abnormal bladder with high voiding pressures.
  * There is no evidence that primary VUR of uninfected urine at normal pressure damages the kidney.
  * There may be associated renal dysplasia—termed 'reflux nephropathy' in the past and frequently due to congenital renal dysplasia, with or without additional acquired infection.
  * VUR is frequently familial, with a 30–50% chance of occurring in first-degree relatives.

Prognosis

* Mild VUR is unlikely to be of significance, either in causing UTI or renal scarring.
* The incidence of renal defects on scanning increases with increasing severity of VUR; however, half of children with renal defects do not have VUR.
* DMSA scans cannot distinguish between renal scars and renal dysplasia (unless there is development of new areas), so abnormalities should be called 'defects'.
* VUR resolves in 10% of cases/year. VUR into dilated ureters is less likely to resolve, particularly if abnormal kidneys.
* Conversely, VUR associated with two normal kidneys is very likely to resolve

UTI: acute management

(See also ➲ Table 16.3.) There should be a high suspicion for UTI during acute illnesses. UTIs should be promptly identified and treated with antibiotics:

- Most children can be treated with PO antibiotics.
- Use IV antibiotics in infants/children who are severely ill, vomiting, or immunosuppressed until the temperature settled; then PO.
- Most laboratories monitor local bacterial resistance patterns and are able to advise prescribers accordingly.
- Asymptomatic bacteriuria should not be treated with antibiotics, either acutely or with prophylactic therapy.
- Antibiotic prophylaxis is not recommended unless recurrent UTIs.

Investigations

NICE guidelines have defined an atypical UTI, which leads to more intensive investigation. Investigation is also dependent on age.

Definition of an atypical UTI
- Seriously ill child.
- Poor urine flow.
- Abdominal or bladder mass.
- Raised plasma creatinine.
- Septicaemia.
- Failure to respond to treatment within 48h.
- Non-*E. coli* UTI.

Imaging studies
Since mild VUR usually resolves spontaneously, and surgery to stop VUR has not been shown to decrease renal scarring, radiological investigations are reserved for infants and children at greatest risk of developing renal scarring (see NICE guidance)[1] (see Tables 8.2–8.4).

Table 8.2 Infants aged <6mth

Test	Responds well to treatment with 48h	Atypical UTI or recurrent UTI
USS during acute infection	No	Yes
USS within 6wk	Yes	No
DMSA 4–6mth after acute infection	No	Yes
MCUG	No	Yes

Table 8.3 Children aged >6mth, but <3y

Test	Responds well to treatment with 48h	Atypical UTI	Recurrent UTI
USS during the acute infection	No	Yes	No
USS within 6wk	No	No	Yes
DMSA 4–6mth after acute infection	No	Yes	Yes
MCUG	No	No	Yes

Table 8.4 Children aged >3y

Test	Responds well to treatment with 48h	Atypical UTI	Recurrent UTI
USS during acute infection	No	Yes	No
USS within 6wk	No	No	Yes
DMSA 4–6mth after acute infection	No	No	Yes
MCUG	No	No	Yes

UTI: long-term management

Prevention of urinary tract infection

General measures to prevent UTI

- High fluid intake to produce high urine output.
- Regular voiding.
- Complete bladder emptying using double micturition to empty any residual or refluxed urine returning to the bladder.
- Prevention or treatment of constipation.
- Good perineal hygiene.
- *Lactobacillus acidophilus*, to encourage colonization of the gut by this organism.

Antibiotic prophylaxis

The use of antibiotic prophylaxis is controversial. UK NICE guidelines do not recommend routine prophylaxis following a first UTI, although this may be considered in those with recurrent UTIs. Prophylaxis is used most in those <2y of age and those with ureters that are dilated up to the renal pelvis. Antibiotics include:

- Trimethoprim (2mg/kg at night).
- Nitrofurantoin (1mg/kg at night).
- Nalidixic acid (7.5mg/kg bd).
- Broad-spectrum, poorly absorbed antibiotics, such as amoxicillin, should be avoided.

Follow-up

- *Routine urine culture* in well children should not be undertaken.
- *No further imaging* is necessary in a child with no or unilateral defects, with no further UTIs.
- Renal defects require *annual BP checks* for life, although hypertension is uncommon.
- Regular *assessment of renal function* and growth using USS and EMU dipstick testing for proteinuria for those with bilateral renal defects who are at risk of progressive CKD.
- Circumcision may benefit boys with recurrent UTIs. It has been estimated ~100 circumcisions are required to prevent one case of UTI.
- Anti-reflux surgery may be indicated if there is progression of scarring with ongoing VUR, but outcome has not been shown to be better than the use of antibiotic prophylaxis. Open re-implantation of the ureters has been replaced by peri-ureteric injection of bulking agents (STING procedure). However, the success rate is less for this procedure than for re-implantation of the ureters and it often needs to be repeated.

- There is no evidence for when antibiotic prophylaxis (if used) should be stopped. This should be considered at the age of 2y (by when maximum renal growth has occurred) or after 1y free of UTIs. Others will discontinue antibiotics once the child achieves daytime continence.
- If there are further symptomatic UTIs, investigations are required to determine whether there are new scars or continuing VUR. New scars are rare in previously unscarred kidneys after the age of 4y, even with VUR.

Asymptomatic bacteriuria

Occasionally bacteriuria may be discovered during investigation of another problem in an asymptomatic child. Although treatment with antibiotics will eradicate the bacteriuria, recurrence is common. Asymptomatic bacteriuria should not be treated, as long-term follow-up studies have shown that it does not cause renal damage in otherwise healthy children and there is a risk of developing infection with antibiotic-resistant organisms.

Renal tubular disorders

The renal tubules (RTs) regulate fluid and electrolytes, and acid–base balance. Abnormalities may occur at any point along the length of the RT and may lead to a disturbance in the equilibrium of any substances handled by it. Consider these disorders when there are any of the following, particularly if there is FTT:

- *Glycosuria, amino aciduria, or impaired ability to concentrate or acidify urine:* RTA, Fanconi syndrome.
- *Stones or nephrocalcinosis:* distal tubular acidosis.
- *Polyhydramnios and FTT in a newborn:* Bartter syndrome associated with hypokalaemic alkalosis.
- *FTT with rickets:* cystinosis, commonest cause of Fanconi syndrome.
- *Rickets with low plasma PO43– levels:* familial hypophosphataemic rickets.
- *FTT with low urine osmolality:* nephrogenic diabetes insipidus (NDI).

Renal tubular acidosis

Proximal RTA

(See also → Unexplained metabolic acidosis, p. 75.)

Reduced proximal tubular reabsorption of HCO_3^-, resulting in urinary HCO_3^- wasting:

- The threshold when urinary HCO_3^- wasting ceases: 15–18mmol/L.
- Because distal HCO_3^- acidification is intact, urinary pH can be <5.
- Proximal RTA may occur as an isolated disorder, with no other abnormalities of tubular function (rare).
- Proximal RTA also occurs as a generalized defect of proximal RT transport: with glycosuria, phosphaturia, amino aciduria, organic aciduria, low-molecular weight proteinuria, and wasting of Na^+, K^+, Ca^{2+}, and uric acid (Fanconi syndrome). Fanconi syndrome may be primary/ secondary to inherited or acquired disease (see Box 8.1).

> **Box 8.1 Causes of Fanconi syndrome**
> - Primary.
> - Secondary:
>   - Cystinosis.
>   - Galactosaemia.
>   - Wilson's disease.
>   - Lowe syndrome.
>   - Vitamin D deficiency rickets.
>   - Hypothyroidism.

Distal RTA

- Deficiency in H^+ secretion by distal tubules and collecting ducts.
- Urine pH cannot be reduced below 5.5.
- Hyperchloraemia and hypokalaemia are characteristic, but less severe than that found in proximal RTA.
- Nephrocalcinosis may be present. Distal RTA may be isolated or a secondary complication of other diseases (see Box 8.2).

Box 8.2 Causes of distal renal tubular acidosis
- Primary.
- Secondary:
  - CKD.
  - Autoimmune disease.
  - Toxins/drugs involving distal tubule/collecting duct.

Diagnosis

Other causes of systemic acidosis (e.g. chronic diarrhoea, lactic acidosis, DKA) should be excluded. Investigations to establish a diagnosis of RTA should include:
- Blood: pH, HCO_3^- (low), K^+ (low), Cl^- (high).
- Urine—early morning sample:
  - pH <5.5 suggests proximal RTA.
  - pH ≥5.5 suggests distal RTA.

If proximal RTA is detected, blood and urinalysis to establish other tubular defects should be undertaken.

Treatment

Correct acidosis and maintain normal HCO_3^- and K^+—achieve with alkali (citrate or HCO_3^-) or K^+-containing solutions.

Bartter syndrome

- Hypokalaemic, hypochloraemic metabolic alkalosis with elevated renin and aldosterone levels, and normal to low BP.
- Polyuria, polydipsia, and salt craving to replace renal losses.
- Maintain serum K^+ >3.0mmol/L with PO K^+ supplement and a K^+-sparing diuretic (e.g. spironolactone) and indometacin (prostaglandin inhibitor).

Nephrogenic diabetes insipidus

- Tubular unresponsiveness to antidiuretic hormone [arginine vasopressin (AVP)], with ↑ volume of dilute urine with polydipsia, polyuria, and FTT.
- X-linked in 90% of cases of NDI.
- To differentiate central DI from NDI, a desmopressin (DDAVP®) test is performed.
- *Treatment:*
  - Reduce the osmotic load, which mainly consists of salts and protein, and free access to water.
  - Thiazides and indometacin.
  - IV fluids should be given as 5% glucose without saline.

Renal calculi

The incidence of renal calculi varies according to geography and socio-economic conditions around the world.

Aetiology

Infective (25%)
- Associated with chronic UTI with *Proteus*—'staghorn' calculi.
- Also UTI with *Pseudomonas, Klebsiella,* and *E. coli.*
- Associated with urinary stasis due to CAKUT.

Metabolic (50%)
- *Hypercalciuria:* i.e. 24h urinary Ca^{2+} >0.1mmol/kg/day or urinary Ca^{2+}:creatinine ratio >0.74mmol/mmol:
  - Prolonged immobilization, hypervitaminosis D.
  - Primary hyperparathyroidism, idiopathic infantile hypercalcaemia.
- *Cystinuria:* typically radiolucent stones.
- *Oxalosis:* primary hyperoxaluria.
- *Uric acid stones:*
  - Myeloproliferative disorders following medication/chemotherapy.
  - For patients with leukaemia and lymphoma.
  - Lesch–Nyhan syndrome.

Idiopathic (25%)

Clinical features

Macro- or microscopic haematuria or renal colic.

Investigations

Urine
- Dipstick analysis, microscopy (pH, cells, crystals).
- Culture (exclude infection).
- Ca^{2+}:creatinine ratio, oxalate:creatinine ratio.
- Amino acid screen.

Blood
- U&E, HCO_3^-, creatinine.
- Ca^{2+}, PO_4^{3-}, parathyroid hormone (PTH).
- Uric acid.

Renal tract US

Other investigations
- AXR:
  - Radio-opaque stones: Ca^{2+}/cysteine/infective.
  - Radiolucent stones: uric acid/xanthine.
- Further radiological imaging may include DMSA or CT scan.
- Renal stone analysis: composition.

Treatment

Acute
- An obstructive stone is an emergency. Persistent obstruction and the potentially associated infection can cause permanent renal damage.
- If an obstructive stone is suspected, perform immediate imaging and liaise with a urologist.

Long-term management
- High fluid intake.
- Treatment of any underlying CAKUT or metabolic disorder.

Nephrocalcinosis

An increase in the Ca^{2+} content of the cortex or medulla. Typically associated with current or previous hypercalciuria.

Diagnosis

- *Hyperechoic medullae:*
  - Prematurity (presumed to furosemide use).
  - Inherited disorders with ↑ Ca^{2+} excretion, e.g. Bartter syndrome, Dent disease, Lowe syndrome, distal RTA.
  - Acquired disorders of ↑ Ca^{2+} excretion, e.g.: hyperparathyroidism, hyper- and hypothyroidism, idiopathic hypercalciuria, immobilization, medications including vitamin D.
- *Dense cortical and medullary nephrocalcinosis:*
  - Hyperoxaluria.

Renal cystic diseases

The unifying aetiology is dysfunction of primary cilia or the centrosome. The commonest renal cystic diseases (and the responsible genes) are:

- Autosomal dominant polycystic kidney disease (ADPKD; *PKD1* and *PKD2*). Cysts progressively increase in number and size. Kidneys are asymmetrical and large; 50% reach ESKD by age 60y.
- Tuberous sclerosis (TS). Contiguous gene syndrome (AD; *TSC2*, and *PKD1*). Large polycystic kidneys with progression in cysts and CKD. Annual screening is recommended.
- Renal cysts and diabetes syndrome (AD; *HNF1β*). Variable renal size, cysts, dysplasia.
- Autosomal recessive polycystic kidney disease (ARPKD; *PKHD1*). Large kidneys with small cysts. Hepatic fibrosis.
- Nephronophthisis (AR; *NPHP*). Polydipsia, anaemia, CKD in childhood. Normal-sized kidneys with small cysts. May be associated with extrarenal abnormalities.
- Bardet–Biedl syndrome (BBS) (AR); obesity, rod–cone dystrophy, polydactyly, cognitive impairment, and GU developmental abnormalities.

Renal dysplasia

- May be unilateral or bilateral.
- Bilateral renal dysplasia is the commonest cause of CKD in childhood.
- The majority of children are diagnosed antenatally, with small, 'bright' kidneys which may contain cysts.
- May occur in association with CAKUT (see Ↄ Congenital abnormalities of the kidneys and urinary tract (CAKUT), p. 328).
- There is a familial incidence, with a recurrence risk of up to 10%.
- Occurs in a variety of genetic disorders.
- Tubular salt handling is particularly affected, so polyuria and acidosis are common.

Hypertension

BP measurement should be part of routine examination. BP can be affected by changes in vessel size and the volume of blood pumped through the arterial system. The latter is affected by cardiac output and blood volume, which is regulated by the kidney:

- Short-term changes in BP are mostly mediated by the heart and blood vessels (key hormones are catecholamines).
- Long-term BP is mediated by the kidney through regulation of salt reabsorption (key hormone, aldosterone).
- All forms of hypertension with defined aetiology are related (directly or indirectly) to altered renal salt handling, establishing the central role of the kidney in BP regulation.

Definition

Defined by reference to sex, age, and height charts (see Fig. 8.1):
- *Stage 1:* BP >95th, but <99th percentile for gender, height, and age, plus 5mmHg.
- *Stage 2:* BP >99th percentile for gender, height, and age, plus 5mmHg.

Measurement technique

- The widest cuff that can be applied to the arm should be used. The length of the inflation bladder should be at least 70%, preferably 90–100% of the circumference of the arm.

NB: small cuff area is a common cause of false +ve high BP.
- After 5min rest (ideally!).
- Sitting position with arm at level of heart (children).
- Supine position in infants.
- On auscultation: first and fifth (disappearance) Korotkoff sounds used for systolic and diastolic values, respectively.

Measurement devices

- *Accoson green light:* validated as comparable with the mercury manometer.
- *Doppler* to magnify the pulse: should be used when <5y of age.
- *Automatic oscillometry:* measures the mean BP and calculates the systolic and diastolic values using proprietary algorithms. Some devices overestimate BP in young children and very few devices have been validated in hypertensive children <5y old.
- *Ambulatory BP monitoring (ABPM):* for 24h profiles. Little normative data for age <5y. Significant hypertension in ≥30% readings above 95th centile.
- *Intra-arterial:* in PICU.

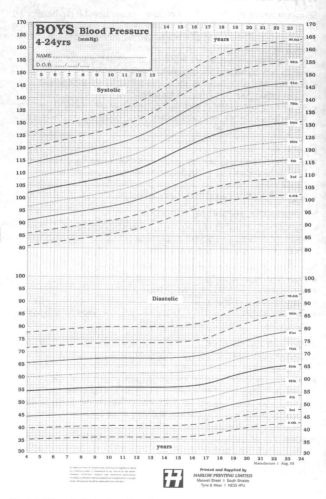

Fig. 8.1 BP centile figures for girls and boys.

Reproduced under Creative Commons Attribution Licence, from Jackson LV, Thalange NKS, Cole TJ. Blood pressure centiles for Great Britain. *Archives of Disease in Childhood* 2007;92:298–303.

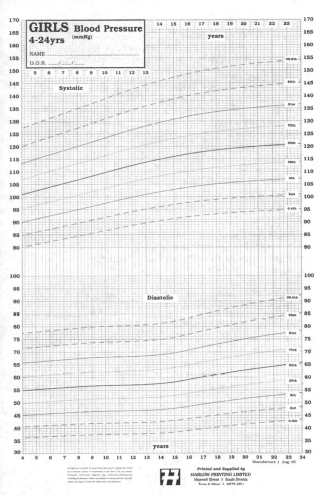

Fig. 8.1 (Contd.)

Hypertension: causes and features

Causes of hypertension

Primary (essential) hypertension
This is a diagnosis of exclusion. High BMI, excessive salt intake, lack of exercise, and family history may be underlying predisposing factors.

Secondary hypertension
- Renal (commonest cause in hospital referral practice):
  - Chronic renal parenchymal disease.
  - PKD.
  - Obstructive uropathy.
  - Acute nephritis.
- Vascular:
  - CoA.
  - UACs/UVCs.
  - Renal artery stenosis.
  - Renal vein thrombosis.
  - Vasculitis.
- Endocrine:
  - CAH.
  - Hyperthyroidism.
  - ↑ steroids (iatrogenic or endogenous).
  - Phaeochromocytoma (BP intermittently raised).
  - Hyperaldosteronism.
- Neurological:
  - Secondary to pain.
  - Raised intracranial hypertension.
- Tumours:
  - Neuroblastoma.
  - Wilms' tumour.
- Medication:
  - Steroids.
  - Aminophylline/caffeine.
  - Oral contraceptive pill.
  - Calcineurin inhibitors, decongestants.
  - Amphetamines, cocaine.
- Others:
  - BPD.
  - ECMO.
  - 'White-coat' hypertension.

Clinical features

Most children are asymptomatic.

Infants

- Vomiting.
- FTT (rare).
- Congestive cardiac failure/respiratory distress (in newborns).

Children

- Headache/nausea and vomiting.
- Visual symptoms.
- Irritable/tired.
- Bell's palsy.
- Epistaxis.
- Growth failure.
- Seizures.
- Altered consciousness.

Examination

- Check fundi.
- Feel abdomen for abdominal masses.
- Listen for renal bruits.
- Feel femoral pulses and compare to radial/brachial pulses (to exclude CoA) and check BP in all four limbs.
- Examination of the heart.

Investigations

A secondary cause is more likely with severe hypertension. Treatment and investigations may need to proceed together.

Urine

- Urinalysis for blood and protein.
- Catecholamines (adrenaline, noradrenaline/metadrenaline, dopamine)-to-creatinine ratio.
- Steroid profile and toxicology.

Blood tests

- FBC, U&E, creatinine.
- HCO_3^-, Ca^{2+}, PO_4^{3-}, albumin.
- Plasma renin and aldosterone.

Other investigations

- ECG and CXR.
- US of urinary tract + Doppler if renal artery stenosis suspected.
- Further imaging will depend upon suspected cause and USS findings, e.g. DMSA, CT scan, arteriogram.
- Specialized tests, e.g. for phaeochromocytoma (see Phaeochromocytoma, p. 604).

Hypertension: management

Hypertensive crises

Severe elevation of BP can result in hypertensive encephalopathy, seizures, and congestive heart failure. It should be treated with IV antihypertensive drugs in a paediatric renal unit or PICU (see → Hypertension, p. 47).

Maintenance antihypertensive therapy

Once daily drugs are preferable. The agent(s) come from the following 'ABCD' groups:
- ACE inhibitor and angiotensin II receptor blocker inhibitors (ARBs).
- β-blocker.
- Calcium channel blocker.
- Diuretic.

Children generally respond better to drugs that block the renin–angiotensin system:
- 'A' drugs (ACE inhibitors and ARBs) and 'B' drugs:
  • If combination treatment is needed, combine A or B with C or D.
  • The third step would be triple therapy with either A + C + D or B + C + D.

The clinical situation, including the presence of any proteinuria (for which ACE inhibition or angiotensin II blockade would be recommended), will determine which group you should start with.

For infants, use shorter-acting agents for flexibility of dosage—propranolol instead of atenolol, and captopril instead of enalapril. Once stable, the patient may be changed to longer-acting antihypertensives.

Treatment of phaeochromocytoma requires α- and β-blockade using propranolol and phenoxybenzamine.

Acute kidney injury

(See also ➔ Renal insufficiency, pp. 76–7.) AKI is a sudden, potentially reversible inability of the kidney to maintain normal body chemistry and fluid balance. It is usually accompanied by oliguria (urine output <0.5mL/kg/h or <1mL/kg/h in a neonate). However, polyuric AKI can also occur.

Classification

Causes are pre-renal, renal (including acute-on-chronic kidney disease), and post-renal (see Box 8.3). A patient may have more than one cause for their AKI.

Box 8.3 Causes of AKI

Pre-renal
- *Hypovolaemia:* GI losses, burns, third-space losses (post-operative, sepsis, and nephrotic syndrome), and excess renal losses (renal tubular disorders).
- *Peripheral vasodilatation:* sepsis.
- *Circulatory failure:* congestive cardiac failure, pericarditis, cardiac tamponade.
- *Bilateral renal arterial or venous thrombosis.*
- *Drugs:* diuretics, ACE inhibitors, NSAIDs.
- *Hepato-renal syndrome.*

Renal
- *Arterial:* embolic, arteritis, HUS.
- *Venous:* renal venous thrombosis.
- *Glomerular:* acute GN.
- *Tubular:* established ATN due to prolonged pre-renal AKI, ischaemia, toxins, or drugs; obstructive (crystals).
- *Interstitial:* tubulo-interstitial nephritis, pyelonephritis.
- *Acute-on-chronic:* decompensation of CKD due to intercurrent illness.

Post-renal
- Obstruction in a solitary kidney.
- Bilateral ureteric obstruction.
- Urethral obstruction.
- Neuropathic bladder.

Obstruction may be congenital (e.g. at the PUJ, VUJ, ureterocele, or PUV) or acquired (e.g. calculi, external compression).

History

The major differential diagnosis of AKI is the first presentation with CKD, which may be either AKI on CKD or previously unrecognized advanced CKD.

Initial assessment, examination, and resuscitation

- Attend to life-threatening features first, i.e. volume status, oxygenation (colour, RR, SpO_2), and electrolyte derangements (see Initial management in Table 8.5).
- Oedema is not be helpful in deciding on fluid replacement, as it may represent intravascular overload or hypovolaemia due to third spacing.

Table 8.5 Assessment and management of intravascular volume status

Hydration status	Clinical features	Initial management
Dehydrated	Tachycardia, cool hands, feet, and nose (>2°C core–peripheral temperature gap), prolonged CRT, low BP (late sign), dry mucous membranes, sunken eyes	Fluid resuscitation 10mL/kg NS over 30min; assess urine output and repeat if necessary
Euvolaemic		Fluid challenge 10–20mL/kg NS over 1h, with furosemide 2–4mg/kg IV, max 12mg/kg/day
Intravascular fluid overload	Tachycardia, gallop rhythm, raised JVP and BP, palpable liver	Furosemide 2–4mg/kg IV, max 12mg/kg/day. Dialysis if no response

Investigations

Urgent USS to look for:
- Obstruction, signs of CKD (small or cystic kidneys).
- In most cases of AKI, the kidneys are enlarged and echo-bright.
- Doppler studies if an abnormality of renal blood flow is suspected.

Urine biochemistry is useful in distinguishing between pre-renal AKI and established ATN; urinary Na^+ (U_{Na}) <10mmol/L (<20 in neonates), fractional excretion of sodium (FeNa) <1% (<2.5% in neonates), and urine osmolality >500mOsm/kg (>400 in neonates) suggest pre-renal AKI.
- *Urine:* for blood, protein, and casts; MC&S.
- *Blood:* U&E, creatinine, plasma HCO_3^-, Ca^{2+}, PO_4^{3-}, and Mg^{2+}, ALP, albumin, LFTs, glucose.
- FBC, including blood film if low platelets (see ➔ Haemolytic uraemic syndrome, pp. 354–5).
- Coagulation screen.
- Blood culture and CRP.
- CXR if respiratory or cardiac signs.

Further additional investigations depend on clinical presentation.
Renal biopsy is indicated as soon as possible when:
- Renal function is deteriorating and the aetiology is not certain.
- Nephritic/nephrotic presentation.

Because these features are suggestive of rapidly progressive crescentic GN, urgent treatment is needed to prevent long-term renal damage.

Monitoring
- Weigh twice daily.
- Hourly input–output recording.
- Hourly observations, including BP and monitoring of toe–core temperature gradient.
- 6-hourly BMs if disease affects blood sugar control (e.g. HUS).
- Neurological observations hourly.
- U&E, creatinine, plasma HCO_3^-, Ca^{2+}, PO_4^{3-}, FBC; frequency determined by clinical picture (may be appropriate to perform up to every 6h).
- If not anuric: urine electrolytes (not if on furosemide).

Management
The patient may require transfer to a paediatric nephrology centre if dialysis looks likely or there is uncertainty about the diagnosis. The following may need emergency management:
- Hyperkalaemia (K^+ >6.5mmol/L) (see ➲ Hyperkalaemia, p. 73).
- Metabolic acidosis (see ➲ Unexplained metabolic acidosis, p. 75).
- Hypertension (see ➲ Hypertension, p. 348).
- Shock (see ➲ Hypovolaemic shock, p. 53).
- Fluid overload (see ➲ Circulatory overload, p. 583).
- Hypocalcaemia (see ➲ Hypocalcaemia, p. 74).
- Hypo-/hypernatraemia (see ➲ Other fluid and electrolyte abnormalities, pp. 72–4).

Medications: adjust drug doses according to level of renal impairment.

Indications for dialysis

- Oligo-anuria with no response to furosemide.
- Hyperkalaemia >6.5mmol/L, with T-wave changes on ECG.
- Severe fluid overload with pulmonary oedema.
- Urea >40mmol/L (consider >30mmol/L in a neonate).
- Severe hypo- or hypernatraemia or acidosis.
- Multisystem failure.
- Anticipation of prolonged oliguria, e.g. HUS, so that space can be made for blood transfusions, if required, and dietary intake.

Acute dialysis—methods
- Peritoneal dialysis.
- Haemodialysis.
- Haemofiltration.

Follow-up of AKI

- Survival and renal recovery depend on the cause of the AKI. Long-term follow-up is necessary, with the exception of children with pre-renal AKI, to detect the development of proteinuria and hypertension which herald CKD, a risk after AKI.
- BP and Ua:Ucr ratio on the first urine of the morning, taken on rising, 12mth after AKI.
- Annual BP and Ua:UCr ratio for life.
- Check creatinine if previous measurement elevated or if proteinuria or raised BP develop.

Haemolytic uraemic syndrome

A triad of microangiopathic haemolytic anaemia, thrombocytopenia, and AKI.

HUS can occur in association with infections

- Enterohaemorrhagic *E. coli* producing shiga toxin (STEC HUS) is the commonest cause.
- *Shigella dysenteriae* type 1 producing shiga toxin.
- *S. pneumoniae* producing neuraminidase [Thomsen Friedenreich antigen ('T antigen')].
- Influenza virus.
- HIV.

Atypical HUS (defined as HUS without coexisting disease)
- Complement alternative pathway dysregulation, due to complement gene mutations and/or anti-complement factor H antibodies.

Other causes of HUS
- In association with malignant hypertension and some medications, cancers, and autoimmune diseases.

STEC HUS

- 90% of HUS in children.
- Occurs mainly in children <3y; almost never in neonates.
- Serotype *E. coli* 0157:H7 is the most frequent.
- The risk of developing HUS in patients with intestinal *E. coli* 0157:H7 infection is 10%.
- Humans are infected from contaminated undercooked ground beef, unpasteurized raw milk or milk products (cheese), contaminated water (well water or lake water swallowed during bathing), fruits, fruit juice, and vegetables. Person-to-person transmission is possible.

Clinical features
- Diarrhoea (bloody) and vomiting.
- Rectal prolapse, intussusception, toxic dilatation of the colon, and bowel perforation.
- The commonest extrarenal manifestation is CNS disturbance, affecting up to 20%.
- Cardiomyopathy.
- Diabetes mellitus.

Investigations
- FBC, platelets, blood film (will show fragmented RBCs).
- Blood glucose monitoring.
- Chemistry, including renal function and LFTs, lactate dehydrogenase (LDH), glucose, urate, lipase, and amylase.
- Clotting screen.
- Group and save blood.
- Stool MC&S.
- STEC serology.
- Direct Coombs' test (DCT) (+ve in pneumococcal HUS).

Treatment
- Early diagnosis and supportive care are of major importance. There is no specific therapy for STEC HUS, although there are ongoing trials of eculizumab.
- Eculizumab is the treatment of choice for atypical HUS (aHUS). This must be administered by a renal unit.

Prognosis
- Acute mortality rate is currently 3–5%.
- After 15y, up to 60% have proteinuria and/or hypertension, with up to 20% having CKD. These problems may appear after several years of apparent recovery.

Chronic kidney disease

CKD should be suspected in any child with:
- Plasma creatinine above the normal range for age.
- Bilateral renal defects on antenatal scans.
- Bilateral renal defects on incidental scans, e.g. for UTI.
- A family history of CKD.
- Persistent proteinuria.
- Previous AKI.
- Hypertension.

Presentation of CKD

~50% of cases are diagnosed antenatally. Other presentations include:
- UTI.
- Decompensation of CKD causing AKI (precipitated by infection or dehydration).
- Polydipsia and polyuria.
- Poor nutritional intake and short stature.
- Pallor (anaemia), lethargy, nausea.
- Bony abnormalities from CKD mineral and bone disorder (CKD-MBD).
- Incidental finding of proteinuria.
- Hypertension.
- Mild cases are frequently asymptomatic.

Staging of CKD

(See Table 8.6.)

Table 8.6 Staging of CKD

Stage	GFR (mL/min/1.73m²)	Features
1	>90	Renal parenchymal disease present
2	60–89	Usually no symptoms but may develop biochemical abnormalities at the lower end of the GFR range
3A	45–59	Biochemical abnormalities and anaemia and, in addition, may develop poor growth and appetite
3B	30–44	
4	15–29	Symptoms more severe
5	<15 or dialysis	Renal replacement therapy will be required

- This staging system does not apply in the first 2y of life when GFR is increasing from intrauterine levels. Plasma creatinine must be compared to age-matched levels.
- Plasma creatinine can remain normal until GFR reduces to <50%.
- GFR can be formally measured by the clearance of a substance that is fully filtered by the glomerulus, but not reabsorbed, e.g. iohexol, although this accuracy is rarely required.
- GFR (mL/min/1.73m^2) may be estimated as: GFR = 36.5 × height (cm)/ creatinine (micromoles/L).

Causes of CKD (in order of frequency)

- CAKUT.
- Renal cystic diseases.
- Nephrotic syndromes.
- Nephronophthisis (isolated or in association with syndromes).
- GNs.
- Vascular events.
- aHUS.
- Renal stone diseases.
- Familial nephropathies.
- Systemic diseases (SLE, vasculitis).
- Following AKI.

Investigations

Renal USS

- *Small kidneys:* dysplasia, vascular events, post-AKI.
- *Normal-sized:* nephrotic syndromes, nephronophthisis, GNs.
- *Cystic:* all renal cystic diseases.
- *Renal calculi.*

Urine stick testing

- *Heavy proteinuria* without significant haematuria suggests nephrotic syndrome.
- *Proteinuria and haematuria* suggest GN or familial nephropathy.
  - *Proteinuria* may rarely be tubular (tubulopathy), e.g. Dent disease—send urine for low-molecular weight proteins such as RBP or β2-microglobulin.
  - *Proteinuria* may result from any cause of CKD because of hyperfiltration.
  - There may be *no proteinuria* with cystic diseases and dysplasias.
- *Further investigations* will depend on likely cause from history, examination, USS, and urine stick testing.
- More and more causes of CKD can be diagnosed by looking for *genetic mutations.*

Management of CKD

Aims

- Slow progression of CKD.
- Prevent biochemical and haematological derangements.
- Maintain normal growth and development.
- Preserve the limb vasculature—when possible, avoid use of:
  - Antecubital veins, as they will be needed for fistula formation.
  - Subclavian veins, stenosis precludes creation of a fistula in that arm.

Outpatient checks in the child with CKD

- Height, weight, and OFC.
- Pubertal stage.
- BP.

Investigations at each clinic visit

- FBC and estimation of iron stores if needing an erythropoiesis-stimulating agent.
- U&Es, HCO_3^-, and creatinine.
- Ca^{2+}, ionized Ca^{2+}, PO_4^{3-}, albumin, ALP, intact PTH.
- Upr:Ucr or Ua:Ucr ratio measured in the first urine of the morning (to standardize measurements and reduce the orthostatic element).

Management

- *Nutrition:* involve a paediatric dietician. Poor appetite leads to malnutrition and poor growth.
- *Growth:* growth retardation occurs in up to 50% of children with CKD stage 3B-5. Children with congenital nephropathies are particularly affected. Renal transplant can normalize growth in some children. Recombinant human growth hormone (rhGH) is used when all other causes of poor growth are resolved.
- *Fluid and electrolyte balance:* CKD due to disorders that predominantly affect the RTs (e.g. CAKUT, nephronophthisis) causes salt, HCO_3^-, and water wasting. Na^+ and HCO_3^- supplementation and free access to water are necessary. Glomerular disease (GNs) causes salt and water retention and hypertension, and may need Na^+ restriction and diuretics. A low K^+ diet may be necessary when GFR <10% normal.
- *Anaemia:* PO iron supplements and erythropoiesis-stimulating agents are usually needed when the GFR falls below $30mL/min/1.73m^2$.
- *CKD-MBD:* CKD leads to abnormal vitamin D, Ca^{2+}, PO_4^{3-}, fibroblast growth factor 23 (FGF23), and PTH metabolism. Nutritional vitamin D intake and blood levels are low and supplements are needed. As CKD progresses, activated vitamin D needs replacing as well. PO_4^{3-} clearance decreases and absorption is restricted by using phosphate binders. Stimulation of PTH, alongside high PO_4^{3-} levels, results in renal bone disease and cardiovascular disease, which is a major cause of death.

Renal replacement therapy

Children should prepare for a living- or deceased-donor transplant once GFR is <15mL/min/1.73m², and it is clear that they are likely to require dialysis in the near future and/or are experiencing significant complications of their CKD. In this way, dialysis may be avoided.

It is preferable to avoid dialysis because:

- Dialysis is disruptive to family lifestyle, schooling, and social interactions, and places huge demands on the family.
- Dietary and fluid restrictions are necessary on dialysis.
- Mortality is higher on dialysis than post-transplant.
- Avoidance of dialysis preserves vascular and peritoneal access sites for future use.
- Dialysis is associated with vascular calcification and risk of cardiovascular events.
- Well-being, growth, and development are improved post-transplant.

Dialysis

Peritoneal dialysis (PD)

- The commonest choice is continuous cycling automated peritoneal dialysis (CCPD) in the patient's home (with mobile machines).

Haemodialysis (HD)

- Vascular access using an arteriovenous fistula (wrist or elbow) is preferable because of ↓ infection risk and better vessel preservation, but many children are dialysed through a tunnelled central line.
- The session is usually for 4h, three times per week, in hospital.
- Home HD is possible if there is a family member to support this.

Renal transplantation

- The minimum weight for transplanting into a child is 10kg.
- The outcomes for living donor are superior to deceased donor, with 10y graft survival of 80% for living donor and 70% for deceased donor.

References

1. National Institute for Health and Care Excellence. (2007, updated October 2018). *Urinary tract infection in under 16s: diagnosis and management.* Clinical guideline [CG54]. Available at. ℔ https://www.nice.org.uk/guidance/CG54.

Neurology

History taking in paediatric neurology

An accurate history contributes the most to a successful diagnosis, particularly in neurology. So when making a medical diagnosis, you need the:
• Clinical history obtained from the patient and parent.
• Signs noticed on physical examination.
• Results of investigations.

General points

Listen carefully and hear what the child or carer are saying, not what you expect or want them to say. It is important to make history taking interactive and to involve the child as much as possible, even when they are of a younger age. Start with open questions and document the exact words used by the child or carer to describe symptoms.

History of presenting complaint

The progress of symptoms may give you the diagnosis—an instantaneous onset may be due to a vascular cause; a gradual onset over days may be due to inflammation, and evolution over weeks may be due to a space-occupying lesion. Paroxysmal episodic phenomena are characteristic of epileptic or migrainous events.

Pain history

Location, quality, intensity, duration, frequency, associated symptoms, aggravating/alleviating factors, and impact on daily activities.

Birth history

Pay particular attention to antenatal scan results, maternal serology, mode of delivery, and the need for perinatal resuscitation.

Past medical history

Comorbidities may be linked to a primary neurological issue.

Drug history

Make note of regular medications, vaccination history, and allergies.

Family history

This is particularly important since many neurological illnesses have a genetic basis. Draw a family tree and ask about consanguinity.

Social history

Ask about home environment and school performance. Pay attention to interaction with peer groups and participation in activities.

Developmental history

All four domains of development need to be assessed. Ask about milestones achieved and do not miss signs of regression or the possibility of a communication disorder.

Diet and sleep

Review the child's growth and plot on a centile chart. Enquire about sleeping habits since sleep-related problems are associated with numerous neurological conditions.

Examination

Children with mental age ≥5 yrs who walk

Full 'adult' neurological examination by making it a game. Pay particular attention to affect, gait and spine, head size, and skin (neurocutaneous signs).

Children with mental age <5 yrs who walk

Examined by stealth. Observe play and note gait, visual acuity, speech and hearing, behaviour, and movements. Examine skin, spine, and OFC. Look at co-ordination and formation of movement.

Cranial nerves (II, III, IV, VI)
- Look at the child's eyes. Do they fix and follow?
- Is there a squint (see ⊃ Squint (strabismus) p. 971).
- Examine the fundi.

Other cranial nerves
- Watch the facial movements (VII).
- Say something while covering your mouth and see if the child responds appropriately (VIII).
- Does the child dribble excessively? Watch them swallow and listen to their speech (IX, X).
- Children love to stick out their tongues and shrug their shoulders (XI, XII).

Neuromuscular and peripheral examination
Children who can walk, run, jump, hop, and spring up from the ground well are unlikely to have an abnormality of the peripheral neurological system. If there is an abnormality do the following.
- Look at the gait. Is there abnormality of posture?
- Observe muscle bulk and joint positions.
- Assess all limbs for joint ranges, tone, and power. Use an adult tendon hammer for reflexes.
- Categorize the pattern of abnormality (e.g. unilateral, bilateral, all limbs, bulbar muscles).

Sensation
If indicated assess sensation. Move around dermatome by dermatome, but move irregularly.

Children <5 yrs who do not walk

This examination relies more on observation of development (see ⊃ Chapter 18), movement, tone, peripheral reflexes, and any primitive reflexes (see ⊃ Primitive reflexes, p. 726).

Epilepsy

Epilepsy (or, more accurately, the epilepsies) is a group of conditions defined by (mostly) unprovoked, recurrent seizures. One per cent of children will have one afebrile seizure by the age of 14y. The majority will be generalized tonic–clonic (GTC) episodes.

Forms of epilepsy

Epilepsies are categorized as involving generalized or focal seizures.

Generalized seizures

These can be described as follows:
- *Myoclonic:* shock-like movement of one or more parts of the body.
- *Tonic:* with sustained contraction and stiffness.
- *Clonic:* rhythmic jerking of one limb, one side, or all of the body.
- *Tonic–clonic:* a combination of the above forms.
- *Absence:* abrupt psychomotor arrest lasting 5–15s in younger children— can be longer in the older child. Can be associated with retropulsion of the head, upward deviation of eyes, or perioral myoclonia.

Focal seizures

These seizures start in one area of the brain and then may spread, and ultimately generalize. If the latter part of the event is witnessed, it may be described incorrectly as being primarily generalized. The *semiology* depends on the locality of the initial electrical activity. 'Typical' seizure semiology includes the following:
- *Occipital:* multi-coloured bright lights spreading from one area of homonymous visual fields.
- *Centroparietal:* sensorimotor phenomena spreading from one limb and marching up one side of the body.
- *Temporal:* feelings of gastric discomfort, strangeness, anxiety, memory disturbances (e.g. familiarity, 'déjà vu'), autonomia (e.g. automatisms such as nose rubbing), and contralateral clonic or dystonic movements.
- *Frontal:* dystonic posturing and strange guttural noises.

Status epilepticus

(See → Status epilepticus, p. 64.) SE can be convulsive with tonic/clonic movements. Alternatively, it can be non-convulsive with impairment of consciousness and often subtle twitching. In SE, we talk about two times:
- 5min (t_1): the time from which treatment should given.
- 30min (t_2): the time after which brain injury may occur.

Epilepsy management

Febrile seizures

These children may have a temperature ≥39°C; however, the temperature may have become normal by the time it is measured.

- Febrile seizures (FS) are common (4% of children between the ages of 6mth and 5y) and do not constitute a diagnosis of epilepsy.
- On presentation, assess for possible meningitis/encephalitis and treat accordingly with antimicrobials if CNS infection is suspected.
- *Simple FS:*
  - Should not be >15min.
  - Should not involve focal or asymmetrical activity.
  - Should not recur within 24h.
  - Should not be associated with focal neurological findings.
- Provided the FS conforms to the above criteria and there is full recovery, carers can be reassured and the child discharged home.
- Carers should be advised of:
  - Recurrence risk (35% over lifetime; 25% during next 12mth).
  - ↑ risk of developing epilepsy in later life (2–5%), compared to the general population (0.5%).
- If a FS is complex (i.e. prolonged, focal, or recurrent <24h), referral to a specialist clinic ± admission and investigations are required.

First afebrile seizure

Since epilepsy is defined as a condition of prolonged recurrent seizures, a single seizure does not usually lead to a diagnosis of the condition and the risk of recurrence is small.

- Children presenting with a first seizure should be resuscitated, as per local guidelines, using an ABC approach.
- Once stable, a detailed history of the event and a thorough clinical examination should be performed.
- All children presenting with a first afebrile seizure should have the following investigations: blood glucose, FBC, biochemistry (U&E, Ca^{2+}, Mg^{2+}, LFTs) and a 12-lead ECG (to exclude long QT syndrome).

If the seizure event is considered to be of epileptic origin and the child is <2y old, the case should be discussed with a paediatric neurologist, especially in the case of suspected infantile spasms. This is because the aetiology of epileptic seizures in this age group is less likely to be benign. Admission to hospital and inpatient investigations are likely to be required (see ➔ Epilepsy syndromes: infantile, p. 371).

If the seizure is deemed to be of epileptic origin and the child is >2y old with full recovery, further management can be conducted as an outpatient at a specialist 'first seizure clinic' (see ➔ First seizure clinic, p. 366).

First seizure clinic

Misdiagnosis of epilepsy in children is common (20–40%) and has long-term consequences for the patient. Hence, every child with a *first epileptic seizure* needs review by an epilepsy specialist. The diagnosis should be reviewed by focusing on the history and the patient's background. Examination and initial investigations should be revisited:

- *If the diagnosis is uncertain:* further investigations or a period of observation may be required.
- *If epilepsy is confirmed:* explain the diagnosis to child and family. Provide additional resources. Outpatient EEG often useful (see ➲ EEG, p. 367).

When epilepsy is newly diagnosed

- *Treatment:* the option of starting antiepileptic treatment should be discussed with the family. Risks, benefits, and side effects should be explained and a joint decision should be made. The child should also be involved in this discussion when possible and appropriate.
- *Care plan:* every child with epilepsy should have a care plan that includes contact details, describes their diagnosis, lists regular medications, and explains what should be done in the event of another seizure.
- *Emergency buccal midazolam:* children with a previous history of prolonged (>5min) or serial (three within 1h) seizures should be issued with emergency buccal midazolam and their carers should be trained on how to use it.
- *Serious injury prevention:* children and carers should be provided with safety advice to help prevent serious injury in a seizure—water safety and risk of drowning for people with epilepsy; other risks include climbing, sport/traffic-related issues, and avoiding burn injury.
- *Related risks:* as appropriate, discuss teratogenicity and sodium valproate, and sudden unexpected death in epilepsy (SUDEP).
- *Psychological impact:* don't underestimate the impact of diagnosis.
- *Specialist epilepsy nurses:* vital in supporting families and professionals during the management of this chronic condition.

Involving a regional paediatric neurology service

- When the child is aged <2y.
- When there is ongoing diagnostic uncertainty.
- When seizures fail to respond to treatment with two different antiepileptic drugs (AEDs) administered in adequate dosage.
- If possible epilepsy-related language, behaviour, or cognitive issues.
- In cases of 'epileptic encephalopathy'.

Epilepsy investigations

EEG

It should be used in a targeted way to help classify, and not to diagnose, epilepsy. It is not a screening tool for the condition because a large percentage of children with epilepsy have a normal EEG between seizures. Also, a significant proportion of the general population who do not have epilepsy may have epileptiform discharges on EEG.

Indications

- After the second afebrile seizure, to provide syndromic classification or to guide future treatment choices after the diagnosis is made.
- After a complex febrile convulsion.
- In monitoring efficacy of AED treatment.
- In acute encephalopathy of unknown aetiology.
- When there is unexplained deterioration in cognitive performance or dementia or specific cognitive decline.
- When a new seizure type becomes apparent or to review the epilepsy syndrome diagnosis.

Depending on the semiology of the seizures, sleep EEG, telemetry, or ambulatory EEG may be more appropriate than a standard recording to increase the chance of capturing ictal activity.

Brain imaging

Brain ± spine MRI for children with epilepsy is indicated in:
- All children with seizures aged <2y.
- All children with focal seizures, except in some cases of benign partial epilepsy with typical clinical and EEG features, e.g. benign epilepsy with centro-temporal spikes (BECTS).
- All children >1 afebrile generalized seizure (not typical childhood absence epilepsy, juvenile myoclonic or juvenile absence epilepsy).
- All children whose epilepsy is resistant to treatment.

Other investigations in a child <2y

Presentation with epileptic seizures
- *Blood:* FBC, U&E, LFTs, acylcarnitines, glucose.
- *Plasma:* amino acids, ammonia, biotinidase, creatine kinase (CK), lactate, Mg^{2+}, Ca^{2+}, TFTs, autoantibodies, urate, ABG.
- *DNA:* arrays and karyotype.
- *Urine:* organic acids.
- *CSF:* MC&S, protein, glucose, lactate; neurotransmitters (after advice from paediatric neurologist).

Table 9.1 Summary of recommended AEDs by seizure type

Seizure type	First line	Second line	Avoid
GTC	Ca, La, Va	Cl, La, Le, Va, To	–
Tonic/atonic	Va	La	Ca, Ga, Vi, Ox
Absence	Et, La, Va	Et, La, Va	Ca, Ga, Vi, Ox, Ph
Myoclonic	Le, Va, To	Le, Va, To	Ca, Ga, Vi, Ox, Ph
Focal	Ca, La, Le, Va	Cl, La, Le, Va, To	–
Childhood and juvenile absence epilepsy	Et, La, Va	Et, La, Va	Ca, Ga, Vi, Ox, Ph
Juvenile myoclonic epilepsy	La, Le, Va, To	Cl, Zo	Ca, Ga, Vi, Ox, Ph
Idiopathic generalized	La, Va, To	La, Le, Va, To	Ca, Ga, Vi, Ox, Ph
Infantile spasms	*Refer to a tertiary paediatric epilepsy specialist (steroids or vigabatrin)*		
BECTS Panayiotopoulos	Ca, La, Le, Ox, Va	Ca, Cl, Ga, La, Le, Ox, Va, To	–
Dravet	*Refer to a tertiary paediatric epilepsy specialist (Va or To, then Cl and/or stiripentol)*		
Electrical status in slow-wave sleep	*Refer to a tertiary paediatric epilepsy specialist*		
Landau–Kleffner syndrome	*Refer to a tertiary paediatric epilepsy specialist*		
Myoclonic astatic	*Refer to a tertiary paediatric epilepsy specialist*		

Where: Ca, carbamazepine; La, lamotrigine; Va, valproate; Cl, clonazepam; Le, levetiracetam; To, topiramate; Ga, gabapentin; Ox, oxcarbazepine; Vi, vigabatrin; Et, ethosuxamide; Ph, phenytoin; Zo, zonisamide.

Epilepsy treatment

Pharmacological treatment for epileptic seizures

(See Table 9.1.)
- Start with a single first-line drug at a low dose and increase slowly.
- If seizures continue on the maximum tolerated dose of the first-line drug, consider adding a second-line drug.
- Management should be guided by clinical response, not drug levels.
- Remember that the dose may need increasing, in line with the child's growth, but may be unchanged if the child is seizure-free.
- In ♀, avoid sodium valproate in view of risk of teratogenicity. Consider only if other treatment has failed, with appropriate counselling. Input from a paediatric neurologist is needed.
- After 2y of seizure freedom while on AEDs. consider whether weaning medications with a view to stopping them is appropriate.

Non-pharmacological treatment options for epilepsy

- Ketogenic diet.
- Vagus nerve stimulation.
- Epilepsy surgery.

Epilepsy syndromes: neonatal

(See also ➔ Neonatal seizures, pp. 114–15; ➔ Seizures/epileptic encephalopathy, p. 502.) Rarely benign and always need to be managed with expert advice. Seizures are not GTC because of cerebral immaturity.

Important points for neonatal seizures

- *History*: should focus on family history of convulsions, consanguinity, and risk factors for perinatal sepsis and hypoxic injury.
- *Examine*: for neurocutaneous stigmata and dysmorphic features.
- *Investigate*: blood and CSF (if not contraindicated), looking for infection, and perform neurometabolic screen.
- *Imaging*: cranial US or MRI can be helpful.

Treatment

- *Treat for sepsis*: with antimicrobials since CNS infection is a major cause for neonatal seizures.
- *Use phenobarbital*: loading dose 20mg/kg IV. Further AED treatment varies, depending on local protocols, cause, and expert advice.
- *Levetiracetam*: has an increasing role in the management of neonatal seizures (low side effect profile and available IV).
- *Pyridoxal phosphate*: should be considered if the infant is unresponsive to phenobarbital. If possible, wait for 48h to assess effect.

Benign familial neonatal seizures

- *Features*: AD inheritance, +ve family history, focal clonic seizures, normal development, resolution by 16mth, with 10–15% developing epilepsy. Need to exclude other causes.

Benign neonatal seizures/fifth day seizures

- *Features*: onset fourth to sixth day of life; brief clonic seizures, becoming more severe and can be associated with apnoeic spells or SE. Diagnosis is by exclusion; good prognosis; 2% develop epilepsy.

Early infantile epileptic encephalopathy/Otahara syndrome

- *Features*: onset in the first 10 days of life, with no previous concerns. Seizures are sustained tonic spasms that can occur in clusters. EEG shows burst suppression pattern during both awake and sleep. Poor prognosis and high incidence of drug resistance.

Early myoclonic encephalopathy

- *Features*: onset during first days of life. EEG shows burst suppression. Frequent, fragmented, migrating, massive myoclonic episodes. Tends to be associated with underlying metabolic disorder.

Epilepsy syndromes: infantile

Epilepsy syndromes are complex and need expert input.

Benign myoclonic epilepsy of infancy

- Myoclonic seizures only, normal interictal EEG, and otherwise normal health and development.
- Usual onset between 4mth and 3y, and commoner in girls.
- Seizures usually affect the trunk and upper limbs.
- No treatment usually indicated, but response to valproate or broad-spectrum AED.

Severe myoclonic epilepsy of infancy/Dravet syndrome

- From first year onwards, prolonged FS, shorter afebrile seizures, focal seizures, atypical absences, and segmental myoclonia.
- EEG: may be normal initially but may develop photosensitivity and generalized discharges once the seizures are frequent.
- Genetics: >70% have a mutation in the *SCN1a* gene.
- Treatment sequence, and add new AEDs if no response. Avoid lamotrigine. Start with sodium valproate, then clobazam; then consider stiripentol if resistant to AEDs (needs expert supervision).

Infantile spasms/West's syndrome

- Onset 4–7mth, can occur in late neonatal period or >12mth.
- Diagnosis based on triad of: infantile spasms, developmental delay or regression, and hypsarrhythmia on EEG (NB: hypsarrhythmia develops with age and may not always be present).
- Exclude TS, and obtain expert opinion for investigations.
- Treatment with adrenocorticotrophic hormone (ACTH)/steroids (prednisolone) or vigabatrin. A UK study suggested steroids more effective at stopping spasm. Research is ongoing.
- Management should be guided by expert opinion.

Myoclonic astatic epilepsy/Doose syndrome

- Characterized by myoclonic astatic seizures, myoclonic jerks, and GTC seizures.
- EEG demonstrates predominantly generalized discharges once seizures are established.
- Treat as for idiopathic generalized epilepsy (see ⊃ Epilepsy: mid to late childhood, pp. 372–3), and consider ketogenic diet early in refractory cases.

Lennox–Gastaut syndrome

- Tonic seizures with trunk flexion (often evolving out of infantile spasms), atonic seizures, myoclonic jerks, and atypical absences.
- Invariably developmental delay once seizures established.
- EEG shows slow spike-and-wave discharges interictally, with a pattern of 10–12Hz paroxysmal fast discharges in sleep.
- Prognosis poor in terms of response to AEDs and development.

Epilepsies: mid to late childhood

The idiopathic generalized epilepsies are better described as genetic epilepsies and include the following conditions.

Myoclonic absence epilepsy

- Typical absences, with short symmetrical jerks of mainly the upper limbs, with abduction and elevation. Onset <5y of age.
- EEG demonstrates generalized discharges of three cycles per second spike-and-wave and, in addition, may have short bursts of polyspikes.
- Poor prognosis; can deteriorate into epileptic encephalopathy, may require treatment with ketogenic diet.

Childhood absence epilepsy (CAE)

- Previously known as 'petit mal'. Onset between 4 and 8y (<3 rare).
- Typical absences only, but very frequent; rarely GTC seizures.
- Absences can be associated with mild myoclonia or automatisms.
- EEG demonstrates regular bursts of 3Hz spike-and-wave pattern.
- Good prognosis, but GTC events may continue.

Juvenile absence epilepsy (JAE)

- Onset towards end of the first and during second decade (peak 12y).
- All have absences, with up to 15–30% also having myoclonic jerks.
- Majority (80%) develop GTC seizures.
- EEG discharges more fragmented and irregular than in CAE.
- Prognosis guarded since relapse common; most respond to AEDs.

Juvenile myoclonic epilepsy

- Onset in the second decade (usual onset 12–18y).
- Myoclonic jerks classically within the first hour of awakening.
- Classic history of dropping objects while preparing breakfast, and awareness maintained during seizures.
- High risk of GTC seizures; up to 80% of adolescent girls will have further GTC seizures if they withdraw medication completely.
- EEG may have absences and photosensitivity; discharges are more fragmented and irregular than in JAE, with bursts of polyspike.

Benign childhood epilepsy with centro-temporal spikes (Rolandic) (also known as benign epilepsy with centro-temporal spikes or BECTS)

- Predominantly nocturnal sensorimotor seizures.
- Onset on one side of face or a hand that may generalize.
- EEG may be relatively normal awake, but in slow-wave sleep or drowsiness, will develop frequent centro-temporal spike-and-wave discharges with an easily recognizable shape and distribution.
- Majority of children suffer infrequent seizures, and treatment is not required. Good prognosis, with 90% achieving remission by 16y.
- If seizures are frequent/prolonged, AED response is excellent.

Benign childhood occipital seizure syndrome (Panayiotopoulos)

- Occurs in young children (aged 1–7y).
- Prolonged (<30min), stereotyped episodes of encephalopathy, often associated with ictal vomiting, headache, and eye deviation.
- Heterogenous EEG abnormalities.
- Good prognosis, with infrequent seizures and most children seizure-free by age 10y. Treatment is rarely indicated.

Landau–Kleffner syndrome (LKS) (acquired epileptic aphasia)

- Rapid onset between ages of 3 and 8y, with loss of language skills.
- Seizure phenotypes include GTC, absences, or motor seizures.
- EEG shows frequent epileptiform discharges, especially in sleep and over temporal areas. There is overlap with electrical status in slow-wave sleep (ESES) (see ➔ Electrical status and slow-wave sleep, p. 373).
- Treatment options include steroids and benzodiazepines.

Electrical status in slow-wave sleep

- A triad of continuous spike-and-wave activity for > 80% of slow sleep, seizures, and developmental regression.
- Onset is usually 4–6y; ♂ more affected than ♀.
- Treatment is often difficult; carbamazepine exacerbates the condition. Options are: benzodiazepines, steroids, sodium valproate, with addition of ethosuximide or levetiracetam in some cases.

Frontal lobe focal epilepsies

- Presents with short, frequent seizures, often arising out of sleep.
- Associated with asymmetric dystonic posturing and brought on by loud noises. Recovery quick.
- EEG assessment can be difficult.

Temporal lobe focal epilepsies

- The seizures affect memory and emotion, with disturbances such as 'déjà vu', fear, abdominal discomfort, and automatisms.

Occipital lobe focal epilepsies

- Associated with simple multi-coloured blobs of light on one side of visual field.
- Often produces headache and vomiting.

Non-epileptic paroxysmal conditions

Up to one-third of children diagnosed with 'epilepsy' actually have non-epileptic events. A misdiagnosis of epilepsy can have profound long-term effects (e.g. limitation of activities such as driving, side effects from medication, etc.). Be aware of other paroxysmal conditions (described below) before diagnosing epilepsy and using AEDs.

Neonates and infants

* *Benign neonatal sleep myoclonus:* single or repetitive episodes of jerking of arms and legs (typically while falling asleep after a feed), sparing the face.
* *Shuddering attacks:* brief, shiver-like movement, usually precipitated by an interesting stimulus.
* *GOR and Sandifer syndrome:* often leads to movements mistaken for epileptic seizures—back/neck arching and head turning. Symptoms settle with anti-reflux medications.
* *Dystonia:* abnormal muscle contraction due to sustained and simultaneous contraction of agonist and antagonist muscles can lead to repetitive and abnormal posture that can be mistaken as seizure activity. It is important to differentiate epilepsy and dystonia since treatment for the two conditions (that often coexist in the same patient) is distinct.
* *Hyperekplexia:* exaggerated startle response due to mutation in glycine receptor gene. Sudden noise or being handled causes whole body stiffening. A wide spectrum, with the most severe forms having life-threatening apnoea.

Older infants and toddlers

* *'Breath-holding attacks' and reflex anoxic seizures:* suddenly going limp, followed by clonic jerking. At least one episode triggered by a noxious stimulus. Typically, a short cry and then the child goes limp, collapses to the floor, and may have brief jerking. Other episodes are characterized by 'blue' breath-holding when the child starts to cry, the crying builds up, and then the child collapses at the end of expiration.
* *Masturbation and other gratification phenomena:* when the child is bored, they indulge in self-stimulation. Sweatiness almost invariably raises the possibility of a tonic seizure and can lead to misdiagnosis.
* *Febrile myoclonus:* short jerks associated with high fever.
* *Benign paroxysmal vertigo:* acute onset of fear, nausea, vertigo, and unsteadiness if forced to walk. May exhibit nystagmus.
* *Benign paroxysmal torticollis:* acute episodes of head tilt, similar to the nystagmus seen in benign paroxysmal vertigo.
* *Night terrors:* common in 3–8y olds; while in deep sleep, about 1–2h after bed, the child suddenly wakes up and is inconsolable. This lasts some 10–20min, and then the child 'wakes', looks confused, rolls over, and sleeps again.

Childhood

- *Daydreaming:* can appear similar to an absence seizure. However, the history of the two conditions is distinct. Daydreaming usually occurs when the child is bored, tired, or watching TV and often the parents have to call the child multiple times before they respond. Absence seizures tend to actively interrupt across normal activity.
- *Tics:* stereotypical movements often associated with tiredness, stress, boredom, or behavioural problems. Usually +ve family history. If associated with vocalizations, consider *Tourette syndrome*.
- *Syncope:* occurs after age 7mth. May be a history of precipitating events (e.g. fright, head bang, sudden standing). Often the child has an aura of loss of vision, tingling, and auditory phenomena, followed by loss of consciousness and posture change (falls over if standing). Not all syncopal events result in a loss of tone. In some, the fall is accompanied by ↑ tone. Myoclonic jerks may follow for a few seconds. Useful for diagnosis: a history of a precipitant, jerking lasting <20s, with movements that may not be rhythmic.

When investigating suspected epilepsy or syncope, always perform a 12-lead ECG to exclude long QT syndrome.

- *Psychologically determined paroxysmal events (PDPEs):* previously described as pseudoseizures, malingering, and factitious or conversion disorders. Due to psychological causes, features suggestive, but not diagnostic, of PDPE include: events triggered by specific situations, thrashing movements that wax and wane ± pelvic thrusting, persistent falls without injury, gain from the situation, and generalized movements, with rapid return to normal.

Management of non-epileptic paroxysmal conditions

Infantile non-epileptic disorders, syncopal episodes, and jerks
Allay the carer's concerns over the diagnosis.

Psychologically determined paroxysmal events
PDPE can be difficult to treat, but these patients do respond to well-organized management. The principal areas include the following:
- Unambivalent diagnosis explained to both the parent and the child/young person.
- Acknowledgement/acceptance by the young person, carers, and all health professionals that these are non-epileptic.
- Stabilization phase where the family is developing an understanding.
- Strengthening coping abilities and removing gain from the behaviour.
- Psychological support is essential. Some families will feel very threatened when the possibility is raised of looking at psychological issues that may have triggered these events in the child.

Primary headaches in children

Two-thirds of children have had ≥1 headache in the past year.

Migraine

This is the most prevalent form of primary headaches in children.

> **International Headache Society Criteria for diagnosis of migraine without aura in children and adolescents**
> At least five headaches of 1–72h, with at least two of the following:
> - Unilateral or bilateral pain.
> - Throbbing pain.
> - Moderate or severe pain.
> - Pain aggravated by routine physical activity.
>   And at least one of the following:
> - Nausea/vomiting.
> - Photophobia/phonophobia.

The paediatric migraine spectrum includes benign paroxysmal torticollis, benign paroxysmal vertigo, cyclical vomiting syndrome, hemiplegic migraine, and abdominal migraine. Treatment options involve:
- *Exclusion of triggers* (diet, dehydration, tiredness, and stress).
- *Acute treatment* choices include ibuprofen, nasal sumatriptan/zolmitriptan, and PO rizatriptan.
- *Antiemetics* can also be helpful.
- *Prophylaxis:* if the migraine is frequent enough to disrupt activity, consider prophylaxis, e.g. topiramate, propranolol, and flunarizine.

Tension-type headache

Poorly researched primary headache. Evidence suggests association with anxiety, depression, stress, and difficulties with relationships.

> **International Headache Society Criteria for diagnosis of tension-type headache in children and adolescents**
> At least ten headaches of 30min for 7 days, with ≥2 of the following:
> - Bilateral pain.
> - Pressing/tightening quality of pain.
> - Mild to moderate pain.
> - Pain not aggravated by physical activity.
>
>   And both of the following:
> - No nausea or vomiting.
> - No photophobia/phonophobia, or one but not the other.

Treatment options for tension-type headaches include:
- Analgesia for only the most incapacitating headaches.
- CBT; healthy physical exercise and sleep routine, manual therapies (e.g. stretching, trigger point release).
- Transcutaneous electrical nerve stimulation (TENS), writing to the school to support classroom participation.

Chronic cluster headache

A rare cause of headache in children and involves:
- Severe, unilateral (around the eye, above the eye, and along the side of the head or face) pain of variable quality that interferes with daily activity.
- Associated with red or watery eye (or both); nasal congestion, constricted pupil, or drooping eyelid on the ipsilateral side.
- Pain typically lasts from 15min to 3h, and the frequency can vary from eight episodes per day to one every other day.

Treatment for acute attacks involves:
- O_2 (100% at flow rate >12L/min with non-rebreathing mask and reservoir bag).
- Subcutaneous (SC) or nasal triptan.

Chronic paroxysmal hemicrania (CPH)

A severe, debilitating unilateral headache, usually affecting the area around the eye. It tends to respond to treatment with indometacin.

Medication overuse headache

A commonly encountered headache in children, which should always be considered as a potential cause of chronic daily headache, especially when analgesia is routinely used for ≥10 days/mth.
  Treatment involves stopping all medications in one step:
- Worsening of symptoms is to be expected in the short term.
- Children with medication overuse headache tend to respond to medication withdrawal within 1mth.
- If this does not happen, the diagnosis needs to be reconsidered.
- Withdrawal of medications may lead to reversal to the original headache type that was originally treated.

Secondary headaches in children

When initially assessing a child with headache, it is important to recognize whether the symptoms are secondary to another condition. Prompt diagnosis of the cause is vital since missing some of the following conditions may lead to serious clinical consequences:

- Brain tumours.
- Trauma.
- Disorders of cranial and/or cervical vessels.
- Infection (e.g. meningitis, sinusitis, otitis media).
- Substance misuse/withdrawal.
- Psychiatric causes.
- Cranial neuralgias (often associated with facial pain).

'Red flag' signs and symptoms suggestive of serious cause of headache

- Persistent and/or recurrent vomiting.
- Persistent and/or recurrent headaches.
- Balance or coordination problems/focal neurological signs.
- Abnormal eye movements, e.g. nystagmus/blurred or double vision.
- Behavioural changes, e.g. lethargy.
- Seizures.
- Increasing head circumference in younger children.
- Delayed or arrested puberty.
- Abnormal head position, e.g. head tilt in younger children.

Raised intracranial pressure

This is a potential cause of headache and will be associated with either or both abnormal coordination examination findings and a short history of severe vomiting, morning headache and visual disturbance. The main concern is a mass obstructing CSF flow, *and therefore* expert opinion and neuroimaging are needed as soon as possible. MRI/magnetic resonance venography (MRV) are recommended if cerebral sinus thrombosis is suspected.

Idiopathic intracranial hypertension (IIH)

A group of patients have raised ICP of unknown cause, and the only sign on examination is papilloedema ± reduced visual acuity (VA), with essentially normal cranial imaging. IIH is associated with obesity, ♀ sex, and adolescence. Diagnosis is confirmed through LP (with CSF opening pressure of >20cmH$_2$O). Management includes:

- Weight loss in obese patients.
- Removing causal medication (e.g. steroids, oral contraceptive).
- Diuretics (e.g. acetazolamide, furosemide).
- Serial LPs and regular monitoring of vision.
- *Steroid treatment* may be effective but can cause rebound problems when withdrawn.

Macrocephaly and microcephaly

Macrocephaly

Macrocephaly is defined as OFC of >99.6th centile. The majority of such children will have a benign and familial cause for this condition. However, hydrocephalus and degenerative disorders need to be considered.

History

Take a full history, including developmental progression.
- Are there any features of autism or degenerative disorders?
- Are there signs of raised ICP?

Examination

- Plot OFC on a growth chart, along with previous measurements.
- Look at the skin for signs of neurofibromatosis (NF).

Findings and investigations

- *Abnormal:* if there are any abnormalities, these will need further investigations, depending on the specific findings.
- *Normal:* if the examination is normal, try and compare the child's OFC with the parents' OFC:
  - If all large, then likely diagnosis is familial macrocephaly.
  - If the parents' OFCs are normal, then probably benign, but appropriate to follow measurements for the next year.
  - If there is crossing of centiles, then perform brain imaging, looking for hydrocephalus or other intracranial cause.

Microcephaly

(See ➲ Microcephaly, p. 153.) Microcephaly is defined as OFC of <0.4th centile. The majority have coexisting developmental and neurological abnormalities.

History

- Take a full history, including developmental progression and antenatal history, and enquire about infection during pregnancy.
- Enquire about newborn screening (to exclude PKU).

Examination

- Plot OFC on a growth chart, along with previous measurements.
- Look for features of craniosynostosis.

Investigations

- Repeat PKU screening.
- Karyotype, plasma lactate, maternal and child's TORCH screen, urine for CMV, plasma and urine for amino acids and organic acids.
- MRI.

Management

- Obtain genetic advice. There may be a recurrence risk of up to 25% (AR microcephaly) if no cause is found.

Hydrocephalus

(See also ⊃ Congenital hydrocephalus, p. 152.) Hydrocephalus may be present, irrespective of whether there is obstruction to CSF flow. The causes are:
- Obstructive (non-communicating): aqueduct stenosis, posterior fossa and other tumours.
- Communicating: meningitis, subarachnoid haemorrhage, IVH.

Clinical features

History
- Older children may present with headache and vomiting.
- Babies usually present because there is concern about head growth (i.e. OFC crossing centiles) and delay in development.

Examination
- Plot OFC on growth chart, along with previous measurements.
- Note macrocephaly or bulging fontanelle in those with open sutures.
- 'Sunsetting' of the eyes or papilloedema; hyperreflexia, spasticity, poor head control—all can be signs of hydrocephalus.

Diagnosis
- Cranial imaging looking for enlarged ventricles.
- Imaging may also reveal associated congenital abnormalities such as Arnold–Chiari malformation.

Treatment
- Urgent neurosurgical referral for placement of ventricular peritoneal shunt system or other intervention.

Children with ventricular shunt drainage systems in place are at risk of shunt blockage, infection (e.g. ventriculitis), and subdural haematoma.

Acute changes in behaviour, new-onset headache, or persistent fever will need to be assessed with these problems in mind. Again, referral to the neurosurgical team for imaging and CSF sampling will need to be carried out.

A shunt-related complication must always be excluded before an alternative diagnosis is reached!

Bell's palsy

Acute paralysis of muscles of facial expression. May be unable to close the eye on the affected side.
- Normally unilateral but may be bilateral lower motor neuron lesion.
- Secondary to oedema of the facial nerve, as it passes through the temporal bone.

Aetiology
- Idiopathic.
- Varicella or other viral cause.
- *Borrelia burgdorferi* (Lyme disease), particularly if bilateral.

Examination
- *Check:* whether other branches of the facial nerve are affected, e.g. hyperacusis.
- *Full systemic examination:* in particular, look for signs of leukaemia and vasculitides.
- *Full neurological examination:* look for other signs, the presence of which would exclude an idiopathic Bell's palsy.

Investigations
- FBC and film (leukaemia).
- Varicella titres.
- *Borrelia* investigation, in suspicious cases, after discussion with microbiology.

Treatment
- *Steroids:* evidence for use of steroids is limited, but the general opinion is to use 2mg/kg (maximum 60mg) prednisolone od for 5 days if the symptoms are <7 days old.
- *Aciclovir:* recent evidence indicates that PO aciclovir for 10 days, irrespective of varicella status, may be useful.
- *Good eye care:* important with lubricating eye drops or ointment and taping of the eyelid to keep it closed during bedtime.

Prognosis
- Most children will either recover fully or recover to a good degree.
- When recovery does not occur after 6mth, referral for facial nerve grafting is appropriate.

Neurocutaneous disorders

Tuberous sclerosis complex (TSC)

- TSC is an AD inherited disorder affecting the brain, skin, heart, kidney, eyes, and lungs (see also ➜ Tuberous sclerosis complex, p. 883).
- Two genes have been identified: *TSC1* and *TSC2*. About one-third of cases are inherited; the others involve *de novo* mutations.
- The clinical disorder relates to hamartomata affecting the above organs, although other neoplasms also occur.

Diagnosis of TSC

The diagnosis is made when a child has either two major or one major and two minor criteria.

Major criteria	Minor criteria
Facial angiofibromas	Pits in dental enamel
Ungal fibroma	Rectal polyps
Hypomelanotic macules (>3)	Bone cysts
Shagreen patch	Cerebral white matter 'migration tracts'
Cortical tubers	
Subependymal nodules	Gingival fibromas
Subependymal giant cell astrocytoma	Non-renal hamartoma
Retinal nodular hamartoma	Retinal achromic patch
Cardiac rhabdomyomata	Confetti skin lesions
	Multiple renal cysts

Management

Treatment is symptomatic, depending on the organ-specific effects. All cases require expert assessment, with common issues being:
- Recurrence risk in family members.
- Symptomatic epilepsies, particularly if West's syndrome occurs.
- Cardiac rhabdomyomata needs to be referred for cardiology support.
- Renal complications are very rare, but biannual renal USS, with regular enquiry for renal function/loin pain, is needed. Polycystic kidney disease can occur.
- Pulmonary lymphangiomatosis occurs very rarely in childhood, and only in girls. Regular screening not indicated, unless symptomatic.
- Ophthalmological hamartomata need to be referred to specialist ophthalmology services.

Neurofibromatosis

There are two distinct AD disorders, characterized by multiple benign tumours of the peripheral nerve sheath. (See also ⟴ Neurofibromatosis, p. 423; ⟴ Neurofibromatosis type 1, p. 882.)

NF1: chromosome 17

The diagnosis is based on having at least two of the following:

- >6 café-au-lait macules: >5mm diameter before puberty, >15mm diameter after puberty.
- Skinfold or axillary freckling.
- One neurofibroma or a plexiform neurofibroma.
- One Lisch nodule in the iris.
- Optic glioma.
- Skeletal dysplasia.
- Affected first-degree relative.

Management of this condition is symptomatic and depends on the local effects of the neurofibroma. However, all cases require expert assessment of:

- Recurrence risk in family members (they need assessment annually).
- Neoplasia and optic gliomata.
- Renal artery stenosis.
- Skeletal dysplasia.
- Cognitive performance.

NF2: chromosome 22

The diagnosis is based on having one major or two minor criteria.

- *Major criteria:* unilateral vestibular schwannoma and first-degree relative with NF2; bilateral vestibular schwannomas.
- *Minor criteria:* meningioma, schwannoma, ependymoma, glioma, cataract.

The management of NF2 is complex—the tumours themselves do not need to be removed when identified in many cases, although they may be symptomatic.

Sturge–Weber syndrome

Leptomeningeal angiomatosis—associated with a port wine naevus in the distribution of the first branch of the trigeminal nerve. Children may be very well but can have:

- Severe focal epilepsies.
- Learning disability.
- Hemiplegia.
- Glaucoma.
- Transient stroke-like episodes and severe headaches.

Diagnosis is based on facial appearance and following CT ± MRI scan.

Neuromuscular disorders

Think about the anatomical site that is affected (see Fig. 9.1).
- Brain, spine, anterior horn cell.
- Peripheral nerve, NMJ, muscle.

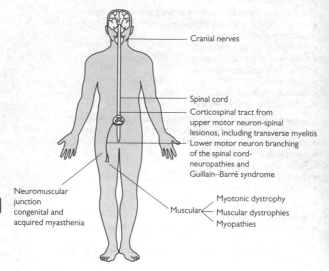

Cranial nerves

Spinal cord

Corticospinal tract from upper motor neuron-spinal lesionos, including transverse myelitis

Lower motor neuron branching of the spinal cord- neuropathies and Guillain–Barré syndrome

Neuromuscular junction congenital and acquired myasthenia

Muscular
Myotonic dystrophy
Muscular dystrophies
Myopathies

Fig. 9.1 Anatomical sites affected in neuromuscular disorders.

Cerebral insult

Any brain insult may make a child unreactive and affect movement. Facial movement and peripheral power are good if the child is able to follow commands. However, they may have low tone in the trunk, with relatively better tone at limb extremities. Reflexes should be present. If there is damage to the upper motor neuron, then there will be spasticity, ↑ tone, and brisk reflexes, e.g. in CP.

Spinal cord lesions

Spinal tumours and transverse myelitis should produce a rough level, beneath which there will be upper motor neuron signs or a sensory level or both. Spinal cord tumours are normally associated with a number of signs, including constipation and urinary symptoms. There are particular signs which should always be investigated (see Box 9.1).

Box 9.1 When to worry about a spinal cord lesion
- Neurological signs, e.g. hyperreflexia, at a level below C1.
- Back pain, with no other signs, in children under 11y.
- Change in urinary function or bowel habit with back pain.

Transverse myelitis
Quick onset of weakness ± anaesthesia ± urinary dysfunction ± bowel disturbance ± back pain, often within 1wk of a viral infection. Acutely, there may be reduced reflexes and power, then upper motor neuron signs. Urgent spinal MRI with gadolinium is required to exclude cord compression and, in many cases, will confirm appearances of myelitis.

Management
Immediate admission for monitoring of respiratory status. Review for urinary and GI disturbance. Feeding/swallowing assessment.
- *Analgesia.*
- *Methylprednisolone:* IV treatment normally used initially.
- *Plasma exchange and immunomodulation:* may be needed if initial therapy with steroids not effective.
- *Rehabilitation:* crucial for a better final outcome. PT and occupational therapy (OT) to avoid joint contracture.

Prognosis
One-third make a full recovery; one third make a partial recovery, and one-third of patients suffer significant long-term impairment.

Anterior horn cell disorders
The disorder here produces flaccid, areflexic limb, with sparing of the face. Polio is now rare but may still be seen following vaccination or in immigrants. In the long term, the limb becomes flaccid and wasted.

Spinal muscular atrophies
Confirmation of these conditions includes fibrillation on EMG and homozygous deletion of survival motor neuron (*SMN*) genes (see ➲ Spinal muscular atrophy, p. 881).
- *Type 0 (neonatal form):* very severe, often with arthrogryposis. Ventilator-dependent at birth.
- *Type 1 (Werdnig–Hoffman):* severe with onset in the first months of life. Typically, there are 'bright eyes', severe hypotonia, 'frog-like posture', areflexia, and weakness that is present more in the legs than in the arms. Previously fatal by 2y, but new therapies evaluated.
- *Type 2:* onset in the first years of life, with low tone, peripheral weakness, absent reflexes, and scoliosis.
- *Type 3 (Kugelberg–Welander):* adolescent onset with progressive weakness and gait disturbance, loss of reflexes, and low tone.

These disorders are very complicated and will need specialist input and multidisciplinary therapy support.

Peripheral neuropathies

Charcot–Marie–Tooth disease (hereditary motor and sensory neuropathies)
A group of disorders with mainly AD inheritance. The hallmark is progressive distal weakness, initially presenting in the lower limbs with peroneal muscle weakness and atrophy. Also, there is reduced coordination and loss of fine motor control. Later, these patients develop sensory disturbances with pins and needles in a glove-and-stocking distribution. The commonest types are:

- *Type 1:* demonstrates reduced conduction velocities on nerve conduction studies due to demyelination.
- *Type 2:* near-normal nerve conduction and symptoms due to axonal degeneration.
- *Type 3:* has a much earlier onset and is sometimes called Dejerine–Sottas syndrome. Characterized by very slowed motor nerve conduction velocities.

Diagnosis
Based on the clinical picture, nerve conduction studies, and genetic analysis of the *P0, PMP22* (AD), and less commonly *Connexin 32* genes (X chromosome). There are now other genetic tests available, including mitofusin 2 and ganglioside-induced differentiation-associated protein (GDAP).

Treatment
Symptomatic, with PT and orthoses to encourage joint mobility and maintain range of movement. Particular emphasis is put on the avoidance of contractures in the hands ('clawing'), as well as peroneal muscle weakness, with foot drop and shortening of the Achilles tendons.

Other neuropathies

Neuropathy may also occur in many systemic disorders, including the following conditions:

- Leukodystrophies.
- Porphyria.
- Diabetes.
- Uraemia.
- Hypothyroidism.
- Vitamin deficiencies (B_1, B_6, B_{12}, and E).
- Autoimmune disorders such as SLE.
- Acutely as part of G-BS.

Guillain–Barré syndrome

G-BS is an acute, potentially fatal demyelinating polyneuropathy. It often follows an intercurrent infection, classically *Campylobacter* enteritis. Initially, there are motor signs that progress up the body. First, there is gait disturbance, then arm involvement, followed by respiratory and bulbar involvement in severe cases.

Causative organisms
- EBV, CMV.
- Measles, mumps.
- Enteroviruses.
- *Mycoplasma pneumoniae*.
- *B. burgdorferi*.
- *Campylobacter*.

Diagnosis
The differential diagnosis includes myasthenia gravis, polio, spinal cord compression/myelitis, and botulism. The diagnostic features of G-BS are:
- *Clinical picture:* muscle weakness, with ascending loss of reflexes.
- *Nerve conduction studies:* demonstrate characteristic features.
- *CSF:* elevated protein, but not at the onset of the illness.
- *Variants:* Miller–Fisher variant includes bulbar cranial nerve involvement, ophthalmoplegia, ataxia, and areflexia.
- *Bladder:* should be spared.

Course
- *Onset:* starts 1–2wk after an antecedent illness.
- *Ascending weakness:* initial deterioration, normally lasts <2wk.
- *Plateau phase:* symptoms are static, normally lasts for 1–2wk.
- *Recovery:* should begin within 2–4wk, in a descending manner, though full recovery sometimes takes a number of months. The reflexes are the last to recover.

Management
- *Immediate admission for monitoring:* respiratory state (use FVC) and autonomic involvement. Dysautonomia leads to tachycardia, fluctuating BP, and GI disturbance. Pain control. Feeding/swallowing assessment.
- Early introduction of *PT and OT* to avoid joint contracture.
- *Analgesia*.
- *Immunoglobulin:* IV treatment (400mg/kg/day for 5 days) is normally used initially, with plasmapheresis reserved for refractory cases. Note risk of transmissible infection and allergic reactions to IVIG.

Neuromuscular junction disorders

Autoimmune myasthenia gravis

The hallmark of this condition is fluctuating, fatiguable weakness. Ptosis in 50–80% of patients. Caused by nicotinic ACh receptor autoantibodies. Normally insidious, sometimes presents with acute, fluctuating weakness of extra-ocular, facial, oropharyngeal, respiratory, and limb muscles.

Diagnosis
- *Clinical picture:* fatiguability of power/reflexes, particularly upward gaze, fluctuating weakness of muscle groups (see above).
- *Electrophysiological assessment* (of the NMJ): in affected muscles.
- *Response to a trial of edrophonium:* do note that response may be brief and video recording may be helpful.
- *ACh receptor antibodies:* present in >50% of cases.

Management
Immediate assessment of respiratory status using bedside measurement of FVC and assessment of bulbar function and swallowing.
- *First line:* cholinesterase inhibitors (pyridostigmine) with steroids.
- *Refractory cases:* may respond to plasmapheresis. Other treatment options include immunosuppression and thymectomy.

Congenital myasthenia gravis (CMG)

Group of AR disorders. Can rarely be caused by passive transfer of maternal antibodies, which have a predilection for fetal NMJ. They are lifelong and cannot be cured completely.

Presentation
Often as neonates, with arthrogryposis ± bulbar/respiratory insufficiency ± facial weakness ± limb girdle weakness. Laryngeal palsy is particularly noteworthy, as this is a rare condition and very likely to be caused by CMG if there are no other ENT problems.

Diagnosis
- Clinical picture, including examination of the mother.
- Electrophysiological assessment of the NMJ in affected muscles.
- Response to a trial of edrophonium.
- ACh receptor antibodies are not present if mother is unaffected.

Several drugs are contraindicated in myasthenic syndromes. Botulinum is absolutely contraindicated. Penicillamine and interferon can trigger autoimmune myasthenia gravis. Aminoglycoside/macrolide antibiotics are relatively contraindicated. Mg^{2+}, calcium channel blockers, and β-blockers can increase weakness.

Management
Specialist input required (see → Management of muscular disorders, p. 391).

Muscular disorders

(See also ⊃ Genetic disorders with neuromuscular features, pp. 880–1.)

Muscular dystrophies

These are a group of congenital disorders that are characterized by dystrophic change on muscle biopsy. They can affect muscles in different patterns and are characteristically associated with raised CK enzyme levels on blood testing.

Duchenne muscular dystrophy

DMD classically presents within the first 4y with delayed motor milestones and mild speech delay. It is an X-linked recessive condition that lies at the severe end of the spectrum of disorders and is due to a molecular abnormality of dystrophin.

Examination

- Waddling lordotic gait.
- Calf hypertrophy.
- Weakness in limb girdles (lower more than upper): Gower's sign +ve on examination.
- Sparing of facial, extra-ocular, and bulbar muscles.

Investigations and diagnosis

- Markedly raised CK.
- Genetic analysis: this does not differentiate between the milder Becker muscular dystrophy (BMD) and the more severe DMD—therefore, expert interpretation is required.

Myotonic dystrophy

AD disorder with expanded CTG trinucleotide repeats on chromosome 19 (anticipation when transmitted from mother).

- Congenital form: severe cases may present in the neonatal period and are almost always of maternal inheritance. Infants present with hypotonia, feeding difficulty, tent-shaped mouth, and respiratory impairment. Treatment is supportive, but notably the symptoms become less disruptive as the child grows.
- Later-onset form: children present with hypotonia, myopathic face, and global developmental delay. Later complications include diabetes mellitus, cataracts, and cardiac involvement. The diagnosis will initially be made by the characteristic clinical picture.

Diagnosis

Confirmation can be made on examination of both parents and DNA analysis. EMG demonstrates the characteristic myotonic discharges but is not essential for diagnosis.

There is a particular risk of malignant hyperthermia during GA for most neuromuscular disorders, so make sure the child, the parents, and all relevant professionals are alerted.

Congenital myopathies

These are a group of mainly AR disorders characterized by:
- Muscle weakness.
- Hypotonia.
- Variable involvement of facial, bulbar, and extra-ocular muscles.

Congenital myopathies can be associated with arthrogryposis, and if present in the neonate, long-term outcome may improve with good management in the first years.

Diagnosis
- Clinical picture.
- EMG and nerve conduction studies.
- DNA analysis.
- Muscle biopsy is used when the commoner disorders (myotonic dystrophy, DMD, and spinal muscular atrophy) have been excluded.

Management of muscular disorders

These disorders are rare, severe, and complicated. They need to be managed with ongoing advice from a specialist centre. Key components of care include:
- Assessment for power, joint ranges, and contractures—with appropriate advice from physiotherapists and occupational therapists.
- Access to speech therapy and dietary assessment.
- Consideration on appropriate management of respiratory, cardiac, and other systemic complications.
- Liaison with allied services, particularly education/social services.
- Genetic counselling for the child and other family members.
- Psychological support for the child and family.

It should be noted that, although a specialist centre will need to be involved, they will fail if they do not liaise and empower a good local service and the child/family with the above key parts. Their advice on the projected trajectory and likely complications for the specific disorder should inform the exact local management plan.

Cerebral palsy

- *Definition:* a chronic disorder of movement and/or posture that presents early (i.e. before the age of 2y) and continues throughout life. It is caused by static injury to the developing brain.
- *Associations:* children with CP are at ↑ risk of impairments, including vision, hearing, speech, learning, nutrition, and psychiatric problems. They are also at ↑ risk of developing epilepsy.
- *Clinical forms:* most children will have a mixed disorder, but some can have pure spasticity, choreoathetosis, or very rarely ataxia.

Spastic CP

This is the commonest label and children can be hemiplegic, diplegic, or quadriplegic. Monoplegic CP is extremely rare. Spasticity is characterized by a velocity-dependent ↑ resistance to passive stretch. It is caused by disruption to the spinal reflex arc by the upper motor neuron. It affects all skeletal muscles and causes:

- ↑ tone and reflexes.
- Clasp knife phenomenon on rapidly stretching tendons (a 'catch').
- *Leg:* ankle plantar flexion and deformity of the foot.
- *Hip:* flexion, limited adduction, and often internal rotation.
- *Wrist:* flexed and pronated.
- *Elbow:* flexed.
- *Shoulder:* adducted.
- *Bulbar muscles:* may be spastic, causing dysphagia and dribbling.

Choreoathetosis

Involuntary movements with chorea (irregular migrating contractions) and athetosis (twisting and writhing). Presents as a four-limb disorder, with greatly ↑ tone while awake, less so during early stages of sleep. These patients do not have the stretch-related response and ↑ reflexes of pure spastic CP. However, there may be combinations of these features in mixed CP. As the child grows, they often develop fixed reduction in joint range of movement, and then the signs will be more difficult to distinguish from those of spastic CP. They almost always have bulbar problems.

Ataxic cerebral palsy

A very rare form of CP, also known as *disequilibrium syndrome*. The ataxia gives marked loss of balance in early years. Mild diplegia also makes this form of CP distinct from other types of CP, in which hypoxia and ischaemia are causal factors.

Investigations of CP

- *History:* the cause may be evident from a good history, in particular for prematurity and periods of hypoxic ischaemia.
- *Imaging:* brain MRI (see Fig. 9.2), with reference to pyramidal tracts in those with spasticity, and to the basal ganglia in others. *When imaging does not confirm static insult, seek expert opinion.*

Management of CP

- Complex and should involve sub-specialists, general paediatricians, community paediatricians, therapists, and education.
- *Multidisciplinary input:* the primary therapists are the child's carers because they provide most of the therapy. In early years, use experts in speech and language, PT, and OT.
- *Posture and movement:* optimize function by improving symmetry, joint ranges, muscle length, and power. Treatments include: stretching exercises, orthoses, and wheelchair for mobility; sleeping and standing systems; and botulinum toxin (Botox) to the gastrocnemius. Surgical options include muscle lengthening and osteotomy.
- *General medical surveillance:* watching for seizures, constipation, malnutrition, and behavioural or psychiatric disturbance.

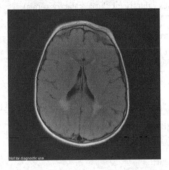

Fig. 9.2 T2-weighted axial images of periventricular leucomalacia.

Subdural haemorrhage

(See also ➔ Physical abuse, pp. 914–15; ➔ Inflicted (abusive) head injury (NAI), p. 987.) Subdural haemorrhage (SDH) in children <2y is an important cause of morbidity and mortality. A significant number will have been caused by purposeful inflicted trauma, and during the investigation of non-accidental head injury (NAHI), it is important to differentiate inflicted injury from other causes of SDH.

Causes of SDH
- Trauma (including traumatic labour).
- Neurosurgical complications.
- Cerebral infections.
- Coagulation and haematological disorders.
- Metabolic causes (glutaric aciduria, galactosaemia).
- Biochemical disorders (hypernatraemia).

Symptoms/signs of acute SDH
- Encephalopathy (irritability, lethargy, focal neurological signs).
- Vomiting, poor feeding.
- Breathing abnormalities, apnoea.
- Pallor, shock.
- Tense fontanelle.
- Seizures (more frequently in inflicted than non-inflicted injury).

Symptoms/signs of subacute or chronic SDH
- Expanding head circumference.
- Vomiting, FTT.
- Neurological deficit.
- Associated conditions

Retinal haemorrhages are strongly associated with NAHI but are not specific for the diagnosis. An ophthalmologist with expertise in eye assessment in children should examine the child.

Skull fractures that are depressed or have branching, crossing, or stellate fracture lines are highly suggestive for NAHI, whereas accidental fractures typically are linear, parietal, and over the vertex.

Coagulation and haematological disorders need to be excluded. Do platelet count, FBC, and blood film. Renal and liver function tests rule out numerous acquired coagulation defects. Extended coagulation screening and factor assays may also be required after discussion with a paediatric haematology specialist.

Glutaric aciduria type 1 (GA1) is associated with spontaneous SDH, and therefore, test for urine organic acids.

Brain imaging in SDH

Initial investigation is likely to be CT, but MRI will also be necessary. (See Fig. 9.3.)

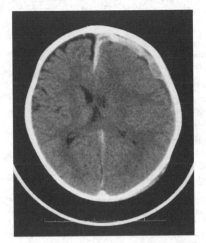

Fig. 9.3 CT head scan of SDH overlying the right frontal lobe, but extending posteriorly and along the falx—highly suggestive of NAHI. The child had extensive retinal haemorrhages, and skeletal survey showed fractures consistent with inflicted injury.

Further management

- Take full social, medical, and family history.
- Skeletal survey.
- Clotting assessment.
- Store urine in case needed for organic acids.
- Arrange ophthalmology assessment.
- *Treat sequelae of SDH:* depends on presentation (e.g. seizures and AEDs) and resuscitation needs.
- *Complete safeguarding procedures:* involve external agencies (e.g. social services, police).
- *Multidisciplinary and specialist follow-up.*

Stroke in childhood

(See also ◑ Cerebral infarction (perinatal stroke), p. 159; ◑ Sickle crises and problems, pp. 550–1.) Cerebrovascular stroke is rare in childhood, but it causes significant morbidity. The aetiology can be arterial ischaemic stroke, haemorrhagic or venous in origin, due to:

- SCD.
- Congenital cardiac defects.
- Cerebral infection.
- Trauma (arterial dissection).

Management

Children with stroke will need initial attention to ABC and treatment of acute conditions, such as mastoiditis/meningitis, before early transfer to a specialist unit.

Initial assessment

- The FAST ('Face, Arms, Speech Time') criteria to determine stroke in children and young people should be used.
- A cranial CT scan should be performed within 1h of arrival at hospital, including CT angiography (CTA).
- Initial scan images should be reviewed on acquisition and, if necessary, discussed with the regional paediatric neuroscience centre.
- In the case of acute arterial–ischaemic stroke, anticoagulation and thrombolysis therapy are currently being introduced in paediatric practice.
- In haemorrhagic stroke, focus on good resuscitation, correct haematological parameters, and liaise with local neurosurgical services.

Treatment

- After *initial assessment and stabilization*, further treatment and investigations should be undertaken in a specialist centre.
- *Subsequent management* would be undertaken with the same team and aims as those outlined for CP.
- *Further specialist input* indicated, depending on cause of stroke.

Investigations for stroke

- *Blood—haematology:*
  - FBC, ESR: polycythaemia.
  - Thrombophilia screen, fibrinogen: thrombophilia.
- *Blood—biochemistry:*
  - U&E, Mg^{2+}.
  - LFTs.
  - CRP: inflammation.
  - Plasma lactate and CSF lactate: mitochondrial disorders.
  - Fasting glucose: diabetes.
  - Fasting lipid screen: hyperlipidaemias.
  - TFTs: Hashimoto's thyroiditis/encephalopathy.
  - Ammonia: urea cycle disorders.
  - Homocysteine (free and total): methyltetrahydrofolate reductase (MTHFR) deficiency can also be picked up by common mutation analysis on the thrombophilia screen and, if symptomatic, has raised plasma homocysteine.
  - Serum iron, total iron-binding capacity (TIBC), ferritin, red cell folate, and vitamin B_{12}: iron deficiency and other nutritional disorders.
  - Plasma amino acids: amino acidurias.
  - Carnitine (acyl, free, and total): β-oxidation defects.
- *Urine:* biochemistry.
- *Urine organic and amino acids:* homocystinuria, MTHFR deficiency.
- *Blood immunology and infection screen:*
  - IgG, IgM, IgA: immunodeficiency.
  - Titres for infection screen of: *Mycoplasma, Chlamydia, Helicobacter, Borrelia,* and *Brucella*; viruses (echovirus, Coxsackie, EBV, varicella, hepatitis B).
  - ASOT, anti DNase B: streptococcal disease.
  - ANA, ANCA, anticardiolipin, and antiphospholipid antibody: SLE and autoimmune disease.
- *Imaging studies:*
  - MRI/MRA of head/neck: vascular disease, particularly dissection and thromboembolism.
  - Echocardiogram: endocarditis and other cardiac disease.

Acute disseminated encephalomyelitis

ADEM is an immune-mediated disease. It usually occurs following a viral infection but may follow other infections or vaccination. It involves autoimmune demyelination; it is similar to multiple sclerosis (MS)—although monophasic. ADEM produces multiple inflammatory lesions in the brain and spinal cord, particularly in the white matter. Usually these are found in the subcortical/central white matter and cortical grey–white junction of both cerebral hemispheres, cerebellum, brainstem, and spinal cord, but other areas, including the basal ganglia, may also be involved.

Presentation

- The average age of onset is around 5–8y.
- Abrupt onset and a monophasic course.
- Symptoms usually begin 1–3wk after infection or vaccination and include fever, headache, drowsiness, coma, and seizures.
- The average time to maximum severity is ~4.5 days.
- Other symptoms: hemiparesis, paraparesis, and cranial nerve palsies.

Diagnosis

Based on finding typical changes on MRI (see above—in the subcortical/central white matter, cortical grey–white junction, cerebellum, brainstem, and spinal cord). The basal ganglia may also be involved. CSF may show mild lymphocytosis, with normal glucose, but there may be a mild rise in protein.

Treatment

Exclude other causes of encephalopathy. Then supportive measures, such as hydration/feeding, and monitoring of bulbar function and respiration should be instituted. Pulsed IV methylprednisolone is widely recommended as definitive treatment and is normally associated with improvement within days.

Multiple sclerosis

MS rarely occurs in childhood but becomes commoner as children approach adulthood. It presents with demyelinating plaques, which differ from ADEM in their distribution (i.e. more periventricular white matter and with much less encephalopathy, seizures, and coma, but more focal neurological signs).

Acute abnormal movements

Ataxia

An abnormality in gait that is wide-based, staggering, and unsteady. May have a number of causes, including: posterior fossa tumours, IEM, poisoning, brainstem encephalitis, post-infectious or autoimmune causes, trauma, vascular disorders, ataxia telangiectasia (AT), Friedreich's ataxia, and conversion disorders.

Clinical review

- *Speech:* ↑ separation of syllables, with varied volume.
- *Neurology:* abnormal proprioception, +ve Romberg, nystagmus.
- *Systemic:* immunodeficiency in AT; hypertrophic cardiomyopathy and diabetes in Fanconi's anaemia (FA).

Investigations

- Cerebral imaging.
- If cause not found: plasma and CSF assessing for varicella, streptococcal, and other infections and for IEM (e.g. urea cycle disorders).

Chorea

Jerk-like movements that may involve the face, arms, or legs. In childhood, the causes are:

- Drugs (anticonvulsants, psychotropics, benzodiazepine withdrawal).
- Systemic illness (Sydenham's chorea, SLE, hyperthyroidism
- Genetic conditions (Huntington's chorea, GA1, other IEM).
- Benign familial chorea.

Streptococcal infection

Sydenham's chorea is often associated with streptococcal infection. It occurs in older children and is frequently misdiagnosed as psychogenic. It is characterized by mild to moderate chorea that is more distal, in a well child. About 20% of rheumatic fever cases include chorea.

Treatment

- High-dose phenoxymethylpenicillin; then daily prophylaxis.
- Sodium valproate is the first-line treatment if IEM is excluded, as it can cause metabolic decompensation.
- Benzodiazepines, phenothiazine, and haloperidol may control symptoms.
- Improvement may occur over weeks to months.

Paediatric autoimmune neuropsychiatric disorder associated with *Streptococcus* (PANDAS)

PANDAS has specific diagnostic criteria and is accompanied by behavioural problems, e.g. obsessive–compulsive disorder (OCD) and tics.

Conversion or 'psychologically mediated' disorders

(See also ⊃ Somatoform disorders and typical consultation-liaison presentations, p. 752.) A high percentage of children older than 7y who present with rapidly progressing neurological symptoms and retained consciousness have a conversion disorder. Diagnosis is by exclusion and examination must be thorough. Video inspection of events can be helpful and it is important not to overinvestigate. Treatment is similar to that of PDPE.

Acute encephalopathy

Encephalopathy is defined as degeneration of brain function, due to different causes. It is thought to denote a process with impaired cognition ± focal neurological signs. It normally is matched by a typical EEG trace with an abundance of slow waves.

Causes

- *Infection:* viral, as well as bacterial, e.g. meningitis.
- *Metabolic:* e.g. mitochondrial dysfunction; check for consanguinity.
- *Autoimmune:* e.g. ADEM, thyroiditis, N-methyl-D-aspartate-receptor encephalitis.
- ↑ *ICP:* e.g. tumours obstructing CSF flow.
- *Lack of O_2 or blood flow:* hypoxia–ischaemia.
- *Trauma.*
- *Toxins:* including solvents, drugs, alcohol, and metals.
- *Radiation.*
- *Nutrition.*

Assessment

Perform a full neurological examination—with particular focus on assessment of the conscious state, GCS score, eye movement, fundi, bulbar control, and upper motor neuron signs.

Management

These children are critically ill and at risk of cardiorespiratory compromise.

- *GCS score <8:* proceed to ETT intubation and MV, and use neuroprotective measures, keeping $PaCO_2$ between 4 and 5kPa.
- *Treat shock:* if present.
- Unless a non-infective diagnosis, treat for meningitis with appropriate antibiotics (e.g. ceftriaxone). Also treat herpes with aciclovir, and M. pneumoniae with clarithromycin.
- *Blood tests:* check FBC, CRP, ESR, glucose, and renal/liver function. If cause unclear, check ammonia, lactate, acylcarnitine profile, and plasma amino acids.
- *Urine:* organic acid profile and store for further assessment as needed, e.g. toxicology.
- Neuroimaging is essential once the child is stable. Always give enhancement; if possible, scan the spine as well, and obtain MRI, rather than CT, although the latter may be easier to obtain.
- Only when stable and neuroimaging shows no contraindication, perform LP. Make sure there is WCC, glucose, protein, lactate, and stored sample for subsequent viral analysis/immunology as needed.
- Further therapy will depend on the case and should only happen within a centre with a paediatric neurology service and PICU.

Further reading

Appleton RE, Marson AG. *Epilepsy: the facts*, third edition. Oxford University Press, Oxford; 2009.

Carville S, Padhi S, Reason T, Underwood M; Guideline Development Group. Diagnosis and management of headache in young people and adults: summary of NICE guidance. *BMJ* 2012; **345**: e5765.

Epilepsy Action. Available at: ℘ https://www.epilepsy.org.uk.

Epilepsy Society. Available at: ℘ https://www.epilepsysociety.org.uk.

Forsyth R, Newton R (eds). *Paediatric Neurology* (Oxford Specialist Handbooks in Paediatrics), second edition. Oxford University Press, Oxford; 2012.

Hampton JR, Harrison MJ, Mitchell JR, Prichard JS, Seymour C. Relative contributions of history-taking, physical examination, and laboratory investigation to diagnosis and management of medical outpatients. *BMJ* 1975; **2**: 486–9.

HeadSmart, Early Diagnosis of Brain Tumours. Available at: ℘ https://www.headsmart.org.uk.

Healthy London Partnership and Young Epilepsy. (2018). *London Epilepsy Standards for Children and Young People: Promoting integrated, holistic care for all children and young people affected by epilepsy*. Available at: ℘ https://www.healthylondon.org/wp-content/uploads/2018/05/London-epilepsy-standards-for-children-and-young-people-May-18.pdf.

Howells R. Headache in childhood and adolescence. *ACNR* 2010; **10**: 27–9.

Lissauer T, Clayden G. *Illustrated Textbook of Paediatrics*, second edition. Mosby, London; 2001.

National Institute for Health and Care Excellence. (2012). *Epilepsies: diagnosis and management.* Clinical guideline [CG137]. Available at: ℘ https://www.nice.org.uk/guidance/cg137.

Royal College of Paediatrics and Child Health. (2017). *Stroke in childhood: clinical guideline for diagnosis, management and rehabilitation*. Available at: ℘ http://www.rcpch.ac.uk/stroke-guideline.

Endocrinology

Obesity

Obesity is a major global public health problem, reaching epidemic levels. Obesity in childhood strongly predicts obesity in adulthood. It is a risk factor for disease in later life, including type 2 diabetes mellitus (T2DM), hypertension, cardiovascular disease, and cancer.

Definition and diagnosis

Obesity implies ↑ central (abdominal) fat mass. Body mass index (BMI) is a convenient indicator of body fat mass.

$$BMI = weight(kg)/[height(m)]^2$$

- *Overweight:* BMI >91st centile, weight <98th centile.
- *Obese:* BMI >98th centile.

Other measures of obesity include waist circumference and waist:hip ratio, less frequently used in paediatric practice.

Epidemiology

Risk factors include:
- Parental/family history of obesity.
- Afro-Caribbean and Indian–Asian ethnic origins.
- *Catch-up growth (weight) in early childhood (0–2y):* infants born SGA who demonstrate significant weight catch-up (>2 SDs) in the first 2y of life are at significant risk of obesity.

Causes

Idiopathic (or 'simple') obesity accounts for ≥95% of cases and is multi-factorial in origin. It represents an imbalance in nutritional–environmental–gene interaction:
- Genetic predisposition (energy conservation).
- Sedentary lifestyle (energy expenditure).
- Increasing consumption and availability of high-energy foods.

Endocrine (rare)
- Hypothyroidism.
- Cushing's syndrome/disease.
- GH deficiency.
- Pseudohypoparathyroidism.
- Polycystic ovarian syndrome (PCOS).
- Acquired hypothalamic injury, i.e. CNS tumours and/or surgery.

Genetic
(See also ➔ Obesity, p. 885.)
- Prader–Willi syndrome (PWS).
- BBS.
- Monogenic causes: leptin deficiency (rare); melanocortin 4 receptor gene (5–6% of all causes).

Obesity: management

Evaluation and investigations, including a detailed history
- Birthweight (NB: SGA).
- Feeding habits/behaviour: hyperphagia may suggest a genetic cause.
- Weight gain/growth pattern (check previous health records).
- Physical activity.
- Neurodevelopment, school performance.
- Screen for comorbid factors (see ➲ Complications and comorbid conditions, p. 407).
- Family history: obesity, T2DM, cardiovascular disease.

Laboratory investigations are directed at excluding causes and detecting complications:
- *Blood biochemistry*: TFTs, cortisol, LFTs, lipid profile.
- Genetic studies (e.g. PWS).
- OGTT (see ➲ Obesity and oral glucose tolerance testing, p. 407; ➲ Diagnosis, p. 480).

Complications and comorbid conditions
Severe obesity is associated with the following complications in childhood:
- *Psychological*: low self-esteem, depression.
- *ENT/respiratory*: OSA, obesity–hypoventilation syndrome, pulmonary hypertension.
- *Orthopaedic*: leg bowing, slipped femoral epiphysis, osteoarthritis.
- *Metabolic*: impaired glucose tolerance/T2DM, hypertension, dyslipidaemia, PCOS.
- *Hepatic*: non-alcoholic steatohepatitis.

Obesity and oral glucose tolerance testing
Consider an OGTT if the following risk factors are present:
- *Severe obesity*: BMI >98th centile.
- *Acanthosis nigricans*: pathognomonic of insulin resistance.
- *Symptoms of diabetes* (polyuria ± polydipsia).
- +ve family history of T2DM.
- *Ethnic origin*: Asian/Afro-Caribbean/African-American.
- PCOS.
- Hypertension.

Management
Treatment requires a multidisciplinary approach.
- Nutrition and lifestyle education/counselling: important.
- Decreasing calorie intake/increasing exercise.
- Behaviour modification and family therapy strategies.
- Drug therapies (currently limited, not licensed for children): appetite suppressants.
- Obesity (bariatric) surgery (rarely).
- Family or population-based intervention and prevention strategies may be more effective than approaches targeted at the obese individual.

Goitre

A goitre is an enlargement of the thyroid gland. It may be congenital or acquired. Enlargement is usually secondary to ↑ pituitary secretion of TSH but could be due to an infiltrative process that may be inflammatory or neoplastic.

Congenital goitre

The commonest causes are due to transplacental transmission:
- Maternal antithyroid drugs.
- Maternal iodine exposure.
- Maternal hyperthyroidism (Graves's disease).

Other rare causes include:
- Thyroid teratoma.
- Endemic iodine deficiency.
- Thyroid hormone biosynthetic defects (e.g. Pendred syndrome).

Acquired goitre

- Simple (colloid) goitre.
- Multinodular goitre.
- Acute thyroiditis.
- Graves's disease.
- Antithyroid drugs: lithium, amiodarone.

Simple (colloid) goitre

A euthyroid, non-toxic goitre of unknown cause. It is not associated with inflammation or neoplasia. TFTs and radioisotope scans are normal. It is commonest in girls during or around the peripubertal years. Treatment is not needed. Follow-up is recommended.

Multinodular goitre

- Rare. A firm goitre with single or multiple palpable nodules.
- TFTs usually normal, although TSH and antithyroid antibody titres may be elevated.
- Abnormalities on thyroid US and areas of reduced uptake on radioisotope scanning may be seen.

Solitary thyroid nodule

Uncommon pre-puberty. ~25% may be associated with underlying thyroid cancer. Requires careful evaluation.

Causes

- Benign adenoma.
- Thyroglossal cyst.
- Ectopic, normal thyroid tissue.
- Single median thyroid gland.
- Thyroid cyst or abscess.
- Thyroid carcinoma.

Investigations

Should include radioisotope (^{99m}Tc) scan. Cold nodules or nodules that feel hard on palpation or are rapidly growing should raise suspicion of thyroid cancer—consider biopsy.

Thyroid carcinoma

Rare in childhood. Many thyroid carcinomas in the past were associated with previous irradiation to the head and neck for other conditions. Characteristics are:

- Histologically classified as being papillary, follicular, or mixed.
- Usually slow-growing.
- Girls are affected twice as often as boys.
- Presentation is usually with a painless thyroid nodule.
- Cervical lymph node involvement is often evident at diagnosis.
- Asymptomatic lung metastases may be seen radiologically.
- Diagnosis is established by biopsy.
- Radioisotope scans (^{123}I or ^{99m}Tc) demonstrate reduced uptake.
- TFTs are usually normal.

Treatment and prognosis

Thyroidectomy (subtotal or complete) is indicated. Radioiodine therapy after surgery is often given. Post-ablative PO thyroid hormone replacement therapy is needed. Prognosis is usually very good, even with the presence of cervical node and/or metastases at diagnosis.

Congenital hypothyroidism

Congenital hypothyroidism occurs in ~1/2000–3000 births. It is twice as common in girls than in boys.

Aetiology

- *Thyroid dysgenesis (85%)*: usually sporadic; thyroid aplasia/hypoplasia, ectopic thyroid (lingual/sublingual).
- Iodine deficiency (rare in the UK, but common worldwide).
- *Congenital TSH deficiency (rare)*: associated with hypopituitarism.
- 10–15% are due to thyroid dyshormonogenesis; seven genes are known to be associated: *SLC5A5* (NIS), *TG, DUOX2, SCL26A4* (PDS) (e.g. Pendred syndrome), *DUOXA2, TPO*, and *IYD* (DHEAL1).
- Hypothyroidism can be permanent or transient.

Clinical features

Usually non-specific, often difficult to detect in first month of life:
- Hypotonia and poor feeding.
- Prolonged jaundice.
- Constipation.
- Dry skin and coarse facies.
- Delayed neurodevelopment.
- Umbilical hernia.
- Hoarse cry.

Diagnosis

- National neonatal screening programmes exist in many countries—in first week of life, blood spot test detects elevated TSH level.
- Laboratory confirmation with both TSH and free T4 levels should be performed ASAP.
- Thyroid US to identify thyroid structures.
- Radionucleotide scanning (^{99}Tc or ^{131}I) to identify thyroid position.

Treatment

Prompt treatment is important to prevent adverse sequelae:
- Neurodevelopmental delay and mental retardation.
- Poor motor coordination, ataxia.
- Poor growth and short stature.

Monitoring therapy

Monitor serum TSH and T4 levels: every 1–2mth in first year; every 2–3mth at age 1–2y; every 4–6mth at age >2y. Maintain T4 level in upper half of normal range, TSH in lower end of normal range.

Transient hyperthyrotropinaemia

- Uncommon (may be detected by neonatal screening).
- Characterized by slightly elevated TSH, but normal serum T4.
- Due to transfer of transplacental maternal thyroid antibodies.
- Does not need treatment but must be monitored.
- If TSH remains elevated after a few months or T4 is low, treat with PO levothyroxine.

Thyroiditis

Autoimmune thyroiditis (Hashimoto's)

The commonest cause of thyroid disease in childhood:
* Lymphocytic infiltration of the thyroid gland and early thyroid follicular hyperplasia, leading to eventual atrophy and fibrosis.
* Associated with a family history of thyroid disease. ↑ risk of other autoimmune disorders, e.g. T1DM.
* 4–7 times commoner in ♀ than in ♂.
* Children with Down's or Turner's syndrome are at ↑ risk.
* Peak incidence is in adolescence, although may occur at any age.

Presentation
* Usually insidious with a diffusely enlarged, non-tender, firm goitre.
* Most children are asymptomatic and biochemically euthyroid.
* Some present with hypothyroidism.
* A few may have initial hyperthyroidism, i.e. 'Hashitoxicosis'.
* Variable clinical course: goitres may become smaller and disappear or persist. Many who are initially euthyroid develop hypothyroidism within months/years of presentation.
* Periodic follow-up is necessary.

Investigations
* Thyroid biochemistry may be normal or abnormal.
* Thyroid peroxidase antibody titres are usually raised, whereas anti-thyroglobulin titres are ↑ in only ~50%.

Treatment
Only required for hypothyroidism or hyperthyroidism if present.

Acute suppurative thyroiditis

* Uncommon infection of the thyroid gland. Often preceded by respiratory tract infection.
* Organisms include *Staphylococcus aureus*, streptococci, *Escherichia coli* (rarely fungal).
* Presents with painful, tender swelling of the thyroid. TFTs are usually normal; hyperthyroidism may occur.
* Recurrent infection suggests presence of a thyroglossal tract remnant.
* Treatment: antibiotics and surgical drainage of abscess if present.

Subacute thyroiditis (de Quervain's)

* A self-limiting condition of viral origin.
* Tenderness and pain overlying the thyroid.
* Symptoms of thyrotoxicosis may be present initially; hypothyroidism may develop later.
* Treatment: non-steroidal anti-inflammatory agents, corticosteroids if severe. β-blocker therapy may help control thyrotoxic symptoms.

Resistance to thyroid hormone (RTH)

* Mutation in the *THR* gene, leading to defect in thyroid hormone receptor.
* RTH β—variable phenotype, may be thyrotoxic.
* RTH α—very rare 'hypothyroid' phenotype.

Acquired hypothyroidism

Estimated prevalence of 0.1–0.2%. Incidence in girls is 5–10 times greater than in boys.

Aetiology

Primary hypothyroidism (raised TSH; low T4/T3)
- Autoimmune (Hashimoto's or chronic lymphocytic thyroiditis).
- Iodine deficiency: commonest cause worldwide.
- Subacute thyroiditis.
- Drugs (e.g. amiodarone, lithium).
- Post-irradiation thyroid.
- Post-ablative (radioiodine therapy or surgery).

Central hypothyroidism (low serum TSH; low T4)
Hypothyroidism due to pituitary or hypothalamic dysfunction.
- Intracranial tumours/masses.
- Post-cranial radiotherapy/surgery.
- Developmental pituitary defects (genetic, e.g. *PROP-1*, *Pit-1* genes): isolated TSH deficiency; multiple pituitary hormone deficiencies.

Clinical features

Symptoms and signs are often insidious and can be extremely difficult to diagnose clinically. A high index of suspicion is needed.
- *Goitre:* primary hypothyroidism.
- ↑ weight gain/obesity.
- ↓ growth velocity/delayed puberty.
- Delayed skeletal maturation (bone age).
- *Fatigue:* mental slowness, deteriorating school performance.
- *Constipation:* cold intolerance, bradycardia.
- *Dry skin:* coarse hair.
- *Pseudo-puberty.*
- *Slipped upper (capital) femoral epiphysis:* hip pain/limp.

Diagnosis

- TFTs: high TSH/low T4/low T3.
- Thyroid antibody screen. Raised antibody titres: antithyroid peroxidase, anti-thyroglobulin, TSH receptor (blocking type).

Treatment

- PO levothyroxine.
- Monitor TFTs every 4–6mth during childhood.
- Monitor growth and neurodevelopment.

Hyperthyroidism (thyrotoxicosis)

- *Thyrotoxicosis:* the clinical, physiological, and biochemical findings that result when the tissues are exposed to excess thyroid hormones.
- *Hyperthyroidism:* denotes those conditions resulting in hyperfunction of the thyroid gland, leading to a state of thyrotoxicosis.

Causes of thyrotoxicosis

Due to hyperthyroidism
- Excessive thyroid stimulation:
  - Graves's disease.
  - Hashimoto's disease.
  - Neonatal (transient) thyrotoxicosis.
  - RTH β.
  - McCune–Albright syndrome (McAS).
  - hCG-secreting tumours.
- Thyroid nodules (autonomous):
  - Toxic nodule/multinodular goitre.
  - Thyroid adenoma/carcinoma.

Not due to hyperthyroidism
- Thyroiditis:
  - Subacute.
  - Drug-induced.
- Exogenous thyroid hormones.

Clinical features (all causes)
- Hyperactivity/irritability.
- Poor concentration, altered mood, insomnia.
- Heat intolerance/fatigue/muscle weakness/wasting.
- Weight loss despite ↑ appetite.
- Altered bowel habit—diarrhoea.
- Menstrual irregularity.
- Sinus tachycardia, ↑ pulse pressure.
- Hyperreflexia, fine tremor.
- Pruritus.

Investigations
- *TFTs (serum):* raised T4 and T3, suppressed TSH.
- *Thyroid antibodies:* antithyroid peroxidase, anti-thyroglobulin, TSH receptor antibody (stimulatory type).
- *Radionuclide thyroid scan:* ↑ uptake (Graves's disease), ↓ uptake (thyroiditis).

Graves's disease

An autoimmune disorder. Several HLA-DR gene loci (DR3; DQA1*0501) have been identified as susceptibility loci. There is often a family history of autoimmune thyroid disease (girls > boys). Graves's disease occurs due to a predominance of stimulating-type autoantibodies to the TSH receptor.

Clinical features

In addition to those of hyperthyroidism, specific features are:
- Diffuse goitre (majority).
- *Graves's ophthalmopathy*: exophthalmos/proptosis, eyelid lag/retraction, periorbital oedema/chemosis, ophthalmoplegia/extra-ocular muscle dysfunction.
- Pretibial myxoedema.

Diagnosis

- *TFTs*: high T4/high T3/low TSH.
- *Thyroid antibody screen*: antithyroid peroxidase; anti-thyroglobulin +ve, TSH receptor antibody (stimulatory type) +ve; radionucleotide thyroid scan—↑ uptake.

Treatment

Aims to induce remission with antithyroid drugs (carbimazole or propylthiouracil) and, if necessary, to bring the symptoms of thyrotoxicosis (anxiety, tremor, tachycardia) under control using a β-blocking agent (propranolol). Two alternative regimens are practised:
- *Dose titration*: antithyroid treatment titrated to achieve normal thyroid function.
- *Block and replace*: antithyroid treatment maintained at lowest dose necessary to induce complete thyroid suppression. Replacement thyroxine therapy is needed to achieve euthyroidism.

Antithyroid therapy is usually given for 12–24mth, before considering a trial off treatment. Thyroid function (serum-free T4; TSH) should be monitored at regular intervals (1–3mth).

Prognosis

After completion of treatment, 40–75% relapse within 2y. Relapses are treated with antithyroid drugs. Definitive therapy with radioiodine or thyroid surgery may be offered. Following radioiodine or surgery, lifelong thyroxine replacement is required.

Neonatal thyrotoxicosis

- Rare and due to passive transfer of maternal thyroid antibodies from a thyrotoxic mother to the fetus (see also ↪ Thyroid disease, p. 105).
- Affected neonates are irritable, flushed, and tachycardic. Weight gain is poor and cardiac failure may be present.
- Self-limiting. Supportive treatment (e.g. β-blocker therapy) is required.

Adrenal insufficiency

- *Primary adrenal failure:* reduced glucocorticoid (cortisol) and mineralocorticoid (aldosterone) production. ACTH levels are elevated due to reduced −ve feedback drive.
- *Secondary adrenal failure:* reduced corticotrophin-releasing factor (CoRF) or reduced ACTH production (or both) results in reduced cortisol. Mineralocorticoid activity remains normal.

Causes of adrenal insufficiency

Primary

Acquired

- Autoimmune adrenalitis (Addison's disease).
- Adrenal infection, e.g. TB.
- Adrenal haemorrhage/infarction.
- Iatrogenic: adrenalectomy, drugs (e.g. ketoconazole).

Congenital

- CAH.
- Congenital adrenal hypoplasia.
- Adrenoleukodystrophy.
- Familial glucocorticoid deficiency.

Secondary

- Defects of hypothalamus/pituitary structures:
  - Congenital—pituitary hypoplasia.
  - Intracranial masses: tumours (e.g. glioma), craniopharyngioma.
  - Intracranial inflammation: Langerhans histiocytosis.
  - Intracranial infections.
  - Cranial radiotherapy/irradiation.
  - Neurosurgery.
  - Traumatic brain injury.
- Suppression of hypothalamic–pituitary–adrenal axis:
  - Glucocorticoid therapy.
  - Cushing's disease (after pituitary tumour removal).

Clinical features

Clinical features may be subtle and a high index of suspicion is required. Symptom onset may be gradual with partial insufficiency, leading to complete adrenal insufficiency with impaired cortisol responses to stress and illness (adrenal crises):

- Anorexia and weight loss.
- Fatigue and generalized weakness.
- Dizziness (hypotension).
- Salt craving (primary adrenal insufficiency).
- Hyperpigmentation (primary adrenal insufficiency).
- Reduced pubic/axillary hair (primary adrenal insufficiency).
- Hypoglycaemia (neonates/infants).

Diagnosis

Basal serum cortisol and ACTH

NB: random basal cortisol levels are often within the normal range and not reliable. Low cortisol during 'stress' suggests insufficiency. Cortisol level of >550nmol/L usually excludes this diagnosis. Elevated early morning (9 a.m.) ACTH is suggestive of primary adrenal insufficiency.

Adrenal stimulation tests

Establish a diagnosis of adrenal insufficiency. Assesses cortisol responses to stimulation of the adrenal glands.

- *Insulin tolerance test:* serum cortisol response to hypoglycaemia.
- ACTH stimulation (Synacthen®) test: considered the gold standard, serum cortisol is measured at baseline and +30 and +60min after IV/ IM synthetic ACTH (short Synacthen® test). Serum cortisol response of >500nmol/L is considered normal (but check local lab assay used, as threshold varies between labs).

Other investigations

- *Serum electrolytes:* serum Na+ (low) serum K+ (high).
- *Adrenal antibody titres:* Addison's disease.
- *Adrenal imaging:* USS; CT scan.
- *Adrenal androgen profile:* serum/urine.
- *Pituitary imaging:* CT or MRI scan.
- *Serum very long-chain fatty acids (VLCFAs):* X-linked adrenoleukodystrophy.

Adrenal insufficiency: treatment

Primary adrenal insufficiency requires glucocorticoid and mineralocorticoid replacement therapy. Secondary adrenal insufficiency requires glucocorticoid therapy only.

- *Glucocorticoid therapy:* hydrocortisone.
- During illness and stress (e.g. infection, trauma, surgery), increase the daily maintenance dose of hydrocortisone by 2–3 times.
- *Mineralocorticoid therapy:* fludrocortisone. Monitor BP and renin.

Adrenal crises

An adrenal (or Addisonian) crisis is an acute exacerbation of an underlying adrenal insufficiency brought on by 'stresses'. This is a life-threatening emergency and should be treated if there is a strong clinical suspicion, rather than waiting for confirmatory test results. Typical causes include infection, trauma, and surgery. Symptoms include:

- Nausea/vomiting.
- Abdominal pain.
- Lethargy/somnolence.
- Hypotension.
- Characterized by hyperkalaemia, hyponatraemia, and (hypoglycaemia).

Treatment

- Immediate IV bolus of hydrocortisone, followed by 6-hourly repeat injections. IVI fluids/glucose.

Adrenal excess

A state of glucocorticoid (cortisol) excess. The commonest cause of hypercortisolaemia is iatrogenic, due to exogenous steroid therapy.

The term Cushing's disease applies to an ACTH-secreting pituitary tumour (rare). All other causes of glucocorticoid excess are often referred to as Cushing's syndrome.

Causes of adrenal (cortisol) excess

- Iatrogenic.
- *Primary adrenal hyperfunction (ACTH-independent):*
  - Adrenal tumour (carcinoma/adenoma).
  - Nodular adrenal hyperplasia.
  - McAS.
- *Secondary adrenal hyperfunction (ACTH-dependent):*
  - Cushing's disease—pituitary adenoma/hyperplasia.
  - Ectopic ACTH secretion (tumour).

In young children (<5y), adrenal disorders are the commonest non-iatrogenic cause. In neonates and infants, consider McAS. In older children and adolescents, Cushing's disease is the commonest.

Clinical features

- *Obesity:* central adiposity—face, trunk, abdomen.
- 'Moon' facies.
- *'Buffalo hump':* prominent posterior cervical fat pads.
- Muscle wasting.
- Proximal muscle weakness.
- *Skin abnormalities:* thinning (rare in children), easy bruising, striae.
- Hypertension.
- *Growth impairment:* reduced growth velocity, short stature.
- Pubertal delay/amenorrhoea.
- Osteoporosis.

  NB: other signs may be present, depending on the cause.

Investigations

Diagnose hypercortisolism and thereafter differentiate between ACTH-dependent and ACTH-independent causes (see Box 10.1).

Management

Cushing's disease
- Preoperative treatment in order to normalize blood cortisol levels:
  - Metyrapone.
  - Ketoconazole.
- Pituitary surgery: trans-sphenoidal surgery.
- Pituitary radiotherapy.

Adrenal disease/tumour
- Surgery, i.e. adrenalectomy.

Box 10.1 Investigations to determine the following

Is hypercortisolism present or not?
- *Serum cortisol circadian rhythm:*
  - Midnight serum cortisol (NB: patients must be asleep at time of sampling for test to be valid).
  - Loss of normal diurnal variation—raised midnight value observed.
- *Urinary free cortisol excretion:* 24h collection.
- *Dexamethasone suppression test:*
  - Overnight test (1mg dexamethasone at midnight).
  - Low-dose test (0.5mg every 6h for 48h).
  - Failure of suppression of plasma cortisol levels is observed.

Causes of hypercortisolism
- *Plasma ACTH:* high in ACTH-dependent causes.
- *Dexamethasone suppression test:*
  - High-dose test (2mg every 6h for 48h).
  - In Cushing's disease, serum cortisol levels decrease by ~50%. Ectopic ACTH secretion: no suppression.
  - CoRF test.
  - CT scan of adrenal glands.
  - MRI scan of brain.
  - Bilateral inferior petrosal sinus sampling.

Congenital adrenal hyperplasia

A family of disorders characterized by enzyme defects in the steroidogenic pathways that lead to the biosynthesis of cortisol, aldosterone, and androgens. The relative decrease in cortisol production results in ↑ secretion of ACTH and subsequent hyperplasia of the adrenals. CAH is inherited in an AR manner, and the clinical manifestation is determined by the effects produced by the particular hormones that are deficient and by the excess production of steroids unaffected by the enzymatic block.

The causes of CAH include deficiencies in the following steroidogenic pathway enzymes:

- 21α-hydroxylase (*CYP21*).
- 11β-hydroxylase (*CYP11*).
- 3β-hydroxysteroid dehydrogenase.
- 17α-hydroxylase/17–20 lyase (*CYP17*).
- Side-chain cleavage (*SCC/StAR*).

Deficiency of the 21α-hydroxylase accounts for >90% of cases.

21α-hydroxylase deficiency

CAH as a result of defunctioning mutations in the active gene (*CYP21*) located on chromosome 6p. Incidence is ~1/14 000 births.

- *Classic CAH:* includes a severe 'salt-wasting' form that usually presents with acute adrenal crisis in early infancy (usually ♂ at 7–10 days of life), and a 'simple virilizing' form with masculinization of the external genitalia (♀ at birth) or signs of excessive virilization in early life in ♂.
- *Non-classic (late-onset) CAH:* presents in ♀ with signs and symptoms of mild androgen excess at or around the time of puberty.

Diagnosis

'Classic' CAH is diagnosed by:

- Elevated plasma 17-hydroxyprogesterone levels.
- Elevated plasma 21-deoxycortisol levels.
- ↑ urinary adrenocorticosteroid metabolites.

NB: it may be difficult to distinguish elevated androgen levels from the physiological hormonal surge in the first 2 days of life. These tests should be postponed or repeated after 48h of age.

In the 'salt-wasting' form, aldosterone deficiency results in hyponatraemia, hyperkalaemia, and metabolic acidosis. These are not specific findings and can cause diagnostic confusion with children presenting with commoner causes of renal tubular dysfunction.

Treatment

Glucocorticoid replacement therapy

Required in all patients. In addition to treating cortisol deficiency, this suppresses the ACTH-dependent excess adrenal androgen production. During stress and illness, ↑ amounts (e.g. double or triple dose) of glucocorticoid therapy are required.

Mineralocorticoid therapy
For the salt-wasting form of CAH only: fludrocortisone.

Sodium chloride therapy
Resistance to mineralocorticoid therapy is usually seen in infancy. Sodium chloride supplements are often required during this period to maintain normal electrolyte balance. Once a normal solid diet is established, salt supplements may be discontinued.

Urogenital surgery
Reconstructive surgery (clitoral reduction and vaginoplasty) may be performed in ♀ with significant virilization of the external genitalia. Consideration should be given as to whether this could be delayed to enable patient choice in later life.

Long-term management and monitoring

Regular monitoring of patients by a specialist team is required in order to ensure the child's optimal growth and development.

Mineralocorticoid excess

Primary hyperaldosteronism

Characterized by hypokalaemia and hypertension. The renin–angiotensin system is suppressed with low plasma renin. Children may have no symptoms, and the diagnosis made after an incidental finding of hypertension. Chronic hypokalaemia may result in muscle weakness, fatigue, and poor growth.

Causes of primary hyperaldosteronism
- Bilateral adrenal hyperplasia.
- Adrenal tumours.
- Glucocorticoid-remediable hyperaldosteronism.

Secondary hyperaldosteronism

Excess aldosterone production is secondary to elevated renin levels. Hypertension may or may not be present.

Causes of secondary hyperaldosteronism
Associated with hypertension
- Renovascular malformations/stenosis.
- Primary hyperreninaemia.
- Juxtaglomerular tumour.
- Wilms' tumour.
- Post-renal transplantation.
- Urinary tract obstruction.
- Phaeochromocytoma.

No hypertension
- Hepatic cirrhosis.
- Congestive cardiac failure.
- Nephrotic syndrome.
- Bartter's syndrome.
- Anorexia nervosa.
- Syndrome of apparent mineralocorticoid excess: type 1 and type 2 variants.

Mineralocorticoid deficiency

Reduced aldosterone production or activity is rare and may be due to congenital or acquired causes.

Inherited endocrine syndromes

Multiple endocrine neoplasia

A family of endocrine neoplasia syndromes inherited in an AD manner:
- MEN type 1.
- MEN type 2.
- von Hippel–Lindau (VHL) syndrome.

Genetic screening is available. Patients with these conditions require close surveillance and screening (biochemistry, radiology, etc.).

Succinate dehydrogenase (SDH) deficiency

- Hereditary phaeochromocytomas, paragangliomas, and gastrointestinal stromal tumours (GISTs).

McCune–Albright syndrome

Characterized by the following triad of clinical features:
- *Skin:* hyperpigmented (café-au-lait) macules.
  - Classically irregular edge ('coast of Maine' appearance).
  - Do not cross the midline.
- *Polyostotic fibrous dysplasia:*
  - Slowly progressive bone lesion.
  - Any bones, although facial/base of skull bones the commonest.
- *Autonomous endocrine gland hyperfunction:*
  - Ovary most commonly affected.
  - Precocious puberty (gonadotrophin-independent).
  - Thyroid (hyperthyroidism).
  - Adrenal (Cushing's syndrome).
  - Pituitary (adenoma—gigantism).
  - Parathyroid (hyperparathyroidism).

Neurofibromatosis

Two types of NF are recognized. Type 1 (NF1; also known as von Recklinghausen's disease) is an AD condition due to a mutation of the *NF1* gene (see ➔ Neurofibromatosis, p. 383; ➔ Neurofibromatosis type 1, p. 882).
  NF1 may be associated with endocrine abnormalities:
- Hypothalamic/pituitary tumours: optic glioma (15%).
- GH deficiency.
- Precocious puberty.
- Delayed puberty.

Hypocalcaemia

- Hypocalcaemic seizures, muscle spasms, or laryngeal spasm may occur acutely.
- Cardiac conduction abnormalities (prolonged QT interval, QRS and ST changes, and ventricular arrhythmias) may be seen.
- Chronic hypocalcaemia may be asymptomatic.

Causes of hypocalcaemia

Early neonatal causes
- Prematurity.
- Maternal diabetes.
- Maternal pre-eclampsia.

Late neonatal causes
- Cow's milk hyperphosphataemia.
- Maternal hypercalcaemia.
- Congenital hypoparathyroidism.

Causes in infancy
- Nutritional rickets.
- PHP type 1a.

Childhood causes
- PHP type 1b.
- Hypoparathyroidism.

Iatrogenic causes
- Chemotherapy agents, e.g. cisplatin.
- Anticonvulsant agents, e.g. phenytoin.

Investigations

- Plasma Ca^{2+}.
- Plasma PO_4^{3-}.
- Serum PTH. Low/normal PTH implies failure of PTH secretion.
- Plasma vitamin D.
- Plasma Mg^{2+}.
- X-ray of skull. Chronic hypocalcaemia: basal ganglia calcification.

Treatment

Acute treatment
(See ➲ Hypocalcaemia, p. 74.)

Chronic treatment
- Treat the underlying cause.
- PO Ca^{2+} supplements, together with PO vitamin D therapy, in the form of calcitriol (1α-calcidiol) are often required to maintain plasma Ca^{2+} levels within the normal range.

Hypoparathyroidism

- *Failure in parathyroid development (agenesis/dysgenesis):*
  - Isolated defect: X-linked recessive.
  - Associated with other abnormalities, e.g. di George syndrome, Kearnes–Sayre syndrome.
- Destruction of parathyroid glands:
  - *Autoimmune*—type 1 autoimmune polyendocrinopathy.
  - Surgery (post-thyroidectomy).
  - Radiotherapy.
- Failure in PTH secretion: Mg^{2+} deficiency.
- Failure in PTH action: PHP.

Investigations
- *Plasma Ca^{2+}:* low.
- *Plasma PO_4^{3-}:* high.
- *Serum PTH:* low.

Pseudohypoparathyroidism

A genetic disorder with several subtypes, characterized by end-organ re-sistance to the actions of PTH. Other features include learning difficulties, obesity, and shortened fourth and fifth fingers. Lab results show low Ca^{2+}, high PO_4^{3-}, and raised PTH.

Rickets

(See also ➲ Vitamin D deficiency and rickets, p. 687.) A disorder of the growing skeleton due to inadequate mineralization of bone as it is laid down at the epiphyseal growth plates. *Osteomalacia* occurs due to inadequate mineralization of mature bone.

Causes

Calcium deficiency
- Dietary, malabsorption.

Vitamin D
- *Vitamin D deficiency:* dietary, exclusive breastfeeding 6–12mth, malabsorption, lack of sunlight, iatrogenic (e.g. phenytoin therapy).
- *Defect in vitamin D metabolism:* vitamin D-dependent rickets (VDDR) type I (1α-hydroxylase deficiency), liver disease, renal disease.
- *Defect in vitamin D action:* VDDR type II—symptomatic rickets in first year of life, alopecia/sparse body hair.

NB: in the UK, it is advised that all children between 6mth and 5y of age take vitamin D supplements (e.g. 400IU daily as colecalciferol).

Phosphate deficiency
- Renal tubular PO_4^{3-} loss (isolated): hypophosphataemic rickets:
  - X-linked.
  - AR.
  - AD.
- Acquired hypophosphataemic rickets:
  - Fanconi syndrome.
  - RTA.
  - Nephrotoxic drugs.
- Reduced PO_4^{3-} intake.

Clinical features

- Growth delay or arrest.
- Bone pain and fracture.
- Muscle weakness.
- Skeletal deformities: swelling of wrists, swelling of costochondral junctions ('rickets rosary'), bowing of the long bones, frontal cranial bossing, craniotabes (softening of skull).

Diagnosis

- Laboratory (see Table 10.1):
  - Plasma Ca^{2+}/PO_4^{3-}/ALP/PTH; vitamin D metabolites [25-hydroxyvitamin D3 (25-OHD)/1,25-dihydroxyvitamin D3 (1,25-OHD)].
- *Radiological:* X-ray of wrists (osteopenia/widening, cupping and fraying of metaphyses).

There are three characteristic stages in disease progression:
- *Stage 1:* low plasma Ca^{2+}/normal plasma PO_4^{3-}.
- *Stage 2:* normal plasma Ca^{2+} (compensatory hyperparathyroidism).
- *Stage 3:* low plasma Ca^{2+} and PO_4^{3-} (advanced bone disease).

Stages 1 and 2 are biochemically evident. Stage 3 has clinical features.

Table 10.1 Laboratory findings in different types of rickets

	Plasma Ca^{2+}	Plasma PO_4^{3-}	ALP	25-OHD	1,25-OHD	PTH
Vitamin D deficiency	↓	↓	↑	↓	↓	↑
VDDR, type I	↓	↓	↑	↓	↓	↑
VDDR, type II	↓	↓	↑	↓	↑	↑
X-linked hypophosphataemia	↓	↓	↑	↓	↓	↓ or ↑
RTA	↓ or ↓	↓	↑	↓	↓ or ↑	↓

Hypercalcaemia

- Williams syndrome (WS).
- Idiopathic infantile hypercalcaemia.
- Hyperparathyroidism.
- Hypercalcaemia of malignancy.
- Vitamin D intoxication.
- Familial hypocalciuric hypercalcaemia.
- Less common: sarcoidosis/granulomatous disease, chronic immobility, renal failure, hyperthyroidism, Addison's disease, iatrogenic.

Clinical features

- *GI:* anorexia, nausea, vomiting, FTT, constipation, abdominal pain.
- *Renal:* polyuria and polydipsia.
- *CNS:* apathy, drowsiness, depression.

Investigations

- Plasma Ca^{2+} (total and corrected for albumin).
- Serum PTH.
- Vitamin D metabolites.
- U&E/LFTs.
- TFTs.
- Urinary Ca^{2+} excretion [urinary Ca^{2+} (UCa):urinary creatinine (UCr) ratio; 24h UCa].
- Renal USS (screen for nephrocalcinosis).

Treatment

- *Acute treatment* (see ⮕ Hypercalcaemia, p. 614).
- *Chronic treatment:* directed at the underlying cause (e.g. low-Ca^{2+} diet).

Hypopituitarism

Hypopituitarism refers to either partial or complete deficiency of the anterior and/or posterior pituitary function.

Congenital hypopituitarism

Abnormalities in the hypothalamic–pituitary structures and other midline brain structures (e.g. septo-optic dysplasia, optic nerve hypoplasia, absent corpus callosum) are often detected on imaging.

A number of specific inherited genetic defects have been characterized, e.g. mutations in pituitary transcription factor genes (e.g. *HESX-1*, *PIT-1*, *LHX-4*) can result in isolated or multiple anterior pituitary hormone deficiencies.

Acquired hypopituitarism

Potential causes of pituitary hormone deficiency include the following:
• Intracranial (parapituitary) tumours.
• *Cranial irradiation/radiotherapy*: GH axis is the most sensitive to radiation damage, followed by gonadotrophin, adrenal, and thyroid axes.
• Traumatic brain injury.
• *Inflammatory/infiltrative*: Langerhans cell histiocytosis, sarcoidosis.
• Pituitary infarction (apoplexy).
• Intracranial infection.

Investigations

• *Basal hormone levels*: e.g. luteinizing hormone (LH)/follicle-stimulating hormone (FSH); TSH, fT4; prolactin; cortisol (9 a.m.); IGF (insulin-like growth factor) 1.
• *Dynamic endocrine testing*: specific tests to assess secretory capacity of the anterior pituitary gland.
• *MRI scan*: brain.

Treatment

Adequate and appropriate hormone replacement therapy and, where applicable, management of underlying cause.

Posterior pituitary: SIADH

(See also ➲ Hyponatraemia, p. 72.) A heterogenous disorder characterized by inappropriately high ADH secretion, hypotonic *hyponatraemia*, and impaired urinary dilution that cannot be accounted for by a recognized stimulus to ADH secretion. There are many causes of SIADH (see Box 10.2).

> **Box 10.2 Causes of SIADH**
> * *Congenital:* agenesis of corpus callosum.
> * *Acquired:*
>   * *CNS*—traumatic brain injury, cerebrovascular bleeding.
>   * *Tumours*—brain, lung, thymus.
>   * *Infection*—pneumonia, meningitis, encephalitis, TB.
>   * *Neurological*—G-BS.
>   * *Respiratory*—asthma, pneumothorax.
>   * *Drugs*—vincristine, cyclophosphamide.

Up to 15% of children with brain trauma or infection develop SIADH. Clinical features include confusion, headache, lethargy, seizures, and coma.

Symptoms do not necessarily depend on the concentration of serum Na^+, but on its rate of development. Slow, gradual development of hyponatraemia may be asymptomatic.

> **SIADH diagnostic criteria**
> * Hyponatraemia (serum Na^+ <135mmol/L).
> * Hypotonic plasma (osmolality <270mOsm/kg).
> * Excessive renal Na^+ loss (>20mmol/L).
> * No hypovolaemia or fluid overload.
> * Normal renal, adrenal, and thyroid function.
> * ↑ plasma ADH.

Management

Treat the underlying cause. Fluid restriction is the mainstay of therapy.
* Hypertonic (3%) saline solution may be used to correct severe hyponatraemia or hyponatraemia resistant to fluid restriction.
* Correcting hyponatraemia slowly is essential to avoid rapid overcorrection with possible complication of central pontine demyelination.
* Longer-term management/treatment with demeclocycline may be effective for fluid balance by inducing NDI.

Posterior pituitary: diabetes insipidus

DI is inappropriate passage of large volumes of dilute urine (<300mOsm/L). Due to a deficiency in arginine vasopressin (AVP) production (cranial DI) or resistance to its actions at the kidney (NDI). The commonest cause is cranial DI.

> ## Causes of diabetes insipidus
> ### Cranial DI
> *Inherited/familial (various genetic forms of DI)*
> - Wolfram syndrome (also known as DIDMOAD: DI, DM, optic atrophy, deafness).
> - Psychogenic.
> - Dipsogenic (abnormal thirst).
> - Holoprosencephaly.
> - Midline craniofacial defects.
> - Midline tumours/traumatic brain injuries, infection.
>
> ### NDI
> - X-linked recessive: *ADH receptor-2* gene.
> - *Aquaporin-2* gene mutations.
> - Drugs (lithium, cisplatin, amphotericin).
> - Hypercalcaemia.

Clinical features

Children present with polydipsia, polyuria, and nocturia, so commoner differential diagnoses (e.g. diabetes mellitus) should be excluded first. Infants may exhibit FTT, fever, and constipation. Other symptoms may be related to underlying cause, e.g. headache, VA/field impairment.

Diagnosis

- Assessment of 24h urinary volume and osmolality under conditions of ad libitum fluid intake. Serum osmolality, U&E, and blood glucose should also be measured.
- Blood hypertonicity (serum osmolality >300mOsm) with inappropriate urine hypotonicity (urine osmolality <300mOsm) should be demonstrated. Diabetes mellitus and renal failure should be excluded.
- A water deprivation test and assessment of responses to exogenously administered ADH are required to diagnose the type of DI. Other tests to determine the underlying cause of DI will also be needed (e.g. cranial MRI).

Treatment

Cranial DI

- The synthetic analogue of ADH—desmopressin (DDAVP) (which has a longer duration of action)—can be given intranasally/PO.
- Dose varies considerably and must be titrated for each patient.

- The dose and frequency of administration (1–3 times a day) are adjusted to maintain 24h urine output volume within the normal range. Avoid water retention.
- It is essential to educate patients and families about the hazards of excessive water intake. Patients with intact thirst sensation mechanism should achieve this.

Nephrogenic DI

- Correct underlying metabolic or iatrogenic causes, if possible.
- Maintenance of an adequate fluid input is essential.
- Thiazide diuretics (e.g. hydrochlorthiazide), amiloride, and prostaglandin synthase inhibitors (e.g. indometacin) can be effective.

Primary polydipsia

- Treatment is often difficult. Behaviour modification strategies usually required.

Polycystic ovarian syndrome

Affects ♀ of reproductive age. *Diagnostic criteria*: any two of the following three features:
- Oligo- and/or anovulation.
- Clinical/biochemical evidence of hyperandrogenism (provided other aetiologies of androgen excess have been excluded).
- Polycystic ovaries on USS.

Clinical and biochemical features are variable. Typical signs and symptoms develop during or after puberty and may include:
- Oligo-/amenorrhoea.
- Hirsuitism.
- Acne.
- Obesity.
- Acanthosis nigricans.

Laboratory findings include:
- Elevated androgen concentrations, e.g. testosterone, dehydroepiandrosterone sulfate (DHEAS).
- Elevated plasma LH:FSH ratio.
- ↓ sex hormone-binding globulin (SHBG) concentrations.
- Hyperinsulinaemia [fasting, OGTT, IV glucose tolerance test (IVGT) samples].
- ↓ insulin-like growth factor-binding protein 1 (IGFBP1) concentrations.

PCOS is associated with abnormalities that are characteristic of the metabolic syndrome.
   Treatment is directed at the presenting clinical problems and may include:
- Lifestyle modifications (especially if obesity is a factor).
- Metformin (insulin sensitizer).
- Combined oral contraceptive pill (suppresses ovarian hyperandrogenism).
- Spironolactone (anti-androgen).
- Cyproterone acetate (synthetic progesterone—anti-androgen).
- Flutamide (anti-androgen).

Normal growth

Prenatal/fetal growth

- The fastest period of growth.
- Accounts for around 30% of eventual height.
- Factors that determine growth during this period include: maternal size, maternal nutrition, and intrauterine environment.
- Hormonal factors: insulin, IGF 2, and human placental lactogen are important regulators of growth during this period.

Postnatal growth

Infantile period

- Birth to 18–24mth of age.
- Rapid, but decelerating growth rate (growth velocity: 22–8cm/y).
- Growth largely under nutritional regulation during this period.
- Some infants (15–20%) may show significant catch-up or catch-down in length and weight.
- By 2y, height is more predictive of final adult height than at birth.

Childhood period

- 2y until onset of puberty.
- Characterized by a slow, steady growth velocity (range 8–5cm/y).
- Primarily dependent on GH, provided adequate nutrition and health.

Puberty

- Growth dependent on GH and sex steroid hormones (testosterone and oestrogen).
- This induces the characteristic 'growth spurt' of puberty.
- In ♂ and ♀, oestrogen induces maturation of the epiphyseal growth centres in bones, resulting in fusion of the growth plates, cessation of linear growth, and attainment of final height.

Sex differences in growth during puberty

Onset of the pubertal growth spurt is earlier in ♀, compared with ♂. ♀ are, on average, taller than ♂ between 10 and 13y. In ♂, the pubertal growth spurt is greater in magnitude. ♂ are, on average, 12–13cm taller than ♀ at final height.

Normal puberty

Puberty is a well-defined sequence of physical and physiological changes occurring during the adolescent years that culminates in attainment of full physical and sexual maturity.

- Nocturnal pulsatile secretion of gonadotrophin-releasing hormone (GnRH) by the hypothalamus is the first step in the imitation of puberty. This results in the pulsatile secretion of the gonadotrophin hormones LH and FSH by the anterior pituitary gland. LH stimulates sex hormone production from the gonads.
- The age of onset of puberty is earlier in ♀ [mean (range) 10.5y (8.5–12.5y)], compared to ♂ [12.0y (10–13.5y)]. In each sex, puberty progresses in an orderly or 'consonant' manner through distinct stages (see Table 10.2).
- In ♀, the first sign of puberty is breast development, followed by pubic hair growth and growth acceleration. Menarche (the onset of menstruation) occurs, on average, 2.5y after start of puberty.
- In ♂, the first sign of puberty is enlargement of testicular size to >4mL in volume. Pubic hair development and growth acceleration follow.

Pubertal growth spurt

Peak height velocity occurs relatively earlier in girls (Tanner stages 2–3), compared to boys (Tanner stages 3–4; testicular volumes 10–12mL).

NB: the age of onset of puberty varies slightly between children of different races. In Afro-Caribbean and African-American children, the average age of onset of puberty may be earlier, compared with that of white children.

Table 10.2 The normal stages of puberty ('Tanner stages')

Boys

Stage	Genitalia	Pubic hair	Other events
I	Pre-pubertal	Vellus not thicker than on abdomen	TV <4mL
II	Enlargement of testes and scrotum	Sparse long, pigmented strands at base of penis	TV 4–8mL; voice starts to change
III	Lengthening of penis	Darker and curlier, and spreads over pubes	TV 8–10mL; axillary hair
IV	Increase in penis length and breadth	Adult-type hair, but covering a smaller area	TV 10–15mL; upper lip hair; peak height velocity
V	Adult shape and size	Spread to medial thighs (stage VI: spread up linea alba)	TV 15–25mL; facial hair spreads to cheeks; adult voice

Girls

Stage	Breast	Pubic hair	Other events
I	Elevation of papilla only	Vellus not thicker than on abdomen	
II	Breast bud stage: elevation of breast and papilla	Sparse long, pigmented strands along labia	Peak height velocity
III	Further elevation of breast and areola together	Darker and curlier, and spreads over pubes	
IV	Areola forms a second mound on top of breast	Adult-type hair, but covering a smaller area	Menarche
V	Mature stage: areola recedes and only papilla projects	Spread to medial thighs (stage VI: spread up linea alba)	

TV, testicular volume (measured by size comparison with a Prader orchidometer).

Source: Tanner JM (1962) *Growth at adolescence*, 2nd edn. Oxford: Blackwell Scientific Publications.

Assessment of growth

Growth must be measured accurately. The equipment used for weight and height must be maintained, checked, and calibrated. Measurements should be carried out by an auxologist, which will minimize error.

Assessment of height

- From birth to 2y, length is measured horizontally using a measuring board (e.g. Harpenden neonatometer). Two people need to ensure that the child is lying straight, with the legs extended.
- In children aged ≥2y, standing height is measured against a wall-mounted/free-standing stadiometer. A specific technique is required, with the person measuring applying moderate upward neck traction to the child's head, with the child's head in the horizontal plane.
- Measurement of sitting height with a modified stadiometer and calculating leg length (standing height *minus* sitting height) allows an estimate of upper and lower body segments and body proportion.

Growth data interpretation

Weight and height measurement data should be plotted on a sex- and age range-appropriate standard growth centile chart. Measurements should be plotted on specific population growth charts where applicable, e.g. Turner's syndrome, Down's syndrome.

Serial measurements show a growth pattern and determine the growth rate. Height velocity (cm/y) should be taken from measurements at least 6mth apart, ideally from the same equipment and person.

Final height and target height

Final height is reached after completion of puberty and is estimated to be achieved when growth velocity has slowed to <2.0cm/y. This can be confirmed by finding epiphyseal fusion of the small bones of the hand and wrist on assessing the bone age X-ray.

A target final height range can be estimated from parental heights, first by calculating the mid-parental height (MPH).

$$\text{MPH (boys)} = [\text{mother's height (cm)} + \text{father's height (cm)}/2)] + 6.5\text{cm}$$

$$\text{MPH (girls)} = [\text{mother's height (cm)} + \text{father's height (cm)}/2)] - 6.5\text{cm}$$

$$\text{Target height range} = \text{MPH} \pm 10\text{cm}$$

Bone age

Skeletal maturation can be assessed. Conventionally using X-rays of the left hand and wrist, with either compared with standard images (e.g. Gruelich and Pyle method) or assessed using an individual bone scoring system (Tanner–Whitehouse methods).

Bone age may be used as an indicator of the likely timing of puberty, which usually starts when bone age is around 10.5y in ♀ and 11.5y in ♂.

Girls usually reach skeletal maturity at a bone age of 15.0y and boys when bone age is 17.0y. Bone age can be used as an estimation of the remaining growth potential and to predict final adult height.

Short stature

Defined as a height 2 SDs or more below the mean for the population. On a standard growth chart, this represents a height <2nd centile.

NB: abnormalities of growth may be present long before height falls below this level and can be identified earlier by monitoring growth velocity and observing a child's height crossing centile lines.

Causes of short stature

These are summarized in Box 10.3. Just about any chronic illness of childhood can cause growth failure and short stature, so non-endocrine illness must be considered in assessment. The commonest cause is familial where either one or both parents will also be short. Height correlates well with parental height and is probably of polygenic inheritance, but it should be noted that rarely short parents may have a dominantly inherited growth disorder.

Assessment

Antenatal history
• Pregnancy illness/drugs/complications.

Perinatal/infancy history
• Gestational age and complications.
• Birthweight (length and head circumference).
• Feeding and weight gain

Past medical history
• Chronic asthma, renal disease, other chronic illness.

Drug history
• Corticosteroids.

Systematic enquiry
• Headaches/visual disturbance.

Growth history
• Examine previous growth records, if available.

Neurodevelopmental
• Developmental delay, school performance.

Family history
• Short stature/pubertal delay.
• Endocrine disease.

Examination

• Measure height, weight, and head circumference.
• General systems examination.
• Puberty (Tanner) staging.
• Observe for goitre, dysmorphic features, and malnutrition.
• Assess growth velocity over (a minimum of) 6-monthly intervals.
• Measure parent's height and calculate MPH and family height target.

Box 10.3 Causes of short stature

- Familial (genetic) short stature.
- CDGP.
- IUGR.
- GH deficiency.
- Other endocrine disorders, e.g. hypothyroidism, Cushing's syndrome.
- Dysmorphic syndromes:
  - Turner's syndrome.
  - Ns.
  - Down's syndrome.
- Coeliac disease.
- CRF.
- Chronic inflammatory disorders: IBD, rheumatic disease.
- Skeletal dysplasia: achondroplasia/hypochondroplasia.
- Metabolic bone disease: X-linked hypophosphataemic rickets.
- Malnutrition.

Investigations

- U&E (renal function).
- FBC, CRP, and ESR (chronic disease/inflammation).
- Ca^{2+}, PO_4^{3-}, ALP, albumin (bone disorder).
- Karyotype (chromosomal abnormalities, e.g. Turner's syndrome).
- TFTs.
- Serum IGF 1 (and IGFBP3) (GH deficiency).
- Coeliac disease antibody screen.
- Urinalysis.

  Where clinically indicated:
- Bone age X-ray.
- GH provocation test.

Management

Depends on the underlying cause (see later sections of this chapter). The diagnosis of a child with short stature is often a shock to the family, and they should be offered detailed, reliable information about their child's condition and informed where to get additional support and advice. Familial short stature does not require specific treatment.

NB: most short children are psychologically well adjusted. Where there are problems from being teased and bullied at school or poor self-esteem, psychological intervention measures may be needed.

Constitutional delay in growth and puberty

Relative short stature occurs because of a delay in the timing of onset of puberty. It is a variation in the timing of normal puberty. It usually presents in early adolescence and there is often a +ve family history. It is commoner in ♂, although this may reflect a bias in the level of concern.

Features include short stature and delayed pubertal development by >2 SDs. Typically, there is a mild degree of skeletal disproportion, with evidence of a shorter back (sitting height percentile), relative to leg length. There is delay in bone age maturation, which usually remains consistent over time. Height velocity is appropriate for bone age. Laboratory investigations are normal, including GH provocation tests (rarely needed).

Management

Usually no treatment is required, as puberty and the accompanying growth spurt will occur spontaneously and final adult target height is achieved.

Treatment is sometimes indicated in those who have difficulty coping with their short stature or their delayed physical development. Administration of sex steroids (see ⊃ Delayed puberty: management, pp. 450–1) for a period of 3–6mth can be used to induce pubertal changes and accelerate growth rate.

Psychosocial deprivation

Children subjected to physical or emotional abuse may exhibit growth failure. This may be due to reversible inhibition of GH secretion that improves within 3–4wk of being removed from the adverse environment. Catch-up growth is usually dramatic.

Intrauterine growth retardation

A reduction and restriction in expected fetal growth pattern. In placental causes of IUGR, 'catch-up growth' occurs in the majority of infants during the first 1–2y of life, with infants regaining their genetically determined weight and height centiles. In ~15–20% of infants, catch-up growth does not occur and patients are at risk of short stature. Recent studies implicate IUGR in adult onset of hypertension and coronary heart disease and in early-onset obesity, PCOS, and T2DM. GH treatment is indicated if catch-up growth is not complete by age 4y.

Turner's syndrome

(See also $\Rightarrow$ Turner's syndrome, p. 884.) This condition must always be considered in girls with short stature or height below the parental target height range. Karyotype confirms the diagnosis.

The majority of girls with Turner's syndrome will not have the classical phenotype of dysmorphic features and it may be difficult to identify, particularly where there is mosaicism in the karyotype.

- Short stature is frequent. Typically, growth rate begins to falter from age 3–5y and is due to an underlying skeletal dysplasia.
- Ovarian dysgenesis and consequent gonadal failure result in loss of the pubertal growth spurt.
- Mean final height is consistently 20cm below the norm.

Treatment with daily SC injections of high-dose rhGH $1.4\text{mg}/\text{m}^2/\text{day}$ (UK NICE) increases the final height, although individual responses are variable.

Oral oestrogen (ethinylestradiol) or transdermal (17β-oestradiol) patches are used to induce puberty between ages 12 and 14y.

Chronic inflammatory disorders

Poor growth and short stature are common features of long-term inflammatory conditions and other GI disease such as coeliac disease. It may be a presenting feature in CD.

In IBD, short stature occurs due to long-term use of immunosuppressive agents (e.g. corticosteroids) and the generation of inflammatory factors [e.g. interleukin 6 (IL-6)]. Both lead to GH/IGF 1 resistance and suppression of bone growth. Management should be aimed at minimizing inflammation and at immunosuppressive therapy.

Skeletal dysplasias

(See also $\Rightarrow$ Skeletal dysplasia, p. 887.) Include achondroplasia and hypochondroplasia. There is often severe short stature and evidence of disproportion in body segment development. Skeletal survey may identify a specific condition.

Growth hormone deficiency

Causes of GH deficiency

Primary (or congenital) or secondary (acquired) in origin (see Box 10.4).

Clinical features

GH deficiency in infancy

May present with hypoglycaemia. Coexisting pituitary deficiencies in axes may cause prolonged jaundice and micropenis. Size and growth may be normal during the first year of life (not GH-dependent yet).

GH deficiency in childhood

Typically presents with slow growth rate and short stature. Characteristics include ↑ subcutaneous fat, truncal obesity, and ↓ muscle mass. Children with congenital GH deficiency develop relative hypoplasia of the mid-facial bones, frontal bone protrusion, and delayed dental eruption. Delayed closure of the anterior fontanelle.

Box 10.4 Causes of GH deficiency

Primary or congenital causes
- Idiopathic/isolated.
- Congenital hypopituitarism.
- Midline brain anomalies.

Secondary or acquired causes
- Intracranial tumours: craniopharyngioma.
- Cranial irradiation/radiotherapy/traumatic brain injury.
- Psychosocial deprivation.
- Inflammatory/infiltrative disease:
  - Langerhans cell histiocytosis/sarcoidosis.
- Intracranial infection.

Investigations

- *Baseline/random serum IGF 1, IGFBP3*: GH-dependent; may be low in GH deficiency; normal levels do not exclude GH deficiency.
- *GH provocation tests*: tests should be performed in the morning after an overnight fast, and serial blood samples collected. GH provocation test should be performed in experienced centres with appropriate technical and laboratory support.

GH deficiency: management

Treat with rhGH, as a once-daily SC injection. Treatment should be undertaken in experienced centres. Height velocity increase and dose adjustments should be reviewed every 6mth. Catch-up growth optimal if GH therapy is started early.

Transition to GH deficiency care in adulthood

Treatment with rhGH is continued until final adult height is achieved. GH deficiency should then be reconfirmed to assess if ongoing treatment required.

GH insensitivity syndrome

Rarely, short stature may be related not to GH deficiency, but to GH resistance leading to elevated GH levels, often in the context of low IGF 1 levels (multiple genetic variants can occur) and short stature.

Tall stature

Referral for tall stature is much less common than for short stature.

Causes of tall stature

In the majority, tall stature is genetic and inherited from tall parents. Other causes, although rare, need to be considered:

- Early (normal) puberty.
- Obesity.
- *Endocrine disorders:*
  - Precocious puberty.
  - GH excess.
  - Pituitary adenoma.
  - Androgen excess.
  - CAH.
  - Hyperthyroidism.
  - Aromatase enzyme deficiency (very rare).
  - Oestrogen receptor defects (very rare).
- Chromosomal abnormalities: Klinefelter's syndrome (XXY); XYY; XYYY.
- *Syndromes:* MFS, homocystinuria, Soto, BWS.

History

Perinatal/infancy history
- Size at birth, birthweight (OFC).
- Feeding and weight gain.
- Developmental delay.

Systematic enquiry
- For example, headaches/visual disturbance.

Growth history
- Examine previous growth records, if available. Recent growth acceleration. Signs of puberty.

Family history
- Tall stature, early puberty, endocrine disease.

Examination

- *Measure:* height, weight, and head circumference.
- Puberty staging (Tanner).
- Observe dysmorphic features; goitre.
- Assess growth velocity over a minimum of 6-monthly intervals.
- *Measure parents' heights and calculate:* MPH, family target height.

Investigations

- Karyotype (chromosomal abnormalities—Klinefelter's syndrome).
- TFTs/serum IGF 1 (and IGFBP3).
- Sex hormone/LH and FSH levels.
- Androgen levels (DHEAS; 17-OH progesterone).
- Bone age X-ray.
- Where clinically indicated, GH suppression test.

Assessments commonly used in children/adolescents

Pharmacological stimulation tests
- Insulin tolerance test (children aged ≥5y).
- Glucagon stimulation test.
- Clonidine test.
- Arginine test.
- Peak GH levels of >6.5mcg/L generally considered normal.

Physiological tests
- Exercise.
- Overnight or 24h GH serum profiles.
- Random serum IGF 1 and/or IGFBP3 level.

Radiological
- Bone age.
- MRI scan of brain (hypothalamic/pituitary structures).

Management

In familial tall stature, reassurance and information about predicted final height are usually sufficient. Early induction of puberty using low-dose sex steroid to advance the pubertal growth spurt and to cause earlier epiphyseal closure is occasionally considered. However, this produces variable results and there is a theoretical risk of complications (including thromboembolic disease and oncogenic risk). Epiphysiodesis may be considered to cause premature fusion of the growth plate.

Delayed puberty: assessment

The lack of initiation and progress of pubertal development > +2 SDs later than the average age of onset of puberty for the population. In the UK, this equates to >14y for ♀ and >16y for ♂ (see Box 10.5).

History

A detailed history, including age at puberty onset (including menarche in ♀) in other family members.

Examination

- Measure height, weight, and head circumference.
- Puberty (Tanner) staging.
- Review previous growth records, if available.
- Measure parents' heights; calculate MPH and family height target.

Investigations

Blood

- LH and FSH levels.
- *Sex hormone:* oestrogen/testosterone.
- Karyotype (chromosomal abnormalities).
- TFTs.
- Routine biochemistry and inflammatory markers (e.g. CRP).

Radiological

- Bone age X-ray; pelvic US (ovarian morphology).
- Abdominal US (e.g. intra-abdominal testes); MRI brain.

Tests

- hCG stimulation test (3- or 21-day test).
- GnRH [luteinizing hormone-releasing hormone (LHRH)] test.

NB: it is difficult to distinguish constitutional delay in growth and puberty (CDGP) from other causes of hypogonadotrophic hypogonadism (HH) using current tests. In both conditions, basal and stimulated gonado-trophin (LH/FSH) levels are low. Differentiation may only be possible after induction of puberty with sex steroid therapy and attainment of final height, when reassessment of the hypothalamic–pituitary–gonadal axis should be repeated after withdrawal of treatment.

Box 10.5 Causes of pubertal delay

Constitutional delay of growth and puberty (hypogonadotrophic hypogonadism)

Low/undetectable basal and stimulated gonadotrophin levels
- Congenital:
  - KS.
  - Congenital hypopituitarism (e.g. *LHX-3, PROP-1*; see ● Congenital hypopituitarism, p. 429).
  - Isolated LH deficiency.
  - Isolated FSH deficiency.
  - Other causes of gonadotrophin deficiency, e.g. congenital adrenal hypoplasia (*DAX-1* gene).
  - Syndromic associations, e.g. PWS.
- Acquired:
  - Intracranial tumours (e.g. craniopharyngioma).
  - Cranial irradiation.
  - Traumatic brain injury.
  - Langerhans cell histiocytosis.
  - Anorexia nervosa.
  - Excess physical training.
  - Chronic childhood disease, e.g. IBD.

Primary gonadal failure (hypergonadotrophic hypogonadism)

High basal and stimulated gonadotrophin levels
- Congenital:
  - Chromosomal disorders: Turner's syndrome, Klinefelter's syndrome.
  - Gonadal dysgenesis.
  - LH resistance.
  - Disorders of steroid biosynthesis (e.g. CAH: *StAR; CYP17; 3BHSD*).
- Acquired:
  - Chemotherapy.
  - Gonadal irradiation (local radiotherapy).
  - Gonadal infection (e.g. mumps orchitis).
  - Gonadal trauma/gonadal torsion.
  - Cranial irradiation.
  - Autoimmune (ovarian).

Delayed puberty: management

- CDGP may be treated with a short course of sex steroid therapy.
- Children with permanent gonadotrophin deficiency or gonadal failure requiring complete induction of puberty and long-term treatment can have puberty induced with gradually increasing doses of sex steroids over a period of 2–3y.
- Induction of ♂ secondary sexual characteristics: e.g. Sustanon® 250 (1/4 vial, i.e. 75mg) IM injection monthly for 3–6mth initially (then stop if CDGP).
- Induction of ♀ secondary sexual characteristics: e.g. ethinylestradiol 2mcg daily, increasing to 10mcg daily over 2y, or oestrogen patches (e.g. Evorel® 25, 1/4 patch twice weekly, increasing to whole patch twice weekly over 2y). Once menstruation occurs or sexual maturation achieved, maintenance supplementation is usually required (unlike many boys), e.g. with combined oral contraceptive pill (e.g. Microgynon® 30 or Loestrin® 20).
- The aim of long-term sex steroid therapy is maintenance of secondary sexual features, libido, and menstruation in ♀. There are also +ve benefits in terms of bone mineralization and cardiovascular health.

NB: testosterone therapy does not promote testicular growth; testicular size remains pre-pubertal unless spontaneous puberty occurs.

Constitutional delay of growth and puberty

The commonest cause of delayed puberty. Usually observed in boys and reflects a delay in the timing mechanisms that regulate puberty onset. There is often a family history.

- Children presenting with CDGP are invariably healthy.
- Onset and progress through puberty will occur normally with time.
- Children achieve a final adult height in keeping with their predicted familial target range.

There is often evidence of delayed or slow growth in childhood, most pronounced in the peripubertal years due to lack of anticipated growth spurt. There is evidence of delayed skeletal maturation on bone age assessment. No specific therapy is required other than explanation and reassurance that puberty will occur normally. However, children who are experiencing significant social or psychological difficulties may request treatment (see ⮡ Constitutional delay in growth and puberty, pp. 442–3). Any decision to commence therapy, or not, must include the views of the child and their parents who should be part of the decision-making process.

Hypogonadotrophic hypogonadism

Impaired gonadotrophin release from the pituitary gland (see Box 10.3).
   Congenital causes of HH may be characterized by micropenis and undescended testis at birth in boys. In girls, physical signs are absent.

Kallmann syndrome (KS)

A genetic disorder characterized by the association of HH and anosmia. X-linked, AD, and AR modes of inheritance are recognized. The X-linked form of KS results from a mutation in the *KAL* gene (encoding the glycoprotein anosmin-1). It is also characterized by a range of clinical features, including synkinesia (mirror image movements), renal agenesis, and visual problems, as well as craniofacial anomalies, although their expression is highly variable.

Precocious puberty (PP)

Early onset and rapid progression of puberty. In white European children, PP is defined as <8y in ♀ and <9y in ♂.

Classification and causes

Central (true) PP (gonadotrophin-dependent)
- Idiopathic (familial/non-familial).
- *Intracranial tumours.*
- *Other CNS lesions:* hydrocephalus, arachnoid cysts, traumatic brain injury, cranial irradiation.
- *Secondary central PP:* early maturation of the hypothalamic–pituitary–gonadal axis due to long-term sex steroid exposure, e.g. CAH, McAS.

Puberty occurs as a consequence of early physiological (true) activation of the hypothalamic–pituitary–gonadal axis (central). A normal sequence of pubertal development occurs. Central PP may also be idiopathic and familial. In girls, central PP is more likely to be idiopathic, whereas in boys, there is a greater risk of CNS tumours.

Peripheral PP (gonadotrophin-independent)
- *Gonadal:* McAS, ovarian tumours (e.g. benign cyst, granulosa cell tumour), testicular tumour, familial testitoxicosis (LH receptor-activating mutation).
- *Adrenal:* CAH, adrenal tumour (carcinoma, adenoma).
- *hCG-secreting tumours:* e.g. CNS (chorioepithelioma, dysgerminoma).
- Iatrogenic (exogenous sex steroid administration).

The source of sex steroid may be endogenous (gonadal or extragonadal) or exogenous. Endogenous hormone production is independent of hypothalamic–pituitary–gonadal activity. An abnormal sequence of pubertal development is usually observed.

Assessment

History
- Age when first signs of pubertal development observed.
- Features of puberty present, and in what order they appeared.
- Evidence of growth acceleration.
- Family history: age of onset of puberty (including age of menarche in ♀) within other family members.

Examination
- Puberty (Tanner) staging.
- Measure height, weight, and head circumference.
- Review previous growth records, if available.
- Measure parents' heights and calculate MPH/family height target.
- *Skin lesions:* e.g. café-au-lait marks (McAS, NF1).
- Abdominal/testicular masses.
- *Neurological examination:* visual fields, fundoscopy.

Investigations
- Plasma LH and FSH levels.
- *Plasma sex hormone:* oestrogen/testosterone.
- *Other serum androgen levels:* e.g. 17-OH progesterone, DHEAS, androstenedione.

  In addition, undertake the following:
- *Urine:* steroid profile (sex/adrenal steroids).
- Bone age X-ray.
- Pelvic US (ovarian morphology, testicular masses).
- Abdominal USS, e.g. adrenal glands.
- MRI brain.
- *GnRH (LHRH) test.*

Precocious puberty: management

Diagnosis

Diagnosis is based on demonstrating progressive pubertal development and ↑ growth rate, with laboratory evidence of ↑ sex steroid production. Distinguishing central and peripheral PP and PP from other normal variants of pubertal development may be difficult (see Table 10.3). In central PP, there is evidence of consonance in sequence of pubertal development, in keeping with the normal physiological activation of puberty.

Management

Management of PP is aimed at the following:

- *Detection and treatment of underlying pathological causes of PP*: especially important in ♂ where early puberty is invariably due to organic disease.
- *Reducing the rate of skeletal maturation*: skeletal maturation exceeds concomitant growth, thus reducing growth potential. Final adult height is reduced.
- *Reducing and halting, if necessary, the rate of physical pubertal development.*
- *Addressing potential behavioural and psychological difficulties*: sexual and reproductive characteristics advance inappropriately for age, leading to mature appearance.
- It is essential that an explanation for the physiology and physical consequences of PP is given to the parents and the child. The decision on therapy should be made jointly with the parents.

Treatment of precocious puberty

Central PP

- Suppression of the hypothalamic–pituitary–gonadal axis with a long-acting GnRH analogue is the only currently effective treatment for central PP. These work by providing continuous stimulation of the GnRH receptor on the pituitary gonadotrophs, resulting in down-regulation of the receptor, and thus ↓ LH and FSH secretion.
- GnRH analogues are administered by either SC or IM injection monthly (or 3-monthly in depot preparations).
- Treatment efficacy should be assessed by monitoring growth rate and pubertal stage. In addition, serum LH and FSH levels (basal and stimulated) should be measured to ensure hypothalamic–pituitary–gonadal axis suppression.

Table 10.3 Characteristic findings of disorders of pubertal development

	Sequence of pubertal changes	Height velocity	Sex steroids	LH/FSH (basal/ stimulated)	BA
Central PP	Consonant	++	++	++, LH-predominant	++
Peripheral PP	Usually non-consonant	++	++	Pre-pubertal; suppressed	++
Premature thelarche	Breast tissue only	N	N	Pre-pubertal/ FSH +	N
Thelarche 'variant'	Breast tissue only	+	N	Pre-pubertal/ FSH +	N/+
Premature adrenarche	Pubic hair; skin changes only	N	N/DHEAS +	Pre-pubertal; suppressed	N

BA, bone age; N, normal; +, slightly raised or advanced; ++, raised or advanced.

Variants of normal puberty

Premature thelarche

- Isolated premature breast development.
- Typically, ♀ present in infancy, usually by 2y of age.
- Breast development is due to the action of physiological or mild increases in the amounts of circulating oestrogen.

Waxing and waning in breast growth, normal growth (height) rate, and absence of further sexual development. Breast development may be asymmetrical, and there is usually resolution of breast enlargement by age 4–5y.

The condition is benign. Bone maturation, age of onset of menarche, and final adult height are not affected. Management is conservative with re-evaluation of growth and puberty stage 3- to 6-monthly.

Thelarche variant

- An intermediate condition between premature thelarche and central PP.
- A non-progressive form of early pubertal development.

Evidence of breast development, ↑ growth rate, and advanced skeletal maturation on bone age assessment. For most, the tempo of progression of pubertal development is slow and laboratory findings are within normal range for age. Management is usually conservative with regular re-evaluation of growth and pubertal status at 3- to 6-monthly intervals. Decisions to treat (as for central PP) are based on height velocity and final height predictions.

Premature adrenarche

A common variant of normal pubertal development.

- Premature appearance of androgen-dependent secondary sexual hair, acne, and axillary odour.
- May have mild acceleration in height velocity and slight increase in bone age.
- Laboratory investigations: increase in serum DHEAS levels that is appropriate for pubic hair stage, rather than age.
- Serum testosterone and 17-OH progesterone are normal.

Look for signs and symptoms that might indicate another cause (e.g. adrenal tumour, CAH) The latter are characterized by signs of virilization, rapid growth rate, and significantly advanced bone age.

Premature adrenarche is a benign condition. The timing of onset of true puberty is normal and final adult height is unaffected. Management is conservative with reassurance after exclusion of other causes. Symptomatic treatment may be required if adrenarche is pronounced.

Differences in sex development

Terminology

- Previously known as disorders of sex development.

Differences in sexual development

Numerous differences that can result in genital ambiguity and uncertainty about an infant's sex are recognized (see Box 10.6).

Assessment

History

- *Family history:* ambiguous genitalia, disorders/problems of puberty, inguinal hernia.
- *Prenatal history:* maternal health, maternal drugs, maternal virilization during pregnancy.
- History of previous stillbirths or neonatal death.

Examination

- *General examination:* dysmorphic features or midline defects, state of hydration, BP.
- *Are the gonads palpable?* Likely to be testes or ovotestes?
- *Assess the degree of virilization:*
  - Prader stage (see Fig. 10.1).
  - External masculinization score.
- *Measure length of the phallus.*
- *Penis:* presence of chordee.
- *Vagina:* locate opening?
- Appearance of labioscrotal folds.
- Position of urethral opening.
- *Skin—pigmentation of genital skin:* hyperpigmentation with excessive ACTH and opiomelanocortin in CAH.

In preterm girls, the clitoris and labia minora are relatively prominent. In preterm boys, the testes remain undescended until 34wk gestation.

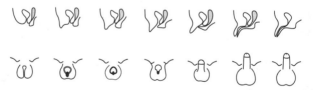

Fig. 10.1 Prader staging: virilization.

Reproduced from Prader A. Der Genitalbefund beim Pseudohermaphroditismus femininusdes krongenitalen Adrenogenitalen Syndromes. *Helv Paediat Acta.* 1954;9:231–48. With kind permission of Schwabe Verlag, Basel.

Box 10.6 Genetic disorders of gonadal determination

46, XY disorder of sex development (DSD)

- Disorder of gonadal development.
- Complete/partial gonadal dysgenesis.
- Testes regression.
- Ovotesticular DSD.
- Disorder of androgen synthesis.
- HSD17B3; SRD5A2 deficiency.
- *StAR; HSD3B2; CYP17A1.*
- Placental insufficiency or endocrine disruption.
- Syndromic causes (Smith–Lemli–Opitz syndrome).
- Disorders of androgen action.
- Complete/partial androgen insensitivity.
- Presistent Müllerian duct syndrome.
- AMH or AMH type 2 receptor (AMHR2) deficiency.
- Unclassified disorders.
- Hypospadius (distinguished from proximal hypospadius with normal gonadal development).

46, XX DSD

- Disorders of gonadal development.
- Ovotesticular DSD.
- Mutations in ovarian development (eg. *NRSA1, WT1*).
- Syndromic forms.
- Disorders of androgen excess.
- Aromatase (CYP19A1) deficiency.
- CAH (*CYP21A2, HSD3B2*, CYP11B1).
- Iatrogenic (maternal androgen exposure).
- Unclassified disorders.

Sex chromosomal DSD

- 45, X.
- Turner's syndrome and variants.
- 47, XXY.
- Klinefelter's syndrome and variants.
- 45, X/46, XY and 46, XX/46, XY.
- Mixed gonadal dysgenesis.

Differences in sex development: management

Investigations

Laboratory

- *Genetic sex determination:* fluorescence *in situ* hybridization (FISH) for Y and X chromosomes; karyotype (takes 3–5 days).
- Serum electrolytes; blood sugar (hypoglycaemia).
- *Adrenal androgens:* plasma testosterone; 17-OH progesterone; urine steroid profile; LH and FSH.
- Molecular genetic studies; blood (DNA).
- Genetic testing—may include whole-genome sequencing.

If ♂/mosaic karyotype is confirmed, further investigations are directed at establishing whether testicular tissue is capable of producing androgens:
- hCG stimulation test.
- Testosterone:dihydrotestosterone ratio.
- Androgen receptor binding studies.
- Anti-Müllerian hormone (AMH) levels.
- Genital skin biopsy (fibroblasts).

Imaging studies

- *USS pelvis:* anatomy of urogenital sinus/vagina/uterus.
- *USS abdomen:* renal anomalies.
- Urogenital sonogram.
- MRI.

Internal examination

- Examination under anaesthesia (± cystography).
- Laparoscopy.
- Gonadal biopsy.

Management

Requires an MDT, including the following:
- Paediatric endocrinologist.
- Neonatologist.
- Paediatric urologist.
- Gynaecologist.
- Clinical geneticist.
- Radiologist.
- Psychologist.
- Clinical biochemist.
- Social worker.

Most infants presenting with a disorder of sexual differentiation will present with ambiguous genitalia at birth.
- Decisions about an infant's sex assignment must be delayed until the MDT has carried out a thorough assessment and discussion with the parents.
- Delay birth registration until this has been completed and an agreement on sex assignment has been made with the parents (see Box 10.7).
- Surgery may be delayed until adolescence/adulthood in order to allow individual consent.

Box 10.7 General principles of sex assignment

Virilized females
- Should be brought up as ♀.
- *Clitoromegaly*: clitoral reduction (clitoroplasty) in infancy/childhood.
- Vaginoplasty is deferred until late childhood/early adolescence.

Under-virilized male

Decision regarding sex assignment is more complex. Depends on the following:
- Degree of sexual ambiguity.
- Underlying cause if known.
- Potential for normal sexual function and fertility.
- *Phallic size*:
  - If >2.5cm, reconstructive surgery more likely to be successful.
  - A trial of IM testosterone or topical dihydrotestosterone cream may improve phallic size.

  Gonadectomy is considered if:
- Dysgenetic testis.
- Complete AIS.
- Decision to raise as ♀.

Hormone replacement therapy
- Testosterone therapy if decision to raise as ♂.
- Oestrogen therapy if decision to raise as ♀.

Psychological support
- Experienced counselling is essential.
- Patient support groups are available.

Issues regarding assignment of gender, timing of reconstructive surgery, and hormone replacement therapy are complex. Current consensus on management is largely based on expert opinion.[1]

1. Cools M, Nordenström A, Robeva R, *et al*. Caring for individuals with a difference of sex development (DSD): a Consensus Statement. *Nature Review Endocrinology* 2018; **14**: 415–29.

Androgen insensitivity syndrome (AIS)

Complete AIS

- ♀ external genitalia, normal clitoris, hypoplastic labia majora, blind-ending vaginal pouch. Müllerian structures are absent. Testes may be located in the abdomen, inguinal canal, or labia.
- Strongly suspect and exclude AIS in ♀ with inguinal hernia.
- Complete AIS often presents with primary amenorrhoea.
- At puberty, serum testosterone and LH are elevated. Conversion of testosterone to oestradiol in the testis and peripheral tissues results in normal breast development.
- Pubic and axillary hair development is absent or sparse.
- Confirm diagnosis with 46, XY karyotype.
- Due to the potential risk of malignant transformation, testes should be removed soon after diagnosis or completion of puberty. After gonadal removal, oestrogen replacement therapy is given.

Partial AIS

Phenotypic expression ranges from ambiguous genitalia to a normal ♂ phenotype presenting with fertility difficulties.

Micropenis

Often an incidental finding on newborn examination.

Evaluation

Penile size
- Measured from pubic tubercle to tip of stretched penis in a term baby. Normal size at birth is usually >3cm. Micropenis <2.2–2.5cm (varies with ethnicity).

General examination
- Dysmorphism.
- Midline craniofacial defects.

Ophthalmic examination
- Optic nerve hypoplasia/septo-optic dysplasia.

Investigations
- US of head for midline defects.
- MRI head.
- *Anterior pituitary hormone levels (basal and stimulated):* ACTH and cortisol; GH (IGF 1, IGFBP3); LH and FSH; TSH and fT4.
- Karyotype.

Management

Referral to a paediatric urologist is often required. If severe micropenis is present, a decision regarding sex assignment will be needed.
- *Treatment:* short course of IM testosterone or topical dihydrotestosterone cream may stimulate penile growth and improve appearances.

Gynaecomastia

Aetiology

(See Box 10.8.)

Pubertal gynaecomastia

The commonest cause in children and adolescents. Usual age of onset is just before puberty (10–12y), peaking during puberty (13–14y); usually involutes after 1–2y and resolves by the end of puberty. Establish the diagnosis by excluding other causes of gynaecomastia by taking a detailed history and examination.

Investigations
- Serum oestrogen, testosterone, LH, FSH.
- Serum prolactin.
- LFTs, TFTs.
- Karyotype.

   Where testicular/adrenal/hepatic tumour is suspected:
- US abdomen/testis.
- MRI abdomen/testis.
- Serum β-hCG levels.

Box 10.8 Classification and causes of gynaecomastia

- Pubertal gynaecomastia.
- Neonatal gynaecomastia.
- *Impaired gonadal function:*
  - HH.
  - Hypergonadotrophic hypogonadism.
- AIS.
- Adrenal tumours.
- *Testicular tumours:*
  - Leydig cell tumour.
  - Sertoli cell tumour.
  - Germ cell tumour.
- *Iatrogenic:*
  - Exogenous hormones, e.g. oestrogen, anabolic steroids.
  - Ketoconazole.
  - Psychoactive drugs, e.g. diazepam, phenothiazine.
- Familial gynaecomastia (aromatase enzyme excess).
- Alcohol excess, cannabis.

Management

Reassurance and explanation for pubertal gynaecomastia. In severe cases where pubertal gynaecomastia is causing significant pyschological distress or persists beyond puberty, surgical resection of excess glandular breast tissue is warranted. The role of medical therapy with aromatase inhibitors or selective oestrogen receptor-blocking agents (e.g. tamoxifen) is currently unclear.

Further reading

Congenital hypothyroidism

Kwak MJ. Clinical genetics of defects in thyroid hormone synthesis. *Ann Pediatr Endocrinol Metab* 2018; **23**: 169–75.

Solitary thyroid nodules

Francis GL, Waguespack SG, Bauer AJ, *et al.* Management guidelines for children with thyroid nodule and differentiated thyroid cancer. *Thyroid* 2015; **25**: 716–59.

Adrenal insufficiency

Bornstein SR, Allolio B, Arlt W, *et al.* Diagnosis and treatment of primary adrenal insufficiency: an Endocrine Society clinical guideline. *J Clin Endocrinol Metab* 2016; **101**: 364–89.

Growth hormone deficiency

National Institute for Health and Care Excellence. (2010). *Human growth hormone (somatropin) for the treatment of growth failure in children.* Technology appraisal guidance [TA188]. Available at: https://www.nice.org.uk/guidance/ta188/resources/human-growth-hormone-somatropin-for-the-treatment-of-growth-failure-in-children-pdf-82598502860485.

Chapter 11

Diabetes mellitus

Childhood diabetes mellitus

Several forms of diabetes mellitus are found in the childhood population and broadly divided into five categories:
1. Type 1 (T1).
2. Type 2 (T2).
3. Monogenic [maturity-onset diabetes of the young (MODY)].
4. Neonatal.
5. Other (e.g. CF-induced diabetes, steroid-induced, etc.).

Diabetes mellitus diagnostic criteria

- WHO definition: raised fasting glucose level of ≥7.0mmol/L.
- Random glucose >11.1mmol/L.
- In practice, OGTTs are reserved for cases of diagnostic doubt. (See also Diagnosis, p. 480.)
- In most instances, a random blood glucose test is quite sufficient.

Type 1 diabetes mellitus

Epidemiology

Aetiology

Demographics

Clinical presentation

Type 1 diabetes mellitus

This is the commonest form of diabetes mellitus in children and adolescents, accounting for 96% of cases in the UK.

Epidemiology

- A disease of any age, but rarely presenting before the age of 1y.
- The incidence of T1DM is increasing globally but shows marked geographical variation (e.g. high rates in Scandinavia).
- Presentation is commonest between ages 5y and 7y, and then another peak in rate occurs just before, or at the onset of, puberty.
- Seasonal variation in presentation of T1DM is also observed, with a peak seen in winter months.

Aetiology

The causes of T1DM involve both genetic and environmental factors. Over 20 T1DM susceptibility genes have been identified. The insulin-dependent diabetes mellitus 1 (*IDDM1*) gene locus, which represents the HLA-DR/DQ locus on the major histocompatibility complex, accounts for the greatest susceptibility. The role of various environmental (e.g. viral) interactions and triggers is controversial.

Pathophysiology

T1DM is a chronic autoimmune condition leading to destruction of the islet of Langerhans β-cells (insulin-producing cells) in the pancreas.

- Immune-mediated inflammation and antibodies against specific β-cell autoantigens are generated.
- T-cell activation leads to β-cell inflammation and subsequent islet cell loss through apoptosis.
- The rate of β-cell loss varies (months to years), and the timing and presentation of symptomatic DM may depend on factors that increase insulin requirements (e.g. puberty).

Clinical presentation

Insulin is not only responsible for blood glucose control but also activates intracellular mechanisms that are key to most anabolic processes. Hence, insulin loss (T1DM) in the acute presentation should not be thought of as solely a 'high glucose' problem. While hyperglycaemia causes the symptoms of polyuria and polydipsia (common to all forms of diabetes mellitus), it is the catabolic effect of insulin deficiency that causes weight loss and potentially life-threatening DKA still seen at presentation in ~30% of newly diagnosed children. In the majority, symptoms evolve over weeks:

- Weight loss (often dramatic).
- Polyuria and polydipsia.
- Nocturia/nocturnal enuresis.
- Signs of DKA: tachypnoea, ketotic breath, vomiting, abdominal pain, ↓ LOC/agitation (see Diabetic ketoacidosis, p. 477).

Other less common symptoms include:
- *Candida* infection (e.g. oral thrush, balanitis, vulvovaginitis).
- Skin infections.

Any child with the above symptoms should have a bedside fingerprick glucose test without delay in primary care.

Failure to recognize these symptoms may result in delayed or late diagnosis and more likely presentation with DKA. There remains a high rate of DKA at diagnosis of T1DM, in particular in younger children who have a shorter prodrome and may present with isolated tachypnoea mistaken as a primary respiratory problem.

Assessment of new patient

Emphasis should be put on:
- *History:* duration of symptoms, any possible infectious triggers.
- *Family history:* of diabetes mellitus or other autoimmune disease.
- *Examination:* ruling out DKA, weight/BMI, infection (e.g. oral/vaginal thrush).

Investigations at diagnosis

(See Box 11.1 for take-home messages.)
- Blood pH (to exclude DKA) (see also ➲ DKA treatment, pp. 80–1).
- Blood ketones (normal <0.6mmol/L).
- Consider requesting diabetes-related autoantibodies: islet cell, anti-insulin, anti-glutamic acid decarboxylase (GAD), anti-islet cell antigen 2 (IA-2), and anti-zinc transporter antibodies.
- Other autoimmune disease screen: TFTs, thyroid antibodies; coeliac disease antibody screen.

Box 11.1 T1DM take-home messages
- *To diagnose:* check fingerprick blood glucose, rather than wait for fasting glucose, HbA1c, and glucose tolerance tests.
- *Always test blood glucose:* in a child with unexplained tachypnoea.
- *Insulin pumps* and CGM: can appear a technical challenge—all manufacturers have 24h helplines to give technical advice.
- Most UK paediatric diabetes teams have 24/7 telephone advice available in case of doubt.
- If pumps are not working, revert to SC injections.
- If a child is acidotic or vomiting persistently, revert to DKA guideline and insulin IVI.

Type 1 diabetes mellitus: management

The initial care and subsequent long-term management of patients with T1DM should be delivered by a specialist paediatric diabetes MDT.

All newly diagnosed patients must start insulin therapy as soon as possible. This treatment usually requires a period of hospital admission at diagnosis to provide education, training, and support.

Diabetes is a lifelong condition that carries an ever-present threat of future complications—the day a child is diagnosed is unlikely to ever be forgotten, so initial education is very important and should include:

- *Principles of insulin therapy:* timing, technique, dosing (see ➔ Type 1 diabetes mellitus: insulin therapy, pp. 471–3).
- *Nutritional management:* carbohydrate counting (see ➔ CHO counting: insulin dose adjustment, p. 472).
- *Monitoring of blood glucose levels:* aiming for at least five times a day (see ➔ Insulin requirement and dose adjustment, p. 472).
- *Avoidance and management of hypoglycaemia* (see ➔ Hypoglycaemia, p. 476).
- *Management of acute illness* and monitoring blood ketone levels: 'sick day rules' (see ➔ Sick-day management, p. 477).

Type 1 diabetes mellitus: insulin therapy

Insulin is administered SC, usually as a bolus injection or as a continuous subcutaneous insulin infusion (CSII) via an insulin pump (see Box 11.2 for typical total daily doses). Insulin injection sites include the subcutaneous tissues of the upper arm, the anterior and lateral thigh, the abdomen, and the buttocks. Intensive multi-dose injection (MDI) insulin therapy is the first-line therapy option for most newly diagnosed patients. In less usual circumstances (e.g. the very young, the child with significant learning difficulties), less frequent insulin injections or CSII with a pump may be considered more appropriate from diagnosis.

> ### Box 11.2 Typical total daily dose of insulin requirements in T1DM
> - At diagnosis: 0.5–0.75U/kg/day.
> - Pre-pubertal: 0.5–1.0U/kg/day.
> - During puberty: 1.2–2.0U/kg/day.
> - Post-puberty: 0.7–1.2U/kg/day.

Insulin regimens

Standard/typical insulin therapy regimens are delivered in a basal bolus fashion in an attempt to mimic physiological insulin secretion.

Multiple daily injections

Low-level background basal insulin provides for fasting and between-meal insulin requirements, and larger acute doses of fast-acting insulin are given to provide for prandial requirements.
- *Basal insulin:* once-a-day intermediate- or long-acting insulin (traditionally at bedtime).
- *Fast-acting insulin:* at mealtimes (i.e. three per day) and with between-meal snacks.

Advantages

- ↑ flexibility with mealtimes/exercise planning.
- Insulin dose adjustment— carbohydrate (CHO) counting.

Disadvantages

- Need for more injections.

CSII

Current insulin infusion pumps are reliable and portable. CSII therapy can be used in children of all ages. Rapid-acting insulin is administered as a continuous insulin infusion. Mealtime boluses and 'blood glucose correction' boluses are administered when required.

Advantages

- No bolus injections/reduced injection frequency.
- ↑ flexibility with mealtimes/exercise planning.
- Small insulin dose adjustment (e.g. <0.5U).

Disadvantages
- No long-acting insulin, so any interruption gives risk of rapid DKA.
- Body image concerns with pump attachment, e.g. with beachwear.

Insulin requirements and dose adjustment
Insulin doses are adjusted based on home blood glucose monitoring. Generally, it is simpler and safer not to alter the basic insulin regimen every time blood glucose levels are outside the target range of 4–7mmol/L (fasting/ before meals) and 5–9mmol/L (after meals). Rather, recorded blood glucose levels should be reviewed and insulin adjustments should be made to correct recurrent profiles that are either too low or too high. Insulin doses are adjusted by 5–10% at a time.

CHO counting: insulin dose adjustment system
Applies the principle that the amounts of fasting/rapid-acting insulin given at mealtimes are adjusted and matched according to the amount of carbohydrate consumed.

Table 11.1 shows the insulin analogue preparations (created by minor amino acid substitutions to the 'native' human insulin molecule).

Table 11.1 Characteristics of insulin analogue preparations

Type	Example	Onset	Peak	Duration
Short-acting	Regular/soluble (Actrapid®)	30–60min	1.5–3h	4–6h
Rapid (analogue)	Insulin lispro (Humalog®)	5–30min	30–90min	3–5h
	Insulin aspart (NovoRapid®)	10–30min	1–3h	3–5h
	Fast-acting aspart (Fiasp®)	5–10min	1–3h	3–5h
Intermediate-acting	NPH	1–4h	10h	10–16h
	Lente	3–4h	6–12h	12–18h
Long-acting	Ultralente	1–4h	8–16h	18–22h
Long-acting (analogue)	Insulin detemir (Levemir®)	2–4h	4–6h	12–20h
	Insulin glargine (Lantus®)	2–4h	3–6h	20–24h
	Insulin degludec (Tresiba®)	2–4h	12h	36–42h

Starting a child on insulin at diagnosis

Although many options exist for the types of insulin and variations in dosing frequency, MDI is usually considered a good starting point. Different calculations are used for initial starting dose calculations and it is important to recognize that these are estimations which will almost inevitably require changing during the physiological adaptation period after diagnosis and frequent recovery of some pancreatic function (often referred to as the 'honeymoon phase').

Steps for starting a child on MDI

(See also Box 11.3 for an illustration of starting SC MDI.)

1. Calculation of the total daily dose (TDD) of insulin:
   a. *Younger children (e.g. <8y):* 0.5U/kg/day.
   b. *Older/obese patients:* 0.75U/kg/day.
2. Calculation of long-acting insulin dose (insulin glargine, e.g. *Lantus*®; insulin degludec, e.g. *Tresiba*®; or insulin detemir, e.g. *Levemir*®) given od at night:
   a. TDD divided by 2 = dose of long-acting insulin per day.
3. Calculation of dose of rapid-acting insulin (e.g. insulin aspart, *NovoRapid*®) to be given for meals:
   a. 300 divided by TDD gives the number of grams of carbohydrate needing 1U of insulin administered.
4. Calculation of dose of rapid-acting insulin (e.g. insulin aspart) to be given to correct a high blood glucose (e.g. ≥12mmol/L):
   a. 100 divided by TDD gives the number of mmol/L that 1U of insulin can be expected to reduce blood glucose level.

Box 11.3 Illustration of starting SC MDI therapy in a child

- An 8y old weighing 24kg might start at TDD of 12U (0.5U/kg/day).
- Half is given as long-acting insulin at night (e.g. 6U of insulin glargine).
- Rapid-acting insulin is given with carbohydrates as a ratio:
  - For example, 1U of insulin aspart for every 25g of carbohydrate consumed.
- Correction doses of rapid-acting insulin aspart with a sensitivity factor of 1U, reducing blood glucose by 8mmol/L.

Evolving technologies and T1DM

T1DM is a relatively simple endocrine disorder, but a complicated condition to live with and control effectively. The range of technological advances aimed at improved quality of life and diabetes control is ever-growing. While popularity with patients is strong, the evidence base for their clinical effectiveness is weak.

Insulin pumps

Insulin pumps are, in essence, simply a portable syringe driver that administers both a continuous infusion (basal rate) and boluses of insulin to meet the patient's demands. The principles of diabetes control are not dissimilar to the 'MDI' regimen described previously. In the case of a pump, the long-acting insulin is replaced by a 24h infusion of rapid-acting insulin, but boluses for meals and corrections are calculated in the same way.

Additional pump functions
- Multiple boluses, needle-free.
- Ability to change basal rate to match metabolic demands of the body (e.g. dawn rise in insulin requirement before waking).
- Ability to suspend insulin administration if trending low blood glucose levels.
- Ability to temporarily increase the rate of insulin administration if running high blood glucose levels (e.g. at menstruation)—known as 'temporary basal rate'.
- Ability to administer very small doses of insulin and fractions of a unit (particularly helpful for small children).
- Ability to prolong boluses of rapid-acting insulin, e.g. over 1h (extended bolus) or in two parts (dual-wave bolus).

SC glucose monitoring systems (continuous glucose monitoring)

- Two system subsets exist that use similar technology: *real-time CGM* (e.g. Dexcom and Medtronic systems) and *intermittently viewed CGM* (e.g. Abbott Libre system).
- Systems that monitor interstitial fluid glucose levels which match blood glucose with ~10–20% margin of error [mean absolute relative difference (MARD)] and a 5–15min lag-time behind changes in blood glucose levels.
- A SC sensor is inserted and must be changed every 1–2wk, depending on the device.
- At times of illness/rapid changes in blood glucose levels, fingerprick glucose levels should still be measured, alongside/instead of interstitial glucose levels. Daily calibration is also required with some devices.
- Frequent sensor usage, downloading of data, and review of the data leading to insulin dose adjustment are important for successful use of CGM.

Real-time CGM offers
- Real-time values on a handheld meter or uploaded to mobile phone apps (e.g. parent-held).
- Alarms if hypoglycaemic or trending towards hypoglycaemia.

Intermittently viewed CGM offers
- A sensor that can be 'swiped' with a meter or mobile phone to give interstitial glucose reading.
- When 'swiped', up to 8h of readings are made available, so a picture of the glucose profile can be built up.

Sensor augmented pump therapy
Combining use of CGM and an insulin pump permits additional functionality, e.g.:
- *Low (or predictive low) glucose suspend function:* whereby if CGM detects low (or nearing low) interstitial glucose levels, it signals to the pump to suspend insulin until recovery of glucose levels.
- *Hybrid 'closed loop' systems:* whereby both reduction and increase in basal insulin delivery by the pump is signalled by the CGM system detecting dropping or rising interstitial glucose levels.

Acute complications of T1DM

Hypoglycaemia

All children with T1DM will experience an episode of hypoglycaemia. Symptoms develop when blood glucose is <4mmol/L. The frequency of hypoglycaemia is higher with more intensive insulin regimens and in younger children. Symptoms and signs include:

- Feeling of hunger.
- Sweatiness.
- Feeling faint/dizzy.
- 'Wobbly feeling'.
- Irritability/confusion/misbehaviour.
- Pallor.

Severe hypoglycaemia is characterized by:
- Third-party rescue.
- Loss of consciousness.
- Seizures.

Nocturnal hypoglycaemia

The frequency is thought to be high in well-controlled T1DM (up to 50%). Nocturnal hypoglycaemia should be suspected when fasting early morning blood sugars are repeatedly high, despite seemingly adequate overnight insulin cover (secondary to hypoglycaemia counter-regulation). Detection and confirmation of nocturnal hypoglycaemia can be achieved by using an SC CGM system (CGMS) device.

Hypoglycaemia: management

Acute episodes of mild to moderate symptomatic hypoglycaemia can be managed with PO glucose (glucose tablets or sugary drink). PO glucose gels applied to the buccal mucosa can be used in the child who is unwilling or unable to cooperate to eat. A simple 'rule of 15' may be a helpful starting point:

1. Give 15g of glucose.
2. Re-check blood glucose after 15min.
3. If blood glucose still <4mmol/L after 15min, repeat step 1.

Severe hypoglycaemia can be managed in the home with an IM injection of glucagon (1.0mg). It is available as an injection kit but requires preparation and skill on the part of the carer who may be at the height of anxiety, so it is often overlooked or not given.

Hypoglycaemia unawareness

Occasionally, sudden-onset hypoglycaemia may result in unconsciousness and seizures. Children experiencing frequent episodes of hypoglycaemia may fail to develop the typical (i.e. counter-regulatory/adrenergic) symptoms of hypoglycaemia. Avoidance of hypoglycaemia for some weeks usually results in restoration of warning symptoms.

Sick-day management

During illness and other physiological stresses (e.g. following injury), insulin requirements dramatically increase in response to the body's ↑ catabolic state. Blood glucose should be monitored more frequently than usual, and insulin doses may need to be ↑. Insulin must be continued at all times, even though oral intake of food and fluids may be ↓. Blood (or urinary) ketones must be monitored and, if elevated, are a sign of ↑ insulin needs and possible impending DKA.

- In the presence of moderate to high ketone levels, doses of soluble/regular insulin must be ↑ (by 25–50%) and supplemental doses may need to be given.
- Carbohydrate and fluid intake should be maintained as much as possible in order to avoid hypoglycaemia and dehydration.

If the child is unable to maintain hydration (e.g. due to excessive vomiting) or cannot take in adequate carbohydrate to avoid hypoglycaemia, then the child should be evaluated by the diabetes or other medical team and consideration given to treatment with IV fluids and insulin infusions (see ➔ DKA treatment, pp. 80–1).

Diabetic ketoacidosis

(See also ➔ DKA treatment, pp. 80–1.)

DKA is caused by a decrease in effective circulating insulin associated with elevations in counter-regulatory hormones (glucagon, catecholamines, cortisol, GH). This leads to ↑ glucose production by the liver and kidneys and impaired peripheral glucose utilization, with resultant hyperglycaemia and hyperosmolality. ↑ lipolysis, with ketone body (β-hydroxybutyrate, acetoacetate) production, causes ketonaemia and metabolic acidosis. Hyperglycaemia and acidosis result in osmotic diuresis, dehydration, and obligate loss of electrolytes. Ketoacid accumulation also induces ileus, resulting in nausea and vomiting and an exacerbation of dehydration.

DKA frequency

- *DKA is most likely to occur at the point of diagnosis:* ~23% of newly diagnosed children present in a state of DKA. In established T1DM, the frequency of DKA is ~1–10% per patient per year.
- *Risk of DKA is ↑ in children with:* poor metabolic control, previous episodes of DKA, peripubertal and adolescent girls, children with mental health disorders (including those with eating disorders), and those with difficult family circumstances.

DKA mortality and morbidity

Mortality rates for DKA are 0.15–0.31%. Cerebral oedema accounts for 57–87% of all DKA-related deaths. Reported mortality from cerebral oedema is high (21–25%), and significant morbidity is evident in 10–26% of all cerebral oedema survivors.

T1DM: long-term complications

The risk of microvascular or macrovascular complications is related to the duration of diabetes and the degree of glycaemic control achieved over time. Patients who achieve and maintain good glycaemic control, i.e. HbA1c ≤48mmol/mol (6.5%), have very low risk. The risk increases almost exponentially, so that improvement of very poorly controlled diabetes has a bigger long-term gain than at the very well-controlled end of the spectrum. Genetic factors may also influence the risk of complications. The conditions outlined in Box 11.4 require screening.

> **Box 11.4 Long-term complications of T1DM**
>
> *Microvascular complications*
> * *Renal*: microalbuminuria, diabetic nephropathy.
> * *Eyes*: retinopathy.
> * *Nervous*: peripheral neuropathy, autonomic neuropathy.
>
> *Macrovascular*
> * Hypertension.
> * Ischaemic heart disease/cerebral stroke.

* *Macrovascular* complications are almost never seen in children and adolescents.
* *Microvascular* complications may be seen during childhood and adolescence with T1DM. The incidence and frequency are low before puberty. Risk factors for the development of early microvasular disease are: duration of diabetes, glycaemic control (long term), and onset of puberty.

Microalbuminuria (MA)
* Rare before puberty.
* May be intermittent and transient.
* May be associated with ↑ BP.
* May require treatment with ACE inhibitor if persistent on three consecutive early morning samples (± hypertension).

Retinopathy
Significant changes are rare before onset of puberty. Background retinopathy (microaneurysms, retinal haemorrhages, soft and hard exudates) may be seen and is reversible. Pre-proliferative or proliferative retinopathy is rare (see ➲ Diabetes mellitus, p. 982).

T1DM: associated illnesses

Patients with T1DM are at ↑ risk of a number of other disorders. The most important of these are the following:
- *Autoimmune thyroiditis:* up to 5% develop hypothyroidism.
- *Coeliac disease:*
  - Prevalence rate 5–10%.
  - Usually atypical symptoms or asymptomatic.
- *Adrenal insufficiency:* rare.
- *Vitiligo:* 1–7% of patients affected.
- *Short stature:* associated with poor glycaemic control.

Screening and long-term monitoring

Glycaemic control
- Glycated haemoglobin index (HbA1c) measured every 3–4mth.

Growth and development
- Height/weight/BMI (regularly at clinic).
- Puberty stage (annual).

Associated conditions
- Coeliac disease: annual measurement of IgA, TTG, and endomysial antibodies (EMA) from diagnosis.
- Thyroid: annual measurement of TSH and free T4 from diagnosis.

Microvascular complications
- All screening for microvascular complications begins at 11y.
- MA screening:
  - Urine dipstick test (regularly at clinic).
  - Early morning Ua:Ucr ratio.
- Retinopathy screening: retinal photography.
- Neuropathy (rare).
- Diabetic foot: annual foot check for signs of sensory neuropathy from diagnosis.
- Dislipidaemia: as an additional risk factor for cardiovascular disease, early detection (e.g. annual screening) of raised cholesterol (LDL) and treatment may reduce the risk of cardiovascular disease in adult life.

Type 2 diabetes mellitus

T2DM is a multifactorial and heterogenous condition in which the balance between insulin sensitivity and insulin secretion is impaired. The condition is characterized by hyperinsulinaemia; however, there is relative insulin insufficiency to overcome underlying concomitant tissue insulin resistance.

Epidemiology

T2DM is emerging as a significant health problem with increasing incidence in most developing countries. The increasing frequency of T2DM parallels the upward trend in childhood obesity in these populations. In the UK, T2DM remains an uncommon, but emerging, disease, while in the United States, T2DM now accounts for up to 45% of the new cases of diabetes diagnosed in childhood.

Aetiology

T2DM is not an autoimmune disease. There is no association with HLA-linked genes; however, there is a strong genetic basis, which is thought to be polygenic. The known risk factors for the development of T2DM are as follows:
- Obesity.
- Family history of T2DM.
- *Ethnic origin:*
  - Asian.
  - African-American.
  - Afro-Caribbean.
  - Pacific-Islander.
  - Mexican-American.
  - Native American.
- PCOS.
- SGA.

Clinical features

Clinical presentation ranges from mild incidental hyperglycaemia to the typical manifestations of insulin deficiency. Presentation with DKA may occasionally be seen. Frequent clinical findings include evidence of obesity and acanthosis nigricans.

Diagnosis

Box 11.5 summarizes the OGTT criteria for abnormal response. The current diagnostic criteria for T2DM are the presence of an abnormal test and:
- The presence of T2DM risk factors.
- Lack of absolute/persistent insulin deficiency.
- The absence of pancreatic autoantibodies.

Not infrequently, the distinction between T1DM and T2DM at initial presentation may be difficult.

Box 11.5 Oral glucose tolerance testing

- *Conditions:* performed in the morning after 8–10h fast.
- *Dose:* glucose 1.75g/kg to a maximum of 75g, drunk after first blood samples taken.
- *Sampling:* blood glucose at 0min and 120min.

Fasting insulin and C-peptide levels may be taken (raised levels indicating insulin resistance).

- *Interpretation:* see table below.

	Blood glucose (mmol/L)	
	At 0min	At 120min
Normal	<6.0	<7.8
IGT	6.0–7.0	7.8–11.1
Diabetes mellitus	>7.0	>11.1

Hyperosmolar hyperglycaemic state (HHS)

Formerly known as HONK (hyperosmolar non-ketotic), it is a rare complication of DM in childhood and characterized by a relatively low ketotic response with very high blood glucose level. It has a higher mortality rate than isolated DKA, but both HHS and DKA may occur simultaneously. More commonly occurs in T2DM in the adolescent age group.

Features

- Serum osmolarity >320mOsm/L [to estimate, use: osmolality = $(2 \times Na^+)$ + urea + glucose].
- Marked hyperglycaemia, e.g. >40mmol/L.
- Absence of marked ketonaemia, e.g. blood ketones <3.0mmol/L.
- Relatively mild acidosis, e.g. pH >7.3, HCO_3^- >15mmol/L.
- Commoner in T2DM.
- Extremely high glucose levels lead to massive diuresis and dehydration.
- Hyperosmolar state leads to reduced GCS score and inability to replace lost fluid PO.
- Degree of dehydration may not be apparent clinically due to high osmolality and relatively well-retained intravascular volume.
- Risk of cerebral oedema and thrombosis.
- May coexist with DKA: suspect when the degree of acidosis/ketosis is not in keeping with severity of clinical features or GCS score.

Management goals

- More rapid and larger volumes of fluid replacement needed than DKA.
- Haemofiltration may be helpful.
- Slow correction of hyperglycaemia: delay starting insulin until initial improvement in glucose concentration rate slows to <3mmol/h. Then start with slower rate (e.g. 0.025–0.05U/kg/h); aim for 3–4mmol/L reduction in blood glucose per hour.
- Slow correction of hypernatraemia: use NS initially, and aim for reduction of 0.5mmol/h.

Type 2 diabetes mellitus: management

All patients with T2DM require the same type and degree of educational support and clinical follow-up as for patients with T1DM. Long-term management goals are the same as for T1DM (see ➲ Type 1 diabetes mellitus: management, p. 470). Specific treatment goals should also include the following:

- Increase in regular and sustained physical exercise.
- Reduction in portion sizes and carbohydrate-containing foods.
- Screening and management of T2DM comorbidities such as hyperlipidaemia and hypertension.

Mild (incidental) T2DM should initially be managed with lifestyle interventions aimed at lowering caloric intake (low-fat, reduced-CHO diet) and increasing physical activity. When these interventions fail, pharmacological therapy is added:

- *Metformin* is the first-line therapy for children and acts by improving cellular sensitivity to insulin action. Modified-release formulations may be better tolerated (common side effect of GI upset).
- *Insulin therapy* may seem contradictory, given that fasting insulin levels are typically high at diagnosis. However, there is a relative pancreatic dysfunction with longer-standing insulin resistance in T2DM, and insulin therapy is commonly required either as just long-acting od or as an MDI regime.
- *Alternative hypoglycaemic agents* are not licensed for use in younger children but may be considered in adolescents when metformin/insulin has failed or not been tolerated:
  - PO sulfonylureas (e.g. gliclazide, glibenclamide) stimulate insulin secretion from pancreas.
  - Glucagon-like peptide 1 (GLP-1) receptor agonists (e.g. exenatide, liraglutide) stimulate insulin release and suppress glucagon secretion and gastric emptying.
  - Dipeptidyl peptidase 4 (DPP-4) inhibitors (e.g. sitagliptin): novel agent with similar effects to GLP-1 agonists, but as PO preparations.
  - Sodium–glucose co-transporter 2 (SGLT-2) receptor inhibitors (e.g. dapagliflozin): lower the renal threshold for glucose excretion and also aid weight loss, but risk of euglycaemic DKA.
- *Bariatric surgery:*
  - Reserved for severe obesity with no response to conventional interventions, and comorbidities such as T2DM.
  - High 'cure' rate for T2DM in adulthood, with more than half of patients no longer symptomatic of diabetes post-surgery. Longer-term outlook for young patients remains undetermined.

Box 11.6 Monogenic forms of diabetes mellitus

HNF1α *mutations*
- 70% of MODY cases.
- Mutation in the *HNF1α* gene (12q24) causes decreasing insulin secretion from pancreas over the first two decades of life.
- Usually presents during adolescence/early adulthood with asymptomatic (normoglycaemic) glycosuria.
- Progresses to symptomatic hyperglycaemia.
- Often responds well to PO sulfonylureas (e.g. gliclazide).
- Microvascular complications: frequent/high risk.

HNF4α *mutations*
- 5% of MODY cases.
- Mutation in the *HNF4α* gene (20q).
- Presents/onset at adolescence: <25y age.
- Severe hyperglycaemia.
- Often history of high birthweight and/or neonatal hypoglycaemia.
- Treatment with PO sulfonylureas (e.g. gliclazide) often effective.
- Microvascular complications: frequent/high risk.

Glucokinase mutations
- 10% of MODY cases.
- Heterozygous for mutation in the glucokinase gene (7p).
- Altered glucose sensing by pancreatic β-cell leads to mild hyperglycaemia, not progressive.
- Presents in childhood and often an incidental finding with absence of diabetes symptoms.
- Complications: rare.
- Treatment: not required.

IPF-1 *mutations*
- Rare.
- Heterozygous for mutation in the *IPF-1* gene (13q).
- Onset post-pubertal.
- Moderately severe diabetes.
- Microvascular complications: rare.

HNF1β *mutations*
- Mutation in the *HNF1β/TCF2* gene (17cen-q21.3).
- Onset post-pubertal.
- Severe diabetes.
- Associated renal cysts are clue to diagnosis.
- Microvascular complications: unknown.

Other forms of diabetes mellitus

Monogenic forms of DM

Also known as *maturity-onset diabetes of the young* (MODY)—heterogenous disorder with AD inheritance. Family history is usually present, and suspicion raised if lack of evidence of autoimmune disease or atypical response to usual diabetes treatments. (See Box 11.6.)

Neonatal diabetes mellitus

Rare (1/400 000–500 000 live births). Defined as hyperglycaemia requiring insulin therapy, occurring in the first few weeks of life; transient (50–60%) and permanent forms are recognized; 85% have an identifiable gene mutation. Molecular genetic testing for neonatal diabetes is recommended in all infants with diabetes mellitus in the first 6mth of life.

Transient neonatal diabetes mellitus (TNDM)
• Often IUGR is evident at birth.
• Hyperglycaemia occurs in first 1–2wk of life.
• Most patients achieve remission and insulin independence <1y.
• Chromosome 6 abnormalities are observed in many (paternal duplications, paternal isodisomy, methylation defects).

Permanent neonatal diabetes mellitus (PNDM)
Rare, often associated with clinical syndromes, e.g.:
• Immune dysregulation, polyendocrinopathy, enteropathy, X-linked (IPEX) syndrome: diffuse autoimmunity; severe pancreatic hypoplasia associated with *IPF-1* mutation.
• Walcott–Rallison syndrome: diabetes mellitus, developmental delay, risk of liver failure later in life.

KCNJ11-related diabetes mellitus
Typically presents in infancy and requires insulin initially. Later, treatment with oral sulfonylurea is possible. Association with DEND (developmental delay, epilepsy, and neonatal diabetes) syndrome.

Cystic fibrosis-related diabetes (CFRD)

Prevalence of CFRD increases with age (9% between ages 5 and 9y; 25% between ages 10 and 19y). It is primarily due to a defect in pancreatic insulin secretion, although modest insulin resistance is also recognized. Insulin replacement is recommended in all CFRD patients.

Severe insulin resistance syndromes

Rare genetic mutations resulting in insulin receptor and post-receptor signalling defects cause severe insulin resistance. Features include: hyperinsulinaemia, acanthosis nigricans, and ovarian hyperandrogenism in ♀ (hirsutism, irregular/absent menstruation). Examples include:
• Type A insulin resistance (suspect in T2DM, but absence of obesity).
• Rabson–Mendenhall syndrome (abnormal nails and dentition).
• Partial lipodystrophy (often onset in infancy).

Further reading

For UK and DKA algorithms

Association of Children's Diabetes Clinicians (ACDC). UK ACDC's endorsed guidelines (e.g. sick-day rules, surgery, CGM). Available at: ℵ http://www.a-c-d-c.org/endorsed-guidelines/.

British Society for Paediatric Endocrinology and Diabetes. Guidelines. Available at: ℵ https://www.bsped.org.uk/clinical-resources/guidelines/.

Diabetes Genes. Information regarding monogenic forms of diabetes. Available at: ℵ http://www.diabetesgenes.org.

International Society for Pediatric and Adolescent Diabetes. For broader international guidelines on most aspects of childhood diabetes—consensus guidelines. Available at: ℵ http://www.ispad.org/?page=ISPADClinicalPract.

National Institute for Health and Care Excellence. (2015). *Diabetes (type 1 and type 2) in children and young people: diagnosis and management.* NICE guideline [NG18]. Available at: ℵ https://www.nice.org.uk/guidance/ng18.

Inherited metabolic disease

Introduction

The classic and somewhat oversimplified model of an inherited metabolic disease (IMD) involves a genetic defect (any mode of inheritance) that causes an enzyme in a cellular cycle to be dysfunctional or absent. This abnormality, in turn, causes a 'block' in a metabolic pathway, resulting in a lack of product from the pathway and/or a build-up of an intermediate compound that is toxic to the cell.

Defects in intermediary metabolism (small molecules usually involved in energy metabolism such as breakdown of protein, fat, and glucose) may present acutely with metabolic 'decompensation'. This decompensation can occur in the first few days of life after an initial period of apparent well-being or later in life (infancy through to adulthood) when it is triggered by illness and/or fasting. Examples include organic acidaemias (OAs), urea cycle defects (UCDs), and fat oxidation defects.

IMDs can also affect the metabolism of complex molecules, which tend to cause chronic multisystem disorders. Examples of defects in the production of complex molecules include Smith–Lemli–Opitz syndrome (cholesterol biosynthesis) and congenital disorders of glycosylation (glycan biosynthesis). Conditions involving abnormal breakdown of complex molecules include lysosomal storage disorders.

Other classes of IMDs include mitochondrial disorders, defective transport of molecules, and disorders of neurotransmission.

Individually IMDs are rare diseases. The commonest IMDs, such as PKU and medium-chain acyl-coenzyme A dehydrogenase deficiency (MCADD), have an incidence of around 1/10 000. However, the incidence of total IMDs is estimated to be between 1/200 and 1/800, depending on the criteria used to define this group of disorders. There are >1000 defined IMDs, a number that continues to increase.

The aim of this chapter is not to provide long lists of differential diagnoses, but to increase awareness of common IMDs and to highlight when to suspect IMDs and how to commence investigations and treatment.

IMDs that have specific and effective treatments are particularly important to diagnose early to improve prognosis.

The acutely unwell child

An IMD should be considered in the differential of any acutely unwell child who has not received a definitive diagnosis (and even those who have but are not responding to standard therapy). The acute presentation of decompensating IMDs is often non-specific and initially mistaken for sepsis. Symptoms in the neonatal period include lethargy, poor feeding, and vomiting. This is similar in older children but may also include abnormal behaviour, altered LOC, and cyclical vomiting. The following circumstances should increase the suspicion of an IMD:

- Neonatal presentation with a period (few days) of well-being/feeding prior to presentation (see → Inborn errors of metabolism, p. 169).
- Episodes triggered by illness/fasting (including cyclical vomiting).
- Change in diet precipitating presentation (e.g. weaning).
- +ve family history and/or presence of consanguinity.

It is important to remember that the 'severe' forms of IMDs that commonly present as a neonatal intoxication also have attenuated forms that can present for the first time from infancy through to adulthood (see Table 12.1).

Table 12.1 Classes of commonly decompensating IMDs

	Common features	Important examples
Organic acidaemia (OA)	Encephalopathy Severe ketoacidosis Moderate hyperammonaemia Ketonuria in neonate*	Methylmalonic acidaemia (MMA) Propionic acidaemia (PA)
Cerebral OA	Encephalopathy ± mild acidosis ± mild hyperammonaemia Ketonuria in neonate*	Maple syrup urine disease (MSUD) GA1
Fatty acid oxidation defect (FAOD)	Encephalopathy Cardiomyopathy/arrhythmia Liver dysfunction Hypoglycaemia/↑ CK Lactic acidosis Mild hyperammonaemia	Long-chain 3-hydroxyacyl-CoA dehydrogenase deficiency (LCHADD)
Urea cycle defect (UCD)	Encephalopathy Severe hyperammonaemia ± mild acidosis ± liver dysfunction	Ornithine transcarbamylase (OTC) deficiency Citrullinaemia

* Ketones in the urine during the neonatal period is highly unusual and should raise suspicion of an organic acidaemia.

Suspected IMD: initial investigations

(See ➔ Metabolic investigation, p. 510.) If an IMD is suspected, it is imperative to discuss the case *urgently* with an IMD centre. Prompt recognition and treatment can have a significant impact on outcome. Investigations should include point-of-care testing for acid–base balance (including lactate), glucose, and blood (or urine) ketones. Further tests to assess intermediary metabolism should include:

• Ammonia.
• LFTs.
• CK.
• Plasma amino acids.
• Acylcarnitine profile.
• Urine organic acids.
• Consider DNA and skin biopsy if a child may not survive.

Point-of-care testing and initial biochemistry may point towards a specific group of disorders (see Table 12.1). Further metabolic testing has a longer turnaround time and is less useful in guiding immediate management but is essential to identify an exact metabolic diagnosis. Advances in mass spectrometry allow the detection of hundreds of metabolites from one blood sample (requiring as little as 50 microlitres of plasma). This technology is slowly entering routine clinical laboratories.

Initial management

(See ➔ Chapter 3; ➔ Therapy, p. 82). Children presenting with acute metabolic decompensation need prompt assessment and initial resuscitation, in accordance with standard paediatric guidelines. Significant acidosis and renal losses mean they are very susceptible to hypovolaemia and significant fluid resuscitation is often required.

Sepsis is an important differential (and may coexist), so antibiotic treatment should be started. The presence of infection does not exclude IMDs—it can be the trigger for metabolic decompensation.

Three main principles guide initial management:
1. Stop feeds: intoxicating substrate will usually be fat or protein from feeds. Only re-introduce feeds on advice of IMD centre.
2. Promote anabolism: ensuring adequate energy intake pushes the patient towards anabolism and away from using the defective pathway. Initially give 10% dextrose (always with appropriate electrolytes) at maintenance rates. If hyperglycaemia ensues, consider insulin (also anabolic in action), rather than decreasing the dextrose infusion. Fluids can be subsequently tailored (see Table 12.2) as a guide for carbohydrate infusion rate (many children in the PICU setting will require fluid restriction, so higher concentrations of dextrose may be needed to achieve the same dextrose provision).
   • *Tip for glucose infusion calculations:*

Glucose infusion rate (GIR) $(mg/kg/min) = $ (infusion speed in mL/h $\times$

%dextrose concentration of infusion fluid)$/6 \times$ weight in kg)

Table 12.2 Suggested carbohydrate intake to promote anabolism

Age (y)	Minimum carbohydrate infusion (mg/kg/min)	10% dextrose requirement (mL/kg/day)
0–2	10	150
2–6	8	120
>6	6	90

3. Use of nitrogen 'scavengers': in acute hyperammonaemia, nitrogen scavengers, such as sodium benzoate and sodium phenylbutyrate, can be used to help excretion of nitrogen. They conjugate with glycine and glutamate, respectively, and are excreted in the urine. This provides an alternative pathway for the excretion of ammonia.
   - Sodium benzoate is usually the first choice, as sodium phenylbutyrate should be used with caution in OAs and fatty acid oxidation defects (FAODs) due to the theoretical risk of glutamate depletion.
   - Patients who are naïve to nitrogen scavengers are given an IV loading of 250mg/kg over 90min, followed by a continuous infusion, with a maximum daily dose of 500mg/kg/day. Patients already received nitrogen scavengers should not receive a loading dose.

In acute acidosis, levocarnitine can be used to help the excretion of abnormal organic acids in children with OAs (up to 200mg/kg/day, divided in four doses, either IV or PO). Levocarnitine is contraindicated in fat oxidation defects—it is recommended to discuss with an IMD centre before commencing these therapies.

PICU therapy: patients presenting with an IMD for the first time will often require intensive care support. Early intervention with ETT intubation is often warranted to help support energy-deplete organ systems, as well as prompt transfer to PICU. Children with IMDs presenting with severe acidosis or hyperammonaemia will often need access to further treatment modalities such as haemofiltration.

The British Inherited Metabolic Disease Group publishes disease-specific guides to aid the initial acute management of IMDs, including information on prescribing fluids and drugs (available at: ℰ http://www.bimdg.org.uk).

Hyperammonaemia

Hyperammonaemia is a medical emergency and Table 12.3 is a guide to interpreting ammonia levels. Hyperammonaemia causes cerebral oedema and raised ICP, with outcome being determined by the degree and duration of hyperammonaemia. Unfortunately, delayed recognition of hyperammonaemia is common and can lead to severe neurological disability and death. Prompt measurement of blood ammonia level is very important in all children presenting with unexplained drowsiness or encephalopathy.

Table 12.3 Interpretation of ammonia levels

Neonate	Normal	<100 micromoles/L
	Secondary to non-specific illness (and prematurity)—ensure repeat sampling	<150 micromoles/L
	Suspect metabolic disease	>150 micromoles/L
After neonatal period	Normal	<50 micromoles/L
	Suspect metabolic disease	>100 micromoles/L

Signs and symptoms of hyperammonaemia include lethargy, vomiting, and altered LOC that progresses to coma. Ammonia is a respiratory stimulant, so patients will often be tachypnoeic in early stages with respiratory alkalosis. If systemically compromised, acidosis may be present at later stages—the absence of alkalosis does not exclude hyperammonaemia.

NB: respiratory alkalosis in an unwell child, especially with altered LOC, warrants immediate ammonia measurement.

Signs and symptoms of hyperammonaemia include lethargy, vomiting, and altered LOC that progresses to coma. Ammonia is a respiratory stimulant, so patients will often be tachypnoeic in early stages with respiratory alkalosis. If systemically compromised, acidosis may be present at later stages—the absence of alkalosis does not exclude hyperammonaemia.

NB: respiratory alkalosis in an unwell child, especially with altered LOC, warrants immediate ammonia measurement.

Causes of high blood ammonia levels

Blood ammonia levels are tightly regulated, with ammonia being converted to urea in the liver by the urea cycle.

Artefact

Difficult venepuncture and inappropriate sample handling can cause significantly raised ammonia levels:

- Samples should be free-flowing and ideally uncuffed.
- Capillary samples should not be used.
- It is advisable to discuss with the receiving laboratory prior to sending the sample to ensure prompt handling—some laboratories may require special bottles/transport on ice.

Non-metabolic causes

- Liver failure: ammonia may be significantly raised in acute liver failure and is thought to play a role in hepatic encephalopathy.
- Urease +ve infection (UTI, sepsis): bacteria release ammonia by metabolizing urea. Rare.
- Drugs: valproate, chelation agents.
- Transient hyperammonaemia of the neonate: typically occurs in premature/low-birthweight (LBW) infants. Ammonia can be very high and needs prompt management. Thought to be secondary to patent ductus venosus.

Metabolic causes

Primary urea cycle defect

An enzyme in the urea cycle is absent/defective. Classical presentation is acute neonatal intoxication with ammonia rapidly rising (>1000 micromoles/L) in the first few days of life. Commonest—ornithine transcarbamylase (OTC) deficiency (X-linked).

Organic acidaemias

Production of abnormal organic acids causes secondary inhibition of the urea cycle. Ammonia typically <500 micromoles//L but can be much higher, as seen in UCDs. Main distinguishing feature is severe metabolic acidosis and severe ketosis.

Fatty acid oxidation defects

Mild hyperammonaemia in acute illness, typically <250 micromoles/L. Associated with liver dysfunction, rhabdomyolysis, and hypoglycaemia.

Others

Citrin deficiency, lysinuric protein intolerance, hyperinsulinism–hyperammonaemia syndrome.

Hypoglycaemia

Hypoglycaemia: plasma glucose concentration low enough to cause signs and symptoms of impaired brain function. Historically, a value of ≤2.6mmol/L has been used, but bedside tests are inaccurate at low values and treatment should not be delayed in the symptomatic child while awaiting confirmation on a laboratory sample.

Causes of hypoglycaemia

Inappropriately low glucose can occur:
1. In any very sick child (e.g. sepsis, liver failure).
2. When artefactually low from poorly perfused peripheral samples.
3. In disorders of glucose signalling/control (endocrine disorders—see
   ➔ Chapter 10).
4. In IMDs that affect pathways that supply glucose or are glucose-
   sparing. Hypoglycaemia caused by an IMD is usually precipitated by
   fasting. Fasting tolerance can be as little as 90min, e.g. glycogen storage
   disease type 1 (GSD1), or be relatively normal—only becoming a
   problem when fasting is extended beyond normal such as occurs with
   intercurrent illness (e.g. fat oxidation defects).

NB: a normal response to fasting involves the production of ketones by the liver as a by-product of fat oxidation. A useful way to approach hypoglycaemia is to consider the body's response to fasting in terms of ketone production (see Table 12.4).

Metabolic investigations

Obtain suitable investigations at the time of hypoglycaemia. However, this should not delay the emergency management of the acutely hypoglycaemic child (see ➔ Hypoglycaemia, pp. 78–9). Endocrine investigations (such as insulin, cortisol, and GH) should be considered at the same time as the following metabolic investigations:
- Laboratory venous glucose.
- 3β-hydroxybutyrate (or bedside ketone measurement).
- Free fatty acids, lactate, LFTs*.
- Urine ketones**, urine organic acids*.
- Acylcarnitine profile*, plasma amino acids*.

Further investigation of hypoglycaemia may involve biochemical profiling/controlled fasting in an inpatient setting. This can help obtain a diagnosis but is used more to define safe fasting limits and should be done in a regional IMD service (because of risk of hypoglycaemia).

* If sampling not achieved during episode, ensure these are subsequently completed.

** If the opportunity of blood ketone measurement at the time of hypoglycaemia is missed, catching the first urine will reflect recent ketone status.

Fat oxidation defects should always be excluded (by analysis of acylcarnitine profile) before fasting a child with an unknown cause of hypoglycaemia.

Table 12.4 Differential diagnosis of hypoglycaemia

Non-ketotic hypoglycaemia	Hyperinsulinism	Endocrine
	Fat oxidation defects	Liver impairment ± cardiomyopathy ± elevated CK ± lactic acidosis NB: presence of ketones does not exclude FAOD
	Disorders of ketone body synthesis	± liver impairment ± acute acidosis
	Drugs	Insulin Oral hypoglycaemics
	Liver failure	Multiple causes
Ketotic hypoglycaemia	Idiopathic ketotic hypoglycaemia	(See ⊃ Idiopathic ketotic hypoglycaemia, p. 498)
	Other endocrine causes	For example, adrenal insufficiency
	Hepatic GSD (types 1, 6, 9)	Poor growth Central obesity Hepatomegaly ± lactate
	GSD type 0	Poor growth ± lactate
	Ketolysis defects	Severe ketoacidosis
Hypoglycaemia with significantly elevated lactate (± ketones)	Hepatic GSD1	Poor growth Central obesity Hepatomegaly
	Fructose-1,6-bisphosphatase (F-1,6-BP) deficiency	Severe lactic acidosis triggered by fasting Transient hepatomegaly

Idiopathic ketotic hypoglycaemia

Often referred to as ketotic hypoglycaemia (KH), this usually occurs for the first time in infancy and most often presents during a prolonged fast caused by intercurrent illness (e.g. gastroenteritis).

Patients have an exaggerated ketotic response to fasting and if they continue fasting, they can develop hypoglycaemia. This is thought to be caused by an immature response to fasting (in particular, a reduced rate of gluconeogenesis), although some patients labelled with idiopathic KH may well have mild forms of GSD.

Patients will usually grow out of the propensity to excessive ketosis/hypoglycaemia by the age of 6y.

Treatment is to avoid fasting by providing a prescribed energy drink during times of illness/fasting (often referred to as emergency regimen).

Idiopathic KH is a diagnosis of exclusion—if any of the following RED FLAGS are present, an alternative diagnosis should be considered:
• Short fasting tolerance or no obvious fasting trigger for episode.
• Early presentation <6mth of age.
• Poor growth (weight >> height, consider GSD/endocrine causes).
• Hepatomegaly—chronic (GSD) or transient (FAOD, F-1,6-BP deficiency).
• Hyperpigmentation (adrenal insufficiency).
• Abnormal biochemistry—especially raised lactate or liver dysfunction (GSD/FAOD).

Any ♂ child presenting with adrenal insufficiency should have VLCFAs measured to rule out X-linked adrenal leukodystrophy—a severe neurodegenerative condition that is treatable if caught prior to onset of neurological symptoms.

Initial management

Acute hypoglycaemia should be managed, as per standard paediatric guidelines (see ◆ Hypoglycaemia, pp. 78–9). If a glucose bolus is used, ensure adequate ongoing glucose intake (good PO intake or IV 10% dextrose with appropriate additives) to avoid rebound hypoglycaemia. If an IMD is suspected, prompt discussion with an IMD centre to ensure safe management is warranted.

Elevated lactate

Raised lactate is a common finding, and it is important to consider common non-metabolic causes thoroughly. However, it can be a marker for an underlying defect of energy metabolism.

Causes

- *Tissue hypoxia or underperfusion:* by far the commonest cause. Consider sepsis, hypoxia, seizures, underlying cardiac dysfunction, and GI pathology (e.g. NEC).
- *Artefact:* lactate is commonly raised due to difficult venepuncture or poor sample handling. If unexpectedly raised, repeat using the best possible blood sample (ideally uncuffed). Also consider concurrently measuring plasma amino acids (genuinely raised lactate is associated with raised alanine/proline) and urine organic acids (raised blood lactate will cause ↑ urinary lactate if exceeding renal threshold).
- *Metabolic decompensation:* many of the IMDs already described previously can present with raised lactate, in association with other metabolic derangements such as hypoglycaemia or hyperammonaemia. This is due to secondary dysfunction of energy pathways.
- *Primary (or congenital) lactic acidosis:* persistently raised lactate (see Table 12.5).
- *Other:* drugs (salbutamol, ethanol), thiamine deficiency.

Table 12.5 Primary lactic acidoses

	Common features	Comments
Mitochondrial disorders (>100 indiviual disorders defined)	Diverse multisystem phenotypes. Commonly have disturbed lactate metabolism	Multisystem work-up, including neurological, cardiac, renal, and endocrine. Muscle biopsy and/or genetic work-up required. Few effective treatments
Disorders of biotin metabolism	For example, biotinidase deficiency. Neonatal or infantile presentation, including developmental delay, skin lesions, and seizures	Measure biotinidase activity and organic acids. Effectively treated with biotin
Disorders of pyruvate metabolism	For example, pyruvate dehydrogenase deficiency. Developmental delay, seizures ± structural brain abnormalities (absent corpus callosum)	Measure pyruvate dehydrogenase activity. Occasionally responds to thiamine. Ketogenic diet can improve outcomes

Metabolic acidosis

(See also ⊃ Unexplained metabolic acidosis, p. 75.) Unwell children are commonly acidotic. Metabolic acidosis can be defined as pH <7.35, with low HCO_3^-. This section outlines a simple approach to metabolic acidosis and highlights features that should raise suspicion of an IMD. Most children presenting with metabolic acidosis *do not* have an IMD.

$$\text{Anion gap } (AG) = (Na^+) - (HCO_3^- + Cl^-)$$

(Normal range: 10–12mmol/L; check with laboratory)

- *Normal AG acidosis:* typically caused by loss of HCO_3^-. Unlikely to be IMD.
  - *Intestinal loss:* common in infants presenting with diarrhoeal illness. Exacerbated by administration of Cl^- in fluids. Resolves with appropriate fluid management.
  - *Renal loss:* consider investigating for renal tubulopathy (see ⊃ Renal tubular disorder, pp. 338–9). Some IMDs can cause renal tubulopathy (e.g. mitochondrial disorders, tyrosinaemia, OAs).
- *Raised AG acidosis:* caused by the accumulation of acid such as lactic acid, ketones, or abnormal organic acids in the case of IMD. Always consider RED FLAGS (see ⊃ Idiopathic ketotic hypoglycemia, p. 498).
  - *Most commonly caused by systemic insult:* such as hypoxia or hypovolaemia. Excess acid is lactic acid from anaerobic respiration and ketosis from catabolism.
  - *DM:* associated with significant hyperglycaemia and ketosis. Disorders of ketolysis can masquerade as DKA, but levels of hyperglycaemia are only moderate and there is no ongoing insulin requirement.
  - *Exogenous acid:* e.g. methanol, salicylate.
  - *IMD:* acidosis is caused by a combination of abnormal organic acid, lactic acid, ketones, and mitochondrial dysfunction. Commonly seen in OAs, fat oxidation defects, ketolysis disorders, and mitochondrial disorders.

Acute rhabdomyolysis

Acute rhabdomyolysis presents with muscle pain and myoglobinuria and, if severe, may cause acidosis and renal impairment.

Episodes of acute rhabdomyolysis are most commonly caused by trauma or infection (e.g. benign acute childhood myositis) but can be caused by IMD (see Table 12.6).

Recurrent episodes triggered by fasting, intercurrent illness, or exercise are particularly suspicious of an IMD.

Table 12.6 IMDs causing recurrent rhabdomyolysis

Disorders	Common features	Investigations and treatment
FAODs [e.g. moderate forms of VLCADD, carnitine palmitoyltransferase 2 (CPT2) deficiency]	Recurrent myalgia, myoglobinuria ± hypoglycaemia, liver dysfunction, cardiomyomyopathy	Acylcarnitine profile, fat oxidation studies (fibroblasts) Treatment: ensure adequate carbohydrate intake during fasting or illness
Muscle glycogenoses [e.g GSD5 (McArdle disease)]	Myalgia on initiation of intense exercise. Can display 'second-wind' phenomena ± myoglobinuria	Muscle biopsy, generally superseded by genetic testing Forearm exercise test (rarely used in children) Treatment: exercise conditioning, oral carbohydrate pre-exercise
Lipin-1 (LPIN1) deficiency	Recurrent and potentially catastrophic rhabdomyolysis triggered by fasting or illness (estimated ~10% of recurrent childhood rhabdomyolysis)	No specific biochecmical test. If FAOD ruled out (normal acylcarnitine profile), consider LPIN1 genetics

Systems—neurological

Abnormal neurology can be the presenting feature in many IMDs, although reaching a diagnosis in such patients is a major challenge as symptoms are not specific and the differential is wide. Presenting features can include seizures, developmental delay, and abnormalities in tone. The following red flags should increase the suspicion of an IMD:

- +ve family history.
- Progressive symptoms/developmental regression.
- Intermittent acute attacks or fluctuation of symptoms.
- Symptoms not following a neuroanatomical pattern.
- Multiorgan involvement.
- Dysmorphic features.

Developmental delay

(See also ➲ Chapter 18.) (See Table 12.7.) Children presenting with global developmental delay (GDD) traditionally have not been considered for significant metabolic work-up unless suspicious features were present. However, the increasing availability of metabolic testing and the recognition that some 'treatable' IMDs can present solely with GDD are changing practice. A revised UK guideline for first-line investigation of GDD has been recently proposed.

Regression

True developmental regression (as opposed to failure in progression) is rare and should prompt urgent referral to specialist neurology services. IMDs that can present with isolated regression include the lysosomal storage disorders [in particular, mucopolysaccharidosis type III (MPS III), neuronal ceroid lipofuscinoses, and sphingolipidoses], X-linked adrenoleukodystropy, and mitochondrial disorders.

Seizures/epileptic encephalopathy

(See also ➲ Epilepsy syndromes: neonatal, p. 370.) (See Table 12.8.) Seizures are a common feature of IMDs. They usually occur as a consequence of abnormal brain physiology due to an accumulating substrate and/or abnormal energy metabolism. They can also occur due to CNS damage secondary to a previous acute decompensation. IMDs presenting with seizures can be categorized by age of presentation, varying from neonatal epileptic encephalopathy (NEE) to discrete seizures starting in older children. Some of these conditions are responsive to co-factor supplementation. In the case of NEE, empirical trials of the co-factors pyridoxine, pyridoxal-5-phosphate, and biotin may be warranted.

Table 12.7 Some IMDs whose presenting feature can be GDD, with emphasis given to 'treatable' conditions

	Common features/treatments	Investigations
Creatine disorders	Speech and intellectual delay; behavioural difficulties ± seizures Clinical improvement with supplement ± dietary modification	Urine creatine* and guanidinoacetate (GAA)*
Disorders of biotin metabolism	Global delay ± skin lesions; seizures, acute acidosis, hearing difficulties Responds well to biotin supplementation	Biotinidase activity Urine organic acids* Acylcarnitine profile
Homocystinuria	Speech and intellectual delay; marfanoid features ± thromboses Responds well to dietary therapy if treated early	Plasma total homocysteine* Plasma amino acids*
Lysosomal storage disorders (many subtypes)	GDD; regression may be evident: ± dysmorphism; skeletal abnormalities, organomegaly, cardiomyopathy Some subtypes respond to enzyme replacement therapy and/or bone marrow transplant (BMT)	Urine glycosaminoglycans* + oligosaccharides* Vacuolated lymphocytes Specific enzyme assays (sometimes referred to as white cell enzymes)
Late-onset OAs and UCDs	± history of acute episodes suggestive of decompensations ± abnormal diet—protein avoidance	Urine organic acids* Plasma amino acids* Ammonia
Disorder of purine and pyrimidine synthesis	Global delay ± seizures; deafness, dysmorphic features, abnormal tone, anaemia, renal involvement	Urine purine* and pyrimidines* Urate

* Investigations that are included in the proposed UK guideline.

Table 12.8 IMDs commonly presenting with seizures

Neonatal period to early infancy	Pyridoxine-dependent epilepsy and pyridoxamine-5′-phosphate oxidase (PNPO) deficiency	Drug resistant NEE ± lactate (PNPO)	Measure urine α-aminoadipic semialdehyde (AASA) Highly responsive to pyridoxine or pyridoxal phosphate (PNPO)
	Molybdenum co-factor deficiency	HIE mimic—consider history carefully	Low urate, measure urinary purines and sulfocysteine. No effective treatment
	Glucose transporter type 1 (GLUT1) deficiency	Epileptic encephalopathy ± microcephaly	Low CSF:plasma glucose
	Non-ketotic hyperglycinaemia	Hypotonia, seizures followed by apnoeas, profound lack of development	Raised CSF:plasma glycine No effective treatment
	Biotinidase deficiency	± GDD, rash, lactic acidosis	Low biotinidase activity, abnormal organic acids Highly responsive to biotin
	Menkes disease	Brittle hair, hyperelastic skin, hypotonia	Low copper/caeruloplasmin Early treatment with copper–histidine can improve outcome
	Peroxisomal disorders	Hypotonia, dysmorphism, liver dysfunction	VLCFAs No effective treatment
Infancy	Creatine synthesis disorders	GDD, behavioural difficulties	Urine creatine/GAA Dietary modification and creatine supplementation can improve outcome
	Neuronal ceroid lipofuscinoses	Developmental regression, loss of vision, microcephaly	EM, enzyme studies. No effective treatment
Later childhood	Mitochondrial disorders, including myoclonic epilepsy with ragged red fibres (MERRF) and mitochondrial encephalopathy, lactic acidosis, and stroke-like episodes (MELAS)	Various features, including myopathy, stroke-like episodes, raised lactate, and retinopathy	Multisystem work-up, DNA studies ± skin biopsy No effective treatments

Systems—hepatic

The liver plays a central role in many metabolic pathways and is commonly affected in IMDs. This can be transient as part of an acute decompensation (e.g. fat oxidation defects, UCDs) or manifest as chronic liver disease. A list of differential diagnoses for liver disease in IMDs would be very long, but some important examples of IMDs presenting primarily with liver disease, either as hepatocellular dysfunction or isolated hepatomegaly, are given below.

Hepatocellular dysfunction

(See Table 12.9.) This can manifest with transaminitis, coagulopathy, cholestasis, or more severely as cirrhosis or frank liver failure. The latter may present with signs of encephalopathy such as vomiting and coma. Hepatomegaly is also common in this group.

Table 12.9 IMDs presenting with hepatocellular dysfunction

	Common features	Investigations/treatment
Galactosaemia	Vomiting, diarrhoea, jaundice, coagulopathy Onset in first week of life Renal tubulopathy ± cerebral oedema (acute)	Enzyme assay [galactose-1-phosphate uridyl transferase (Gal-1-PUT)]. Urine-reducing substances not reliable Effective treatment—galactose-restricted diet. This should be started empirically if diagnosis suspected. Can be serendipitously suspected on newborn screening
Tyrosinaemia type 1	Acute liver failure in neonatal period or chronic cirrhosis, renal tubulopathy, and neurological crises	Urine organic acids—succinylacetone highly specific. Effective treatment with nitisinone and tyrosine-restricted diet
Hereditary fructose intolerance	Vomiting, FTT, hypoglycaemia, and liver dysfunction on introduction of solids (contain fructose)	Trial of fructose elimination from diet diagnostic Enzyme assay requires liver tissue. Confirm with genetic studies

Isolated hepatomegaly

(See Table 12.10.) Isolated hepatomegaly (i.e. without evidence of hepatocellular dysfunction) is generally caused by excess accumulation of substrate.

Table 12.10 IMDs commonly presenting with hepatomegaly

	Common features	Investigations/treatment
Lysosomal storage diseases	Hepatomegaly without hepatocellular dysfunction ± splenomegaly; dysmorphism, skeletal dysplasia, cardiomyopathy, developmental delay; adenotonsillar hyperplasia	Urine oligosaccharides/ glycosaminoglycans Vacuolated lymphocytes Specific enzyme assays Enzyme replacement therapy/ BMT may improve outcomes, depending on subtype and age of diagnosis
GSDs	Presenting feature may be hepatomegaly ± splenomegaly, poor growth, fasting intolerance, hypoglycaemia. Neutropenia (type 1b)	Lactate, glucose, and ketone profiling Enzyme or genetic subtyping. Effective treatment with dietary modification

Systems—cardiac

(See Table 12.11.) Many IMDs that affect energy production in muscle or involve accumulation of substrate in muscle impact the heart. This can manifest as cardiomyopathy, rhythm disturbance, or abnormal valve function. Children with IMDs need cardiac assessment.

In children with cardiac dysfunction, features such as multisystem involvement, dysmorphism, skeletal myopathy, skeletal dysplasia or short stature, and neutropenia should all raise suspicion of an IMD.

Table 12.11 IMDs with cardiomyopathy as the presenting feature

	Common features	Investigations/treatment
Infantile Pompe disease	Hypertrophic cardiomyopathy, severe hypotonia, respiratory failure, macroglossia. Raised CK	Urine oligosaccharides, vacuolated lymphocytes, enzyme assay. Enzyme replacement therapy can be effective
Fat oxidation defects (LCHADD, carnitine disorders)	Cardiomyopathy, arrhythmias ± liver dysfunction, hypoglycaemia, rhabdomyolysis	Acylcarnitine profile Dietary modification and aggressive illness management can be very effective
Mucopolysaccharidosis (type I or Hurler)	Cardiomyopathy, valve dysfunction, coarse features, developmental delay, organomegaly, skeletal dysplasia	Urine glycosaminoglycans, enzymology. BMT ± enzyme replacement therapy can be effective
Barth syndrome	Cardiomyopathy (non-compaction type), skeletal myopathy, developmental delay, cyclical neutropenia	Cardiolipins, urine organic acids (3-methylglutaconic aciduria) No effective treatment
Mitochondrial disorders (various)	Cardiomyopathy and arrhythmias may be presenting features. Other systems often involved—CNS, skeletal muscle, liver, renal	Multisystem work-up required No effective treatments

Systems—dysmorphism

(See Table 12.12.) IMDs are not usually associated with dysmorphic features. There are, however, some notable exceptions affecting the breakdown or synthesis of complex molecules and that are associated with multisystem disease. Some defects in energy metabolism can also be associated with dysmorphic features.

Table 12.12 IMDs commonly presenting with dysmorphic features

	Common features	Investigations/treatment
Peroxisomal disorders (Zellweger spectrum disorders and rhizomelic chrondrodysplasia punctata)	Neonatal presentation. High forehead, wide fontanelle, skeletal dysplasia, including stippled epiphyses (patella), hypotonia ± seizures, liver dysfunction	VLCFAs, plasmalogens, bile acids, enzyme studies. No effective treatment
Lysosomal storage disorders	Coarse facies ± hepatosplenomegaly, adenotonsillar hypertrophy, cardiomyopathy, developmental delay/regression, skeletal dysplasia	Urine glycosaminoglycans/oligosaccharides. Vacuolated lymphocytes. Specific enzyme assays. Treatment depends on subtype—enzyme replacement therapy/BMT may improve outcomes, depending on subtype and age of diagnosis
Smith–Lemli–Opitz syndrome (disorder of cholesterol biosynthesis)	Microcephaly, anteverted nares, micrognathia, ptosis, 2/3 Y-shaped toe syndactyly. Cardiac/renal defects. Developmental delay, behavioural difficulty	Plasma sterols (raised 7-dehydrocholesterol). Cholesterol supplementation may help with skin manifestations and behaviour
Homocystinuria	Marfanoid features. Lens dislocation. Learning difficulties. Thromboembolism	Raised homocysteine. Included in UK newborn screening. Good outcomes with dietary modification if started early. May be pyridoxine-responsive
Congenital disorders of glycosylation (>100 individual disorders described—phosphomannomutase deficiency CDG-1a commonest)	Multisystem manifestation. Hyperinsulinaemic hypoglycaemia. Structural brain abnormalities. Abnormal fat distribution with buttock atrophy. Inverted nipples	Transferrin isoelectric focusing. Genetic studies. Mostly symptomatic therapy. Mannose therapy for CDG type 1b

Metabolic investigations

The main diagnostic tools in inherited metabolic medicine are biochemical tests characterizing analytes or enzyme activities There are currently a wide range of tests available and it is important to choose the correct test to get meaningful results. Although the 'metabolic screen' (all potential analytes of interest measured in one test) with mass spectrometry is starting to become a reality in the research lab, this is not clinically available. A brief description of some of the more commonly used biochemical tests is below.

Advances in genetic testing are also changing the way IMDs are being diagnosed. Until recently, a diagnosis would be suspected on clinical and biochemical grounds and a single gene would be interrogated to confirm the diagnosis. Single-gene tests are now rarely used, with next-generation sequencing being employed to look at larger gene panels, exomes, or genomes. Many IMDs are being discovered in this manner, some of which do not have specific biochemical markers.

Commonly used biochemical tests

- *Acylcarnitine profile:* uses plasma or bloodspot to detect a wide range of activated fatty acids and organic acids that are conjugated with carnitine. They are important in the diagnosis of FAODs and some OAs. A low level of free carnitine (caused by IMD or poor diet) can make this test unreliable.
- *Urine organic acids:* this is a qualitative test that can detect many hundreds of analytes in urine. An experienced clinical scientist is required to interpret the results to recognize abnormal patterns of analytes that can be disease-specific.
- *Plasma amino acids:* quantitates individual amino acids in plasma. Important in the diagnosis of disorders of amino acid metabolism (e.g PKU) and useful for assessing other metabolic perturbations such as raised lactate (high alanine) and raised ammonia (high glutamine). Very useful in monitoring dietary therapies.
- *VLCFAs:* these metabolites are initially chain-shortened in the peroxisome. Used as a screen for peroxisomal disorders.
- *Urine glycosaminoglycans and oligosaccharides:* used as an initial screen for lysosomal storage disorders. Further testing includes vacuolated lymphocytes and specific enzyme assays—discussion with the metabolic centre and laboratory is recommended if ordering these tests.

Newborn screening

(See also ⊃ Biochemical screening, p. 120.) The purpose of newborn screening is to identify newborns at risk of a modifiable disease. If an individual condition is to be screened, there should be a robust test available and evidence that a +ve screen will result in an altered outcome. The UK is relatively conservative in the choice of screened conditions—a total of six IMDs are currently screened for, in contrast to most states in the United States that screen for >50 IMDs. A further three conditions are also included in the screening programme: congenital hypothyroidism, CF, and SCD.

Parents of all babies born in the UK are offered newborn screening. The screening sample is collected between day 5 and day 8 of life via heel prick on a Blood Spot Card (formerly known as the Guthrie Card) by a midwife, sent by post to the regional newborn screening laboratory, and analysed on the following day.

Annually, there are around 750 000 births in the UK and analysis of newborn screening samples from these babies is carried out across 16 regional specialist laboratories.

The clear majority of samples (>99%) are screened –ve and are reported back to the parents via the Child Health Department and health visitors.

Any screen +ve results for one of the IMDs are reported immediately to metabolic specialist services, which have the responsibility of contacting the parents and arranging an urgent clinical review for further evaluation and confirmatory testing. This may occur in a tertiary IMD centre or with local paediatric services.

Previously unscreened infants (e.g. immigrants) who move into a primary care area are offered screening for the same conditions included in the newborn screening programme.

Comprehensive resources for health professionals and the public about the screening programme, including downloadable patient information leaflets about individual conditions, are available from the UK NHS newborn blood spot screening programme (available at: ℛ https://www.gov.uk/government/collections/newborn-blood-spot-screening-programme-supporting-publications).

Further reading

British Inherited Metabolic Diseases Group. Contains useful information regarding emergency management protocols. Available at: ℘ http://www.bimdg.org.uk.

Hoffmann GF, Zschocke J, Nyhan WL (eds). *Inherited Metabolic Diseases. A Clinical Approach*, second edition. Springer-Verlag, Berlin Heidelberg; 2017.

Lemonde H, Cleary MA, Chakrapani A. Newborn screening for inborn errors of metabolism. *Paediatr Child Health* 2015; **25**: 49–57.

Lemonde H, Rahman S. Inherited mitochondrial disease. *Paediatr Child Health* 2015; **25**: 133–8.

Mithyantha R, Kneen R, McCann E, Gladstone M. Current evidence-based recommendations on investigating children with global developmental delay. *Arch Dis Child* 2017; **102**: 1071–6.

Saudubray JM, Baumgartner MR, Walter J (eds). *Inborn Metabolic Diseases: Diagnosis and Treatment*, sixth edition. Springer Berlin, Heidelberg; 2016.

Zschocke J, Hoffmann GF. (2011). (Based on the third English print edition) *Vademecum Metabolicum*, third revised edition, Milupa Metabolics GmbH, Friedrichsdorf. ℘ http://www.nutricia-metabolics.info (see ℘ http://www.vademetab.org for a downloadable app for iOS and Android, containing a practical guide for IMDs).

Chapter 13

Allergy

Allergy: terminology and tests

Terminology in paediatric allergy

- *Allergy*: a disordered reaction by the immune system to a non-toxic antigen.
- *Atopy*: the predisposition to produce allergic responses.
- *Allergic disease*: includes eczema, food allergies, asthma, and allergic rhinitis. Atopic diseases are common—worldwide 1 in 8 children have asthma, 1 in 13 eczema, 1 in 12 food allergies, and 1 in 8 allergic rhinitis.
- *Allergic reactions*: either IgE-mediated (type I hypersensitivity reactions) or from a mixture of other inappropriate hypersensitivity reactions (labelled 'non-IgE-mediated' for practical purposes due to the complexity of unpicking the precise immune mechanisms in a child).
- *IgE-mediated reactions*: allergen-specific IgE antibodies bind to mast cells via their Fc receptor. Soluble antigens (allergens) bind to the specific IgEs (sIgEs). This results in IgE cross-linking and mast cell degranulation with histamine release.
- *Intolerance*: a non-immune (i.e. not allergic) set of symptoms to noxious substance, e.g. lactose-inducing loose stools and flatulence after a bout of gastroenteritis.
- *Sensitization*: the presence of circulating sIgE for a given antigen which may or may not then lead to allergic reactions.
- *'Allergic March'*: refers to the progression and general evolution of allergic diseases throughout childhood. Eczema (infancy) → food allergy (early childhood, age 1–2y) → asthma (childhood, age 5y onwards) → allergic rhinitis (later childhood, 7+y).

Allergy tests

- The two main tests available are blood-specific IgEs and SPT; both are equally valid means of testing IgE levels to a specific antigen.
- These tests should only be performed after a detailed allergy history is taken, which will help direct what allergens to test against and determine a pre-test probability of the test confirming genuine allergy.
- The tests should be interpreted by clinicians with competencies in the field.
- Presence of a +ve test merely indicates *sensitization* to the allergen *and in isolation does not confirm clinical allergy*.

Specific IgE levels

- sIgE levels are measured in serum, a test usually accessible from primary care. Many hundreds of antigens can be tested.
- Positive predictive values (PPVs) of 95% are used as reference (see ➐ Allergy testing in food allergy, pp. 518–20). NB: high variability between antigens and variation with age of the child.
- A high sIgE level makes an allergy more likely but does not always correlate to the *severity* of the allergic response. It therefore should not be used as a predictor of anaphylaxis risk.

Skin prick tests
- This involves placing a droplet of allergen containing solution on the skin, then using a small lancet to prick the epidermis.
- After 15min, the skin is inspected for the presence of a wheal, and the average diameter of the wheal calculated.
- A +ve (histamine) and –ve (saline) control are used.
- The test is painless and can be performed from infancy onwards.
- PPVs of 95% for SPT are given (see ➋ Allergy testing in food allergy, pp. 518–20).
- Oral antihistamines must be stopped 3 days before testing.
- Contraindications include dermatographism and moderate to severe skin disease.
- Testing should only be performed by trained personnel, in facilities equipped to manage a possible anaphylactic reaction (very rare).
- Prick-to-prick testing (pressing the lancet into the food prior to pricking) can be used if an allergen solution is not available.

A large wheal makes an allergy more likely but does not correlate with the severity of the allergic response. It therefore cannot be used as a predictor of anaphylaxis risk.

Food allergy

(See also ⦿ Adverse reactions to food, p. 284–6.) Food allergy in childhood is common, affecting 6–8% of children aged <3y. The commonest food allergies in early childhood are milk and egg. One to 3% of young children have cow's milk allergy. In later childhood, allergies to peanuts and tree nuts predominate. Other common allergens are fish, shellfish, wheat, and soy.

Food allergy versus food intolerance

Food intolerance is a non-immunologically mediated adverse reaction to food. It includes:
- Enzyme deficiencies, e.g. lactase deficiency.
- Pharmacological, e.g. tachycardias in heavy tea/coffee drinkers due to caffeine.
- Sensitivity to vasoactive amines in food, causing localized reactions such as lip swelling, e.g. cured meats, cheeses, fish, ripe bananas, oranges, tomatoes, strawberries.
- Toxin-mediated, e.g. scrombroid poisoning (histamine from spoilt fish), food poisoning.
- Chemical effects (gustatory rhinitis with hot/spicy foods).
- Irritant reactions.
- Infectious syndromes, e.g. food poisoning or acute urticaria with viral illness.

Taking a food allergy history

Careful history taking is important in a diagnosis of allergic disease, because it helps to differentiate allergic from non-allergic reactions, to identify potential triggers, and to direct investigations.
- Presenting symptoms: focus on gut, skin, and respiratory systems to differentiate IgE from non-IgE-mediated reactions (see Table 13.1).
- Timing of the reaction from ingestion.
- Previous exposure to the allergen and severity of reactions.
- Detailed feeding history, including breastfed/bottle-fed; weaning; foods avoided and why.
- Exposure to other common allergens (see Table 13.2): if they are being consuming regularly, there is no need to test for those allergens.
- Whether the reaction was preceded by exercise, viral illness, or alcohol consumption (as these can lower the threshold for reaction).
- History of other atopic diseases, including infantile eczema, asthma, and allergic rhinitis.
- Family history of atopy.

Table 13.1 IgE- and non-IgE-mediated symptoms in food allergy

	IgE-mediated	Non-IgE-mediated
Onset	Acute	Slower, chronic changes
Skin	Urticaria, angio-oedema (facial), pruritus, erythema	Erythema, pruritus, urticaria
GI	Oral pruritus, vomiting, diarrhoea, colicky abdominal pain	Stools: loose, frequent, or offensive; constipation; blood or mucus in stool Other: GOR, food aversion
Respiratory	Upper airway: nasal itching, rhinorrhoea, hoarseness of voice Lower airway: wheeze, SOB	

Table 13.2 Common food allergens

Common allergen	Additional exposure
Cow's milk	Infant formula, breast milk (if mother consumes dairy), cheese, yoghurt. Baked milk in cakes, biscuits, etc.
Egg	Scrambled, omelette, quiche, meringue. Baked egg (cakes, biscuits, muffins, egg pasta, etc.)
Peanuts	Peanut butter, peanut-containing snacks
Tree nuts (e.g. hazelnut, cashew, almond, walnut, etc.)	Nut butters, nut-containing snacks, chocolate spreads (can contain hazelnuts), pesto (pine nuts)
Wheat	Bread, pasta, certain cereals
Soya	Soya milk, tofu, soya beans
Sesame	Sesame on burger buns and bread, tahini paste, hummus
Other legumes (beans, lentils, chickpeas, peas)	Hummus (chickpeas), dhal (lentils), chapattis (chickpea)

Allergy testing in food allergy

IgE levels to a specific food allergen are influenced by three key factors which must be borne in mind when interpreting the results and using them to estimate if true allergy exists or not:

• Age of the child.
• Length of time since last exposure.
• Type of allergen.

Common examples of the effects of type of allergen and age are shown in Table 13.3, as well as the cut-off values that determine a 95% +ve prediction of true allergy existing.

Table 13.3 95% PPV for serum specific IgEs and SPTs

	Specific IgE level (IU/mL)	Wheal size on SPT (mm)
Egg	≥7	7
Egg (<2y)	≥2	5
Milk	≥15	8
Milk (<2y)	≥5	6
Peanuts	≥15	8
Tree nuts	≥15	8
Fish	≥20	n/a

Other investigations

The use of multiplex allergen testing (e.g. ImmunoCAP ISAC 112) is not re-commended in routine practice outside a specialist allergy clinic. Component testing is useful for stratification of risk of anaphylaxis and/or confirmation of oral allergy syndrome by experts (see ⊃ Component–resolved diagnosis, p. 528). Newer testing techniques, such as the basophil activation test, are limited to research laboratories.

Complementary and alternative medicine allergy tests, including kinesiology, serum specific IgG and Vega tests, are ineffective and have no place in the diagnosis or management of food allergy.

Diagnosis of non-IgE-mediated food allergy

There is no single diagnostic test for non-IgE-mediated food allergy:

• Use a 4wk *exclusion period* and assess symptom resolution.
• Then *re-introduce* any of the suspected allergens into the diet, even if improvement in symptoms is seen.
• Allergy is then confirmed and diagnosed if symptoms recur.

Food allergy: initial management

Key to initial management is *dietary exclusion* of the allergenic food (see also Box 13.1). Practical, individualized advice should be provided on allergen avoidance and dietary alternatives:

- Levels of exclusion depend on the child; some children may tolerate trace amounts or a cooked form (e.g. baked egg or milk).
- Parents, carers, and children should be educated on allergen avoidance, allergy recognition, and treatment. A *written personal management plan* should be provided (see ➔ Management at discharge, p. 525).
- Children with multiple food allergies or young children with cow's milk allergy should have dietetic input to avoid nutritional deficiencies.
- Monitor growth as children with multiple food allergies are at risk of nutritional deficiencies.
- Ensure antihistamines are prescribed and assess the need for an adrenaline autoinjector (see ➔ Adrenaline autoinjector, p. 525).

Box 13.1 'May contain' food labels

Indicate that although the food has not been deliberately included, the manufacturer cannot guarantee the food is completely allergen-free. Some families opt to avoid these foods completely, which is the safest approach but can be very restrictive. Simple rules to help risk-assess these food labels are:

- Check the product every time as ingredients can change.
- Particularly avoid 'may contain' products when unwell (illness lowers the threshold for anaphylactic reactions).
- Only consume these foods when able to easily access help.
- Only consume these foods when rescue medication is available.
- Do not consume these foods if a previous severe (anaphylactic) reaction has occurred to the index food.
- Do not consume if suffering from uncontrolled asthma.

Long-term follow-up

Milk, egg, wheat, and soy allergies are most likely to be outgrown. Eighty per cent of milk and 60% of egg allergies will resolve by age 5y, so yearly follow-up is appropriate. For peanuts and tree nuts, resolution rates are lower (20% by age 5y), so follow-up every 2–3y is sufficient. Follow-up should be focused around key transition points, e.g. school changes, teenage years.

- At follow-up, review if any accidental exposure has occurred and any reaction confirming ongoing allergy.
- Review the need for medications and retrain in adrenaline autoinjector use if needed.
- Assess and optimize management of associated conditions, e.g. eczema and asthma.
- Egg allergy and immunization (see Box 13.2).

Allergy resolution

- For non-IgE-mediated allergy, re-introduction can occur at home, using a staged plan (e.g. see Fig. 13.1 and link to milk ladder in → Further reading, p. 538).
- For IgE-mediated allergy where resolution is suspected (no history of reactions and significant reduction in specifc IgE/SPT), a hospital-based oral food challenge should usually be undertaken as the risk of anaphylaxis is higher.

Oral food challenges

The gold standard for allergy diagnosis is a double-blind, placebo-controlled challenge. They can also be used to assess if resolution of an allergy has occurred. They are, however, time- and resource-intense and open food challenges are routinely used in practice.

- Open food challenges involve graded exposure to increasing amount of the allergenic food over a few hours.
- Graded exposure minimizes the risk of a severe reaction and allows determination of the threshold dose of reactivity.
- Children should be well prior to the challenge, and these should be conducted in departments able to deal with anaphylactic reactions.

Box 13.2 Egg allergy and immunization

- All egg-allergic children can be immunized with MMR (measles, mumps, and rubella) vaccine in primary care.
- Seasonal influenza vaccine is safe for egg-allergic children, except those with anaphylaxis to egg which required intensive care. It can be administered in primary care or schools.
- Children with severe anaphylaxis to egg should be referred to hospital for vaccination with an inactivated vaccine with very low ovalbumin content.
- Yellow fever vaccine is indicated in all, except if there is a history of anaphylaxis to egg.

Cow's milk protein allergy

(See also → Cow's milk protein allergy, p. 286.) Two to 3% of infants will suffer from an allergy to cow's milk. Non-IgE-mediated allergy is commoner than IgE-mediated.

Symptoms suggesting non-IgE-mediated allergy

- Early onset (<6mth): persistent eczema poorly responsive to treatment.
- GI symptoms, including: colic, GORD, vomiting, loose stools, constipation, and stool blood/mucus in an otherwise well infant.
- Non-specific rashes and pruritus.
- Failure to gain weight in severe cases.

Management

- Exclusion of all dairy from diet (i.e. cow, goat, sheep milk).
- If exclusively breastfed, mother needs to be dairy-free (and to ingest daily vitamin D and Ca²⁺ supplement).
- For formula-fed infants, trial of an extensively hydrolysed formula (e.g. Nutramigen®, Pepti®).
- If symptoms persist, then consider trial of an amino acid formula (e.g. Neocate®).
- After 2–4wk of dairy exclusion, assess for symptom improvement and challenge with re-exposure to cow's milk.
- Recurrence of symptoms then confirms the diagnosis.
- Child to remain dairy-free until 9–12mth of age and for at least 6mth.
- Dietician support is required for weaning.

Resolution

In a well child with no history suggestive of IgE-mediated allergy, a planned home re-introduction under dietetic or medical supervision can be performed. The most commonly used is the iMAP milk ladder (see Fig. 13.1), a six-step ladder which gradually introduces baked milk, then cheese, yoghurt, and finally milk back into the diet.

There is an increasing body of scientific evidence that early introduction and regular consumption of high-risk allergens reduce the risk of developing (or recurrence if previous allergy) allergy in the future.

THE iMAP MILK LADDER

To be used only in children with Mild to Moderate Non-IgE Cow's Milk Allergy
Under the supervision of a healthcare professional
PLEASE SEE THE ACCOMPANYING RECIPE INFORMATION

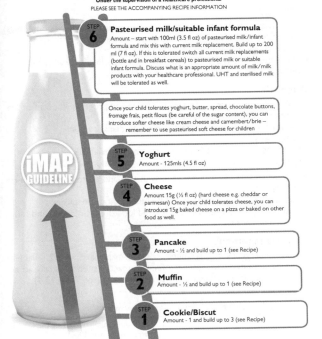

STEP 6 — Pasteurised milk/suitable infant formula
Amount – start with 100ml (3.5 fl oz) of pasteurised milk/infant formula and mix this with current milk replacement. Build up to 200 ml (7 fl oz). If this is tolerated switch all current milk replacements (bottle and in breakfast cereals) to pasteurised milk or suitable infant formula. Discuss what is an appropriate amount of milk/milk products with your healthcare professional. UHT and sterilised milk will be tolerated as well.

Once your child tolerates yoghurt, butter, spread, chocolate buttons, fromage frais, petit filous (be careful of the sugar content), you can introduce softer cheese like cream cheese and camembert/brie – remember to use pasteurised soft cheese for children

STEP 5 — Yoghurt
Amount - 125mls (4.5 fl oz)

STEP 4 — Cheese
Amount 15g (½ fl oz) (hard cheese e.g. cheddar or parmesan) Once your child tolerates cheese, you can introduce 15g baked cheese on a pizza or baked on other food as well.

STEP 3 — Pancake
Amount - ½ and build up to 1 (see Recipe)

STEP 2 — Muffin
Amount - ½ and build up to 1 (see Recipe)

STEP 1 — Cookie/Biscuit
Amount - 1 and build up to 3 (see Recipe)

Fig. 13.1 iMAP milk ladder for home re-introduction of milk.

Reproduced under Creative Commons Attribution 4.0 International License from Venter C, Brown T, Meyer R et al. Better recognition, diagnosis and management of non-IgE-mediated cow's milk allergy in infancy: iMAP—an international interpretation of the MAP (Milk Allergy in Primary Care) guideline. *Clin Transl Allergy* 7, 26 (2017). https://doi.org/10.1186/s13601-017-0162-y.

Anaphylaxis

Anaphylaxis is a severe life-threatening systemic hypersensitivity reaction of rapid onset. (See also ⊃ Anaphylaxis, p. 52.)

Aetiology

- Anaphylaxis can be IgE-mediated (e.g. secondary to food, venom, drugs) or non-IgE-mediated (e.g. idiopathic, exercise-induced, or related to temperature changes).
- In children, food is the commonest trigger: milk in infancy and nuts (e.g. peanuts, brazil, and cashew nuts) in school-age.

Diagnosis

Anaphylaxis has occurred if there is sudden and progressive onset of life-threatening symptoms, including:
- Airway problems (pharyngeal/laryngeal oedema, stridor, hoarseness), *OR*
- Breathing problems (tachypnoea, wheeze, hypoxia), *OR*
- Cardiovascular problems (tachycardia, hypotension, ↓ GCS score).

These are usually (80%) associated with skin and mucosal changes (urticaria/angio-oedema):
- Skin and mucosal changes alone DO NOT indicate anaphylaxis.
- Mast cell tryptase levels will be elevated for 12h post-reaction and can help aid diagnosis.

Early management

(For full emergency management, see ⊃ Anaphylaxis, p. 52.) Patients should be admitted and observed for late reactions; 8h is usually an adequate period. IM adrenaline is key to management (see Table 13.4).

Table 13.4 Adrenaline autoinjector doses by age/weight

Patient age and weight	Dose and volume using 1mg/mL adrenaline (= 1 in 1000)
Age >12y and bodyweight >30kg	0.5mg (= 0.5mL)
Age 6–12y and bodyweight >30kg	0.3mg (= 0.3mL)
Age <6y or bodyweight <30kg	0.15mg (= 0.15mL)

Management at discharge

All children with suspected anaphylaxis at initial discharge should:
- Be prescribed antihistamines and adrenaline autoinjectors (see Tables 13.4 and 13.5). Two autoinjectors are recommended, one for home and one for school.
- Receive appropriate training (with their family) in how to use these devices.
- Have a written allergy action plan (see Fig. 13.2).
- Receive allergen avoidance advice, and
- Every child with suspected anaphylaxis should be referred to an allergy clinic.

Adrenaline autoinjectors

Adrenaline autoinjectors should be prescribed for all those at higher risk of anaphylaxis (see Table 13.5). These include:
- History of previous anaphylactic reaction.
- Previous allergic reaction to trace amounts of allergens.
- Reactions to hard-to-avoid allergens, including venom and certain foods (e.g. nuts, cow's milk, soya milk).
- Idiopathic anaphylaxis.
- Teenagers (greater risk-taking behaviour).
- Comorbidities, especially asthma.
- Patients living in remote locations.

Table 13.5 Comparison of available autoinjectors

Device	Mechanism	Dose (mg)	Needle length (mm)	Needle (G)	Cost (£)	Shelf-life (mth)
EpiPen®	Cartridge	0.30	15	21	26.45	18
EpiPen® Junior	Cartridge	0.15	13	21		18
Jext® (300)	Cartridge	0.30	15	21	23.99	18
Jext® 150	Cartridge	0.15	13	21	23.99	18
Emerade®	Pre-filled syringe	0.50	25	23	26.99	30
Emerade®	Pre-filled syringe	0.30	25	23	25.99	30
Emerade®	Pre-filled syringe	0.15	16	23	25.99	30

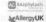

bsaci improving allergy care www.bsaci.org   **RCPCH** Royal College of Paediatrics and Child Health

Allergy Action Plan

AnaphylaxisCampaign   AllergyUK

THIS CHILD HAS THE FOLLOWING ALLERGIES:

Name:

DOB:

Photo

Emergency contact details:

1)
☎

2)
☎

Child's Weight: Kg

PARENTAL CONSENT: I hereby authorise school staff to administer the medicines listed on this plan, including a 'spare' back-up adrenaline autoinjector (AAI) if available, in accordance with Department of Health Guidance on the use of AAIs in schools.

Signed: _____

(PRINT NAME)

Date: _____

Mild-moderate allergic reaction:
- Swollen lips, face or eyes
- Itchy / tingling mouth
- Hives or itchy skin rash
- Abdominal pain or vomiting
- Sudden change in behaviour

ACTION:
- Stay with the child, call for help if necessary
- Locate adrenaline autoinjector(s)
- Give antihistamine:
- Phone parent/emergency contact   (if vomited, can repeat dose)

Watch for signs of ANAPHYLAXIS
(life-threatening allergic reaction)
Anaphylaxis may occur without skin symptoms: **ALWAYS consider anaphylaxis in someone with known food allergy who has SUDDEN BREATHING DIFFICULTY**

AIRWAY:	Persistent cough, hoarse voice difficulty swallowing, swollen tongue
BREATHING:	Difficult or noisy breathing, wheeze or persistent cough
CONSCIOUSNESS:	Persistent dizziness / pale or floppy suddenly sleepy, collapse, unconscious

If ANY ONE (or more) of these signs are present:
1. **Lie child flat:**
   (If breathing is difficult, allow child to sit)
2. **Use Adrenaline autoinjector** (eg. Epipen) **without delay**
3. **Dial 999** for ambulance and say ANAPHYLAXIS ("ANA-FIL-AX-IS")

*** IF IN DOUBT, GIVE ADRENALINE ***

After giving Adrenaline:
1. Stay with child until ambulance arrives, do **NOT** stand child up
2. Commence CPR if there are no signs of life
3. Phone parent/emergency contact
4. If no improvement after 5 minutes, give a 2nd adrenaline dose using a second autoinjector device, if available.

You can dial 999 from any phone, even if there is no credit left on a mobile. Medical observation in hospital is recommended after anaphylaxis.

How to give EpiPen®

1
Form fist around EpiPen® and PULL OFF BLUE SAFETY CAP

2
SWING AND PUSH ORANGE TIP against outer thigh (with or without clothing) until a click is heard

3
HOLD FIRMLY in place for 10 seconds

4
REMOVE EpiPen®. Massage injection site for 10 seconds

©The British Society for Allergy & Clinical Immunology, 09/2017

Additional instructions:

This is a medical document that can only be completed by the child's healthcare professional. It must not be altered without their permission. This document provides medical authorisation for schools to administer a 'spare' back-up adrenaline autoinjector if needed, as permitted by the Human Medicines (Amendment) Regulations 2017.

This plan has been prepared by:

SIGN & PRINT NAME: _____

Hospital/Clinic: _____

☎ _____   Date: _____

Fig. 13.2 Example allergy action plan.
Reproduced from 🔗 www.bsaci.com

Oral allergy syndrome (OAS)

Oral allergy syndrome (OAS)

OAS is due to allergen cross-reactivity in people with pollen allergy. An antibody to a specific pollen allergen (e.g. the birch pollen allergen *Bet v1*) reacts to a structurally similar food allergen. Some 76% of people with pollen allergy have OAS to at least one food. The commonest cross-reactions are shown in Table 13.6.

Table 13.6 Pollen/food cross-reactivity

Pollen/plant	Cross-reactivity with fruits/vegetables
Birch	Apple, cherry, apricot, carrot, potato, kiwi, pear, hazelnut, celery, peanut, soybean
Ragweed	Melon, banana
Grass	Kiwi, tomato, watermelon, potato
Mugwort	Celery, fennel, carrot, parsley
Latex	Banana, avocado, chestnut, kiwi, fig, apple, cherry

Symptoms of OAS

- Symptoms tend to be confined to the lips, mouth, and throat (e.g. perioral rash, oral pruritus and tingling, mild swelling).
- Systemic reactions are rare.
- The cross-reactive allergens are heat-labile, so reactions tend to occur only to raw fruit and vegetables.

Diagnosis of OAS

- sIgEs to pollen allergens can be tested, and prick-to-prick SPT with the suspected fresh fruits/vegetables can be performed (SPT using allergen solutions can lead to false −ves as fruit allergens lose their potency).
- A history of typical reactions must also be present.

Component-resolved diagnosis

This promising new diagnostic tool identifies the presence of sIgEs to much more specific proteins within an allergen, rather than the whole allergen, including those that cross-react between pollens and fruit or nuts.

- In the example of OAS due to birch tree allergic rhinitis, symptoms of oral itch and lip swelling on ingestion of peanuts may be confused with systemic peanut allergy with a risk of anaphylaxis.
- On component testing, detection of the presence of sIgE to the peanut protein *Ara h2* is strongly associated with systemic allergy (and therefore a risk of anaphylaxis). In contrast, +ve IgE to the *Ara h8* component is instead commonly seen with OAS and a lower risk of anaphylaxis.
- Differentiating between the various target allergens can therefore help clarify diagnosis and management (see Table 13.7).

Table 13.7 Common food allergen components

	Cross-reactive component (LTP/PR-10 family)	Storage protein
Peanut	Ara h8; Ara h9	Ara H2
Hazelnut	Cor a1; Cor a8	Cor a9; Cor a14
Kiwi	Act d8	Act d13

Presence of sIgE to cross-reactive plant components tends to be associated with milder symptoms/OAS; presence of sIgE to storage proteins is associated with more significant reactions.

Management of OAS

- For children with mild to moderate symptoms, cooking raw fruit and vegetables will be sufficient to denature the proteins and avoid a reaction.
- Children with a more severe syndrome should avoid the allergenic foods and be prescribed an adrenaline autoinjector.

Food protein-induced enterocolitis syndrome (FPIES)

FPIES is a rare non-IgE-mediated food allergy occurring classically in infants and young children.

- Acute FPIES occurs a couple of hours post-food ingestion and is characterized by repeated vomiting, lethargy, pallor, and hypothermia.
- 15% are at risk of hypovolaemic shock.
- Sepsis is a possible differential, and it is not uncommon for these children to be treated repeatedly for sepsis before diagnosis.
- Acute management is focused on aggressive fluid rehydration.
- Common allergens are cow's milk, wheat, rice, and soybean.
- Chronic FPIES is rare and presents with repeated vomiting, loose stool, FTT, iron deficiency anaemia, and hypoalbuminaemia.
- A trial elimination diet results in improvement of symptoms, as no diagnostic tests are available.
- Oral food challenges can be performed to either confirm the diagnosis or assess for FPIES resolution.
- Oral food challenges are high risk and must be physician-supervised and IV fluids must be readily available.

Eczema

(See ➜ Atopic eczema, pp. 782–5.)

Eczema is often the first atopic disease to present in childhood and a miserable condition for children to suffer with. Parents will often request allergy testing in a bid to eliminate any triggers. There is a strong link with respiratory and food allergy. Children with eczema have a 70% chance of developing asthma or allergic rhinitis later in life. Combine eczema with food allergy and the risk increases even further.

It is important to note that in most cases of eczema, food allergy does not play a role and routine IgE testing is not indicated. However, an underlying food allergy should be suspected in infants with early-onset (<6mth) severe eczema that is poorly responsive to treatment.

- 30–50% of these infants may have an associated food allergy, milk and egg being the most likely allergens.
- Allergy testing can be carried out, although SPTs are difficult to interpret if eczema is severe and false +ves can occur.
- An exclusion diet is required to diagnose a non-IgE-mediated food allergy (see ➜ Management of suspected food allergy or intolerance, pp. 285–6).

Drug allergy

Drug allergy is an immune-mediated hypersensitivity reaction to a medicinal product. In children, prevalence of a self-reported drug allergy is between 3% and 7%. Up to 95% of children with a plausible history of drug allergy are, in fact, able to tolerate the drug on re-challenge. Drug allergies should be investigated as they can lead to lifetime use of less effective and more costly treatments:

- Children with chronic conditions requiring regular antibiotics, e.g. CF, are at higher risk of sensitization and allergy.
- Atopy is not a risk factor for a drug allergy per se but may lead to more severe reactions.
- Cutaneous reaction is the most commonly reported sign, but often due to the underlying illness, rather than the drug administered.
- β-lactam compounds and NSAIDs are the most encountered drug allergies, with penicillin accounting for 75% of fatal drug-induced anaphylaxis cases.

Diagnosis

Detailed history taking is key to focusing on drug formulation, route and dose, time course and pattern of reaction, and history of relevant previous exposure:

- If an anaphylactic-type reaction is witnessed, a serum tryptase sample should be taken 1–2h after onset of reaction.
- SPT can be performed if IgE-mediated allergy is suspected using the specific drug implicated. SPT may be falsely −ve in up to 30% of penicillin allergies.
- sIgE is available for certain drugs (e.g. penicillins). It is useful if +ve, but results are usually −ve and hard to interpret.
- Intradermal or patch testing can confirm a delayed/T-cell-mediated reaction, e.g. drug reaction with eosinophilia and systemic symptoms (DRESS) or SJS, but are difficult to perform in children.
- Drug provocation testing can be performed, but only by experienced personnel in adequate facilities. Intradermal inoculation at tiny doses (e.g. 1/1000 dose) can be used if an IV drug allergy is suspected. It can exclude drug sensitivity or confirm a diagnosis. For possible delayed reactions, a prolonged course of the drug should be given for several days following an in-hospital challenge.

Management

- Manage the immediate reaction by stopping the culprit drug and administering any required treatment.
- Provide written information to the patient and all health care providers regarding which drug to avoid.
- Ensure drug allergy is highlighted in hospital and GP notes.
- Engraved allergy-bracelets can be used.
- Adrenaline autoinjectors are not routinely prescribed if the causative drug has been identified and is easily avoided.

Venom allergy

Allergy to *bee* and *wasp* venom is a common cause of anaphylaxis and may result in death. In general, children have less severe reactions than adults.

- All children with a systemic reaction to venom should be referred to an allergy specialist.
- Large local reactions are common and do not indicate venom allergy, but rather the local histamine response to venom inoculation.
- Family members of bee-keepers have sensitization rates of 30–60% to bee venom.
- Venom allergy is not commoner in atopic individuals.
- In suspected cases, sIgE to both venoms should be tested. If a double +ve result is obtained, SPT can help clarify the responsible species.
- Baseline tryptase levels should be checked, as higher levels are associated with more severe reactions.

Management

- Insect avoidance measures (wear light-coloured clothing; ensure skin is covered when outside; avoid strong perfumes; don't leave food uncovered outside, and exercise caution in outdoor areas).
- Children with a history of systemic reactions or elevated basal tryptase should have a written allergy management plan and be prescribed adrenaline autoinjectors.
- Children with a history of severe systemic reactions should be referred to a specialist allergy service for venom immunotherapy.

Asthma

Asthma diagnosis and management are covered in detail in ➲ Asthma, pp. 232–3. Asthma affects 15% of children, and there is frequently a strong atopic component. Avoidance of aeroallergens is important, as is adequately treating any allergic rhinitis.

Allergy testing for aeroallergens is therefore indicated in severe or hard-to-control asthma. The commonest allergens in childhood are house dust mite and tree and grass pollens. Less common are cat, dog, horse, and moulds (e.g. *Alternaria* species).

Allergic rhinitis

(See also → Allergic rhinitis, p. 250.) Allergic rhinitis (AR), or rhinoconjunctivits, is the commonest allergic disease in older children, affecting 15% of young teenagers.

- Poorly controlled AR is associated with a significant −ve impact on quality of life, school attendance and performance, and sleep disturbance.
- AR is a risk factor for asthma development.
- AR and asthma often coexist, with up to 75% of older asthmatics reporting rhinitis symptoms.
- AR impairs asthma control, and therefore, management of AR should be optimized in asthmatics.

Symptoms

- *Nasal:* rhinorrhoea (clear or yellow), nasal congestion and obstruction, itching, sneezing, nasal voice, snoring.
- *Ocular:* itching, lacrimation, redness, lid oedema.
- *Lower respiratory tract:* cough, wheeze, SOB.

Diagnosis: taking an aeroallergen history

History should focus on elucidating symptoms and their impact on life, atopic family history, and the presence of other atopic disorders. An aeroallergen history should focus on:

- *Seasonal variation:* perennial symptoms suggest house dust mite allergy; symptom onset in early spring suggests tree pollen allergy, and late spring/summer symptoms suggest grass pollen allergy.
- Presence of a furry pet (within the household, but also regular exposure elsewhere).
- Exposure to moulds (household/rural environments).
- Change in symptoms on exposure to new environments (e.g. on holiday).

Examination

- Presence of 'allergic salute' (i.e. with horizontal nasal crease), allergic shiners.
- Chronic mouth-breathing.
- Presence of nasal polyps.

Investigations

These are usually limited in nature, but SPT/sIgE testing may be appropriate to help determine the responsible allergen.

Management

Allergen avoidance

- *House dust mite:* encasing bedding in hypoallergenic covers; removing carpet, soft furnishings, and soft toys from the bedroom; humidity reduction in the bedroom; regular hovering.
- *Pollen:* minimize outdoor activity when high pollen counts—early morning and early evening; keeping windows closed; showering after exposure; wearing sunglasses; applying nasal balms.
- *Pets:* removal of the pet or minimize contact.
- Nasal saline irrigation is of benefit, if tolerated.

Pharmacotherapy

- Intranasal steroids and intranasal antihistamines are recommended first-line treatment. Fluticasone and mometasone are preferred because of minimal systemic bioavailability.
- Administration technique should be reviewed.
- Regular use of second-generation non-sedating antihistamines, e.g. cetirizine or fexofenadine (least sedating).
- Commencing treatment 2wk before a known allergen season improves treatment efficacy.
- For severe nasal congestion, short-term use of nasal decongestant, alongside intranasal steroids, can improve drug penetration.
- Leukotriene receptor antagonists can be used as add-on therapy.
- Topical treatment with antihistamines or chromones is indicated for conjunctival disease.
- For severe cases, allergen immunotherapy can be considered.

Acute urticaria

(See also ➲ Chronic urticaria, p. 790; ➲ Angioedema, p. 791.) *Acute urticaria* is common, affecting up to 5–15% of children at some stage. It is caused by mast cell histamine release and characterized by itchy wheals. It can occur together with angio-oedema, which is non-histamine-mediated deep tissue swelling that is not itchy.

Causes

- *Allergic:* ingested or injected allergens, e.g. food, drugs.
- *Infections:* commonly viral infections, EBV, hepatitis B, Lyme disease, cat-scratch disease, parasitic infections.
- *Contact urticaria:* e.g. from plants or insect bites.
- *Physical:* sunlight, pressure (dermatographism), aquagenic, heat, cold—familial or acquired (e.g. *Mycoplasma*).
- *Autoimmune and vasculitic conditions:* e.g. coeliac disease, HSP.

Diagnosis

- Detailed history, focusing on triggering events and family history.
- Assess for dermatographism (e.g. gently scratch the volar aspect of the forearm and look for a matching wheal after a few minutes).
- Physical provocation tests can be performed in clinic (e.g. with ice).

Management

- Avoidance of triggers (especially for physical urticaria). (See also ➲ Chronic urticaria, p. 790.)

Mastocytosis

Includes a range of disorders characterized by accumulation of mast cells:
- *Cutaneous mastocytosis:* urticaria pigmentosa—itchy brown macules, with urticaria developing on scratching these (Darier's sign).
- *Systemic mastocytosis:* involves the gut, bone, and bone marrow and can present with abdominal symptoms, flushing, palpitation, headaches, SOB, and malaise. Differential diagnosis includes phaeochromocytoma and carcinoid.
- Can be associated with *haematological disorders:* leukaemia, lymphoma, myelodysplasia.

Diagnosis
- Mast cell tryptase.
- Skin/bowel/bone marrow biopsy.
- Exclusion of differentials.
- Assessment for underlying haematological malignancy.

Treatment
- High-dose antihistamines.
- Leukotriene antagonists.
- Sodium cromoglicate.
- Beware use of drugs which activate mast cells (e.g. opiates).

Hereditary angio-oedema

(See also ➔ Angioedema, p. 791.) Due to mostly hereditary C1-esterase inhibitor deficiency:
- AD, so family history may be present.
- Attacks begin in later childhood and can be precipitated by trauma, infections, hormonal changes, and emotional stress. It does not cause urticaria.
- Typically, C4 and C2 levels are low between attacks and undetectable during an attack; C1-inhibitor levels can also be low.
- Treat major attacks with purified/recombinant inhibitor and supportive care as needed. Prophylaxis can be with modified androgens (e.g. danazol) or anti-fibrinolytics (tranexamic acid).

Further reading

Milk ladder

Allergy UK. (2016). *The iMAP milk ladder* (milk ladder for staged re-introduction of cow's milk protein to diet). Available at: ℅ https://www.allergyuk.org/assets/000/001/297/iMAP_Final_Ladder-May_2017_original.pdf?1502804928.

Specific IgE

Stiefel G, Roberts G. How to use serum-specific IgE measurements in diagnosing and monitoring food allergy. *Arch Dis Child Educ Pract Ed* 2012; **97**: 29–36.

Guidelines and websites

Allergy UK. Available at: ℅ https://www.allergyuk.org.

Anaphylaxis Campaign. Available at: ℅ https://www.anaphylaxis.org.uk.

British Society for Allergy and Clinical Immunology. Multiple guidelines and further information. Available at: ℅ http://www.bsaci.org/Guidelines/bsaci-guidelines-and-SOCC.

Public Health England. (2013). *Immunisations against infectious disease* (for guidance on vaccination in egg-allergic children). Available at: ℅ https://www.gov.uk/government/collections/immunisation-against-infectious-disease-the-green-book#the-green-book.

ThermoFisher Scientific. *Allergy and autoimmune disease.* Available at: ℅ https://allergyai.com/uk/allergy/.

Chapter 14

Haematology

Peripheral blood film

(See Table 14.1.)

Table 14.1 FBC and blood film abnormalities and their causes

Abnormality	Cause(s)
Acanthocytes	Abetalipoproteinaemia, severe liver disease, vitamin E deficiency in premature neonates, hereditary acanthocytosis
Basophilia	Myeloproliferative disorders, CML, basophilic leukaemia, reactive disorders, e.g. UC, infection
Basophilic stippling	Ineffective erythropoiesis; haemoglobinopathies, recovering bone marrow, lead poisoning
Echinocytes (burr cells)	Renal failure, PK deficiency, liver disease, HUS, burns
Elliptocytes	Hereditary elliptocytosis (see → Hereditary elliptocytosis, p. 548)
Eosinophilia	Parasitic infections, allergic states, e.g. asthma, eczema, drugs, polyarteritis
Fragmented RBCs	Microangiopathic and mechanical haemolytic anaemias, DIC (see → Red blood cell fragmentation, pp. 555), HUS (see → Haemolytic uraemic syndrome, pp. 354–5), renal failure
Heinz bodies (intracellular Hb precipitate)	G6PD deficiency (see → Glucose-6-phosphate dehydrogenase deficiency, p. 549), haemoglobinopathies, post-splenectomy, hyposplenism, Heinz body haemolysis
Howell–Jolly bodies (intracellular DNA fragments)	Normal neonatal blood picture, hyposplenia, post-splenectomy, megaloblastic anaemia
Leucocytosis	Leukaemia (see → Acute lymphoblastic leukaemia, pp. 590–1)
Lymphocytopenia (lymphopenia)	Viral infection, malignancy, stress, vomiting, burns, anorexia, drugs, SLE, CD, immunodeficiency states [severe combined immunodeficiency (SCID), di George syndrome, acquired, e.g. HIV], marrow failure, aplastic anaemia, leukaemia
Lymphocytosis	Viral and non-viral (pertussis, *Mycoplasma*, malaria) infection, leukaemia, atypical lymphocytosis (EBV, CMV, adenovirus), stress, exercise, SE
Macrocytic RBCs	Vitamin B₁₂ or folate deficiency (see → Macrocytic anaemia, p. 547), aplastic anaemia (see → Acquired aplastic anaemia, pp. 556–7), normal neonatal blood picture (see → Neonatal haematology, pp. 174–5)

Table 14.1 (Contd.)

Abnormality	Cause(s)
Microcytic RBCs	Iron deficiency (see ⊃ Iron deficiency anaemia, p. 546), thalassaemia (see ⊃ Thalassaemia, pp. 552–3), anaemia of chronic disease
Monocytopenia	Autoimmune disorders (e.g. SLE), drugs (e.g. corticosteroids), chemotherapy
Monocytosis	Chronic bacterial infection, malaria, typhoid, TB, infective endocarditis, post-chemotherapy
Neutropenia	(See ⊃ Acquired aplastic anaemia, pp. 556–7; ⊃ Immunodeficiency disorders, p. 646)
Neutrophilia	Infection, inflammation, chronic bleeding, post-splenectomy, drugs (e.g. corticosteroids)
Reticulocytosis/polychromatic RBCs	Haemolysis, bleeding, response to haematinics (e.g. iron), marrow infiltration
Sickle cells	Sickle-cell anaemia (see ⊃ Sickle cell disease, pp. 550–1)
Spherocytes	Normal neonatal blood picture, HS (see ⊃ Hereditary spherocytosis, p. 548), immune-mediated haemolytic disease, post-splenectomy
Target cells	Severe iron deficiency (see ⊃ Iron deficiency anaemia, p. 546), SCD, thalassaemia, liver disease, post-splenectomy, asplenia
Thrombocytopenia	(See ⊃ Thrombocytopenia, p. 576)
Thrombocytosis	(See ⊃ Thrombocytosis, p. 575)

Anaemia

- Hb at birth may be as high as 22g/dL.
- Falls rapidly to about 11g/dL by 3mth.
- A mild hypochromic microcytic picture normally seen between 6mth and 6y.
- Sex differences in red cell indices do not appear until puberty.

Symptoms and signs of anaemia

- Fatigue, lethargy, pallor.
- Poor feeding, anorexia, poor growth.
- Dyspnoea on exertion.
- Rarely stomatitis or koilonychia.

Diagnostic approach to anaemia

History

- Familial (sickle cell, thalassaemia).
- Diet (cow's milk, vegan).
- Overt blood loss.
- Duration of symptoms.
- Drug history, e.g. NSAIDs.

Examination

- Height and weight (FTT, malabsorption).
- Dysmorphic features, e.g. micrognathia, cleft palate, abnormal/absent thumbs (FA, Diamond–Blackfan anaemia).
- Jaundice (haemolysis).
- Lymphadenopathy/organomegaly (underlying malignancy).

FBC and film

(See Table 14.2.)

- *Red cell indices:* mean cell volume (MCV), mean cell Hb (MCH), mean corpuscular Hb concentration (MCHC) (anaemia may be microcytic, macrocytic, normocytic, and/or hypochromic).
- *RBCs:* spherocytes, sickle cells, Howell–Jolly bodies.
- *Other cytopenias.*

Table 14.2 Investigations for different anaemia types

Anaemia type	Investigate for
Microcytic anaemia	Iron deficiency, thalassaemias, sideroblastic anaemias, anaemia of chronic disease
Macrocytic anaemia	Bone marrow failure syndromes (reticulocytopenic anaemias; pure red cell aplasia, aplastic anaemia, Diamond–Blackfan anaemia), MDS, megaloblastic anaemia (B_{12}/folate deficiency), dyserythropoiesis, drugs
Normocytic anaemia	Haemolysis, sequestration, anaemia of chronic disease, recent significant bleeding, combined iron and B_{12}/folate deficiency, i.e. severe malnutrition
Haemolytic anaemia	Investigate as described in ⊃ Haemolytic anaemias, p. 544–5

Haemolytic anaemias

- Haemolysis causes reduction in the normal mean RBC survival of 120 days.
- Intrinsic (RBC membrane defects, enzyme defects, or haemoglobinopathies).
- Extrinsic (immune-mediated or mechanical RBC fragmentation).

Diagnosis

History

- *Symptoms:* e.g. headache, dizziness, fever, chills, dark urine, back or abdominal pain (intravascular haemolysis).
- *Possible precipitating factors:* e.g. infection, medications, foods such as fava beans in G6PD deficiency.
- *Ancestry:* e.g. African, Mediterranean, or Arabic ancestry is suggestive of G6PD deficiency in boys.
- *Family history:* e.g. gallstones in spherocytosis.

Examination

- Look particularly for temperature, pallor, jaundice, and splenomegaly.

Investigations

FBC and blood film

↑ reticulocyte count suggests ↑ RBC production in response to haemolysis or blood loss.

- *Platelet count:*
  - Thrombocytopenia with normal clotting suggests HUS and thrombotic thrombocytopenic purpura (TTP).
  - Thrombocytopenia with abnormal clotting suggests DIC.
  - Pancytopenia: consider viral infection, malignancy, hypersplenism.
- *Abnormal blood film:* e.g. spherocytes or RBC abnormalities, malaria parasites, features of RBC fragmentation (schistocytes, burr cells).

Specific tests

- Unconjugated bilirubin: raised level = ↑ RBC destruction.
- LDH: raised activity = ↑ RBC production.
- Free plasma Hb, haemoglobinuria, haemosiderin in urine: all ↑ in intravascular haemolysis.
- Coombs' antiglobulin test to establish if there is immune or non-immune haemolysis.
  - +ve DCT = antibodies on RBC surface.
  - +ve indirect Coombs' test = antibodies in serum.
  - If DCT +ve, screen serum for RBC isoimmune antibodies, e.g. neonatal Rh or ABO haemolytic disease (see ➲ Rh disease (rhesus haemolytic disease), p. 176).
  - If DCT +ve, IgG- and C3-specific reagents suggest warm and cold antibody autoimmune haemolysis, respectively.

- IgM for *Mycoplasma*, CMV, EBV, rubella, for cold antibody autoimmune haemolysis.
- Hb electrophoresis for sickle-cell anaemia, thalassaemias, unstable Hbs, e.g. Hb Koln.
- Flow cytometry for hereditary spherocytosis (HS).
- RBC enzyme assays for RBC enzyme defects, e.g. G6PD.
- If history suggestive, immunophenotyping (CD55 + CD59) for paroxysmal nocturnal haemoglobinuria (PNH).

Iron deficiency anaemia

Commonest nutritional deficiency. Occurs in 10–30% of high-risk patients:
• Preterm, LBW infants, multiple births.
• After exclusive breastfeeding >6mth, delayed introduction of iron-containing solids, excessive cow's milk (protein enteropathy).
• Adolescent ♀ (growth spurt and menstruation).
• Low iron-containing diet due to poverty, fad diets, or strict vegans.

Causes

• *Dietary*: commonest cause, e.g. prolonged, exclusive consumption of cow's/breast milk, with late introduction of iron-containing solids.
• *Infancy and early childhood*: low level of dietary iron, e.g. high milk intake (low iron); GI blood loss, e.g. cow's milk protein enteropathy.
• ↑ *demand in rapid growth*: e.g. after prematurity or puberty.
• *Malabsorption*: e.g. coeliac disease, IBD.
• *Rarely blood loss*: e.g. Meckel's diverticulum, oesophagitis. Bleeding may be occult into cysts; tumours or drugs, e.g. NSAIDs.
• *Intestinal parasites*: e.g. hookworm (in less developed world).

Presentation

Most cases are subclinical. Onset of symptoms of anaemia is usually insidious. Profoundly iron-deficient toddlers usually adapt to their anaemia and tolerate surprisingly low Hb, with pallor, lethargy, poor feeding, and breathlessness (only in severe anaemia).

Symptoms

Neurological effects of listlessness, irritability (infants), mood changes, reduced cognitive and psychomotor performance (can occur in mild/moderate deficiency before anaemia develops), and rarely pica (eating unusual items, e.g. soil, chewing on pencils).

Diagnosis

Iron deficiency anaemia is a sign, not a diagnosis—always look for the underlying cause (usually dietary or GI disease):
• *FBC*: Hb ↓; MCV, MCH, and MCHC ↓ (below normal range for age), platelets often raised.
• *Blood film*: microcytic, hypochromic anaemia.
• *Serum ferritin* ↓ *(indicative of iron stores)*: it may be low before anaemia. Check CRP, as ferritin may be falsely raised due to acute phase reaction (↓ *serum iron and* ↑ *TIBC confirms iron deficiency*).

Treatment

Elemental iron (see *British National Formulary for Children*). Use for 3mth after Hb normalizes to replete body stores. If indices do not improve once Hb is normal, screen for thalassaemia trait.

Prevention in high-risk groups

• Iron supplementation in preterm infants.
• Encourage iron-containing diet: e.g. iron-fortified formulas, breakfast cereals, meat, green vegetables, beans, egg yolk, foods rich in vitamin C (increases iron absorption).
• Avoid prolonged cow's milk consumption to the detriment of solids intake.

Macrocytic anaemia

Vitamin B_{12} deficiency

We get vitamin B_{12} (cobalamin) from animal products. Vegans or those on other diets lacking meat are most at risk. Alternatively, defective absorption due to intrinsic factor deficiency (congenital AR or juvenile autoimmune pernicious anaemia), defective B_{12} transport (transcobalamin II deficiency), diseases causing malabsorption (ileal resection, IBD, coeliac disease), or small bowel bacterial overgrowth.

Folate deficiency

A common nutritional deficiency worldwide. Causes include:
- *Malnutrition* (marasmus, kwashiorkor), goat's milk feeding.
- *Malabsorption:* e.g. coeliac disease, IBD, other small intestinal disease.
- ↑ *requirements:* e.g. rapid growth, chronic haemolytic anaemias (give daily folic acid prophylactically), hypermetabolic states (infection, hyperthyroidism), severe skin disease.
- *Drugs:* e.g. phenytoin, valproate, trimethoprim, nitrofurantoin.
- *Disorders of folate metabolism:* Lesch–Nyhan syndrome, orotic aciduria.

Presentation of folate or vitamin B_{12} deficiency

- Insidious onset of pallor, fatigue, anorexia, glossitis, developmental delay, and hypotonia.
- Severe cases, subacute combined degeneration of the cord (rare in children): paraesthesiae of hands/feet, ataxia, loss of vibration sense.

Diagnosis of macrocytic anaemias

- *Macrocytic anaemia:* Hb ↓, MCV ↑ (above normal range, i.e. >82, 1y; >90, 6–12y; or >125fL as a newborn).
- *WBC:* ↓, hypersegmented neutrophils, platelets ↓, bilirubin ↑.
- ↓ *serum B_{12} or ↓ folate level:* red cell folate level is more reliable than serum folate, which reflects recent intake.
- *Bone marrow:* if indicated, shows megaloblastic appearance. Rarely, intrinsic factor autoantibodies or test for B_{12} absorption.

Treatment

- Improve diet, depending on whether vitamin B_{12} or folic acid deficiency:
  - *B_{12} deficiency:* IM hydroxocobalamin—usually response is within 1wk. Watch K^+ level as it may fall. Treat three times/wk until Hb normal; then give 2- to 3-monthly if underlying problem persists (must know cause).
  - *Folate deficiency:* daily PO folic acid.
    - Look for underlying cause (usually GI).
    - Never treat with folic acid alone, unless serum B_{12} level is normal, as subacute combined degeneration of the cord can be precipitated.

RBC membrane defect anaemias

Hereditary spherocytosis

- AD in 75%. Incidence ~1/5000 (Northern European). Various RBC membrane skeletal defects occur; commonest involves ankyrin (~50–60%).
- Mild to moderate anaemia in compensated cases. Anaemia can be severe, with transfusion requirement.
- Splenomegaly is usually present.
- Infection exacerbates haemolysis, with worsening jaundice.
- Aplastic (red cell) crisis can occur with parvovirus B19 infection. Severity depends on degree of baseline haemolysis (worst in those with high reticulocyte counts due to sudden decompensation).
- Folate deficiency can occur with massively ↑ RBC turnover, so PO supplementation with 5mg/day folic acid.
- Laboratory investigations include: ↑ reticulocytes, very high spherocytes on blood film; red cell indices may be slightly low, but the clue is MCHC which is raised (i.e. hyperchromic due to spherical RBCs). DCT –ve (excludes autoimmune causes).
- Diagnosis can be made based on clinical and haematological indices, reticulocytes, and blood film. Diagnosis in difficult cases can be made by flow cytometry but is usually not clinically warranted.
- Provide supportive treatment, e.g. folic acid supplementation; blood transfusion if anaemia severe during aplastic crises.
- Ideally, if splenectomy is indicated, it is best performed after 5y of age, but before puberty. Consider if: anaemia is not compensated and child is not thriving physically, socially, or educationally or chronic haemolysis with gallstone formation; persistent jaundice is a rare indication for cosmetic reasons. Splenectomy requires preoperative vaccination against *Pneumococcus, Haemophilus influenzae* (HiB), and *Meningococcus* (MenC), as well as post-operative 5-yearly boosters, annual influenza vaccination, and lifelong phenoxymethylpenicillin prophylaxis.

Hereditary elliptocytosis (HE)

- Heterogenous group of disorders.
- Mainly AD inheritance.
- Incidence 1/25 000.
- Severity varies, from asymptomatic chronic compensated haemolysis (majority) to transfusion dependence.
- Presentation and management similar to HS.
- Blood film shows elliptical RBCs.

RBC enzyme defect anaemias

Glucose-6-phosphate dehydrogenase deficiency

G6PD deficiency is X-linked recessive—the disease occurs in heterozygous ♂ and homozygous ♀, with variable expression in heterozygous ♀. It is endemic in the Mediterranean, South East Asia, West Africa, and the Middle East. Over 400 enzyme variants. African (A–) (10–60% enzyme activity) and Mediterranean (3% activity) are the most clinically relevant.

- RBC G6PD levels fall rapidly as cells age, with impaired elimination of oxidants and reduced cell integrity.
- Intermittent acute haemolytic episodes (intravascular haemolysis) are associated with febrile infections (commonest), oxidant drugs (antimalarials, sulfonamides, dapsone, aspirin, phenacetin, ciprofloxacin), foods (fava beans), and chemicals (naphthalene).
- May present as neonatal jaundice or chronic haemolytic anaemia.

Laboratory investigations
- Normal during non-haemolytic state.
- During haemolysis, findings of RBC destruction [bite cells and Hb puddling (ghost cells)], ↑ RBC production (raised reticulocyte count), spherocytes and Heinz bodies on blood film, DCT –ve.
- *Definitive diagnosis:* reduced G6PD enzyme activity (may be falsely normal during acute haemolysis; repeat 6wk later).

Management
Avoid oxidant drugs and foods; maintain good urine output with fluids; transfuse if required; give folate supplements in chronic haemolysis or in patients recovering from acute episodes; treat hyperbilirubinaemia in newborns.

Pyruvate kinase (PK) deficiency

Rare congenital AR condition. Chronic haemolytic anaemia results from deficiency of PK. Enzyme deficiency leads to ↓ RBC adenosine triphosphate (ATP) generation and ↑ 2,3-diphosphoglycerate (DPG) production [shifts oxyhaemoglobin (HbO_2) dissociation curve to the right].

- Severity is variable. Neonatal jaundice is common. Patients can have persistent, severe hyperbilirubinaemia.
- Parvovirus B19 infection can cause aplastic crisis.

Laboratory findings
↑ RBC destruction and production, ↓ PK enzyme level. Blood film pre-splenectomy not very informative.

Management
- PO folate supplements.
- Blood transfusion if symptomatic anaemia.
- Support of aplastic crisis, e.g. blood transfusion.
- Splenectomy in severe cases.

Sickle-cell disease

- AR. Mutation in codon 6 of *β-globin* gene (chromosome 11) with single amino acid substitution (glutamine for valine).
- Most severe form homozygous sickle Hb HbSS; less severe disease in compound heterozygotes, e.g. HbSC, HbSD, HbSB0, or HbSB+ thalassaemia.
- The Caribbean, Africa, the Middle East, the Mediterranean, India: in Jamaica (10% carriers) HbSS 1/300 births; HbC carriers 3.5%. HbS heterozygous carriers have some resistance to malaria, and high gene prevalence in malarial regions. In UK, SCD 1/2000 live births.
- Disease from vaso-occlusive crisis/disease (VOD) and haemolysis. ↑ blood viscosity and low flow in small vessels → infarction. Premature destruction of RBCs → haemolytic anaemia.

Clinical features

Spectrum of disease, ranging from asymptomatic to severe, frequent crises, and organ damage. Usually presents between 3mth and 6y.

- *Infancy:* high HbF is protective in the first month of life.
- *Common problems:* dactylitis, splenic sequestration and pneumococcal sepsis (if not vaccinated and no phenoxymethylpenicillin prophylaxis).
- *Young children:* risk of pneumococcal sepsis greatest <3y. Infection from encapsulated organisms (if not vaccinated or no phenoxymethylpenicillin prophylaxis) or parvovirus; VOD in long bones, UAO, stroke.
- *Older children:* VOD, avascular necrosis, stroke.

Sickle crises and problems

- *VOD crises:* with excruciating pain in bones and joints, often hands and feet, and more central with age. Dactylitis is an early manifestation; precipitated by cold, dehydration, infections, and hypoxia.
- *Acute chest syndrome:* precipitated by chest infection, with SOB, cough, chest pain, and falling SpO_2. CXR changes may be late and progress within hours. Prompt treatment essential.
- *Sequestration:* organs trap sickled RBCs. Splenic sequestration commoner in first year; later, liver and lung sequestration. Rapid fall in Hb may be fatal. Recurrent episodes warrant splenectomy.
- *Stroke:* mostly in 5–10y olds; by 20y, up to 20% will have silent stroke. Untreated, mortality 20%; recurrence rate 70% within 3y. Treat promptly with exchange transfusion (ET) to reduce HbS <20%. UK children >2y need annual transcranial Doppler (TCD)—if high-flow velocity, serial ET to prevent stroke.
- *Infections:* patients are functionally hyposplenic by 1y, resulting in high risk of infection from *Pneumococcus, Meningococcus,* and *H. influenzae* (HiB). Ensure vaccination is up-to-date, and give phenoxymethylpenicillin prophylaxis.
- *Aplastic crises:* typically, after infection with parvovirus B19. Reticulocytes and consequently Hb falls. Spontaneous recovery usually occurs in 10 days. The patient may require transfusion.

- *Priapism:* 3–5% of pre-pubertal and 30–40% of post-pubertal boys. Acute fulminant (painful, >3h) or minor 'stuttering' priapism (<3h, self-limiting). May result in erectile dysfunction. Major episodes require urgent urology assessment. (See also ➲ Priapism, p. 843.)
- *Avascular necrosis:* hip joint, humerus, or any bone.
- *Renal impairment:* hyposthenuria (urine concentration defect), high urine output, and susceptibility to dehydration. Enuresis common. Papillary necrosis causes haematuria. CRF later.
- *Retinopathy:* small vessel occlusion → neovascularization → vitreous haemorrhage → resorption → fibrous strands → retinal detachment. Commoner in HbSC disease. Surveillance needed. Treat with photocoagulation (see ➲ Sickle-cell disease, p. 982).
- *ENT problems:* adenotonsillar hypertrophy is common and may lead to nocturnal hypoxia precipitating crises. Ask about 'snoring'.
- *Leg ulcers:* uncommon in childhood.
- *Growth and development:* generally delayed; final height is normal.

Diagnosis

- *Clinical suspicion:* required in unscreened population. Routine screening of Afro-Caribbean children prior to anaesthesia.
- *Haematology:* Hb 5–9g/dL, reticulocytes ↑, sickle cells on blood film. Hb electrophoresis [high-performance liquid chromatography (HPLC)] is definitive test.
- *Prenatal:* on fetal RBCs/fibroblasts or newborn screening (UK).

Management of acute crises

- *Investigations:* CXR, Hb (low), reticulocytes (raised), blood culture, U&E, creatinine, LFTs, CRP (up in sickling/infection), group and save.
- *Hydration:* aim for 150% normal maintenance (PO or IV).
- *Analgesia:* titrate to severity. Initially treat at home with simple analgesia, e.g. paracetamol, NSAIDs; give opiates if required.
- *Antibiotics:* broad-spectrum cephalosporin, after blood culture if fever >38°C. Add a macrolide if atypical pneumonia.
- *O_2:* to maintain SpO_2 >95%. Keep warm.
- *Blood:* transfusion for aplastic crisis, sequestration, or anaemia; ET for sequestration, chest syndrome, or stroke.

Maintenance treatment

- *Avoid precipitators:* hypoxia (air travel), cold, dehydration.
- *Vaccination:* see ➲ Immunization, p. 652.
- Lifetime PO phenoxymethylpenicillin prophylaxis and daily PO folic acid.
- *Hydroxycarbamide (hydroxyurea):* may reduce crises and need for blood. Rise in MCV shows compliance, and myelosuppression is commonest adverse effect. Use in moderate to severe disease.
- *BMT:* if successful, is curative.
- *Serial ET to prevent stroke:* for those >2y with high-velocity TCD flow detected on annual screening.

Thalassaemia

Inherited defect in synthesis of one or more globin chains (globin chain linked to haem group = Hb) resulting in imbalanced globin chain production → ineffective erythropoiesis → precipitation of excess chains → haemolysis → variable-severity anaemia.
- At birth, the major Hb is HbF ($\alpha 2 \gamma 2$).
- By the end of the first year of life and into adulthood, the major Hb is HbA ($\alpha 2 \beta 2$); 72.5% is HbA2 ($\alpha 2 \delta 2$), and only 1–2% is HbF.

HbA ($\alpha 2 \beta 2$) comprises two α-globin chains that are encoded by two α-globin genes on each chromosome 16 (i.e. each cell has four α-globin genes), designated as ($\alpha \alpha / \alpha \alpha$). The two β-globin chains are encoded by only one β-globin gene on each chromosome 11, designated (β / β). HbF has two α-globin chains combined with two γ chains ($\alpha \alpha / \gamma \gamma$). HbA2 has two α chains combined with two δ chains ($\alpha \alpha \delta \delta$).

The severity of anaemia and clinical picture are related to the number and nature of gene mutation and deletions and consequent imbalanced globin chain production. Thalassaemia is common in malaria-affected regions of the world (the trait is probably protective), i.e. parts of Africa, the Mediterranean, the Middle East, India, and Asia.

α-thalassaemia

- Silent α-thalassaemia ($\alpha \alpha / \alpha-$): one α-gene deletion. Asymptomatic.
- α-thalassaemia trait ($\alpha \alpha / - -$) or ($\alpha - / \alpha -$): two α-gene deletions. Asymptomatic with microcytic, hypochromic picture (Hb may be low, MCV low, MCH low). May mimic iron deficiency, if RBC >5.0 × 10^{12}/L, with microcytic, hypochromic film, then thalassaemia trait more likely.
- HbH disease ($\alpha - / - -$): three α-gene deletions or equivalent. Variable chronic anaemia with mild hepatosplenomegaly and jaundice. Hypochromic anaemia with target cells and reticulocytes ↑. HbH inclusions (tetramers of β-globin) are seen on special staining. Folic acid supplements required, and occasionally transfusions. Splenectomy may be beneficial.
- Hb Bart's hydrops fetalis ($- - / - -$): four α-gene deletions. Causes hydrops fetalis, leading to stillbirth or early neonatal death. Hb analysis shows mainly Hb Bart's ($\gamma 4$). Most often seen in South East Asia where frequency of ($\alpha \alpha / - -$) carriers is high.

β-thalassaemia

This disorder is not obvious until γ-chain production falls off at around 6mth of age and HbF ($\alpha \alpha / \gamma \gamma$) levels fall.

β-thalassaemia trait

($\beta o / \beta$) or ($\beta + / \beta$). Asymptomatic with mild Hb ↓, MCV low, MCH ↓. HbA2 characteristically ↑ on Hb electrophoresis to >3.5%. No treatment required, but important to detect for genetic counselling, especially if partner also has haemoglobinopathy.

β-thalassaemia major

Presentation

- Presents in first year to 18mth as HbF drops, but no HbA is made, leading to anaemia.
- Severe anaemia (3–9g/dL); markedly low MCV and MCH, ↑ reticulocytes, target cells, and nucleated RBCs.
- Secondary growth and development failure.
- Extramedullary haematopoiesis causes skeletal deformity (frontal bossing of skull, maxillary swelling) and hepatosplenomegaly in older children who are not adequately transfused.
- Hb electrophoresis shows mainly HbF, but no HbA.

Management

- Regular transfusions (every 3–4wk) to maintain Hb level that suppresses extramedullary haematopoiesis and sustains growth and development.
- Iron overload is a major problem, with haemosiderosis affecting the heart, liver, endocrine organs, and pancreas.
- Chelation of iron starts when ferritin level >1000mcg/L (usually following 10–20 transfusions). PO iron chelator or desferrioxamine by SC infusion (side effects include: cataracts, hearing loss, and *Yersinia* gut infections).
- Splenectomy may help if massive splenomegaly or ↑ transfusion requirements.
- BMT is the only cure and is usually successful when carried out as a planned procedure in a unit that specializes in the procedure and in well-chelated patients with no end-organ damage. The procedure carries significant risks.

Immune haemolytic anaemia

RBCs react with autoantibody ± complement, leading to their destruction by the reticuloendothelial system. Drugs can induce antibody-mediated haemolysis, e.g. penicillins, cephalosporins, ibuprofen, antimalarials, rifampicin, antihistamines. Mechanisms are variable. Can be divided into isoimmune and autoimmune forms.

Isoimmune

(See → Rh disease (rhesus haemolytic disease), p. 176.) Sensitization induces maternal RBC antibodies that cross the placenta and haemolyse fetal and neonatal RBCs. Usually, DCT +ve.
- Rh haemolytic disease.
- ABO incompatibility.
- Other blood group incompatibilities, e.g. Kell, Duffy, blood groups.

Autoimmune

Warm antibody type—mostly IgG
- Rare.
- Majority idiopathic.
- Other causes: drugs (e.g. penicillin), lymphoid malignancies, autoimmune diseases (e.g. SLE, IBD).
- Variable haemolytic anaemia, mild jaundice, splenomegaly, DCT +ve.
- Warm autoantibodies—often non-specific.

Treatment: give PO prednisone. If no response, give rituximab (anti-CD20 antibody). Consider splenectomy if severe or poorly responsive to immunosuppression.

Cold antibody type—mostly IgM
- Very rare in children, except paroxysmal cold haemoglobinuria (PCH).
- RBC antibody reacts most actively at <32°C to cause intravascular RBC haemolysis.
- Idiopathic or secondary to EBV or *Mycoplasma* infection.
- Acrocyanosis in cold, splenomegaly.
- Chronic haemolytic anaemia, DCT –ve for IgG, +ve for C3.
- IgM autoantibodies react best at 4°C.

Treatment: rarely needed. Warmth, immunosuppression, plasma exchange, and splenectomy may help. Usually, the condition is self-limiting if there is an infectious cause.

Paroxysmal cold haemoglobinuria
Often due to infections (varicella, measles, syphilis) and vaccinations.
- Acute onset of intravascular haemolysis, after fever and chills.
- Due to a biphasic antibody—the Donath–Landsteiner antibody.
- Antibody attaches to cells in cold peripheries and lyses in central warmth of the body—protect from cold.

Treatment: transfuse as required. Condition is self-limiting.

Red blood cell fragmentation

Causes

- *Microangiopathic haemolytic anaemia (MAHA):* includes—HUS, TTP, giant capillary haemangioma (Kasabach–Merritt syndrome), and DIC.
- *Infection:* e.g. meningococcal, pneumococcal, malaria (black water fever—intravascular haemolysis), viral haemorrhagic fevers (VHFs), *Clostridium perfringens.*
- *Burns.*
- *Mechanical:* e.g. prosthetic heart valves, March haemoglobinuria.
- *Hereditary acanthocytosis:* rare genetic condition of abetalipoproteinaemia with mental retardation, ataxia, RP, and steatorrhoea.
- *Envenomation* from venomous snakes, spiders, etc.

Clinical features

- Depends on underlying cause and anaemia severity.

Laboratory investigations

- Hb ↓.
- Blood film: reticulocytes, nucleated RBCs high, RBC fragmentation, schistocytes, irregularly contracted cells, microspherocytes, acanthocytes.
- Possible platelet decrease or clotting prolongation with consumption.
- In malaria, visible parasites on thick/thin blood film.

Treatment

- Treat underlying disease.
- Correct haematological abnormalities, e.g. blood ± platelet transfusion, FFP to correct clotting abnormalities.
- Iron or folate supplements if required.

Acquired aplastic anaemia

Due to severe bone marrow suppression of RBCs, WBCs, and platelet precursors (pancytopenia). Rare. Acquired or congenital.

Acquired causes

Idiopathic commonest. Rarely, owing to: radiotherapy, chemotherapy, idiosyncratic reaction to drugs or chemicals (chloramphenicol, carbamazepine, phenytoin, NSAIDs, mesalazine, several solvents), or viral (hepatitis A, B, and C; CMV; EBV; parvovirus—commoner in adults). NB: bone marrow invasion (e.g. malignant cells, osteopetrosis) displaces normal marrow; causes pancytopenia, not aplastic anaemia.

Presentation

Features of pancytopenia
- Anaemia: due to very low RBC production.
- Infection: particularly bacterial and fungal. Due to WCC depletion, particularly if neutrophils $<0.5 \times 10^9$/L [severe aplastic anaemia (SAA)] and $<0.2 \times 10^9$/L [very severe aplastic anaemia (VSAA)].
- Mucosal bleeding, purpura, and bruising. Due to very low platelet count.

Investigations

- FBC: WBC low, platelets $<20 \times 10^9$/L, reticulocytes $<20 \times 10^9$/L.
- Bone marrow aspirate and trephine: aplasia (marrow cellularity <25%).
- CD55/CD59 immunophenotyping to exclude PNH (see ➲ Paroxysmal nocturnal haemoglobinuria, p. 557).
- Cytogenetics and chromosomal breakage studies to detect myelodysplastic syndrome (MDS), FA, or dyskeratosis congenita.

Treatment

- Remove or treat underlying cause, e.g. drugs.
- Depending on severity: RBC ± platelet transfusion.
- BMT may be curative.
- Immunosuppression, e.g. rabbit anti-thymocyte globulin followed by ciclosporin, is best second-line therapy for those with no BMT donor.

Prognosis

Depends on underlying cause. Some patients recover spontaneously. Most will progress to more severe disease, PNH, or leukaemia. Long-term survival is unlikely in severe disease without good response to immunosuppressive therapy or BMT.

Paroxysmal nocturnal haemoglobinuria

Rare acquired clonal disorder of marrow cells deficient in glycosyl phosphatidylinositol (GPI) anchors that protect against complement lysis. Usually associated with background aplasia, allowing PNH clone a +ve selective advantage. Complement lysis leads to chronic haemolytic anaemia, with intermittent haemoglobinuria, but persistent haemosiderinuria. Urine is Hb +ve. High risk of recurrent and fatal venous thrombosis, e.g. Budd–Chiari, venous thrombosis, cerebral sagittal sinus.

- FBC: ↑ reticulocytes, ↓ WBC, and low platelets.
- Bone marrow is hypoplastic with erythropoietic islands.
- Flow cytometry detects CD55- and CD59-deficient cells.

Treatment
- Blood transfusion.
- Iron replacement (rarely) or iron chelation.
- Warfarin (anticoagulant therapy).
- Immunosuppression (e.g. with steroids). Eculizumab (anti-complement antibody) may reduce severity.
- BMT can be curative of both PNH and aplasia. Otherwise, median survival is 8–10y. Death is due to thrombosis or complications of pancytopenia.

Inherited and congenital bone marrow failure syndromes

Fanconi's anaemia

Rare, AR condition → progressive bone marrow failure affecting all three haematopoietic cell precursors. Associated with chromosomal fragility and defective DNA repair.

Presentation

May present at any age, but typically at 4–10y.
- Usually presents with bruising, purpura, or insidious-onset anaemia.
- Short stature (80%); café-au-lait spots (75%); skeletal abnormalities, particularly upper limb and thumb (66%); renal malformations (30%); microcephaly (40%); cryptorchidism (20%); mental retardation (17%); deafness (7%); abnormal facies.

Investigations

- FBC: pancytopenia, or just thrombocytopenia initially.
- Bone marrow: hypoplastic, dyserythropoietic, or megaloblastic.
- Chemically induced cultured lymphocyte chromosomal breakages.
- Investigate to detect renal abnormalities or hearing loss.
- Most of the 12 FA genes are cloned and can be screened in families with a known mutation. Diagnosis is essential, as standard BMT conditioning is fatal and appropriate modifications are essential.

Treatment

- Supportive, e.g. RBC transfusion, hearing aids, orthopaedic.
- Immunosuppression: corticosteroids/androgens (oxymetholone).
- Successful BMT curative for haematological defects, but problems post-BMT as FA is a constitutional and multiorgan disorder.

Prognosis

Most respond to steroids/androgens, but treatment is long term. Patients not responding to immunosuppression usually die within a few years due to complications of pancytopenia or acute leukaemia.

Shwachman–Diamond syndrome

Rare AR disorder. Most have mutations in the *SBDS* gene on 7q11. Affects bone marrow, pancreas, and skeleton. Neutropenia occurs more than thrombocytopenia and anaemia → infections due to immunocompromise. Exocrine pancreatic enzyme insufficiency → diarrhoea and FTT. Skeletal effects: metaphyseal dysostosis and dental problems.
- Bone marrow examination is diagnostic ± pancreatic testing.
- *SBDS* genotyping can be helpful.
- Treatment is supportive, e.g. pancreatic enzyme supplements.
- BMT is an option, but survival is relatively poor (i.e. order of 50%).

Dyskeratosis congenita

Very rare condition with dystrophic nails, skin pigmentation, and mucous membrane (oral) leukoplakia. Bone marrow shows hypoplastic/aplastic changes. Treatment is BMT.

Failure of red cell production (pure red cell aplasia)

Causes

- Transient erythroblastopenia of childhood (TEC).
- Diamond–Blackfan syndrome.
- Drugs.
- Viral, e.g. parvovirus B19.
- Isoimmune haemolytic disease in newborn, e.g. anti-Kell.
- Congenital dyserythropoietic anaemia.
- Megaloblastic anaemia (aplastic phase).

Diamond–Blackfan syndrome (congenital red cell aplasia)

Hereditary condition of variable genetic inheritance; unknown defect leads to a specific reduction in bone marrow RBC production. The genetic basis remains unclear; however, mutations in the gene which codes for RPS19, a small ribosomal protein on chromosome 19q13.2, are found in ~25% of patients. The familial form (AR) accounts for 10–20% of cases. The rest are sporadic.

Presentation

Presents in the first year in 95% (25% with severe anaemia <6mth). Occasional late presentations with variable phenotypes can occur and 15–25% of cases undergo remission. The syndrome is associated with:

- Dysmorphic features: cleft palate, hypertelorism (Cathie's facies).
- Thumb abnormalities (10–20%): triphalangeal thumbs; absent radii.
- Deafness, renal defects (>50%), CHD.
- Musculoskeletal defects, short stature, and growth retardation.

Investigations

FBC shows normochromic anaemia, with ↓ reticulocytes (<0.2%). WCC and platelet counts are usually normal. Bone marrow aspirate and trephine show absent red cell precursors but are otherwise normal.

Treatment

Trial of PO prednisolone and wean over several weeks. ~70% have an initial response, but most will need, but often cannot tolerate, a maintenance dose. Give regular monthly RBC transfusion with iron chelation if unresponsive to steroids. BMT can be curative.

Prognosis

Twenty per cent spontaneously resolve, but significant mortality and morbidity in the remainder from steroid treatment and blood transfusion-related complications (e.g. iron overload).

Polycythaemia

Defined as an increase in the total red blood cell mass (RCM) above age-specific normal. As normal ranges of RCM are lacking in children, a raised Hct/PCV above age-specific normal is used instead.

- Commonest in the newborn: venous or arterial Hct >65%.
- Polycythaemia–hyperviscosity syndrome diagnosed in infants when Hct >65–75% and may require partial exchange to reduce to ~55%.
- Very rare in childhood, but seen in teenagers with early-onset myeloproliferative disorders, which should be suspected if Hct is 3–4 SDs above age-specific mean.

Causes of polycythaemia

Neonatal causes

(See also ➔ Polycythaemia, p. 174.)

- Hypertransfusion: delayed cord clamping, twin-to-twin transfusion syndrome, maternal–fetal transfusion.
- Endocrine: infant of a diabetic mother, CAH, neonatal thyrotoxicosis.
- Chronic hypoxia: IUGR, placental insufficiency, high altitude.
- Maternal disease: pregnancy-induced hypertension, cyanotic heart disease.
- Syndromic: Down's syndrome, BWS.
- Relative polycythaemia: due to reduced plasma volume as a result of dehydration, diuretic therapy.

Causes in older children

- Primary: polycythaemia rubra vera (very rare).
- High O_2-affinity polycythaemic Hb variant (familial polycythaemia).
- Secondary to ↑ erythropoietin production:
  - Compensatory increase occurs in cyanotic CHD, severe chronic respiratory disease, chronic OSA, chronic alveolar hypoventilation, e.g. gross obesity, high altitude, abnormal Hb with high O_2 affinity.
  - Inappropriately ↑ production with cerebellar haemangioblastoma, renal disease (renal cysts and carcinoma), HCC.
- Relative: dehydration or diuretic therapy.

Presentation

- Asymptomatic plethora occurs in most patients, particularly newborns.
- Jaundice (newborn): due to ↑ red cell turnover.
- Hypoglycaemia (newborn): due to ↑ red cell glucose consumption.
- Hyperviscosity syndrome in newborns: hypotonia, congestive cardiac failure, tachypnoea, seizures, abnormal renal function, NEC.
- CNS: cerebral irritability, seizures, strokes, cerebral haemorrhage.
- Respiratory distress, pulmonary hypertension, e.g. PPHN.
- Congestive cardiac failure.
- Thrombosis: e.g. renal venous thrombosis.
- Miscellaneous: cyanosis (PaO_2 usually normal), hepatomegaly.

Management

- Diagnosis is often obvious, e.g. cyanotic CHD.
- FBC: ↑ Hct, ↑ red cell count (RCC), blood film.
- Exclude low serum glucose or Ca^{2+}, or ↑ bilirubin (newborn).
- Investigate for cause if not obvious.
- In neonates: if symptomatic or PCV >70%, urgent discussion needed with neonatal specialist to decide if partial (dilutional) ET is needed.

Prognosis

Generally good, unless severe hypoglycaemia or thrombotic complications occur.

Abnormal bleeding or bruising

Causes

- Coagulation factor deficiencies: likely if there is excessive blood loss following surgery or dentistry, recurrent bruises >1cm, muscle haematomas, or joint haemarthroses.
- Platelet deficiency or dysfunction: presents as purpura, petechiae, mucosal bleeding, e.g. recurrent epistaxis, menorrhagia, or GI or GU tract haemorrhage.
- Microvascular abnormalities: palpable purpura suggestive of vasculitis, i.e. not a haematological cause.

Detailed history

- Nature of bleeding.
- History of recent trauma.
- Concurrent disease.
- Age, e.g. haemorrhagic disease of the newborn several days after birth.
- Any maternal disease (if newborn), including maternal ITP.
- Diet.
- Drug history.
- Family history.

Examination

- Is the child well or unwell?
- Hepatosplenomegaly: suggests haemolysis or hypersplenism.
- Dysmorphic signs: e.g. absent radius in thrombocytopenia-absent radius (TAR) syndrome.
- Signs of anaemia: e.g. prolonged blood loss, bone marrow failure syndrome.
- Pattern of purpura or bruising: e.g. extensor and lower limb pattern of HSP.
- Palpable purpura in vasculitis: e.g. HSP.
- Associated features: e.g. arthritis (HSP), albinism (Hermansky–Pudlack syndrome), haemangioma (Kasabach–Merritt syndrome), eczema (Wiskott–Aldrich syndrome).

Investigations

Initially perform coagulation screen [PT (INR), APTT], FBC and film, U&E, LFTs, and CRP/ESR. Depending on presentation, also consider: fibrinogen, TT (presence of heparin).

- If clotting screen abnormal, i.e. prolonged: perform a 50:50 mix to exclude an inhibitor, and if suggestive, request lupus anticoagulant screen and anticardiolipin antibody screen. If 50:50 mix suggests a coagulation factor deficiency, then request factor assays according to whether PT or APTT, or both, prolonged.

- *If clotting screen is normal, perform*:
  - Platelet function assay (PFA); if indicated, formal platelet function studies (need fresh blood, so test is best done near to a laboratory that can perform these assays).
  - von Willebrand's screen should be performed if history suggestive (mucosal bleeding), even if APTT normal (although usually slightly prolonged).
  - Autoantibody screen—antiplatelet antibodies (rarely useful!).
  - Bone marrow aspirate and trephine are rarely required for diagnosis of ITP, but if TAR or bone marrow failure syndrome is suspected, then it is indicated.

Treatment

- Supportive: e.g. colloid/blood transfusion if significantly hypovolaemic or anaemic. NB: send off all blood tests before any transfusion, including blood for viral serology and sufficient samples for coagulation factor assays.
- Correct known coagulation or platelet abnormalities if required.
- If there is catastrophic bleeding without diagnosis, treat with blood, FFP (20mL/kg) ± platelets (10–20mL/kg), as indicated, until the precise defect is known.
- Avoid IM injections, arterial puncture, and NSAIDs.
- If the patient is a young ♂ bleeding post-circumcision, then usually diagnosis is haemophilia or, rarely, some other clotting factor deficiency.
- Important to involve haematologist and blood bank early in presentation to get appropriate expert help.

Outcome

Outcome depends on the cause and severity of the bleed, but generally, bleeding from whatever cause can be controlled by platelet or coagulation factor transfusion, resulting in a low risk of death or permanent morbidity.

Coagulation studies

(See Table 14.3.)

- *APTT:* principally assesses the 'intrinsic' path of the coagulation cascade.
- *PT or INR (monitoring warfarin therapy):* assesses 'extrinsic' pathway.
- *Thrombin time (TT):* only used to differentiate among heparin contamination, dysfibrinogenaemia, and DIC. This test is not used routinely and needs to be requested specifically.
- *Serum fibrinogen:* useful if DIC or haemophagocytic lymphohistiocytosis (HLH) is suspected.
- *PFA: in vitro* test of platelet function. This test is easy to perform, provided platelet count >100 × 10⁹/L. Ranges in children have been produced.
- *Bleeding time:* tests platelet function. Now virtually obsolete.
- *Fibrin degradation products (FDPs):* Components released into blood following clot degradation. Levels rise after any thrombotic event. Can be used to test for DIC. The most notable subtype of FDPs is D-dimer.
- *D-dimer:* principally used to screen adults for thrombotic disorders, e.g. deep vein thrombosis (DVT). Rarely used in children, except possibly to help monitor management of DIC (possibly along with FDPs). NB: DIC is a clinical diagnosis and is not made by measuring D-dimers or FDPs.
- *Other specific tests:* include screening tests of coagulation inhibitor, e.g. lupus anticoagulant, or individual clotting factor level.

Table 14.3 Common causes of deranged coagulation tests

Test	Cause(s)
PT and APTT normal	Normal child, platelet abnormality, vasculitis, e.g. HSP, heparin
PT ↑, APTT normal	Deficiency of coagulation factor VII: vitamin K deficiency (common in toddlers due to poor diet), warfarin therapy, liver disease
PT normal, APTT ↑	Deficiency of factors VIII, IX, XI, and XII (haemophilia A or B, vWD, heparin therapy)
PT and APTT ↑	Deficiency of common pathway factors II, V, and X, fibrinogen (rare factor deficiencies, DIC, toxic doses of warfarin and heparin, profound vitamin K deficiency)
TT ↑	Fibrinogen defect, heparin, DIC
Fibrinogen ↓	DIC, hypo-/dysfibrinogenaemia, HLH
FDPs or D-dimers ↑	DIC
PFA ↑	vWD, platelet dysfunction, drug effect

NB: most clotting times are longer in healthy neonates, particularly in preterm infants. Always refer to appropriate age-specific ranges.

Disseminated intravascular coagulation

DIC is the pathological activation of blood coagulation pathways that occurs in response to a variety of severe diseases. All, or some, of the following may simultaneously occur:
- Consumption of platelets and clotting factors → abnormal bleeding.
- Activation of intravascular thrombosis with both macro- and microthrombi formation, leading to end-organ damage.
- Widespread activation of fibrinolysis, leading to further bleeding.
- MAHA ('RBCs destroyed in fibrin mesh').

Causes in neonatal period
- Common: severe asphyxia, sepsis.
- Less common: severe IUGR, RDS, aspiration pneumonitis, NEC, Rh isoimmunization, dead twin, severe haemorrhage, purpura fulminans, profound hypothermia.

Causes in older children
- Common: septicaemia (60%), severe trauma, and burns.
- Less common: profound shock, hepatic failure, anaphylaxis, severe blood transfusion reactions.

Presentation
- DIC usually occurs in the setting of a profoundly sick child.
- Oozing and bleeding from venepuncture sites, wounds, mucosal membranes, and GI, pulmonary, and GU tracts.
- Microthrombi causing renal impairment, cerebral dysfunction, and localized skin necrosis.
- ARDS.
- MAHA.

Investigations
Platelets ↓, PT ↑, APTT ↑, TT ↑, fibrinogen ↓ (<1g/L), FDPs ↑ (>80mg/mL), or D-dimers (non-specific, but useful in monitoring progress).

Management
- *Immediately:* identify and vigorously treat underlying cause.
- *Supportive care:* O_2, IV volume for shock, blood transfusion.
- *Platelet transfusion:* if uncontrolled bleeding or pre-procedure, but not for oozing. Indiscriminant IV platelets 'fuel the fire' → cause more thrombosis.
- *Coagulation factor replacement:* to control bleeding, e.g. FFP, cryoprecipitate if fibrinogen <500mg/L.
- *ET:* may be beneficial, e.g. sepsis, rhesus isoimmunization, or polycythaemia (removes causative toxins or antibodies, and replaces clotting factors).
- Use of heparin is controversial but may be needed if there is large thrombi or significant organ damage from microthrombi. Seek expert advice from a paediatric haematologist.

Prognosis
There is high mortality, due to either the underlying disease or DIC-related haemorrhage or thrombosis.

Acquired haemorrhagic disorders

Haemorrhagic disease of the newborn

- Due to vitamin K deficiency.
- Rare early presentation occurs within 24h of life with serious bleeding, including intracranial haemorrhage (mothers may be completely vitamin K-deficient).
- More classical presentation occurs in first week of life in breastfed infants with GI bleeding, widespread bruising, and occasionally intracranial haemorrhage.
- Late presentation occurs > first week, again in breastfed infants, and usually associated with a variety of diseases that compromise or reduce availability of vitamin K, e.g. CF with diarrhoea, α1-antitrypsin deficiency, liver diseases.

Coagulation factor deficiencies secondary to liver disease

- DIC (see ➲ Acute hepatitis, pp. 310–11; ➲ Chronic liver disease, pp. 312–13; ➲ Disseminated intravascular coagulation, p. 566).

Haemophilia A

Haemophilia A is a congenital bleeding disorder due to defective production of factor VIII (FVIII); X-linked recessive inheritance. Incidence is 1/10 000–14 000 ♂. One-third have no family history. Carrier ♀ are rarely symptomatic but may have a low FVIII level. Genetic testing may be necessary to confirm carrier status.

Severity depends on degree of FVIII deficiency:

- <1% activity = severe disease, with 'spontaneous' haemarthroses; significant bleeding if cut; mucosal bleeds; and lumpy (pea-sized) bruises as infants. Most require prophylaxis with FVIII concentrate (see ➔ Management, p. 569).
- 2–5% = moderate disease. Bleeding rarely occurs and tends to involve muscles and soft tissues, secondary to trauma. Requires FVIII concentrate when bleeding occurs, but no prophylaxis.
- 5–20% = mild disease. Rarely bleed. May present after surgery or trauma. Prophylaxis with desmopressin (DDAVP) or FVIII concentrate for surgery. Desmopressin (DDAVP) stimulates release of von Willebrand's factor (vWF)—resulting in ↑ FVIII survival from vWF complexing.

Presentation

- *Rare in the neonate:* severe forms present in infancy with intracranial bleeds or after circumcision—most present as they start to mobilize.
- *Easy bruising:* in younger children, often get pea-sized, lumpy bruises.
- *Bleeding into joints (haemarthroses):* knees > ankles > elbows > hips > wrists. The joint is painful, swollen, tender, and warm, with severe limitation of movement ± inability to support weight. Uncontrolled recurrent bleeding can lead to degenerative joint disease.
- *IM bleeds:* can be difficult to differentiate between muscle strain and bleed. May lead to compartment syndrome, nerve compression, or ischaemic contracture.
- *Intracranial bleeds:* may be extradural, subdural, or intracerebral. Usually follows minor head trauma. All patients should seek medical attention, and those with severe disease need immediate FVIII.

Investigations

- APTT ↑ and FVIII ↓ (PT, vWF, and PFA all normal).
- Perform cranial CT scan if any suspicion of intracranial bleed.
- USS are useful for possible joint bleeds and muscle haematomas.

Management

- *Prophylaxis:* in severe disease, most require prophylaxis with alternate-day IV FVIII concentrate to prevent spontaneous bleeds. Children with moderate or mild disease do not require prophylaxis.
- *Major bleeds:* treat with recombinant FVIII product, except in those with FVIII inhibitors. The dose depends on bleeding site, child's weight, and serum half-life of FVIII (usually ~10h). In those with severe disease on prophylactic therapy, regular screens are made to assess exactly how much FVIII is required to treat a joint or a major bleed. The dose for joint bleed aims to get FVIII to 40–50%, while for head injury to 100%, i.e. treat intracranial bleeds with twice the dose used for a joint bleed.
- *Major surgery:* haematologist to plan timing/dose of factor. Give analgesia as required, but not NSAIDs (↓ platelet function).
- *Minor surgery or persistent bleeds:* IV, SC, or intranasal desmopressin (DDAVP) in those with moderate/mild haemophilia may suffice.
- *Mouth bleeding:* tranexamic acid suspension/tablets (20–25mg/kg tds).
- *Avoid IM injections:* including vitamin K at birth, if disease suspected (give IV). All vaccinations should be given SC.
- *Educate family:* about PRICE guidelines for supportive care of a bleed: Pressure dressing, Ice (bag of frozen peas), Rest (non-weight-bearing), Compress (cold if possible), Elevation of limb.
- *Daily PT:* following a bleed is important to avoid muscle weakness or contractures once joint bleeding has resolved.
- *Home FVIII treatment:* parents and, in due course, the boys themselves should be trained to give IV FVIII concentrates. Central venous 'ports' are used when peripheral access is impossible.

Complications

- *Chronic arthropathy:* owing to recurrent joint bleeds.
- *Transmission of hepatitis B, hepatitis C, HIV:* now rare since virally inactivated plasma concentrates and recombinant FVIII concentrate are given. All children should be vaccinated against hepatitis B.
- *FVIII inhibitor development:* is suggested by bleeds not responding to treatment. Measure FVIII inhibitor titre. Difficult to treat, but most are started on immune tolerance induction with high-dose FVIII. Acute bleeds are treated with ↑ FVIII dose or other products, e.g. recombinant FVIIa or FEIBA® (formulated with multiple active coagulaton factors that induce thrombin generation).

Prognosis

Excellent. Life expectancy is now normal with current recombinant therapy (prophylaxis and treatment).

Haemophilia B

- Previously known as Christmas disease.
- X-linked recessive disease caused by defective production of factor IX (FIX).
- Indistinguishable from haemophilia A, although patients may be slower to bleed.
- It is five times less common than haemophilia A.

Investigations

Same as for haemophilia A, except FIX activity is deficient, rather than FVIII.

Management

The principles are the same as for haemophilia A, except that DDAVP is of no use.

- Prophylaxis in patients with severe disease is with recombinant FIX therapy, usually twice a week (FIX plasma half-life is 25h). Generally, 1mcg/kg FIX raises the plasma level by 0.7–1%.
- Complications and prognosis are similar to haemophilia A.

von Willebrand's disease (vWD)

vWF functions as the carrier protein for factor VIII procoagulant (factor VIIIC), protecting it from degradation, which facilitates platelet adhesion to damaged endothelium. Deficiency in vWF leads to reduced FVIII activity and impaired platelet function.

- vWD is an inherited bleeding disorder due to deficiency or abnormal function of vWF.
- Incidence ~1/5000.
- ♂ = ♀.

The three main subtypes are:
- Type I: AD; 70% of cases. Mild to moderate severity.
- Type II: AD or AR; 25% of cases. Mild to moderate severity. In type IIb, there is usually thrombocytopenia.
- Type III: AR. Near-complete absence of vWF; <5% cases. Severe.

Presentation

Presentation is very variable. Type III usually has severe mucosal bleeding, but when FVIII level is very low, the picture is similar to haemophilia A. Other types may vary, from virtually asymptomatic to easy bruising with associated excessive bleeding from dental surgery, trauma, surgery, and menorrhagia (always screen for vWD in any ♀ with menorrhagia or iron deficiency owing to menorrhagia).

Investigations

APTT is usually ↑ (if FVIII activity is low); PT normal; platelet count usually normal, except in type IIb; PFA ↑; factor VIIIC ↓; vWF antigen levels reduced and function ↓.

NB: vWF is an acute phase protein, as is FVIII, and may be raised to normal immediately after birth and following trauma, illness, or traumatic venepuncture (hence difficult to make a diagnosis of mild vWD in a child!).

Management

- Avoid NSAIDs and IM injections.
- Minor bleeding may respond to local pressure or tranexamic acid (locally with mouthwash or systemically 20–25mg/kg tds for ~4–5 days).
- More significant bleeds or minor surgery may respond to desmopressin (DDAVP) (avoid if type IIB, as further reduces platelet count).
- Severe bleeding or severe disease requires virally inactivated plasma-derived FVIII concentrate, combined with vWF (no recombinant product currently available). Manage as for severe haemophilia A.

Complications

Mainly occur in undiagnosed cases. May be profoundly anaemic, owing to chronic blood loss and iron deficiency. If receiving plasma-derived products, there is a low, but present, risk of infection with blood-borne pathogens. Acute joint involvement is rare, except in type III. In severe disease, complications are otherwise similar to haemophilia A.

Prognosis

Patients with type I and II disease rarely have severe bleeds and generally have normal life expectancy and quality of life, especially in men (no periods). Severity seems to improve with age. Knowledge about how to manage bleeds improves with age. Even those with type III, if properly managed, should have normal life expectancy.

Other congenital clotting factor deficiencies

Deficiency of every coagulation factor exists, but most are very rare.

All have AR inheritance. Most patients present with bleeding after surgery (e.g. circumcision, trauma, or dental extraction), rather than spontaneous bleeding or haemarthrosis.

- Severe forms may present in neonatal period with cord hemorrhage or intracranial bleeds.
- Any boy with unexplained bleeding in infancy or as a toddler with isolated raised APTT must be considered to have haemophilia until proven otherwise.
- Unless bleeding is catastrophic, send blood for urgent factor assays and treat with appropriate factor, rather than with FFP.

Platelet function disorders

Congenital causes

All are rare and AR. They are due to the following:

- Defective platelet membrane-specific glycoproteins → defective adhesion to fibrinogen, e.g. Glanzmann disease (thrombasthenia), Bernard–Soulier syndrome (BSS), vWD (usually AD) (see ➲ von Willebrand's disease, pp. 572–3).
- Defective or deficient platelet granules (normal release induces coagulation cascade, vasoconstriction, and platelet aggregation), e.g. TAR syndrome, Chediak–Higashi syndrome.

Acquired causes

- Drugs (e.g. NSAIDs, corticosteroids, antihistamines), renal disease, liver disease, and diets rich in garlic, ginger, and Indian spices.

Presentation

- Easy bruising and purpura, mucocutaneous bleeding, menorrhagia.
- +ve family history is common (although in most AR syndromes, both parents are unaffected).

Investigations

- *Usually normal platelet count* (except in BSS which usually has mild thrombocytopenia).
- ↑ *platelet size*, e.g. giant platelets in BSS.
- *Prolonged PFA:* if congenital platelet functional disorder suspected, perform PFA, followed by formal platelet aggregation studies using ristocetin, collagen, adenosine diphosphate (ADP), arachidonic acid, and adrenaline; and platelet:nucleotide ratios. Interpretation is complex, so seek haematologist help.

Treatment

- Control bleeding, e.g. apply pressure in mild cases.
- Correct underlying abnormality or stop responsible drug.
- Give tranexamic acid for minor bleeding, e.g. mouthwashes or systemically.
- Give platelet transfusion if bleeding severe or to cover for surgery. NB: need to give HLA-matched platelets to avoid HLA-specific antiplatelet antibody formation, if child likely to need frequent transfusions.
- Avoid platelet function inhibitors, e.g. NSAIDs and IM injections.
- Consider oral contraceptives in teenage girls with menorrhagia.

Prognosis

Prognosis is generally good, with normal life expectancy. Serious bleeding is rare but can be difficult to manage, particularly in children with multiple antiplatelet or anti-HLA antibodies.

Thrombocytosis

Normal platelet count <450 × 10⁹/L; platelet counts >1000 × 10⁹/L may cause thrombosis or bleeding if dysfunctional platelets.

Causes

Almost always, thrombocytosis in infants and children is reactive.

Increased production
- Acute or chronic infection.
- Acute or chronic haemorrhage.
- Trauma or surgery.
- KD.
- Iron deficiency anaemia.
- Certain malignancies, e.g. Wilms' tumour.
- Any inflammatory disease, e.g. UC.
- Primary myeloproliferative disorder, e.g. essential thrombocythaemia or in association with chronic myeloid leukaemia (CML).

Decreased destruction
- Post-splenectomy.

Examination

Look for signs of iron deficiency anaemia, bruising or bleeding, spleno-megaly, and signs of KD (see ➔ Kawasaki disease, pp. 630–1) and general ill health. Most commonly, the child is well, having recovered from an acute infection, and a follow-up FBC shows a raised platelet count.

Investigations

- FBC: e.g. WCC ↑ in infection or signs of iron deficiency anaemia.
- CRP/ESR: ↑ in inflammatory/malignant conditions.
- Bone marrow aspirate is only ever indicated if primary myeloproliferative disorder such as essential thrombocythaemia is suspected (which is very rare).

Management

- Treat underlying cause.
- Watch and wait in reactive cases, as requires no treatment.
- Give aspirin in KD.

Prognosis

Reactive thrombocytosis generally has an excellent prognosis. Primary causes are very rare and have a variable prognosis.

Thrombocytopenia

(See also ➔ Thrombocytopenia, p. 175.) Defined as platelets <150 × 10⁹/L. As platelet count decreases, the risk of bleeding and bruising increases. Risk of bleeding is moderately high if platelets <20 × 10⁹/L, and likely if <10 × 10⁹/L.

Causes

Decreased platelet production
- *Selective megakaryocyte depression:* viral (HIV, parvovirus, EBV) or more substantial bacterial infection, drugs, and poisons.
- *Marrow failure:* aplastic anaemia, Fanconi's syndrome, severe IUGR, severe maternal pre-eclampsia, neonatal sepsis.
- *Marrow infiltration:* leukaemia, neuroblastoma, osteopetrosis.
- *Marrow depression:* radiotherapy, cytotoxic drugs, drug reaction.
- *Hereditary:* Wiskott–Aldrich syndrome (X-linked recessive: boys with early thrombocytopenia, eczema, and immunocompromise due to immunoglobulin abnormalities), BSS, TAR syndrome.
- *Nutritional deficiency:* vitamin B₁₂ or folate deficiency.

Increased destruction
- *Immune:* ITP (most commonly child, rarely mother), NAIT, SLE, drugs [penicillin/heparin-induced thrombocytopenia (HIT)], infection (e.g. malaria or HIV).
- *Non-immune:* DIC, giant haemangioma (Kasabach–Merritt syndrome), HUS, cardiac disease (prosthetic valves or cardiopulmonary bypass surgery).
- *Hypersplenism:* platelets pool in enlarged spleen from whatever cause— effect is dilutional, rather than destructive.

History, examination, and investigations

- *History:* drug history, family history, preceding viral illness.
- *Examination:* signs of bleeding, lymphadenopathy, hepatosplenomegaly, concurrent infection.
- *FBC and blood film.*
- *Serology:* antiplatelet antibodies [e.g. anti-human platelet antigen 1 (HPA1)] if NAIT suspected, autoimmune antibodies in those with chronic ITP, viral serology (CMV; EBV, along with Monospot if infectious mononucleosis suspected; or HIV if unusual unexplained thrombocytopenia).
- *Bone marrow aspirate and trephine:* very rarely required in cases of unexplained thrombocytopenia.
- *Cranial CT scan:* if any possible intracerebral haemorrhage.

Treatment

- Treat underlying cause if possible.
- Platelet transfusion: very low platelet count (prophylaxis, guided by haematologist, except for ITP) or life-threatening bleeding.
- Splenectomy, e.g. chronic ITP, hypersplenism.
- BMT used in some inherited bone marrow failure syndromes.

Acute immune thrombocytopenia

ITP is caused by IgG autoimmune antibody to platelet cell membrane antigens, leading to platelet destruction in the spleen and liver.

Presentation

- Most present between ages of 2 and 5y but can occur at any age.
- 60% have preceding viral infection, e.g. URTI.
- Bruising, purpura, petechiae, mucosal bleeding, menorrhagia.
- Intracranial bleeds very rare (<0.5%); often associated with trauma.

Physical examination

Otherwise usually normal, e.g. no splenomegaly.

Investigations

- *FBC:* platelet count markedly low, commonly platelet size ↑ due to compensatory megakaryocytosis.
- *Blood film:* platelet fragments.
- *Bone marrow:* in ITP normal, apart from ↑ megakaryocytes. Generally, bone marrow aspirate not indicated if the child is otherwise well, unless concurrent pancytopenia, hepatosplenomegaly, lymphadenopathy, or abnormally ↑ blasts on FBC, suggesting alternative diagnosis (e.g. aplastic anaemia, acute leukaemia, SLE in adolescent girls, or bone marrow failure syndrome).

Management

Do not treat the platelet count; treat the patient! The aim of treatment is to stop the bleeding, not to 'cure' the disorder, which resolves in its own time. Moderate bleeding can be controlled with tranexamic acid 20–25mg/kg tds for <5 days, provided haematuria is not present. Active treatment is required if patient experiencing significant bleeding, mucosal haemorrhage, or haematuria, as all are associated with ↑ risk of internal bleeding.

- First-line therapy: prednisolone.
- Second-line therapy: IV IgG.
- *If bleeding life-threatening or intracranial:* give 15–20mL/kg of platelets; start prednisolone and IV IgG, and consider emergency splenectomy. *Always discuss with haematology.*
- *Splenectomy for chronic ITP:* is indicated if disease is not steroid-responsive and >5y.
- *For chronic severe ITP:* rituximab has been used.
- *Educate parents:* regarding ITP, including signs and symptoms that should prompt immediate return to hospital.
- *Child can carry on with normal activities:* but should avoid contact sports and NSAIDs when platelet count is low.

Prognosis

Acute ITP in childhood is a self-limiting disorder, and >80% spontaneously remit within 6–8wk. Presentation >10y, or ♀ sex increases chance of chronic disease.

Thrombophilia

Haemostatic disorders predispose to venous or arterial thrombosis. They may be inherited or acquired:
- *Adult:* most inherited thrombophilias are asymptomatic or present in adult life.
- *Childhood:* in children, most thrombophilias present in the *newborn* period or following thrombogenic events (trauma, surgery, or pregnancy). However, newborns requiring intensive support often have multiple thrombotic risk factors, including sepsis, dehydration, polycythaemia, and central vascular lines.
- Inherited thrombophilia should be considered when there is an unexplained arterial or venous thrombosis, neonatal venous thrombosis, or +ve family history.

Inherited causes

Activated protein C (APC) resistance or factor V Leiden (FVL) deficiency
- Commonest inherited form of venous thrombophilia.
- APC is an anticoagulant formed in the vascular epithelium and limits haemostasis with co-factor protein S.
- >90% of APC resistance is due to FVL deficiency (a polymorphism present in 2–5% of population). Adults heterozygous for FVL deficiency have 5–10 times the risk of venous thrombosis, and homozygotes 30 times the risk.
- Homozygous FVL deficiency will often present in children; heterozygous children are unlikely to experience a significant risk, unless an additional prothrombotic risk factor is also present.

Protein C deficiency
- Thromboembolism is rare in childhood.
- Severe deficiency can cause life-threatening massive thrombosis in newborns, resulting in skin bruises that may become necrotic (purpura fulminans).

Protein S deficiency
- AD inheritance.
- Clinically similar to protein C deficiency; less likely to cause thromboembolism in children.

Acquired causes

Acquired thrombophilia is most commonly associated with:
- Septicaemia.
- Use of central lines.
- Takayasu's arteritis.
- KD.
- PNH.
- Polycythaemia.
- SLE, antiphospholipid antibody.
- Development of anti-protein S antibodies post-varicella-zoster virus (VZV) infection; can cause (as with congenital deficiency) necrotic skin bruises.

Newborns, especially if preterm, are most at risk. In the newborn, arterial or aortic thrombosis because a UAC may lead to bowel infarction, NEC, buttock or leg infarction, and renal arterial thrombosis. Commonest venous thrombosis involves the renal vein.

Investigations

- FBC (polycythaemia or infection).
- ESR/CRP (infection or inflammation).
- LFTs (protein C and S and prothrombin are vitamin K-dependent factors).
- Standard coagulation screen.
- Thrombophilia 'screen'. Guided by laboratory and haematologist.

Treatment

- *Acute venous thrombosis:* anticoagulation with SC low-molecular weight (LMW) heparin (or sometimes IV unfractionated heparin) and then warfarin if prolonged anticoagulation required.
- *Recurrent thrombosis:* treatment depends on severity, presentation, coagulation defect, and risk factors. Long-term anticoagulation with warfarin may be appropriate (aim for INR of 3–4).
- *Major vessel or catheter-related thrombosis:* can be treated with fibrinolytic agents, e.g. tissue plasminogen activator (TPA), urokinase.
- *Prophylaxis:* use SC heparin during surgery or trauma in patients with established prothrombotic defects and +ve personal history. Alternatively, antithrombin III or protein C concentrate may be given if relevant.

Blood transfusion

(See also ➜ Haematological support, p. 615.)

Red blood cell transfusion

Packed RBC are preferred to whole blood. In the UK, small-volume QUAD or Octapus packs are preferred for newborns because multiple aliquots can be dispensed as required from a single unit to reduce donor exposure (within a 28-day period).

Platelet transfusion

Indicated for bleeding due to significant thrombocytopenia or as prophylaxis in patients receiving myelosuppressive chemotherapy or with bone marrow failure when platelet count $<10 \times 10^9/L$.

Albumin

Albumin 20% is indicated to correct significant hypoproteinaemia.

Fresh frozen plasma

The indications for FFP are:
- DIC or acute blood loss.
- In an emergency to correct non-specific coagulation failure.
- To correct coagulation deficiencies when no specific concentrate is available.

    Volume = 10–20mL/kg (as guided by coagulation results).

Cryoprecipitate

Rich in clotting factors VIII, XIII, fibrinogen, and vWF. The main indication is to correct clotting defects induced by massive transfusion or DIC, especially if fibrinogen $<1.0g/L$.

Intravenous immunoglobulin

Normal immunoglobulin is predominantly IgG and is obtained from pooled serum of >1000 blood donations. The indications include:
- Hypogammaglobinaemia, e.g. X-linked hypogammaglobinaemia.
- Prophylaxis (rarely) following infectious contact in immunocompromised, e.g. CMV, hepatitis A, measles, chickenpox.
- Immunomodulation, e.g. ITP, NAIT.
- Specific IgGs, e.g. ZIG for prevention of life-threatening chickenpox in immunocompromised children.

Special requirements

CMV-negative blood components

These are required for:
- Intrauterine transfusion.
- Neonates and infants up to 1y.
- CMV-seronegative recipients of allogeneic BMT.

Irradiated blood products (inactivates T-lymphocytes)

These are required in:
- Intrauterine and neonatal exchange transfusions.
- Patients undergoing stem cell harvest for autografts (a week before until 3–6mth afterwards).
- Patients undergoing allogeneic haematopoietic stem cell transplant (a week before and indefinitely thereafter).
- Patients with suspected and confirmed Hodgkin's lymphoma.
- Patients receiving purine analogues, such as fludarabine, clofarabine, etc., indefinitely.
- di George syndrome and other congenital T-cell immunodeficiencies.
- Granulocyte transfusion.
- Patients being treated for aplastic anaemia with anti-lymphocyte globulin (ALG) and ciclosporin.

Blood transfusion reactions

Major blood incompatibility

An example is group A blood being transfused to a child with blood group O. Signs and symptoms of intravascular haemolysis may appear after only 5–10mL of blood infusion with:

• Pain at venepuncture site.
• Agitation, flushing; chest, abdominal, and flank pain.
• Fever, hypotension, haemoglobinaemia, haemoglobinuria, renal failure.

Treatment

• Stop transfusion immediately.
• Keep IV line open with saline.
• Monitor vital signs and urine output.
• Re-check patient and blood unit ID number.
• Give supportive care. Watch for hypotension and respiratory and renal failure.
• *Inform blood bank.*

Minor incompatibilities (i.e. group O+ blood given to an O– child) will not cause intravascular haemolysis but will cause sensitization and problems for future transfusions, in particular in ♀ during later pregnancies.

Bacterial infected blood products

Most serious reactions are seen with platelets (kept at room temperature where bacteria can multiply and produce toxins). At its most severe, there is sudden hypotension, fever, rigors, systemic collapse, and DIC.

Treatment

• *Give IV broad-spectrum antibiotics* (unlikely to help as the reaction is toxin-mediated but will stop the development of further sepsis), inotropic support, and PICU support as required.
• *Delayed reaction after a platelet transfusion*, i.e. not immediate, but within a few hours, must raise the suspicion of an infected product, requiring immediate blood cultures and broad-spectrum antibiotics.
• *Alert the blood bank immediately.*

Transfusion-related acute lung injury (TRALI)

Rapid-onset cough and SOB occur (may mimic fluid overload). TRALI is caused by donor antibodies to recipient leucocytes, leading to ARDS-like picture, with bilateral infiltrates on CXR. ETT intubation and MV likely required.

Febrile, non-haemolytic reactions

Due to recipient anti-HLA or granulocyte antibodies, or cytokines in infused blood product. Reactions are secondary to red cell alloimmunization. Less frequent since universal leucodepletion of blood products. Fever and rigors occur within few hours of starting or completing the transfusion.
- *Treatment:* slow transfusion rate, paracetamol, and antihistamines.

Circulatory overload

Results in pulmonary oedema, dyspnoea, headache, venous distension, and signs of cardiac failure.
- *Treatment:* slow transfusion rate, IV furosemide.

Transfusion-associated graft-versus-host disease (TaGVHD)

Occurs in patients with impaired cellular immunity. Lymphocytes in donor unit 'engraft', leading to rash, diarrhoea, liver impairment, and bone marrow failure.
- *No effective treatment.*
- Prevention by prior irradiation of blood products (see ➔ Special requirements, p. 581).
- Mortality is >90%.

Further reading

Blood Components Smartphone App (by NHSBT). Useful app for transfusion guidelines. Available at: ℜ https://www.hma.co.uk/insights/blood-components-app-now-available/.

NHS Blood and Transplant (NHSBT). Available at: ℜ https://www.nhsbt.nhs.uk/how-you-can-help/get-involved/download-digital-materials/.

Chapter 15

Oncology

Epidemiology of childhood cancer

- Childhood cancer (age <16y) accounts for around 1% of all cancer.
- ~1800 new cases of childhood cancer occur in the UK every year.
- The annual incidence in children under 15y of age is 1/10 000.
- *Causes of cancer in childhood:*
  - Environmental factors do not appear to be clearly linked with childhood cancer. An inherited predisposition applies to a minority of tumours.

Of all cases of cancer in children, we see:
- Leukaemia as the most commonly diagnosed cancer, accounting for around one-third of cases (31%).
- CNS and intracranial tumours account for around one-quarter of cases (26%).
- Lymphomas account for one in ten cases (10%).

Clinical assessment: history

Include specific questions about:
- Fevers, night sweats, anorexia, weight loss, pallor, bruising, and abnormal bleeding.
- Family history, including malignancy and inherited conditions.

Childhood malignancy may present with a variety of clinical features and so special attention should be paid to the following:

Respiratory symptoms
- In particular from mediastinal mass or lymphadenopathy.

Bone and joint pain/swelling, back/hip pain
- Persistent back or hip pain should not be dismissed as innocent in young children. It may reflect bone pain of bone marrow expansion (leukaemia or bone marrow metastases) or a spinal tumour.

Abdominal mass
May be:
- Painless and isolated (e.g. Wilms' tumour, ovarian teratoma).
- Associated with general malaise (e.g. B-cell lymphoma, neuroblastoma).
- Pelvic [e.g. rhabdomyosarcoma (RMS)].

Raised intracranial pressure
The commonest presenting features of brain tumours are:
- Headache (typically on waking up).
- Vomiting.
- Ataxia.
- Papilloedema.
- Deteriorating conscious level.

Growth and endocrine disturbances
Midline CNS tumours are less common but may result in disturbance in the hypothalamic–pituitary hormone axes and present with:
- Poor feeding or FTT (diencephalic syndrome).
- Polyuria and polydipsia (DI).
- Poor growth and short stature (GH deficiency).
- Hypoglycaemia (ACTH deficiency).

Clinical examination

Thorough general examination is required, including:
- *All lymph node stations:* neck, axillae, inguinal regions.
- *Skin:* assess pallor, petechiae, bruising, mucosal bleeding, and signs of infection.
- *Masses:* measure dimensions of any mass and organomegaly.
- If *leukaemia/lymphoma* suspected: assess testes for swelling and optic fundi.

Specific diagnoses or concerns may be indicated by the following findings.

Lymphadenopathy

Malignancy accounts for a small proportion of cases of persistent lymphadenopathy in children. Possible diagnoses include acute leukaemia, non-Hodgkin's lymphoma (NHL), Hodgkin's disease, and metastases from neuroblastoma or sarcoma.

Features of enlarged lymph node that should raise concern
- Diameter >2cm.
- Persistent or progressive enlargement.
- Non-tender, rubbery, hard, or fixed.
- Supraclavicular or axillary position.
- Associated with other features, e.g. pallor, lethargy.
- Hepatosplenomegaly.

Unexplained mass—at any site

The following features should raise suspicion of malignancy:
- Non-tender.
- Progressive and/or rapid enlargement.
- Diameter >2cm.
- Associated lymphadenopathy.

The following should raise suspicion of a brain tumour:
- Cranial nerve deficits from direct tumour involvement.
- Unexplained focal seizure.
- *False localizing signs:* cranial nerve III and VI palsies (mass effect from raised ICP).
- Cerebellar signs (e.g. ataxia).
- *Visual field* and/or acuity defects, abnormal eye movements.
- Gait abnormalities.
- Motor or sensory abnormalities.
- Behavioural disturbances, deteriorating school performance, or neurodevelopmental milestones.
- Increasing head size (OFC, infants).

Key investigations

If malignancy is suspected, the following tests are used in diagnosis, staging, and assessment for prognosis, and as a baseline before starting treatment. They should be directed towards those relevant for the type of tumour suspected, and advice may be sought from the regional paediatric oncology unit regarding local protocols.

Laboratory tests

- FBC and film.
- Coagulation studies.
- Group and cross-match blood.
- Electrolytes; renal, bone, and liver profile; urate; LDH.
- CRP, ESR.
- Ferritin and neuron-specific enolase (if neuroblastoma likely).
- Blood cultures.
- Thiopurine methyltransferase assay—in case of suspected ALL.
- Urine catecholamines (neuroblastoma, phaeochromocytoma).
- LP for cytospin, cell count, and cytology.

Imaging

Sedation or GA may be needed in young children when performing these procedures. The choice of imaging depends on the likely diagnosis and may include:

- CXR.
- CT scan chest and/or abdomen.
- MRI scan (better than CT for soft tissue swellings and brain).
- Bone marrow aspirate and/or trephine.
- Technetium (^{99}Tc) bone scan.
- Meta-iodo-benzylguanidine (MIBG) scan (neuroblastoma, phaeochromocytoma).

Other investigations

These depend on the treatment being planned and may include:

- *EDTA*: GFR (nephrotoxic chemotherapy, nephrectomy).
- Audiology assessment (platinum chemotherapy, radiotherapy).
- Echocardiogram (anthracycline, pulmonary radiotherapy).
- Lung function (bleomycin, pulmonary radiotherapy).
- Pituitary function (suprasellar tumours, CNS surgery, or radiotherapy).

Acute lymphoblastic leukaemia

This is the commonest malignancy in childhood. It arises from malignant proliferation of 'pre-B' (common ALL) or T-cell lymphoid precursors. The cause is unknown, but in a minority, it is associated with chromosomal aberrations.

- ALL accounts for 25% of all childhood malignancies.
- Commonly presents in young children aged 2–6y.

Presentation

Typically, there is a fairly short history (days or weeks) of symptom progression. Symptoms and signs reflect pancytopenia, bone marrow expansion, and lymphadenopathy seen in ALL (i.e. petechiae, bruising, pallor, lethargy, bone/joint pain/swelling, limp, lymphadenopathy, respiratory compromise).

Specific diagnostic tests

- Bone marrow: morphology, immunophenotype, cytogenetics.
- CSF for cytospin (CNS rarely involved at first diagnosis).
- Clinical examination of testes in boys for inappropriate swelling.
- CXR for mediastinal mass.

Outline of 'standard' treatment

Induction (4wk)
- Steroids (dexamethasone) throughout induction.
- Weekly IV vincristine.
- IM asparaginase.
- IV daunorubicin (in intermediate- and high-risk cases).
- Intrathecal (IT) methotrexate (MTX).

NB: tumour lysis syndrome (see ⊃ Tumour lysis syndrome, p. 614) is a significant risk.

Consolidation (CNS-directed therapy)
Maintenance: continuation treatment for 2y for girls, 3y for boys.
- Daily 6-mercaptopurine (6MP), weekly PO MTX (doses titrated according to blood count).
- 4-weekly vincristine IV bolus and 5-day pulses of PO dexamethasone.
- 12-weekly IT MTX.

NB: children were randomized during the UKALL 2011 trial to different treatment groups.

Prognosis

Overall survival is ~92% with current treatment. Adverse prognostic factors include:
- ♂ sex.
- Age <2y or >10y.
- High WCC at diagnosis.
- Unfavourable cytogenetics: Philadelphia chromosome—t(9;22); *MLL* gene rearrangements, e.g. t(4;11) in infants; *AML1* amplification.
- Poor response to induction and failure to remit by day 28.
- High level of minimal residual disease (MRD) at 28 days.

Relapsed ALL

Extramedullary relapse (mainly CNS, testes) may present without bone marrow disease. Treatment is stratified according to risk factors, which include:
- Time from first diagnosis (risk reduces with time).
- Extramedullary relapse (lower risk, particularly if isolated).
- MRD status after re-induction (–ve status reduces risk).

Treatment
- Intensive re-induction and consolidation for all risk groups.
- BMT.

Acute myeloid leukaemia

AML accounts for 15% of childhood leukaemias and 5% of all childhood cancers. AML results from malignant proliferation of myeloid cell precursors.

Presentation

- Symptoms and signs of bone marrow replacement (see ➋ Presentation, p. 590).
- Lymphadenopathy less prominent than in ALL.
- Intrathoracic extramedullary disease less common than in ALL.
- Acute promyelocytic leukaemia may have coagulopathy from proteolytic enzyme activity.
- Solid deposits (chloroma) occasionally seen in AML with maturation, acute myelomonocytic leukaemia, or acute monocytic/monoblastic leukaemia.

Cytogenetics

Analysis shows characteristic abnormalities which can be used to guide prognosis.

Treatment

In AML, prolonged continuation therapy is not used:
- Four courses of intensive myeloablative chemotherapy.
- High-risk cases, including those who fail to achieve complete remission after two courses, are usually offered BMT in first remission.

Prognosis

Overall survival is >60%.

Chronic myeloid leukaemia (adult type)

Classically associated with Philadelphia chromosome +ve disease (t(9;22) translocation). Rare. In the chronic phase, there are non-specific symptoms (fever, night sweats, and hepatosplenomegaly). Some benefit from interferon alfa therapy. BMT is usually required.

Leukaemia and Down's syndrome

The risk of developing acute leukaemia is ↑ 20–30 times. Commonly either a pre-B (common) ALL or AML. Response to chemotherapy is good, and better relapse-free survival is found in those with AML. Children with Down's syndrome-associated leukaemia experience more complications of treatment.

Juvenile myelomonocytic leukaemia

Classified with myelodysplasias, it is also known as juvenile CML. It is rare (<1% of childhood malignancy). Age of onset mostly <2y.

Associated with monosomy 7, NF1, and NS. Response to chemotherapy is poor and only BMT offers a cure.

Lymphoma

Non-Hodgkin's and Hodgkin's lymphoma are distinct disease entities that differ in regard to natural history, presentation, and management. Both are commoner in boys than girls.

Non-Hodgkin's lymphoma

Accounts for 60% of lymphoma in childhood. Majority are high-grade tumours that are divided into categories, using histology, immunophenotyping, and cytogenetics (see Box 15.1).

> **Box 15.1 Classification of NHL**
> - *Lymphoblastic (90% T-cell, 10% pre-B):* 30% of all NHLs. Most have anterior mediastinal mass. Disease may be in bone, bone marrow, skin, CNS, liver, kidneys, and spleen. Cases with >25% blasts in bone marrow are regarded as leukaemia (ALL). Terminal deoxynucleotidyl transferase (TdT) positivity is usually observed. Translocations t(1;14) or t(11;14) may be observed.
> - *Mature B-cell (Burkitt or Burkitt-like):* 30% of childhood NHLs. Occurs in abdomen, head and neck, bone marrow, and CNS. May grow rapidly. Endemic/African Burkitt's associated with early EBV infection and frequently affects the jaw. Expresses surface immunoglobulin and translocations t(8;14), t(8;22), or t(2;8).
> - *Large cell lymphoma:* 15–20% of childhood NHLs. Subtypes—diffuse large B-cell (BLCL) like Burkitt's; anaplastic large cell lymphoma (ALCL) involves extranodal sites (skin and bone). Lymphadenopathy often peripheral and painful. CNS or bone marrow disease is rare. ALCL has CD30 expression and t(2;5).

NHL staging (St Jude system)
- Stage I: single site or nodal area (not abdomen or mediastinum).
- Stage II: regional nodes, abdominal disease.
- Stage III: disease on both sides of the diaphragm.
- Stage IV: bone marrow or CNS disease.

Investigations
- Tissue: bone marrow aspirate; LP; pleural and abdominal (peritoneal) fluid aspirate; exclusional biopsy.
- Imaging: CT and positron emission tomography (PET) scans.

Treatment
- Lymphoblastic (T-cell, pre-B cell) lymphoma: ALL treatment protocol.
- Mature B-cell disease: short series of dose-intensive courses of chemotherapy. Risk of tumour lysis (see ➲ Tumour lysis syndrome, p. 614) is high.

Prognosis
Overall survival rate is 88%.

Hodgkin's lymphoma

40% of childhood lymphomas. The incidence of Hodgkin's lymphoma (HL), or Hodgkin's disease, is very low at <5y and rises with age. It is commoner in patients with previous EBV infection. The histology shows Reed–Sternberg cells in an apparently reactive lymph node infiltrate.

Presentation

Progressive, painless lymph node enlargement. Commonest sites are cervical (80%) and mediastinal (60%). Dissemination to extranodal sites is less common (e.g. lungs and bone marrow). Fever, night sweats, and weight loss (>10%) constitute 'B' symptoms and are common in advanced stages.

Subtypes

Two subtypes:
1. Classical HL includes nodular sclerosing (commonest), mixed cellularity, and lymphocyte-depleted histology.
2. Nodular lymphocyte-predominant HL is characterized by its distinctive histology and favourable prognosis.

Staging (Ann Arbor system)

- Stage I: single site.
- Stage II: >1 site and on one side.
- Stage III: on both sides of the diaphragm.
- Stage IV: disseminated disease.

Investigations

- CT of neck, chest, abdomen, and pelvis.
- Fluorodeoxyglucose-PET (FDG-PET) scan.
- Bone marrow aspiration and trephine.
- EBV serology.
- Isotope bone scan (generally done with stage IV disease, evidence of bone pain, or B symptoms).

Treatment

- Low-stage disease may be cured with involved field radiotherapy alone.
- Chemotherapy usually includes alkylating agents, vinca alkaloids, anthracyclines, and steroids. PET scanning is used in monitoring of disease and determination of therapy.

Prognosis

5y survival >90% (stage IV, 70%; stage I, 97%).

Relapse

Cure is still possible with second-line therapy, including autologous stem cell transplant.

Central nervous system tumours

Brain tumours are the second commonest cancer in children and account for 25% of all childhood malignancies (see Box 15.2 for classification).

> **Box 15.2 Classification of CNS tumours**
> - *Infratentorial tumours (>50%):* present with raised ICP, headaches and vomiting, and cerebellar ataxia.
> - *Supratentorial tumours:* present with raised ICP, focal neurology, hypothalamic/pituitary dysfunction, and visual impairment.
> - *Primary spinal tumours (rare):* may present with cord compression/focal neurology.
> - *CNS metastases:* of extracranial tumours (rare).

Initial management

Diagnostic imaging
- CT is quick and readily available. It provides essential information for emergency management of hydrocephalus.
- MRI gives tumour definition, and spinal MRI used for staging.

Raised intracranial pressure
This requires prompt treatment:
- Referral and transfer to a paediatric neurosurgical unit.
- Control tumour swelling with high-dose steroids (usually dexamethasone, but discuss with oncologist).
- CSF drainage: initial surgery may involve CSF diversion only or combined with biopsy/resection, depending on tumour location.

Low-grade glioma (grade I, 45% of CNS tumours)

Most are pilocytic astrocytoma. Cerebellum and optic pathway are commonest sites. Outcome depends on site. Posterior fossa lesions can be cured with surgery alone, whereas optic pathway tumours are relatively inaccessible and morbidity is high.

Neurofibromatosis type 1 (NF1)
(See ⮞ Neurofibromatosis, p. 383.)
- 50% of optic pathway low-grade gliomas.
- Visual outcome better.
- Radiotherapy contraindicated—↑ risk of second tumours.

High-grade glioma (grades III/IV, 10% of CNS tumours)

Predominantly occur in older children and teenagers. Supratentorial sites predominate. Difficult to manage since complete resection, essential for good outcome, is difficult to achieve.

Diffuse brainstem glioma

Glioma in the region of the pons, usually high-grade and inoperable. Radiotherapy is the mainstay of treatment. Median survival <1y.

Primitive neuroectodermal tumours (PNETs) (25% of CNS tumours)

- Commonest malignant brain tumours of childhood.
- Majority occur in the cerebellum (medulloblastoma).
- Peak incidence is <5y.
- Tumour metastases (mainly via the CSF) in 10–15%.
- 70% of localized cases can be cured.
- Significant long-term morbidity from radiotherapy.

Treatment
Treatment includes excision, craniospinal radiotherapy, and chemotherapy.

Ependymoma (10% of CNS tumours)

Periventricular sites. Usually present with obstructive hydrocephalus; 10% metastasize to the spine. Treated by surgical excision and involves field radiotherapy. Chemotherapy used in younger patients to delay radiotherapy. >70% survival if complete excision.

CNS germ cell tumours (GCTs) (5% of CNS tumours)

Rare and commoner in teenage ♂. In the midline (suprasellar or pineal)—60% of malignant cases are germinomas, and 40% non-germinomatous (secreting) malignant GCTs. Mature teratomas seen more in younger patients.
- *Secreting tumours:* raised markers (AFP/hCG) in serum or CSF.
- *Primary surgery for teratoma:* chemotherapy and radiotherapy for other tumour types.

Cure in 70% of secreting tumours and >90% of germinomas/teratomas.

Craniopharyingioma (10% of CNS tumours)

Slow-growing suprasellar, midline epithelial tumours from 'Rathke's pouch'. *Treatment* is complete resection in 80%, and partial resection with focal radiotherapy in the remainder. Complications include damage to hypothalamic–pituitary structures and visual and behavioural disturbances.

Retinoblastoma (3% of all tumours)

Sporadic or familial (40%) forms that are unilateral or bilateral (30%) on presentation. Present with absent or abnormal light reflex (leucocoria), squint, or visual deterioration. *Treatment* includes surgery, chemotherapy, and focal therapy. >90% 5y survival, but inherited form is at risk of second primary malignancy.

Neuroblastoma

Malignant embryonal tumour with multiple, variable presentations.

It represents 5% of all childhood malignancies. Median age of presentation 2y. Sites of involvement include:
- Adrenal glands (46%).
- Sympathetic chain.

May be locally invasive; surrounds, rather than displaces, vessels and other structures. May metastasize to bone, bone marrow, liver, CNS, lungs, and skin (especially infants).

Presentation

Non-specific and variable, but commonly:
- Palpable mass (may be painless).
- Compression of nerves of spinal cord, airway, veins, and bowel.
- Bone: pain and/or limp.
- Lymphadenopathy and signs of pancytopenia.
- Sweating, pallor, watery diarrhoea, and hypertension.

Specific diagnostic tests

- Urine catecholamine [VMA or homovanillic acid (HVA)]-to-creatinine ratio, which is raised in >80% cases.
- ^{131}I-MIBG uptake scan: usually +ve.

Treatment

Biological factors, such as *MYCN* gene amplification and 17q gain, strongly influence prognosis and treatment:
- Completely resected localized neuroblastoma may need no further treatment.
- Incompletely resected stage 3 tumours require chemotherapy and possibly adjuvant radiotherapy.
- Stage 4 (disseminated) and *MYCN* +ve stage 3 tumours require induction chemotherapy, surgery, high-dose chemotherapy with autologous stem cell rescue, radiotherapy, and differentiation therapy. Targeted antibody treatment is used. The exception is young (<18mth old) stage 4 patients with favourable biological features (disease restricted to bone marrow, liver, and skin), with disease that may resolve spontaneously, or who receive moderately intensive chemotherapy and surgery only.

Prognosis

Disseminated neuroblastoma only cured in 20–30% of cases, despite intensive treatment. Survival in low-risk cases (low stage, infants) is >90%.

Wilms' tumour (nephroblastoma)

An embryonal tumour causing 90% of renal tumours in children. Up to 75% present at 1–3y of age. Most causes are sporadic, but 1% have an affected family member. Wilms' tumour may be associated with:
- GU abnormalities, e.g. horseshoe kidney, hypospadias.
- Hemihypertrophy syndrome.
- Aniridia.
- BWS.
- *WAGR complex:* Wilms', aniridia, gonadal dysplasia, and retardation,
- Denys–Drash syndrome (nephropathy and genital abnormalities).
- Perlman syndrome.

Mutations of the *WT1* tumour suppressor gene on chromosome 11p13 detected in Wilms' tumours, and abnormalities of 11p15 are also implicated, associated with BWS.

Presentation

Visible or palpable abdominal mass, haematuria, and hypertension. Bilateral cases are unusual, and extrarenal Wilms' tumours are very rare. Metastases in 10%, most commonly pulmonary.

Investigations
- Abdominal USS.
- CT scan of abdomen ('claw' sign in involved kidney).
- CXR or CT.
- Urine catecholamines to exclude neuroblastoma.
- FBC, U&E, and coagulation studies.

Treatment
- Surgical excision required.
- Chemotherapy is used for all tumours.
- Stage I disease (complete resection of tumour without breach of renal capsule) is curable with vincristine.
- Vincristine and dactinomycin used for stage II disease.
- In higher-stage disease, doxorubicin is added.
- *Local/abdominal radiotherapy* in incomplete resection (stage III).
- If metastases (stage IV), surgery to primary tumour is delayed until resolution with chemotherapy, and radiotherapy is also added.

Prognosis

Overall survival 90%.

Relapse

Follow-up includes regular CXR, as well as abdominal USS, as pulmonary relapse is twice as common as local recurrence.

Bone tumours

(See also ➲ Benign bone tumours, p. 686; ➲ Malignant bone tumours, p. 672.) These tumours are rare in childhood (4% of all paediatric malignancies).
- Incidence peaks in teenage years.
- Majority of cases are osteosarcoma (OS) or Ewing's sarcoma (ES).
- Sarcomas associated with Li–Fraumeni syndrome (familial mutation of *p53*). Patients cured of familial retinoblastoma are at high risk of OS.

Osteosarcoma

OS presents with localized pain and swelling, pathological fracture, and rarely erythema. Most affect the long bones around the knee (67%) and the humerus. The metaphysis is a commoner site than the mid shaft. Delay in diagnosis is common.

Metastases
Seen at diagnosis in 15–25% of cases.
- Lungs commonest site, followed by bones.

Diagnostic investigations
- Plain X-rays of bony lesion.
- Biopsy (for definitive diagnosis).
- MRI of primary site.
- CT chest.
- Isotope bone scan.

Treatment
Chemotherapy, followed by surgery and then further chemotherapy. The aim is to perform limb-preserving surgery whenever possible.

Prognosis
Worse if inability to resect primary tumour or poor response to induction chemotherapy.

Relapsed OS
Mostly isolated pulmonary metastases. Surgical resection can result in long-term survival in 20–30% of patients.

Ewing's sarcoma of bone and soft tissues

ES usually occurs in bone but may also occur in soft tissues. ES and peripheral PNETs (NB: not the same as CNS PNETs) share immunophenotype. Both tumours belong to the Ewing's family of tumours.

Presentation
Localized pain and swelling, and sometimes pathological fracture. Diaphysis of long bones more commonly affected than metaphysis. Axial skeleton involved more often than in OS, with pelvis the commonest site. Metastases to lungs and bone are commoner at diagnosis than in OS.

Diagnostic investigations
- Plain X-rays of bony lesion.
- Biopsy (for definitive diagnosis).
- MRI of primary site.
- CT chest.
- Isotope bone scan.
- Bone marrow aspirates and trephines (bilateral).

Treatment
Chemotherapy, followed by surgery and then further chemotherapy. For extremity sites, limb-preserving surgery is the aim whenever possible. Radiotherapy is an effective adjunct.

Prognosis
Adverse outlook associated with:
- Large primaries.
- Axial sites (spine, sacrum, pelvis, scapula, clavicle, rib cage).
- Poor response to induction chemotherapy.
- Metastatic disease.

Bony metastases confer a particularly grave prognosis, with <20% long-term survivors.

Rhabdomyosarcoma

RMS is the commonest soft tissue sarcoma in childhood (51% of all soft tissue sarcomas). It accounts for 6% of all childhood malignancies (commonly aged <10y). Mostly embryonal or alveolar (more aggressive) subtypes. Botryoid (good prognosis) and spindle cell types are also recognized. A small number of cases are associated with Li–Fraumeni syndrome.

Presenting features

- Mass, pain, and obstruction of: bladder, pelvis, nasopharynx, parameningeal, paratestis, extremity, orbit, intrathoracic.
- Lymph node involvement is common.
- Distant metastases are rare.

Diagnosis and staging

- Imaging of primary site: CT or MRI.
- Biopsy for histological, molecular, and cytogenetic analysis.
- CT scan of chest.
- Bone marrow aspirates and trephines.
- Isotope bone scan.
- LP (if parameningeal primaries).

Treatment

- Chemotherapy: ifosfamide or cyclophosphamide, dactinomycin/ actinomycin, vincristine, anthracyclines.
- Surgery is reserved for accessible sites (paratesticular, extremities).
- Radiotherapy.

Prognosis

Ranges from <10% survival for bony metastatic disease to >90% for excised paratesticular tumours. Favourable features are:

- Younger age at diagnosis.
- Botryoid or embryonal histology.
- Paratesticular or superficial head and neck sites.
- Absence of nodal involvement or distant metastases.

Relapse

- Second-line chemotherapy.
- Radiotherapy may be employed at sites not previously irradiated.

  Outcome for relapse and recurrence is poor.

Germ cell tumours

Heterogenous group of neoplasms, often with mixed histology. Arise from primordial germ cells in gonads or, following aberrant germ cell migration, in midline extragonadal sites, including sacrococcygeal, mediastinal, or CNS sites. GCTs are rare, occurring in 3–5 per million children <15y of age, with peak incidence seen in children aged <3y.

- Mature teratoma is benign.
- Immature teratoma may disseminate locally.
- Malignant GCTs:
  - *Germinoma* is totipotent.
  - *Teratoma, yolk sac tumour* (YST), choriocarcinoma (CHC), and embryonal carcinoma (EC) represent more differentiated forms.
- Secreting tumours (YST, CHC, some immature teratomas, and mixed tumours) characterized by secretion of AFP and/or hCG, which may be used for diagnosis, monitoring of treatment response, and detection of recurrence.

Presenting symptoms

- *Site-dependent:* testicular masses are usually painless. Ovarian tumours present as either painful or painless abdominal mass.
- *Metastases:* rarely present at diagnosis.

Diagnosis and staging

- Measurement of AFP and β-hCG in serum (in CSF for CNS disease).
- Imaging and biopsy of primary: USS, CT, or MRI.
- CT scan of chest and abdomen, bone marrow, and isotope bone scan to look for metastases.

Prognosis

Survival >90% for malignant extracranial GCTs.

Other rare tumours

Primary liver tumours

(1% of all childhood cancers)

- Hepatoblastoma (HBL) is the commonest primary paediatric hepatic tumour (81% of cases), with two-thirds of cases in the first year of life. Serum AFP levels are raised in >80% HBL.
- HCC, embryonal (undifferentiated) sarcoma, 18% of primary liver tumours.

Treatment

- Chemotherapy for HBL.
- Good surgical result is critical for long-term survival. Liver transplant is indicated if local resection not possible.

Prognosis

Long-term survival for HBL is 86%. Survival for HCC is significantly lower (<30%)

Malignant melanoma

Most cases arise on healthy skin and may be related to sun exposure. Risk factors include:

- Pre-existing conditions.
- Giant congenital naevi, dysplastic naevus syndrome.
- Xeroderma pigmentosum.
- Albinism.
- Immunosuppressive diseases.

Rhabdoid tumours

Highly aggressive tumours that arise in the kidneys or CNS. In the CNS, they appear histologically similar to PNETs but sometimes are associated with tumours outside the CNS. Treatment includes surgery, chemotherapy, and radiotherapy. Long-term survival is rare.

Phaeochromocytoma

Tumours of adrenal medulla and sympathetic ganglia. Usually sporadic but may occur with VHL disease and MEN types IIa and b (see ● Multiple endocrine neoplasia, p. 423). Search for endocrine manifestations (e.g. hypertension, excessive sweating) or a mass. <10% of phaeochromocytomas are malignant.

Investigations

- Plasma/urine catecholamines are usually raised.

Treatment

- Surgery after α-adrenergic antagonists to control sympathetic symptoms.

Other carcinomas

These carcinomas are rare.
- Thyroid (predominantly the papillary variant and associated with exposure to radiation). May present with asymmetrical nodular goitre (see ➲ Solitary thyroid nodule, p. 409; ➲ Thyroid carcinoma, p. 409).
- Adrenal carcinoma (seen in young adults, with occasional occurrences in older children). May present with precocious puberty, inappropriate virilization in ♀ (see ➲ Peripheral precocious puberty, p. 452).

Langerhans cell histiocytosis (LCH)

Disorder of unknown cause with a range of presentations. Non-malignant, but may behave like malignancy in the most severe forms. LCH results from monoclonal proliferation/accumulation of histiocytes, with Langerhans cells, in skin, bone, pituitary, CNS, lungs, intestines, spleen, or bone marrow. Single-system disease confined to bone (occasionally skin) and seen more in older children. Natural history varied with spontaneous resolution, repeated recurrence, or death.

Incidence
- ~1/200 000 children affected each year.

Presentation
Depends on site of disease but may include:
- Pain or lump associated with isolated bony disease (commonest).
- Skin rash (widespread macular–papular or mimicking seborrhoeic dermatitis of the scalp).
- Discharge from the ear.
- DI.
- Systemic disturbance (fever, malaise, anorexia, and FTT).

Diagnosis
Biopsy with confirmation of Birbeck granules (or +ve CD1a or S100 immunohistochemistry). Diagnosis can be made without biopsy in the presence of characteristic pituitary/hypothalamic abnormality, where biopsy is considered too hazardous, or biopsy of lytic bone lesions with clinical features suggesting spontaneous resolution.

Further investigation
- Skeletal survey.
- Abdominal USS.
- EMU for osmolality.
- FBC and film, coagulation studies, and LFTs.

Treatment
- Single-system LCH (usually bone or skin) frequently resolves spontaneously or following biopsy/surgical curettage, but may require topical or intralesional steroids in persistent or recurrent cases.
- Multisystem LCH, seen mainly in young patients (aged <2y), requires treatment with steroids and chemotherapy (vinblastine, etoposide, or MTX).

Prognosis
>80% survive long-term without significant sequelae. Survivors of multisystem or CNS disease may have lasting disabilities.

Haemophagocytic lymphohistiocytosis

Rare condition that may be primary [familial haemophagocytic (FHL)/erythrophagocytic lymphohistiocytosis (FEL)] or secondary to infection (sHLH). Characterized by accumulation of phagocytic mononuclear cells, rather than dendritic or antigen-presenting cells, as seen in LCH.

- *Presenting features include:* fever, splenomegaly, and cytopenia (two out of three cell lines—red cells, white cells, and platelets).
- *Neurological symptoms:* relating to ↑ CSF cell counts and protein sometimes seen.
- Lymphadenopathy, skin rash, jaundice, oedema, and hepatic dysfunction.
- *Biochemistry:* shows raised triglycerides and low fibrinogen, sometimes raised serum transaminases and ferritin levels.
- *Other investigations to consider:* viral, immunological, and genetic testing.

Treatment

Recovery may be spontaneous in sHLH with resolution of infection, but FHL is fatal without treatment:

- Steroids, etoposide, and IT MTX may stabilize the disease.
- Allogeneic BMT is required for cure.

Prognosis

Overall survival is >50%.

Chemotherapy

Given as adjuvant treatment (following surgery) or neoadjuvant treatment (before surgery). Drug combinations used to increase efficacy, reduce development of resistance, and limit single-organ toxicity. Maximizing dose intensity (treatment frequency) increases efficacy.

- *Short-term side effects:* vomiting, myelosuppression, alopecia, and mucositis (inflammation of mucous membranes).
- *Long-term effects:* on organ function (kidneys, gonads, hearing, heart).

Safe administration of chemotherapy

Chemotherapy should only be given by individuals fully trained in the avoidance and management of complications, working in centres fully equipped and accredited to support chemotherapy.

Route

- IV: CVL is preferred. Risk of extravasation from peripheral access greatest with vinca alkaloids and anthracyclines.
- IT: usually for treatment or prophylaxis of CNS disease in leukaemia, NHL, and some CNS tumours—safety arrangements for IT treatment are paramount.

Dosage

Usually calculated according to body surface area. IV fluid to prevent tumour lysis syndrome (see ➜ Tumour lysis syndrome, p. 614) for certain drugs (e.g. ifosfamide, cisplatin, MTX). Mesna is given with cyclophosphamide and ifosfamide to protect from bladder inflammation.

Monitoring

The type and level of monitoring depend on agents used. This may include peripheral blood cell counts, GFR measurement, and echocardiogram before and between courses of chemotherapy.

Structural analogues of chemicals found in intermediate steps in synthesis of nucleic acids and proteins

- 6MP: 6-thioguanine (6TG), cytarabine (ara-C), fludarabine (used in leukaemia, NHL).
- MTX used in leukaemia, NHL, and OS.

Side effects include renal toxicity (MTX), myelosuppression, hepatotoxicity, and mucositis.

Anti-tumour antibiotics

Originally isolated from bacteria and fungi, they have antibiotic and anti-tumour activity.

- Anthracycline: daunorubicin, doxorubicin, idarubicin, mitoxantrone, and epirubicin used in leukaemia, NHL, HL, neuroblastoma, Wilms' tumour, and sarcoma. *Side effects*—myelotoxicity, alopecia, mucositis, cardiotoxicity.
- Bleomycin used in Hodgkin's disease and GCTs. *Side effects*—include pulmonary toxicity.
- Actinomycin D (dactinomycin) used in Wilms' tumour, soft tissue, and ES. *Side effects*—myelotoxicity (mild), hepatotoxicity.

Epipodophyllotoxins—semi-synthetic analogues of podophyllotoxin

They stabilize normally transient DNA–protein complexes by inhibition of topoisomerase I or II:

- Etoposide (VP16): inhibits topoisomerase II. Used in leukaemia, NHL, neuroblastoma, sarcoma, GCTs, CNS tumours, palliative chemotherapy (low dose). *Side effects*—include hypotension, myelotoxicity, alopecia, hepatotoxicity, mucositis, and secondary leukaemia.
- Topotecan and irinotecan inhibit topoisomerase I. Used in neuroblastoma, sarcoma, and CNS tumours.

Vinca alkaloids

Bind to tubulin, interfering with mitotic spindle:

- Vincristine. Used in leukaemias, NHL, Hodgkin's disease, CNS tumours, Wilms' tumour, and sarcoma. *Side effects*—include neurotoxicity.
- Vinblastine. Used in Hodgkin's disease, anaplastic large cell lymphoma. *Side effects*—include myelotoxicity and mucositis.

Alkylating agents

Covalent binding to DNA, to prevent replication and transcription:

- Cyclophosphamide, ifosfamide: used in leukaemia, lymphoma, sarcoma, neuroblastoma, high-risk Wilms' tumour, and CNS tumours.
- Melphalan, busulfan: conditioning for BMT.
- Chlorambucil (Hodgkin's disease).
- Lomustine (CCNU): used in CNS tumours.

Side effects include: myelosuppression, alopecia, mucositis, tubular nephropathy (ifosfamide), bladder toxicity (cyclophosphamide), encephalopathy (ifosfamide), late effects on fertility, and secondary leukaemia (CCNU).

Platinum compounds

- Cisplatin and carboplatin in sarcoma, neuroblastoma, and CNS tumours.

Side effects include: high emetogenicity, nephrotoxicity, ototoxicity, neurotoxicity (mainly cisplatin), and myelotoxicity (carboplatin).

Other therapeutic agents

- Steroids: as well as symptom control and reduction of oedema, particularly around CNS tumours, have direct anti-tumour effects in haematological malignancies.
- L-asparaginase: depletes pool of asparagine, needed by some malignancies, e.g. ALL. *Side effects*—hypersensitivity, coagulopathy, and rarely pancreatitis.

Stem cell transplant

High-dose therapy

This involves the delivery of myeloablative doses of chemotherapy and/or radiotherapy, followed by rescue with haematopoietic stem cells. The latter may be autologous (from patient) or allogeneic (from sibling or unrelated donor, or haplo-identical from parent).

Indications for use in treatment of childhood malignancy:

• Selected high-risk leukaemia and relapsed ALL (from allogeneic donor).
• High-risk solid tumours, including metastatic neuroblastoma, and high-risk ES (autologous).

Stem cells are harvested from bone marrow or peripheral blood by leucopheresis, following 'mobilization' with granulocyte colony-stimulating factor (G-CSF).

Conventional BMT is used for allografts. Peripheral blood stem cell transplants (PBSCTs) are favoured for autografts. This offers advantages, including less risk of tumour contamination, more rapid engraftment, less severe infections, and avoidance of anaesthetic. Conditioning for BMT involves myeloablative radiotherapy or chemotherapy. The aim is to achieve a state of complete remission prior to conditioning. Monoclonal antibodies are used to suppress immune function of donor T-lymphocytes against recipient.

Outcome

Allografts carry greater risk, with ~10% procedure-related mortality. Morbidity and mortality from stem cell transplant are due to:

• Graft failure.
• Infection secondary to profound immune suppression.
• Mucositis.
• Veno-occlusive disease of the liver.
• Multiorgan failure related to the conditioning regimen.

Graft-versus-host disease

(See also ➜ Transfusion-associated graft-versus-host disease (TaGVHD), p. 583.) GVHD occurs when WBCs in the donor bone marrow/blood/stem cells recognize the recipient as foreign and attack the recipient. GVHD can be acute or chronic. Risk increases if the donor is HLA-mismatched as T-cells from the donor attack the transplant recipient's cells/tissues. GVHD may affect any organ system, but commonly the skin, liver, and GI system. Ciclosporin or tacrolimus are given as prophylaxis, and steroids, monoclonal antibodies, and other immunosuppressants may be used in treatment.

Radiotherapy

In the use of ionizing radiation to kill cancer cells, dose and fractionation (number of treatments to deliver a total dose) vary according to the nature of the tumour and tolerance of the tissue. Strategies to increase therapeutic success include:

- Conformal radiotherapy: matching beam to three-dimensional shape of target, and so sparing surrounding tissue.
- Hyperfractionation and acceleration.
- Targeted radiotherapy with specific isotopes, e.g. ^{131}I-MIBG for neuroblastoma.
- Radiosurgery (high-dose single fraction), brachytherapy (direct application of radionuclides to tumour).
- Proton-targeted beam therapy (reduced dose to non-target tissues).

Indications

- Selected cases of Hodgkin's disease, neuroblastoma, Wilms' tumour, soft tissue and ES, and most subgroups of CNS tumours.
- Limited benefit in OS, extracranial GCTs, and NHL.
- In leukaemia, limited to treatment of CNS and testicular disease and to conditioning for BMT.
- Symptom control in palliative care, e.g. bony metastases, spinal cord compression.

Preparation for radiotherapy

- Planning, by combination of CT and MRI scanning.
- Immobilization using masks/shells and tattoos as markers; sedation or GA for youngest children.
- Protection of surrounding tissues, e.g. gonads, using lead shields.
- Play therapists have a central role in this process.

Side effects

- Acute effects include nausea and vomiting, cutaneous erythema and desquamation, diarrhoea, myelosuppression, pneumonitis, and hepatitis. Toxicity is potentiated by actinomycin D (dactinomycin) or anthracyclines.
- Late effects on growth, endocrine function, CNS, heart, lungs, kidneys, and liver (see ⊃ Principles of follow-up, pp. 616–17).
- Risk of second malignancy, particularly bone tumours.

Surgery

Surgical interventions for solid tumours include the following:

- Resection, primary or following chemotherapy. Completeness of excision influences subsequent adjunctive treatment, e.g. bone tumours, Wilms' tumour, hepatoblastoma, and most CNS tumours.
- Raised ICP and spinal cord compression.
- Tunnelled CVLs for chemotherapy.

Acute care of infection risk

All paediatric oncology centres have clear guidelines for supportive management, which should be used. *This section is not a substitute for such guidelines.* Of note:

- Neutropenic fever is an emergency.
- Immunocompromised children may succumb to overwhelming sepsis within hours.
- Greatest risk is associated with the nadir in WBC (typically at around 10 days) for most regimens.
- In the absence of neutropenia, CVL infection should be considered, particularly if there are symptoms (e.g. rigors) on line flushing.

Febrile neutropenia/neutropenic sepsis

Fever (temperature >38.5°C) with neutrophil count <0.5 × 10⁹/L, leading to ↑ risk of bacterial infections.

Causes

- Skin or GI bacterial flora.
- Greatest risk from Gram –ve organisms, including *Pseudomonas*.
- Gram +ve organisms may be associated with CVL/CVC.

Examination

Include inspection of the skin, mouth, IV line sites, surgical sites, and the perianal area.

Investigations

- FBC and differential count, CRP.
- Culture of blood, urine, stool, swabs of throat, nose, suspicious skin lesions, or CVL exit sites.
- CXR/AXR if indicated by symptoms or signs.

Treatment

- Start broad-spectrum antibiotics without delay because infection with Gram –ve bacilli *may be fatal within hours*.
- Antibiotic choice will vary by institution and local resistance patterns but must include adequate cover for *Pseudomonas* and Gram +ve organisms. Include anaerobic cover in the presence of abdominal pain, diarrhoea, or mucositis. Appropriate agents include:
  - Piptazobactam, ceftazidime, ciprofloxacin, meropenem, gentamicin, amikacin (Gram –ve cover).
  - Vancomycin, teicoplanin (Gram +ve organisms, including coagulase –ve staphylococci).
  - Metronidazole, meropenem (anaerobic cover).
- Review antibiotic choice according to culture results.

Specific infections

Viral infections in immunocompromised patients

- VZV: if in contact and non-immune, give prophylactic aciclovir or ZIG. Active chickenpox or shingles should be treated aggressively with IV aciclovir.
- HSV: may cause painful oral ulceration; treat early with aciclovir.

Other viruses

- CMV, RSV, and adenovirus may all cause pneumonitis, associated with high morbidity and mortality, especially in BMT patients.

Fungal infections

(See also ➲ Candidiasis, p. 650; ➲ Aspergillosis, pp. 650–1.)

- Consider in prolonged febrile neutropenia and treat promptly. Mortality remains high but is reduced with newer therapeutic agents.
- Clinical spectrum includes pulmonary aspergillosis, hepatic candidiasis, and abscess formation.
- Risk is highest during intensive chemotherapy with prolonged neutropenia, such as AML treatment, re-induction for relapsed leukaemia, and following BMT.
- Treatment includes fluconazole (limited cover), itraconazole, amphotericin (liposomal formulation for reduced toxicity), voriconazole, and caspofungin. Prophylaxis is used in high-risk treatment regimens (e.g. AML).

Pneumocystis jiroveci pneumonia (PJP)

(See also ➲ Pneumocystis jiroveci pneumonia, p. 651).

- *Interstitial pneumonitis:* associated with prolonged immunosuppression; presents with tachypnoea, dry cough, and low SpO_2.
- *Prophylaxis (patients on chemotherapy lasting over 6mth):* co-trimoxazole, monthly pentamidine nebulizers, or dapsone.
- *Treatment:* high dose co-trimoxazole, steroids in severe cases.

Biochemical crises in oncology care

Tumour lysis syndrome

Lysis of malignant cells on starting chemotherapy releases intracellular contents, exceeding renal excretory capacity and physiological buffering mechanisms with abnormalities, including:
• Hyperuricaemia.
• Hyperkalaemia.
• Hyperphosphataemia and reciprocal hypocalcaemia.
• Dehydration, leading to risk of ARF.

Mostly seen in ALL, NHL (especially B-cell); occasionally in AML; rarely in solid tumours (e.g. GCT, neuroblastoma). Occurs spontaneously or precipitated by single dose of steroids or chemotherapy. Risk is ↑ with high WCC, bulky disease, and pre-existing renal impairment or infiltration.

Management
Key is prevention and monitoring.
• *Hyperhydration:* e.g. IV 5% dextrose with 0.45% saline at 2–3L/m^2/day, started before treatment and continued until stable biochemical parameters. Avoid added K$^+$.
• Ensure good renal output, with cautious diuretic (furosemide) if necessary.
• Allopurinol reduces urate precipitation; use urate oxidase in high-risk cases.
• *Hyperkalaemia:* may need treatment with salbutamol, calcium resonium (polystyrene sulfonate), dextrose/insulin, and haemofiltration (see ➋ Hyperkalaemia, p. 73).
• *Hyperphosphataemia/hypocalcaemia:* increase fluids; haemofiltration in extreme cases; avoid Ca^{2+} unless symptomatic (tetany, seizures).

Other biochemical disturbances

(See ➋ Other fluid and electrolyte disorders, pp. 78–9; ➋ Hypercalcaemia, p. 428.)

Hypercalcaemia
Rarely complicates malignancy (usually disseminated), e.g. RMS. Manage with hyperhydration (NS) and furosemide; bisphosphonates more effective than steroids or calcitonin.

Renal toxicity
Due to chemotherapy or antibiotics, and particular care needed when any of these drugs are used in combination:
• Cisplatin (glomerular function, Mg^{2+} loss), ifosfamide (tubular losses of Mg^{2+}, PO$_4$$^{2+}$, HCO$_3$$^-$), high-dose MTX.
• Amphotericin (glomerular toxicity and heavy K$^+$ loss), aminoglycosides, vancomycin.

Other acute oncology care problems

Acute abdomen

Possible causes in the oncology patient include the following.

- *Gastric haemorrhage:* secondary to gastritis or ulceration. Risk factors include high-dose steroids and raised ICP.
- *Pancreatitis:* especially with steroids or L-asparaginase treatment.
- *Neutropenic enterocolitis or typhlitis:* bacterial invasion (*Clostridium, Pseudomonas*) leads to inflammation, full-thickness infarction, and perforation. It is associated with leukaemia. *Symptoms of pain ± fever may be masked by concomitant steroids.* The key to management is early, appropriate antibiotic cover on first suspicion and early involvement of surgeons. Mortality is high.

Haematological support

Blood products should be leucodepleted to reduce viral transmission and incidence of reactions. Irradiated products should be used in some patients to prevent TaGVHD, e.g. around the time of stem cell harvesting, following BMT.

- *Threshold for red cell transfusion:* usually Hb <70g/L, but teenagers are often symptomatic at higher levels (caution if high-count leukaemia, long-standing anaemia, or heart failure).
- *Platelets:* should be >10 × 10^9/L if well, >20 × 10^9/L if febrile or for minor procedure (e.g. LP), >30 × 10^9/L if brain tumour, and >50 × 10^9/L after significant bleed or for major surgery. These thresholds are overridden when there is active bleeding.

Nausea and vomiting

Chemotherapy varies in its emetogenicity—PO antimetabolites and vincristine require no prophylaxis; cisplatin and ifosfamide require multiple agents. Aim to prevent severe symptoms.

- *First-line:* domperidone or metoclopramide.
- *Second-line:* ondansetron (5HT antagonist).
- *Dexamethasone:* useful adjunct, but not in ALL/NHL induction or CNS tumours.
- *Other agents:* hyoscine, cyclizine useful in CNS tumours. In severe cases, nabilone, methotrimeprazine, and prochlorperazine can help.

Nutrition and mucositis

Good nutrition is essential for recovery from malignancy, the direct effects of treatment, mucositis, and infection:

- A dietician is central to successful nutrition.
- Chemotherapy-induced mucositis → oral ulceration, pain, and diarrhoea. Good mouth care (basic oral hygiene and antiseptic mouthwashes) helps prevent some infective complications. Prompt analgesia allows maintenance of oral intake for as long as possible.

Principles of follow-up

Follow-up after completion of treatment is focused on disease recurrence and long-term adverse effects of cancer and its treatment.

Monitoring for disease recurrence

This involves clinical review, combined with imaging or laboratory testing, to pick up pre-symptomatic recurrence, which may be amenable to further attempts at curative treatment. For example:
- CXRs and abdominal US: Hodgkin's disease.
- MRI scans: CNS tumours.
- Urine VMA and HVA: neuroblastoma.
- Serum AFP and hCG: GCTs.
- Peripheral blood counts: leukaemia.

Monitoring for late effects of treatment

Late effects of radiotherapy

May occur months to years after treatment. Sequelae usually progressive and irreversible, and depend on sites, dose, mode, and age at treatment.

Growth sequelae
- Direct effects on epiphyseal plates.
- GH deficiency from hypothalamic/pituitary damage.
- Muscle damage and avascular necrosis of bone.

CNS sequelae
- Somnolence and tiredness.
- Hypothalamic and pituitary damage.
- Intellectual effects: reduced numeracy and short-term memory.
- Radiation myelitis.
- Eyes: cataracts, retinal damage.

Other organ system sequelae
- Gonads: infertility/hypogonadism.

'Second' primary malignancies
- Risk of 4–6% of occurrence within radiotherapy field. Common second malignancies include solid tumours occurring in the field of radiotherapy.

Late effects of chemotherapy

Sequelae depend on age at the time of exposure, drugs, and doses. Well-recognized long-term toxicities include:
- Cardiotoxicity following anthracyclines.
- Nephrotoxicity following platinum drugs and alkylating agents.
- Pulmonary fibrosis following bleomycin.
- Impaired fertility following alkylating agents.
- Ototoxicity following platinum drugs and gentamicin.
- Second malignancies: leukaemia and MDS associated with topoisomerase II inhibitors and alkylating agents.

Fertility

Affected by gonadotoxic chemotherapy and radiotherapy fields that impinge on the gonads. The younger the patient when treated, the better the prognosis for future fertility. More spermatic recovery is seen after chemotherapy than after radiotherapy. Risk of gonadotrophin deficiency greatest for radiotherapy directed towards suprasellar and nasopharyngeal tumours, but fertility may be preserved with aid of pulsatile GnRH therapy.

Quality of survival

The long-term effects of treatment go beyond the purely physical consequences of treatment, and this is an evolving area of clinical research. Cancer survivors (and their family members) are at ↑ risk of impaired psychosocial well-being. Risk is not clearly associated with a specific cancer type or treatment and is likely to be multifactorial in origin. Survivors are also at ↑ risk of needing special education and, as they enter adulthood, of unemployment or underemployment.

Palliative care

Around 30% of children with cancer will die, mostly from progressive disease. Death from complications of treatment is more likely to be swift, with limited opportunity for preparation. Palliative care is the active total care of patients whose disease is no longer curable. It needs to embrace the physical, emotional, social, and spiritual needs of children and their families. Chemotherapy, radiotherapy, and surgery may still be used for palliation and control of symptoms.

Breaking bad news

It is extremely important to be honest with an open approach, avoiding false hope. What to tell the child is always difficult; many families tend to be over-protective. This risks loss of their child's trust when the truth can no longer be hidden.

Organization of care

Paediatricians specializing in palliative care lead care:
- *Location:* most children die at home, through family preference; some prefer a hospice, and a minority the acute hospital ward.
- A *multiprofessional* approach is required and will vary according to needs and organization of local health care.
- *Bereavement support* should be considered as part of the role of the palliative care team and may be provided by various disciplines within the team, depending on local arrangements.

Symptom control

Anticipated symptoms will depend on the diagnosis. Symptom control measures may be pharmacological or non-pharmacological. Aim to correct the underlying cause, e.g. constipation, infection. Good communication and consideration of psychosocial and spiritual factors will contribute to good control.

Pain

(See also ➔ Pain management, p. 932.)

- PO route is effective for most, until the terminal phase, when SC infusion, often in combination with antiemetics, sedatives, and AEDs, may be preferred. Transdermal route is used for some agents.
- Treat and recognize different types of pain, e.g. inflammatory and neuropathic pain, muscle spasm, and raised ICP. Combining different agents is more effective than escalating the dose of one.
- Adjuvants (additional drugs) in pain management include:
  - Analgesics for specific circumstances such as gabapentin for neuropathic pain, anti-spasmodics (hyoscine, glycopyrronium), muscle relaxants (diazepam), corticosteroids, and bisphosphonates.
  - Drugs for adverse analgesic effects, e.g. laxatives, antiemetics.

Other symptoms

- *Nausea, vomiting:* domperidone, cyclizine (particularly for raised ICP), methotrimeprazine, haloperidol, ondansetron, metoclopramide.
- *Convulsions, cerebral irritation:* diazepam, midazolam.
- *Spinal cord compression:* dexamethasone, radiotherapy, bladder and bowel management.
- *Terminal restlessness:* midazolam.
- *Dyspnoea:* non-pharmacological measures (position, play therapy, fan), opioids, benzodiazepines, O_2, steroids.
- *Excess secretions:* hyoscine, glycopyrronium.
- *Anxiety, depression:* diazepam, methotrimeprazine, amitriptyline.
- *Constipation:* anticipate and prescribe laxatives when starting opioids (use fentanyl as least constipating); may need high enemas.
- *Bowel obstruction:* anti-spasmodics, stool softeners, rectal preparations to reduce impaction; octreotide to reduce secretions and vomiting.
- *Sweating, from advanced disease, fever, or drugs:* cimetidine, NSAIDs.
- *Pruritus:* cimetidine if due to disease, antihistamine if opiate-induced.
- *Haematological (anaemia, haemorrhage, bruising):* transfuse (RBCs ± platelets) only for symptomatic improvement and quality of life; topical tranexamic acid or adrenaline for troublesome mucosal bleeding.

Further reading

Association for Paediatric Palliative Medicine. Available at: ℘ http://www.appm.org.uk.
HeadSmart. Information on brain tumours. Available at: ℘ http://www.headsmart.org.uk.

Infectious diseases

The child with fever

In children <5y, the body temperature should ideally be measured using a digital thermometer under the armpit. Other methods like chemical dot or tympanic thermometers are also in use. Normal temperature for younger children is around 36.4°C, but it may vary from child to child.
- A temperature of ≥38°C is generally regarded as a fever.
- Babies <4wk of age may not mount a significant febrile response to an infection and sometimes present with hypothermia.

Differential diagnosis

Most children with fever have a self-limiting viral infection. However, always consider other diagnoses, especially in high-risk groups:
- <6wk of age.
- Premature infants.
- Known comorbidity (e.g. congenital cardiac condition, trisomy 21, bronchiectasis, diabetes mellitus, etc.).
- Immunodeficiency, whether confirmed or suspected.
- Immunosuppression (e.g. receiving chemotherapy, PO/systemic steroids, immunomodulating agents, etc.)

Antipyretics

(See also ➔ Fever, p. 933.) Potential measures (see ℜ http://www.nhs.uk/conditions/fever-in-children/):
- Tepid sponging/underdressing is *not recommended*.
- Regular paracetamol/ibuprofen is *not recommended*.
- Limit antipyretic use to children who are distressed with fever.

When there is no apparent cause of infection [pyrexia of unknown origin (PUO)], establish the body location of likely cause of infection, as well as potential treatments. Common diagnoses for febrile illness include:
- URTI (see ➔ Upper airway infection, p. 251).
- UTI (see ➔ Urinary tract infection, pp. 330–1).
- Bacteraemia (see ➔ Sepsis, p. 634).
- LRTI (see ➔ Pneumonia, pp. 258–9).
- Meningitis and encephalitis (see ➔ Meningitis, p. 634; ➔ Encephalitis/meningoencephalitis, p. 637).
- Osteomyelitis (see ➔ Septic arthritis and osteomyelitis, pp. 670–1).
- Bacterial gastroenteritis (see ➔ Bacterial gastroenteritis, p. 307).
- Endocarditis (see ➔ Infective bacterial endocarditis, pp. 212–13).
- Malaria (see ➔ Malaria, p. 644).
- TB (see ➔ Tuberculosis: presentation and diagnosis, pp. 639–40; ➔ Pulmonary tuberculosis, p. 262).
- Post-vaccination fever (diagnosis of exclusion).

Fever assessment

When assessing a child with a fever, a thorough history and examination are essential. The key priorities are:

- *History:* take parental concerns and perception of fever seriously. Ask about ill contacts and immunization, including travel vaccines and travel history. Cases suggestive of infection/exposure to a droplet or airborne infection should be isolated.
- *Measurements:* make sure that temperature, HR, RR, and CRT are measured, as this will determine the order of your priorities and identify the need for active resuscitation.
- *Signs and symptoms:* assess the child for the presence or absence of symptoms and signs indicating serious illness.

Table 16.1 summarizes the UK NICE *traffic light system* for the assessment of disease severity, based on presenting features with: green—low risk, amber—moderate risk, and red—high risk of severe disease.

Table 16.1 Classification of clinical features according to risk of disease

	Green	Amber	Red
Colour	Normal	Reported pallor	Pale/mottled/cyanosis
Activity	Normal	Sleepy, less active, poor social response	Difficult to rouse, high-pitched cry, no social response
Breathing	Normal	Mild distress, tachypnoea, crackles, SpO_2 ≤95%	Moderate to severe distress
Circulation/ hydration	Normal	Tachycardia, CRT ≥3s, dry membranes, poor feeding, reduced urine	Reduced skin turgor
Other	Nil amber/ red features	≥39°C, age 3–6mth, fever ≥5 days, rigors, limb swelling, not weight-bearing	≥38°C, age <3mth, non-blanching rash, bulging fontanelle, neck stiffness, focal neurology, seizures

Fever management

Children with solely *green* features are unlikely to require hospital admission. However, the following factors should be considered:
- Social circumstances and parental anxiety/concerns.
- Child's contact with serious illness/travel history.

If a child is discharged home, give parents clear verbal/written instructions about what to look for and when to call for medical help, e.g. online advice available at ℘ https://www.nhs.uk/conditions/fever-in-children/.

Children with *red/amber* features are likely to require observation/admission. Those with *red* features may have life-threatening illness and need urgent stabilization and treatment (see Table 16.1).
- In hypoxic children or those in shock, follow the emergency care outlined in Box 3.7.
- If there is no apparent source of infection, despite fever, then investigations should include the following:
  - *Blood:* culture, FBC, CRP, U&E, LFTs. EDTA sample for bacterial PCR (e.g. suspected meningococcal/pneumococcal septicaemia).
  - *Urine:* for UTI (dipstick and MC&S for <3y; MC&S if dipstick +ve in >3y).
  - *Throat swab:* bacterial and viral.
  - *LP:* low threshold <3mth; consider in older child with suspected meningitis if no contraindications (see ➔ Lumbar puncture, p. 30; ➔ Lumbar puncture, p. 63; ➔ Lumbar puncture, p. 635).
  - *CXR:* consider if high WBC or unwell with respiratory distress.
  - *Stool:* for MC&S and ova, cysts, parasites if history of foreign travel (specify areas visited). Virology only relevant for immunosuppressed/unwell patients (request extended enteric panel). Do not routinely test for *Clostridium difficile* in <2y, unless clinical concerns or suggestive history.

Infections characterized by rash

Childhood infections often have a rash. Most rashes are non-specific and not pathognomonic (see also ⊃ Exanthematous eruptions, p. 792). Therefore, the history and clinical picture as a whole are paramount. Common exanthemata are described in Box 16.1.

Box 16.1 Common classical exanthemata

Measles virus (rubeola)
- *Incubation:* 6–19 days (median 13 days).
- *Isolation:* until 4 days after the rash appears.
- *Features:* prodromal high fever, upper respiratory tract symptoms, conjunctivitis. Then morbilliform maculopapular rash 2–4 days later; starts on the face and spreads. Koplik spots (1mm small bluish white spots on buccal mucosa) rarely seen, but pathognomonic.
- *Complications:* otitis media, pneumonitis/bacterial pneumonia, encephalitis, ITP, subacute sclerosing panencephalitis (SSPE).
- *Diagnosis:* clinical, salivary measles PCR.
- *Differentials:* other viral exanthems, streptococcal disease, KD.
- *Treatment:* supportive.
- *Prevention:* MMR vaccination. Notifiable.

Group A Streptococcus (scarlet fever)
- *Incubation:* 2–5 days.
- *Isolation:* until 24h of appropriate treatment.
- *Rash:* fine papular rash on flushed skin, sandpaper texture, often followed by desquamation.
- *Features:* sore throat, strawberry tongue, rash, lymphadenopathy. Can cause invasive disease, including pneumonia, empyema, and endocarditis. Rheumatic fever/heart disease common, following missed/delayed treatment, in resource-poor countries.
- *Treatment:* phenoxymethylpenicillin for scarlet fever. IV benzylpenicillin/amoxicillin for invasive disease (liaise with infectious diseases specialist). Invasive disease notifiable.

Parvovirus (fifth disease/erythema infectiosum)
- *Incubation:* 4–14 days.
- *Isolation:* not recommended.
- *Rash:* slapped cheek appearance, erythema infectiosum.
- *Features:* 3–7 days prodrome, then rash for 1–4 days; then evanescent rash over 1–3wk, followed by arthropathy. Self-limiting. Congenital infection gives red cell aplasia and hydrops fetalis.
- *Treatment:* supportive. If congenital infection, fetal transfusion; IVIG in neonates with severe disease.

(Continued)

Box 16.1 (Contd.)

Human herpesvirus 6 (sixth disease/roseola infantum/exanthem subitum)
- *Incubation:* 10 days.
- *Isolation:* not recommended.
- *Rash:* maculopapular.
- *Features:* temperature for 3 days, improvement of fever with appearance of rash.
- *Treatment:* supportive.

Rubella virus (German measles)
- *Incubation:* 14–21 days.
- *Isolation:* from 7 days before to 7 days after the rash.
- *Rash:* maculopapular, rapidly spreads and fades.
- *Features:* enlarged lymph nodes at the back of the neck and ears. Congenital infection associated with retinopathy and cardiac defects.
- *Treatment:* supportive.
- *Prevention:* MMR vaccination, screening in pregnancy.

Lyme disease
- *Cause:* spirochaete *Borrelia burgdorferi*, transmitted by *Ixodes* species tick bite.
- *Incubation:* 3–20 days (median 12 days).
- *Rash—erythema migrans (EM):* painless, non-pruritic, erythematous, circular lesion spreads outward from the site of the bite, occasionally with central clearing. Commonest presenting feature in children typically presents 7–14 days after the bite (3–30 days).
- *Early localized disease (weeks):* symptoms of EM, fever, headache, myalgia, arthralgia, and lymphadenopathy fluctuate over several weeks.
- *Early disseminated disease (weeks):* may present with cutaneous dissemination with multiple EM lesions. Other manifestations are facial nerve palsy, meningitis, papilloedema, and myocarditis (rare).
- *Late disease (months):* large joint arthritis, peripheral neuropathy, CNS manifestations. Rare if received treatment early.
- *Diagnosis:* localized—history and clinical; bloods tests not recommended. Disseminated/late—ELISA antibody screening, followed by confirmatory western blot if +ve.
- *Treatment:* <8y, amoxicillin (azithromycin if definite penicillin allergy); ≥8y, doxycycline; cardiac/CNS: ceftriaxone. Early/disseminated: treat for 2–3wk; late disease: 3–4wk.

Chickenpox (VZV)
Member of the herpesvirus family. Primary infection known as chicken pox; occurs between the ages of 1–6y. Spread occurs by respiratory droplets or direct contact with lesions.
- *Incubation:* 10–21 days. School exclusion until all lesions crusted.
- *Rash:* starts at head and trunk. Progresses from red macules to papular, vesicular, pustular, and crusting stages.

Box 16.1 (Contd.)

- *Features:* fever, headache, anorexia, signs of URTI, itching. High-grade fever after appearance of rash is uncommon and may suggest secondary bacterial infection.
- *Diagnosis:* clinical. Vesicular fluid, blood, CSF VZV PCR, and blood VZV serology may be done in immunocompromised to confirm.
- *Treatment:* supportive; varicella-zoster immunoglobulin (VZIG). (For exposed at-risk individuals, refer to the *Green Book*, chapter 34, available at: ℘ https://www.gov.uk/government/publications/varicella-the-green-book-chapter-34.) IV aciclovir is used in encephalitis, pneumonia, neonatal infection, and immunocompromised patients. Vaccination is provided as part of the national schedule in many countries.
- *Complications:* bacterial infection, e.g. with GAS: infected lesions, cellulitis, necrotizing fasciitis, TSS. Others: pneumonitis, purpura fulminans, cerebrovascular stroke, and encephalitis. Complications common in infants and immunocompromised patients.

Herpes zoster (shingles)

Following primary infection, the virus remains dormant in the dorsal root ganglion, to reactivate later along a dermatomal distribution, known as shingles. Reactivation of latent infection may occur, leading to vesicular lesions in the distribution of a sensory nerve. Commoner in the immunosuppressed host.

Infectious mononucleosis (glandular fever)

Infectious mononucleosis is caused by EBV (90%) and CMV. The source is oropharyngeal secretion. The virus infects B-lymphocytes in pharyngeal tissue and spreads to the rest of the lymphoid system.

- *Incubation:* 4–6wk.
- *Features:* flu-like illness, lethargy, exudative pharyngitis; generalized lymphadenopathy; hepatosplenomegaly; maculopapular rash, especially if inadvertently treated with ampicillin (in 30%).
- *Diagnosis:* atypical lymphocytosis, low platelets, hepatitis, Paul Bunnell/Monospot test in older children (*low sensitivity*), +ve EBV, CMV PCR in early disease, +ve serology later.
- *Treatment:* supportive; avoid contact sport if splenomegaly noted.
- *Complications:* splenic rupture, meningoencephalitis, lymphoma, orchitis, myocarditis, pneumonia, G-BS.

Skin and soft tissue infection

Impetigo

- *Cause:* staphylococcal or streptococcal skin infection.
- *Age group:* infants and young children.
- *Features:* erythematous macules (later vesicular/bullous) on face, neck, hands; often associated with prior skin lesions (eczema).
- *Infectivity:* nasal carriage is often the source of infection. Auto-inoculation occurs and lesions are infectious until dry.
- *Antibiotics:* topical antimicrobials often *not useful*; in younger, if treatment required, PO antibiotic (amoxicillin, co-amoxiclav).

Boils (furuncles)

- *Cause:* *Staphylococcus aureus*.
- *Age group:* any age.
- *Features:* infection of hair follicles or sweat glands.
- *Infectivity:* nasal carriage—often source in recurrent boils.
- *Antibiotics:* flucloxacillin.

Periorbital cellulitis

(See ➔ Periorbital cellulitis, p. 981.)

- *Cause:* GAS, *S. aureus*, *Streptococcus pneumoniae*, rarely *Haemophilus influenzae* type b (HiB) in unimmunized children.
- *Age group:* any age.
- *Features:* fever with unilateral erythema, tenderness, and oedema of the eyelid, often following local trauma to the skin. Complications include local abscess, meningitis, and cavernous sinus thrombosis.
- *Investigations:* if severe (eye movements are not visible or complete ptosis), refer to ENT or ophthalmology and perform cranial CT scan.
- *Antibiotics:* IV co-amoxiclav for preseptal disease. IV ceftriaxone + metronidazole if concerned about orbital or intracranial involvement or poor response to IV co-amoxiclav in 24–48h.

Scalded skin syndrome

- *Cause:* exfoliative staphylococcal toxin, occasionally *Streptococcus*. (See also ➔ Staphylococcal scalded skin syndrome, p. 796.)
- *Age group:* infants and young children.
- *Features:* fever and malaise with a purulent, crusting, localized infection around the eyes, nose, and mouth. Later diffuse erythema and skin tenderness leading to separation of the epidermis through the granular cell layer. Nikolsky's sign is epidermal separation on light pressure, with no subsequent scarring after healing.
- *Antibiotics:* IV flucloxacillin 50mg/kg qds ± clindamycin.

Necrotizing fasciitis

- *Cause:* GAS, less common *S. aureus, Clostridium perfringens*.
- *Age group:* any age.
- *Features:* SC infection of tissue down to fascia and muscle. Symptoms may be due to shock, systemic illness, and severe pain.
- *Antibiotics:* IV piptazobactam + clindamycin, surgical debridement.

Toxic shock syndrome

(See Box 16.2.)

Box 16.2 Toxic shock syndrome

Cause
- Toxin-producing staphylococci or streptococci.
- Multisystem disease due to staphylococcal toxin.

Signs and symptoms
- Systemic illness with high fever.
- *GI:* vomiting, watery diarrhoea.
- Shock and hypotension, altered conscious level.
- *Neuromuscular:* occasional severe myalgia.
- *Skin rash:* red mucous membranes and diffuse macular rash; 10 days after infection, desquamation of the palms, soles, fingers, and toes.

Investigations
- *Haematology:* thrombocytopenia, coagulopathy.
- *Biochemistry:* abnormal LFTs and kidney function.

Diagnostic criteria for staphylococcal TSS
- Temperature ≥39°C.
- sBP <90mmHg.
- Rash (may or may not include desquamation).
- Involvement of three or more of GI, musculoskeletal, renal, hepatic, CNS, blood, and mucous membranes.

Diagnostic criteria for streptococcal TSS
- Isolation of GAS.
- Hypotension.
- Involvement of two or more of coagulopathy, ARDS, soft tissue necrosis, rash with desquamation, and renal or hepatic involvement.

Treatment
- IV fluids and resuscitation.
- Antibiotics against staphylococci and streptococci (e.g. flucloxacillin + benzylpenicillin or ceftriaxone). Clindamycin often added to antibiotic regime due to anti-toxin activity *in vitro*.
- IVIG.

Kawasaki disease

KD is a vasculitis with a predisposition to involving coronary arteries. Worldwide, the highest incidence is in Japan (138/100 000), and in the UK it is 8.1/100 000 in children <5y. Aetiology is unknown, and differential diagnoses are shown in Box 16.3. Multidisciplinary (i.e. cardiology, infection, rheumatology) care is needed.

> **Box 16.3 Differential diagnoses**
> • Streptococcal and staphylococcal toxin-mediated diseases.
> • Adenovirus and other viral infections (enterovirus, EBV, measles).
> • Drug reactions or SJS.
> • Leptospirosis.
> • *Yersinia* pseudotuberculosis infection.
> • Rickettsial infection.
> • Reiter's syndrome.
> • IBD.
> • Post-infectious immune complex disease.
> • Sarcoidosis.

Diagnostic criteria

Fever ≥5 days and four of the five following criteria. KD may be diagnosed with fewer than four features if any coronary abnormalities are seen on echocardiography:
• Bilateral, bulbar, non-purulent conjunctivitis.
• Changes in lips/oral mucosa: cracked lips, 'strawberry' tongue, oropharyngeal erythema.
• Change in extremities: oedema, erythema, or desquamation.
• Polymorphous rash, no vesicles or crusts.
• Cervical lymphadenopathy ≥1.5cm.

Incomplete KD is common in infants and diagnosed with ≤4 of the additional features (see ➲ Associated features, pp. 630–1). *Atypical KD* is diagnosed when there are additional inflammatory features (in >9y olds and <6mth olds), e.g. induration or redness at the BCG inoculation site; arthritis, uveitis, aseptic meningitis, pneumonitis, intestinal obstruction, hydrops of the gall bladder, and jaundice; encephalopathy, MAS and SIADH. However, persisting and additional features should raise the possibility of alternative diagnoses.

Associated features

In addition to the diagnostic criteria of KD, the other features of the condition include the following:
• *Urological:* urethritis with sterile pyuria.
• *Musculoskeletal:* arthralgia and arthritis (35% of patients).
• *CNS:* irritability, aseptic meningitis, SN hearing loss.
• *GI:* diarrhoea and vomiting; hydrops of the gall bladder, jaundice.

- *Cardiac:* coronary enlargement/aneurysms, congestive heart failure, myocarditis, pericardial effusion, arrhythmias, mitral insufficiency, ischaemia, acute myocardial infarction within 1y of disease.
- *Haematology:* leucocytosis, thrombocytosis from second week onwards, ↑ coagulability, platelet turnover, and depleted fibrinolysis.
- *Acute phase reactants:* elevated ESR persists beyond the acute febrile period and gradually returns to normal over 1–2mth. CRP may also be elevated but normalizes faster in response to treatment.
- *Biochemistry:* elevated liver transaminases, hypoalbuminaemia. Role of N-terminal pro-B type natriuretic peptide and urinary meprin A and filamin C as biomarkers is unclear.
- *Immunology:* activation of circulating macrophages; B-cells, elevated immunoglobulin production, T-cell lymphopenia.

Treatment

Should be started within 10 days of fever onset because it reduces the risk of coronary artery aneurysm formation to 4–9%. Therapies are:
- IVIG
  - Dose: 2g/kg, administered 12h apart, splitting the dose over 2–4 days if cardiac failure present.
  - IVIG may be given after 10 days if fever persists.
  - IVIG resistance occurs in 10–20% of cases and associated with risk of aneurysm.
  - In many centres, a second dose of IVIG is given to patients in whom fever persists or returns 36h later, along with IV methylprednisolone (30mg/kg, max 1g).
- IV methylprednisolone and infliximab: associated with fewer days of fever and hospitalization, but reduced rate of aneurysms not yet found.
- Aspirin: 30–50mg/kg/day, reduced to 2–5mg/kg/day when fever has settled, and continued for a minimum of 6wk. Stopped if echo is normal.
- Antiplatelet agents (clopidogrel and dipyridamole): considered when risk of thrombus. Warfarin added in the presence of giant aneurysms.
- Cardiology follow-up: initial echo as early as possible (diagnostic), followed by interval echo (<2wk, 6wk, and then as necessary), based on severity of involvement. Lifelong follow-up is recommended if cardiac disease detected.

Coronavirus and COVID-19

Coronaviruses cause up to 15% of common colds (see ➔ Upper airway infection, p. 251). It is not infrequently identified in infants with bronchiolitis. However, two epidemics and one pandemic of previously unknown coronaviruses have resulted in high mortality rates in infected adults:

- Severe acute respiratory syndrome associated coronavirus (SARS-CoV).
- Middle East respiratory syndrome coronavirus (MERS-CoV).
- SARS-CoV-2, COronaVIrus Disease 2019 (COVID-19) pandemic.

Most infected infants and children are asymptomatic or have mild symptoms. Hence, the illness associated with SARS-CoV-2 has not had a major impact on acute morbidity/mortality in paediatrics. Where there is a primarily respiratory presentation, early escalation to PICU and evaluation for an emerging acute respiratory distress syndrome (ARDS) or myocarditis (see ➔ Myocarditis, p. 218) is important. Consideration for minimizing aerosol spread and risk to staff/carers should also be given, avoiding use of high flow oxygen or suction where possible.

Post-infectious systemic inflammation

There is worldwide interest (including a *British Paediatric Surveillance Unit* study; see https://www.rcpch.ac.uk/work-we-do/bpsu) in the small number of children who appear to have a post-infectious systemic inflammatory response during the COVID-19 pandemic. These children present with features shared with other paediatric inflammatory conditions, including:

- KD (see ➔ Kawasaki disease, pp. 630–1).
- Toxic shock syndrome (see ➔ Toxic shock syndrome, p. 629).
- Other occult inflammatory response that must be considered:
  - Sepsis (see ➔ Sepsis, p. 57).
  - Acute abdomen (see ➔ Acute abdomen, p. 615;
    ➔ Acute appendicitis, p. 807).
  - Macrophage activation syndrome (see ➔ Macrophage activation syndrome, pp. 714–15).

Practice guidance

The Royal College of Paediatrics and Child Health (RCPCH) have provided clinical guidance (see https://www.rcpch.ac.uk/resources/covid-19-clinical-management-children-admitted-hospital-suspected-covid-19) but the evidence base at time of this text is limited and subject to change, so refer to the website for updates. The RCPCH guidance includes the following advice:

- Awareness of children with pre-existing conditions (e.g. sickle cell disease) and not to overlook more common disease presentations.
- To not use high flow nasal cannula O_2 therapy if adequate SpO_2 is achieved with low flow O_2.
- Specific antiviral and immune modulation treatments should only be used in the context of a randomized clinical trial.

Approach in post-infectious inflammatory response

In children suspected of having a post-infectious inflammatory response, additional consideration should be given to:

- Supportive care with PICU/specialist transfer.
- Blood: FBC, U&E, LFT, CRP; troponin, ferritin, LDH, coagulation panel and D-dimer.
- Cultures: blood, urine MC&S, respiratory panel PCR.
- Radiology: CXR.
- Multidisciplinary team care: infectious disease, cardiology, rheumatology, and PICU.
- Cardiology follow-up: concerns about coronary artery aneurysm similar to that seen in KD (see ➜ Kawasaki disease pp. 630–1).

Bacterial meningitis and septicaemia

Some definitions:
- *Meningitis* is infection of the meninges.
- *Bacteraemia* or bloodstream infection (BSI) is the presence of bacteria in the blood (confirmed on culture or molecular methods).
- *Sepsis syndrome* encompasses various consensus definitions, dependent on laboratory and clinical features, e.g. *systemic inflammatory response syndrome (SIRS)*, severe sepsis, and septic shock. For simplicity, the term sepsis/septicaemia is used in the chapter to describe any combination of sepsis syndromes. (See also ➔ Sepsis, p. 57 and 'paediatric sepsis 6', Box 3.7.)

Epidemiology

Meningitis

The epidemiology of bacterial meningitis has changed due to the introduction of vaccination against HiB, *Pneumococcus*, serogroup C *Meningococcus*, and more recently serogroup B *Meningococcus*.
- *Neonates*: commonly caused by *S. agalactiae* (GBS), *S. pneumoniae*, *Escherichia coli*, and *Listeria monocytogenes*.
- *Older children >3mth*: *Neisseria meningitidis* is the commonest, followed by *S. pneumoniae* and *H. influenzae*.

Sepsis

- *Age <3mth*: GBS, *E. coli*, and *L monocytogenes* are commoner.
- *Infants >3mth*: commonest organisms are *N. meningitidis*, *S. pneumoniae*, *S. aureus*, and *E. coli*.
- Infection with enteric and opportunistic pathogens is common in surgical and immunocompromised patients, respectively.
- *Meningococcal disease* is rare, but although the incidence is overall decreasing, delayed diagnosis and treatment are associated with a high mortality rate. Meningococcal disease has therefore featured highly in public education; the 'glass test' is used to identify a typical non-blanching purpuric or petechial rash. In the UK, *N. meningitidis* serogroup B is the commonest pathogen, although incidence of serogroup W is on the rise and serogroup B vaccination has been introduced to the national immunization programme. Disease with serogroup C is now rare, following the introduction of vaccination.

Pathogenesis

The sequence of pathology involves:
- Colonization/invasion of the mucosal epithelium (e.g. nasopharyngeal).
- Invasion of the bloodstream and endotoxin release, causing systemic illness with DIC, capillary leak, and shock (*septicaemia*).
- Attachment to, and invasion of, the meninges (*meningitis*).
- Inflammation with leak of proteins, leading to cerebral oedema.
- Alteration in cerebral blood flow and metabolism.
- Cerebral vasculitis.

Symptoms and signs

- *General:* fever, lethargy, vomiting, loss of appetite, rigors, muscle and joint pains.
- *Rash:* initially maculopapular, progressing to petechiae or purpura, suggestive of DIC secondary to septicaemia.
- *Hypovolaemia/shock:* thirst may be the first sign of shock, followed by poor urine output, tachycardia, poor perfusion, and hypotension.
- *Neurological:* altered LOC may be due to shock, rather than meningitis, and respond to initial fluid therapy. Raised ICP is commoner in meningitis presentation (e.g. bulging fontanelle, headache, neck stiffness, irritability, *Kernig's sign, Brudzinski's sign*) than sepsis but may be less apparent in the young. Seizures are associated with meningitis/encephalitis (focal seizures may suggest infarction/subdural collection). Rarely, cranial nerve abnormalities and papilloedema may be present (late).
- *Respiratory:* respiratory distress common with sepsis/shock, and raised ICP. Features of pneumonia or pulmonary oedema may develop, especially following aggressive initial fluid therapy.

Important practice points

- Meningitis and septicaemia can coexist in up to 60% of cases, more often in young children.
- Presentation may be non-specific initially and difficult to distinguish from other causes (e.g. viral illness). It is essential to monitor vital signs and the rate of illness progression, and consider parental concern.
- Fluid resuscitation and antibiotics should be given as early as possible when the diagnosis is suspected.

Diagnostic testing

- *Blood culture and PCR:* for *Meningococcus* and *Pneumococcus*—should be taken before antibiotics are given, for highest yield.
- *LP:* performed before antibiotics, unless it will delay treatment. Ensure sample is sent for MC&S (two pots), protein (one pot), glucose (oxalate bottle), and viral PCR panel (one pot)—rarely required in neonates, unless strong clinical suspicion. A rapid antigen screen and CSF PCR for suspected bacterial organisms are useful when LP done after antibiotics or culture −ve. CSF should be processed as soon as possible (cell count decreases with time), so liaise with the laboratory. Delay the procedure if there are contraindications present, i.e. shock, raised ICP, focal neurology, focal seizures, lumbar skin infection, coagulopathy (e.g. PT >14.3s, APTT >35.2s, platelets <100 × 10^9/L), extensive or spreading purpura.
- *Cranial CT scan:* unreliable for diagnosing raised ICP and not routinely required before LP, unless clinically indicated (e.g. suspected raised ICP or seizures to rule out alternative pathology).

Meningitis and septicaemia treatments

Antimicrobial therapy

Initial choice

Early clinical management and resuscitation in sepsis are covered in Chapter 3 (see ➲ Sepsis, p. 57):

- *Antibiotics:* first-line empirical therapy is ceftriaxone. Cefotaxime is recommended if Ca^{2+}-containing infusions are required and in preterm or jaundiced neonates.
  - Add amoxicillin for children: <3mth to cover for *Listeria*.
  - Add vancomycin if history of travel, suspected resistant *S. pneumoniae* or meticillin-resistant *S. aureus* (MRSA).
  - NB: modify therapy based on culture results and sensitivities.

For term neonates presenting <72h old, benzylpenicillin and gentamicin are recommended, as they are still most likely to have early-onset sepsis (see NICE guideline on neonatal infection, available at: ➾ https://www.nice.org.uk/guidance/cg149). If presenting at >72h, the above antibiotic recommendations are valid.

Duration of antimicrobial therapy (minimum)

- 7 days for *N. meningitidis*.
- 10 days for *H. influenzae*.
- 14 days for *S. agalactiae* (GBS) and *S. pneumoniae*.
- 21 days for *E. coli*.
- For culture –ve clinically suspected cases, recommendation is at least 10 days in those >3mth and 14 days in those <3mth.
- Always seek expert advice for complicated cases.

Steroid therapy

Not recommended in those <3mth. Use for suspected bacterial meningitis, and start dexamethasone ≤4h of antibiotics (no benefit after >12h). The dose is 0.15mg/kg (maximum 10mg) qds for 4 days if LP shows:

- Frank purulent CSF, with CSF WCC >1000.
- Raised WCC, with protein >1g/L.
- Organisms seen on microscopy.

Follow-up

The majority of survivors of meningococcal disease have few or no sequelae. Overall mortality is as high as 10% and survivors may have one or more long-term complications:

- Orthopaedic: damage to digits, bones, and joints (10% need amputation).
- Dermatological: scarring following necrosis.
- Developmental/psychosocial issues/cognition deficits (up to 30%).
- Hearing loss (4%): all children with meningitis should have formal audiology assessment.
- Renal failure: may have CRF following shock.
- Immunology assessment: to rule out complement deficiency if >1 episode of meningococcal sepsis or other septicaemia, or a single episode with vaccine-covered serogroups of *Meningococcus* or *Pneumococcus* (suggesting vaccine failure).

Encephalitis/meningoencephalitis

Viral

Viral encephalitis and/or meningoencephalitis are commoner than bacterial meningitis, but empirical broad-spectrum antibiotics (IV ceftriaxone/ cefotaxime) are usually recommended until a bacterial cause has been ruled out. Common viruses include:

- *Enterovirus species* (including parechovirus), herpesviruses [HSV 1 and 2, EBV, CMV, varicella-zoster virus (VZV), HHV6/7], adenovirus, and influenza.
- Also caused by HIV and measles, but rare.

These infections are usually self-limiting—except HSV—which can cause rapid deterioration and death, especially in congenital infection (where it can present as disseminated disease). Any agent can cause severe disease in immunocompromised hosts.

Treatment

The principles of treatment are similar to those for meningitis/septicaemia in regards to resuscitation and stabilization. Antiviral therapy includes:

- *Prophylaxis:* aciclovir is recommended for prophylaxis in cases of confirmed HSV encephalitis and immunocompromised patients.
- *Treatment:* antiviral treatment is indicated for HSV (IV aciclovir) and influenza (oseltamivir, zanamivir). A minimum of 21 days' treatment is recommended for HSV encephalitis, with repeat LP before discontinuing treatment to ensure viral clearance.
- *Other care:* supportive therapy used for other viral causes. However, specific drug treatments may be available for CMV and EBV when the host is immunocompromised. Seek expert advice.

Other causes

- *Certain bacteria* can cause a meningoencephalitic picture (e.g. TB, neonatal GBS, *Listeria, Borrelia*) and should also be considered.
- *Fungal meningitis* is almost entirely limited to immunocompromised cohorts (neonates, immunodeficiency, transplant or chemotherapy recipients).

Enlarged lymph nodes

Fever associated with enlarged lymph glands is a common presentation. Although the aetiology is usually infectious, a thorough clinical assessment is required to rule out malignancy:

- *Mobile lymph nodes:* ≤1cm in cervical or axillary and ≤1.5cm in inguinal regions—*usually benign* ('reactive' lymph nodes).
- *Enlarging nodes:* palpable nodes in certain areas (e.g. epitrochlear, supraclavicular, popliteal), with associated weight loss and night sweats and non-mobile and generalized, *warrant further investigation*.

Aetiology

Aetiology depends on history, presentation, and pattern.

Infectious causes

- Acute unilateral (usually bacterial lymphadenitis): *S. aureus, Streptococcus pyogenes* (GAS), *Streptococcus agalactiae* (GBS), anaerobes.
- Acute bilateral (usually viral): EBV, CMV, HSV, adenovirus, human herpesvirus (HHV) 6/7, enterovirus, *Mycoplasma*, influenza, measles, etc.
- Chronic/insidious: non-tuberculous mycobacteria (NTM), TB, HIV, cat-scratch disease (*Bartonella henselae*), toxoplasmosis, anaerobes.

Non-infectious causes

- Malignancy, e.g. ALL, lymphoma.
- Periodic fever syndromes.
- KD.
- Sarcoidosis.
- Rarely: Kikuchi disease, HLH.

Investigations

Based on presentation and may include respiratory specimens:

- *Blood:* inflammatory markers, film, serology, PCR, interferon-gamma release assay (IGRA) for TB/NTM.
- *Imaging:* CXR, USS, CT, MRI.
- If fine-needle aspiration (FNA)/biopsy performed, send pus for microbiology, including fungal/anaerobic culture if suspected. Send tissue for histopathology.

Treatment

Specific to likely aetiology:

- Acute pyogenic lymphadenitis suggestive of bacterial cause should be treated with antibiotics: PO/IV, based on severity and presence of abscess, with co-amoxiclav as first-line empirical choice and ceftriaxone ± metronidazole as second line (if severe and unwell).
- Low threshold for drainage as this reduces the duration of illness.
- NTM (see ➲ Non-tuberculous mycobacteria, pp. 642–3).
- TB lymphadenitis (see ➲ Tuberculosis: presentation and diagnosis, pp. 639–40).

Tuberculosis presentation and diagnosis

Mycobacterium tuberculosis is the major human pathogen causing TB. TB is usually spread from an infectious adult (commonly pulmonary TB from sputum +ve contact). TB involves any organ and can be difficult to diagnose in the young, who often do not have classic features and in whom diagnostic sampling is difficult. Since treatment is prolonged (≥6mth), try to get as many diagnostic samples before treatment.

TB disease is the presence of symptoms/signs and/or radiological changes and/or microbiology results. Five to 10% develop primary disease within 12mth after exposure to an infectious adult; higher risk in <4y.

Latent TB infection (LTBI) implies TB exposure, but asymptomatic and non-infectious. Up to 95% of cases. Tuberculin skin test (TST) or IGRA usually +ve; normal examination and radiology. Some reactivate years later.

Common presentations

Pulmonary tuberculosis

(See ➲ Pulmonary tuberculosis, p. 262.) The commonest presentation of reactivation disease in adolescents and adults.

Tuberculous meningitis (TBM)

TBM is the most feared complication of *M. tuberculosis* infection.
- *Timing:* usually occurs within 12mth of first infection.
- *Age group:* most frequently occurs in those <5y of age.
- *Pathology:* initial pathology is occult haematogenous dissemination to cerebral cortex from primary site (e.g. gut, lung) → meninges and subarachnoid space. Thick gelatinous exudate around the brainstem, compromising cranial nerves III, IV, and VI.
- *Clinical course:* onset is insidious, characterized by apathy or disinterest, then intermittent headaches and anorexia. Fever is almost always present and vomiting is common. Hydrocephalus is common. Focal neurological signs, seizures, and altered LOC may occur.
- *CSF:* lymphocytic picture and acid–fast bacilli may be seen. High CSF protein and CSF:serum glucose ratio <0.5; 50% will grow mycobacteria from CSF. TST/IGRA is often +ve; 40–90% have CXR changes of pulmonary disease.

Lymph node disease
- Common presentation with firm, fixed, slowly enlarging nodes (usually supraclavicular/clavicular—indicates secondary spread from lungs).

Miliary disease
- Common in young children and infants; presents as unwell with fever, respiratory distress, hepatosplenomegaly, and CXR changes.

Abdominal disease
- Lymphadenopathy, insidious GI symptoms, weight loss, ascites. Renal disease may occur but is rare in children.

Bone disease
- Vertebral involvement (Koch's spine), chronic osteomyelitis of joints, psoas abscess, paraspinal abscess (Pott's disease).

Congenital TB
- Rare, but well described. *In utero* transfer from mother via placenta.

Diagnosis
Clinical
Have a high index of suspicion in countries with a low incidence because some areas may have higher incidence (e.g. London, Leicester).
- Symptoms and signs may be non-specific in younger children (e.g. fever, poor weight gain, etc.).
- Presentation in adolescents is similar to that of adult multibacillary disease (weight loss, chronic cough >3wk, fever, night sweats).
- Focal chest signs (pleural effusion), lymphadenopathy, hepatosplenomegaly, and neurological signs may be present.

Radiology and other investigations
- CXR: may show pleural effusion, consolidation, cavitation, hilar/other lymphadenopathy, and miliary disease.
- Chest CT: shows extent (e.g. cavitation, endobronchial disease).
- Head CT: used in TBM and tuberculoma.
- Abdominal USS.
- Endoscopy/colonoscopy, bronchoscopy, tissue biopsy.

Tuberculin skin test
Inject 0.1mL of purified protein derivative (PPD) intradermally (left flexor aspect of mid-forearm) and measure induration 48–72h later.
- Rule out active disease if induration ≥5mm, irrespective of BCG history. Treat for latent TB once active disease ruled out.
- False +ve test can occur with history of BCG and infection with non-NTM. False –ve tests are due to poor technique, HIV, immunosuppression, and malnutrition.

IGRA (T spot®/Quantiferon gold®) tests
IGRA tests are done on blood and measure the production of interferon-gamma, following stimulation with TB-specific antigens. Used in conjunction with TST for screening. Both TST/IGRA suggest exposure to mycobacteria and persistence of specific T-cell responses, respectively, but neither can differentiate between active and latent TB.

Early morning sputum samples
For acid–fast bacilli (×3) (auramine, Ziehl–Neelsen stain), culture, and PCR. Use cough swab/NG aspirate/BAL in younger children. *Xpert* MTB/RIF is a newer real-time PCR which is highly specific for detection of MTB and the presence of resistance to rifampicin.

Tuberculosis treatment and complications

The following recommendations are for otherwise healthy children. Those with comorbidities (e.g. HIV, immunosuppression, liver/renal disease) or drug-resistant TB should be managed with expert advice from a tertiary centre with adequate infection control facilities. Prophylaxis with isoniazid for 6mth or with rifampicin for 3mth is recommended for exposed children <2y and offered up to 18y for those who have latent disease.

Anti-TB therapy

Standard therapy for fully sensitive strains is isoniazid (INH or H), rifampicin (R), pyrazinamide (Z), and ethambutol (E), modified by strain sensitivity. UK NICE guidelines' recommended treatment include:
- Non-CNS sensitive TB for 6mth, with 2mth of HRZE and 4mth of HR.
- CNS disease sensitive TB for 12mth, with 2mth of HRZE and 10mth of HR.

Steroids

Recommended for CNS or pericardial disease.

Complications

Overall prognosis is excellent for non-CNS disease in a healthy child with fully sensitive TB. Early treatment results in complete recovery. CNS disease carries very high complication rates in the form of hydrocephalus and poor neurodevelopmental outcomes, especially if focal neurological signs are already present at the time of starting treatment. Drug-resistant disease has a higher rate of complications and mortality.

Non-tuberculous mycobacteria

NTM are a group of environmental mycobacteria which cause local infection or invasive disease. Common pathogens are *Mycobacterium avium* complex (MAC), *Mycobacterium abscessus*, *Mycobacterium chelonae*, and *Mycobacterium kansasii*, amongst others. Infection is from environmental exposure via direct contact, inhalation, or ingestion. NTM are not known to be transmissible from person to person like TB. Most heal with or without treatment but can cause prolonged and severe disease in the immunocompromised host.

Clinical presentation

Lymphadenopathy
- Commonest presentation seen in 1–5y olds, mostly due to MAC.
- Commonly cervical and submandibular, can involve any chain.
- Can have insidious or acute onset, usually >2cm and unilateral.
- Lymph nodes eventually soften, start discharging, or form a sinus prior to healing, which can take months to years.
- Children mostly remain well, with minimal non-specific symptoms.

Respiratory infection
- Mostly a problem limited to those with underlying pulmonary disease, e.g. CF, chronic lung disease, post-lung transplant, other immunocompromised states.
- Can result in disseminated disease, with high fatality.

Disseminated disease
- Common in primary (e.g. SCID) and secondary immunodeficiency (e.g. chemotherapy, HIV), associated with poor T-cell function.
- Systemic symptoms and signs are reported and infection can spread to multiple organs, including CNS, with high mortality.

Diagnosis

Clinical presentation may be sufficient to make the diagnosis:
- *Classically:* red/purple appearance of overlying skin over enlarged glands, minimal systemic symptoms, long course (with poor response to antibiotics).
- *Retrospective diagnosis:* common following histological finding of caseating granulomas with acid-fast bacilli after surgical resection of a lymph node.
- TST (–ve IGRA): may be +ve and no TB exposure history.
- *Specific mycobacterial cultures:* needed for slow-growing species, e.g. cases of central venous catheter infections.
- Cultures from multiple affected sites, including guided biopsy, may be needed in children who are immunocompromised to confirm the diagnosis and decide treatment.
- FNA of localized lymphadenitis is not recommended for diagnosis due to high risk of fistula formation.

Treatment principles

- Wait and watch if minimal symptoms and localized disease.
- Surgical excision of lymphadenitis is usually curative, although recurrence is possible.
- Removal of central venous device may be necessary in immunocompromised children, with further antimicrobial therapy.
- Medical treatment with antimicrobials may be beneficial if surgical resection not possible or recurrence.
- Treatment is recommended with multiple antimicrobials to avoid risk of resistance, especially in immunocompromised children. Often prolonged treatment is required, based on sensitivities.
- Prophylaxis with macrolides is considered in cases of HIV and primary immunodeficiencies.

Tropical infections

Tropical infections may be present in any child returning from the tropics or visiting the UK. The general principles mentioned in → Fever assessment, p. 623; → Fever management, p. 624 should be followed. Additionally, a detailed travel history is important, including:

- *Status*: overseas visitor or returning from holiday (some illnesses more severe in those who are non-immune/partially immune).
- *Itinerary*: mode of travel, stopovers, illness during/prior to travel.
- *Prophylaxis*: travel vaccines, chemoprophylaxis, other measures.
- *Specific exposures*: food, accommodation, water, dairy, animals.
- *Features*: specific symptoms—fever, rashes, GI symptoms, etc.
- *Local outbreaks*: recent outbreaks, disease common to area.

Malaria

- *Agent*: parasitic infection spread by ♀ *Anopheles* mosquito. Commonest type *Plasmodium falciparum*, usually in Africa (also *Plasmodium vivax*, *Plasmodium ovale*, *Plasmodium malariae*, and *Plasmodium knowlesi*).
- *Features*: non-specific flu-like symptoms, fever, diarrhoea, vomiting, jaundice, anaemia, thrombocytopenia. Children with severe malaria can be very unwell and should be managed as an emergency, as for a child with meningitis/septicaemia.
- *Time course*: onset usually occurs 7–10 days after inoculation but may occur after a few months in children.
- *Diagnosis*: thick (parasitaemia) and thin blood film (speciation), rapid diagnostic tests (high sensitivity, especially for falciparum).
- *Supportive investigations*: ABG, glucose, U&E, LFTs, G6PD, clotting, blood culture (concomitant bacteraemia, e.g. *Salmonella* may occur).

Treatment

Low threshold to admit children for observation if confirmed malaria, especially falciparum. Appropriate resuscitation of severe disease and early discussion with PICU/specialists. Refer to the Centers for Disease Control and Prevention (CDC) website for area-specific drug resistance (available at: ℅ https://www.cdc.gov/malaria/malaria_worldwide/reduction/drug_resistance.html):

- *Falciparum (severe)* (see Box 16.4):
  - First-line IV artesunate, second-line quinine + clindamycin.
  - Commence IV broad-spectrum antibiotic (usually ceftriaxone) for possible concomitant sepsis.
- *Falciparum (non-severe)*:
  - Coartem®; second line atovaquone/proguanil (Malarone®).
- *Non-falciparum*:
  - Coartem®/chloroquine + 14 days of primaquine (check G6PD status) for *P. ovale* and *P. vivax*.

Box 16.4 Features of severe malaria

Manage as medical emergency in the presence of ≥1 of the following:
- Reduced GCS, seizures, signs of raised ICP.
- Respiratory distress or acidosis, pulmonary oedema.
- Hypoglycaemia.
- Severe anaemia, bleeding, or jaundice.
- Renal impairment, hyperkalaemia.
- Parasitaemia ≥2%.

Typhoid fever

- *Agent:* Salmonella typhi or paratyphi.
- *Features:* fever, headache, cough, myalgia, GI symptoms, relative bradycardia, organomegaly, 'rose' spots occasionally reported.
- *Complications:* GI perforation, myocarditis, hepatitis, and nephritis.
- *Diagnosis:* blood culture (may need extended incubation), stool.
- *Treatment:* S typhi—empirical first line: ceftriaxone for bacteraemia; 7–14 days recommended. Paratyphoid: usually self-limiting.

Dengue fever

- *Agent:* viral infection spread by mosquitoes.
- *Features:* primary infection produces a fine erythematous rash, myalgia, arthralgia, and high fever. Secondary desquamation follows.
- *Laboratory findings:* anaemia, low platelets, deranged clotting.
- Shock can occur with subsequent infection with a different strain.
- *Treatment:* supportive. Vaccination available, but poor efficacy.

Viral haemorrhagic fevers

- *Agents:* Lassa, Marburg, Ebola, Crimean Congo, and other viruses.
- *Features:* highly contagious, often fatal. Short incubation, fever; DIC ensues.
- *Management:* strict isolation and use VHF personal protective equipment (PPE); seek specialist advice [Public Health England (PHE), microbiologist, and infectious diseases]. Treatment is supportive in intensive care; ribavarin has been shown to be effective in Lassa fever.

Zika

- *Agent:* viral infection spread by Aedes mosquitoes.
- *Features:* usually mild, e.g. fever, rash, headache, myalgia, arthralgia, conjunctivitis. Perinatal, in utero, sexual and transfusion transmission has been reported. Maternal Zika infection has now been confirmed as a cause of microcephaly and fetal brain defects in infants of women infected during pregnancy.
- *Diagnosis:* suspected based on clinical features and history of travel to a Zika-affected area. Antibody, PCR on blood and urine of newborn.
- *Treatment:* babies born to mothers with confirmed infection in pregnancy should be evaluated at birth and appropriately followed up. Generally, the disease course is mild. Severe disease in children or adults is rare, and treatment is supportive.

Immunodeficiency disorders

Immunodeficiency may be due to causes that are:
- *Primary:* intrinsic abnormalities (see Box 16.5).
- *Secondary:* cancer, immunosuppressive agents, HIV infection, splenectomy, nephrotic syndrome, SCD, etc.
- *Suspect if:*
  - FTT.
  - Family history.
  - ≥2 sinus infections or ≥4 ear infections in 12mth.
  - ≥2 LRTIs or deep-seated infections in 3y.
  - Organ abscesses >1.
  - Frequent/persistent thrush.

Investigations

- Immunoglobulin levels, T-cell subsets.
- T-cell responses, vaccine responses.
- Flow cytometry/western blot for protein expression, molecular testing.
- Prenatal testing: chorion villus sampling, amniocentesis, fetal blood test.

Treatment

(See also ➲ Febrile neutropenia/neutropenic sepsis, p. 612; ➲ Specific infections, p. 613.) Therapy is tailored to the specific primary immunodeficiency, and these children are always looked after in liaison with a tertiary centre.

Treatments include:
- Prophylactic antibiotics.
- Supportive care and antibiotics for acute infections.
- Replacement immunoglobulins and additional immunization.
- BMT.
- Gene therapy.

Box 16.5 Primary immunodeficiency

Caused by defects in the following.

B lymphocytes and antibody production
- *X-linked agammaglobulinaemia*: presents in early childhood with severe bacterial infections.
- *Hyper IgM syndrome*: presents with bacterial infection and PCP.
- *IgG subclass deficiency*: minor immunodeficiency that may cause recurrent respiratory infection.
- *Tests*: immunoglobulin levels and functional vaccine responses, as indicated by clinical presentation.

T-lymphocytes and cellular immunity
- *SCID*: presents in first few months; FTT; persistent infection due to viruses and fungi.
- *Tests*: FBC, blood film, lymphocyte subsets and function.

Neutrophil defects
- *Leucocyte adhesion deficiency*: delayed umbilical cord separation, neutrophilia.
- *Chronic granulomatous disease (CGD)*: bacterial/fungal infections, granulomas.
- *Tests*: assessment of chemotaxis, neutrophil surface adhesion molecules, and killing (e.g. oxidative burst test for CGD).

Opsonization and other innate immunodeficiencies
- *Complement deficiency or mannose-binding lectin deficiency*: rare but may present with severe meningococcal disease.
- *Tests*: complement levels, Toll receptor pathway assays (second-line tests directed by clinical presentation).

Multisystem syndromes
- *Ataxia telangiectasia*: skin, neurological, and immune defects.
- *Wiskott–Aldrich syndrome*: eczema, thrombocytopenia, and immunodeficiency.
- *di George syndrome*: hypocalcaemia, branchial arch and heart defects, and immunodeficiency.
- *Duncan syndrome*: X-linked lymphoproliferative disease due to prior EBV infection.
- *Tests*: chromosomal fragility, genetic polymorphisms.

Immune dysregulation
- HLH (haemophagocytic lymphohistiocytosis).
- IPEX (immune dysregulation, polyendocrinopathy, enteropathy).
- APECED (autoimmune polyendocrinopathy, candidiasis, ectodermal dystrophia).
- ALPS (autoimmune lymphoproliferative syndrome).
- Immune dysregulation with colitis.

Human immunodeficiency virus

(See also ⊃ Human immunodeficiency virus, p. 167.) HIV infection in children is caused mainly by the retrovirus HIV type 1.

Vertical transmission of HIV

Children at risk of acquiring the virus are infants of HIV +ve mothers, although this route of acquisition is increasingly rare because of the success of antenatal preventative measures.

- Infants may become infected during labour, in the postnatal period, or rarely *in utero*.
- Rate of transmission is up to 40% without suitable management, but <1% with effective prophylaxis.

Prevention of vertical transmission

- Avoid natural labour and birth canal contact by elective CS (only recommended if high maternal viral load).
- Avoid breastfeeding.
- Use of antenatal, perinatal, and postnatal antiretroviral drugs.

Clinical features

Dormant infection occurs for a short period and has minimal clinical features. Features of paediatric HIV infection are the following:

- *GI:* chronic diarrhoea, FTT.
- *CNS:* delayed development and CP.
- *Recurrent bacterial and viral infections.*
- *Lymphadenopathy and hepatosplenomegaly.*
- *Opportunistic infections:* Pneumocystis jiroveci (formerly Pneumocystis carinii), Candida, herpes, varicella, and atypical mycobacteria.
- *Respiratory distress:* cough, hypoxaemia, bilateral nodular infiltrates on CXR.

Acquired immune deficiency syndrome (AIDS)

Lymphocytic interstitial pneumonitis, *P. jiroveci* (PJP) infection, and *Candida* oesophagitis are 'AIDS-defining' in an HIV +ve child; they signify progression to the AIDS phase.

Diagnosis

The diagnosis of HIV infection depends on demonstrating specific anti-HIV antibodies and/or viral components in blood (PCR):

- Infants infected perinatally have an immune response by 4–6mth of age. However, an uninfected infant of a HIV +ve mother can test +ve for anti-HIV antibodies for up to 12–18mth.
- In babies born to HIV +ve mothers: send HIV RNA PCR at birth, and repeat test at 2 and 6wk after stopping prophylactic treatment. Further interim test on prophylaxis for high-risk cases.
- In children presenting after 18mth, use the HIV antibody test with additional PCR if +ve.

Management principles (always manage with specialist input)
- Babies born to HIV +ve mothers: use prophylactic antiretroviral therapy (usually zidovudine) for 4–6wk, according to birth plan of the baby. Treatment with three drugs may be required, as per national guidelines/ specialist input, in high-risk cases (e.g. poor maternal compliance, unknown maternal HIV status, resistant/high viral load). Commence as soon as possible after birth.
- Prophylaxis against PJP for those >1mth of age with co-trimoxazole.
- Breastfeeding is not recommended.
- Avoid BCG in confirmed or suspected cases. Refer to guidance for specific vaccines (available at: ℡ http://www.gov.uk/government/ publications/immunisation-against-infectious-disease-the-green-book- front-cover-and-contents-page).
- Antiretroviral therapy to suppress viral replication, based on national guidelines and specialist advice.
- Social, psychological, and family support.

Opportunistic fungal infections

(See also ➲ Acute care of infection risk, pp. 612–13.) Opportunistic fungal infections predominantly present as systemic disease and almost entirely are limited to preterm neonates and children with primary or secondary immunodeficiency (e.g. from chemotherapy, BMT, steroids, etc.). The general principles of management of some common opportunistic infections are presented here.

Candidiasis

- Commonest opportunistic fungal infection.
- Caused by *Candida* species; most cases are caused by *C. albicans*.
- Single-celled yeast, normal commensal in mouth, GI tract, skin, and vagina.
- Invasive/multiorgan disease associated with high mortality.
- Common cause of hospital-acquired and health care-associated infection (instrumentation, contaminated materials).
- *Predisposing factors:* immunosuppression, use of broad-spectrum antibiotics, indwelling catheters, CVLs, loss of mucosal integrity, prolonged hospitalization.
- *Sequelae* of candidiasis range from invasive disease, chronic mucocutaneous, oropharyngeal/oesophageal, and vulvovaginitis/cystitis.
- *Diagnosis:* fungal culture swabs, isolation from sterile site confirms infection (e.g. blood, tissue, CSF). Isolation from non-sterile site often represents colonization. Biological markers (e.g. β-D-glucan) and specific fungal PCR help to support diagnostic studies, as yield from culture methods is often poor. Invasive disease requires further investigations (e.g. echocardiography, other imaging, and ophthalmology).
- *Prevention:* infection control measures, antifungal prophylaxis to high-risk groups (extreme prematurity, BMT, chemotherapy). Azoles are the most commonly used agents.
- *Treatment:* start treatment as soon as suspected. First-line empirical therapy for invasive infection is amphotericin for immunocompromised cohorts. Echinocandins (e.g. caspofungin, micafungin, anidulafungin) are being increasingly used. Azoles may be used as first line for stable, immunocompetent patients or non-invasive disease.

Aspergillosis

- Aerobic spore-forming mould, with septate hyphae.
- Natural immunity in healthy people due to ubiquitous presence in environment and food.
- *Sequelae:* encompasses a wide spectrum, mostly caused by *Aspergillus fumigatus*, including invasive aspergillosis, allergic bronchopulmonary aspergillosis, and necrotizing infection. Pulmonary or multiorgan disease usually occurs in the immunosuppressed or if prolonged neutropenia. Allergic disease is mainly seen in those with respiratory conditions, e.g. asthma, PCD, and CF.

- *Diagnosis:* poor yield from fungal microbiology specimens, PCR, and serological testing. Fungal microscopy with silver stain. Provides definitive diagnosis when cultured from sterile site, but this may take weeks. Galactomannan (*Aspergillus* cell wall antigen) assay is useful for early diagnosis and monitoring of response to treatment. It can be performed on BAL fluid or blood. Imaging (CT/MRI) of affected area can provide information on likely fungal aetiology, based on specific appearances (e.g. upper lung lobe involvement, 'halo' sign), extent of disease, and response to therapy. SPT or blood test for specific IgE to *Aspergillus* in those with aeroallergen allergy.
- *Prevention:* maintenance of ventilation systems, use of +ve pressure cubicles, educating about avoiding high-risk environments. Azoles most commonly used agents for prophylaxis in patients with immunosuppression.
- *Treatment:* first-line empirical broad-spectrum therapy used most commonly is amphotericin; voriconazole is first line for invasive aspergillosis. Echinocandins are reserved for refractory disease. Supportive treatments include surgical resection of localized disease, minimizing immunosuppressant use, and G-CSF use in neutropenic patients.

Pneumocystis jirovecii pneumonia

- Atypical fungus, unable to grow *in vitro*, and unlike other fungi, contains cholesterol in the cell wall and is sensitive to many antiparasitic drugs.
- Ubiquitous organism causing asymptomatic or mild respiratory disease in healthy children, colonizing most by the age of 2y.
- Significant disease limited to immunocompromised cohorts with deficient cell-mediated immunity, e.g. HIV, organ/bone marrow transplant and primary immunodeficiencies.
- Airborne or human–human transmission has been suggested, but not established.
- Presents mainly with pneumonitis and other non-specific symptoms, e.g. weight loss, diarrhoea. Eventually causes hypoxia and worsening respiratory function. Associated with high mortality.
- Bronchoscopy with BAL is procedure of choice if patient stable. Nasopharyngeal aspirate or induced sputum are lower yield, but of diagnostic value if +ve. Organism is identified by special stains, immunofluorescence antibodies, and PCR.
- Treatment options include co-trimoxazole (first line), IV pentamidine, steroids (started within 72h of diagnosis), and intensive care for severe cases. Chemoprophylaxis with co-trimoxazole for high-risk cases.

Immunization

- Immunization is a vital part of child health in the community and is one of the most successful public health interventions in medicine. Table 16.2 shows the current UK schedule.
- Maternal vaccination programme in the UK has been a success in preventing pertussis and influenza in infants through passive immunity.
- Immunization should only be delayed if acutely ill (e.g. febrile).
- In those where there is a family history of febrile convulsions, advice should be given about control of fever with antipyretics and when to seek medical assistance.
- Routine use of antipyretics is not recommended, except for serogroup B *Meningococcus* vaccination.
- Frequent boosters are required in infancy due to poor immune response and memory to vaccines in the first year.
- Absolute contraindications include known or previous allergy to vaccine components (see ⊃ Box 13.2).
- Vaccines cannot cause the disease against which they protect, except a mild form of the illness following live attenuated vaccines. Live vaccines in the UK national schedule include BCG, MMR, and rotavirus.

Immunization in immunocompromised children

Some general principles are mentioned here. Expert immunology advice is needed on a case-by-case basis to balance the risk of disease versus severe reactions following live vaccines.

- Live vaccines are generally avoided in those with severe immunodeficiency and those on high-dose immunosuppression. These include BCG, MMR, rotavirus, and live influenza vaccine. Non-live vaccines (inactivated) are safe to give, but their efficacy is doubtful.
- Additional vaccination with varicella is recommended for children 3–4wk before commencing immunosuppressive therapy and members of household of immunodeficient children.
- Children ≥12mth with HIV and di George syndrome can safely have MMR and varicella vaccines if they only have mild to moderate immunocompromise (CD4 ≥15%).
- Children with minor antibody deficiencies can have routine vaccines, as per the national schedule.
- Passive immunization should be provided on exposure to measles and varicella to children with primary severe immunodeficiencies and those on high-dose immunosuppression.
- Palivizumab is indicated for RSV prophylaxis in extremely preterm babies and those with chronic lung disease and complex congenital cardiac disease.

Table 16.2 Routine childhood immunization programme*

When to immunize	Diseases protected against	Vaccine given
2mth old	Diphtheria, tetanus, pertussis, polio, HiB, and hepatitis B Pneumococcal Meningococcal group B Rotavirus	DTaP/IPV/Hib/HepB PCV13 MenB Rotavirus
3mth old	Diphtheria, tetanus, pertussis, polio, HiB, and hepatitis B Rotavirus	DTaP/IPV/Hib/HepB Rotavirus
4mth old	Diphtheria, tetanus, pertussis, polio, HiB, and hepatitis B Pneumococcal Meningococcal group B	DTaP/IPV/Hib/HepB PCV 13 MenB
Around 12–13mth	HiB and meningitis C Measles, mumps, and rubella Pneumococcal Meningococcal group B	Hib/MenC MMR PCV 13 MenB
≥2y	Annual influenza from September	Live attenuated influenza vaccine*
3y 4mth to 5y old	Diphtheria, tetanus, pertussis, and polio Measles, mumps, and rubella	DTaP/IPV MMR
12–13y old girls	Human papillomavirus	HPV two doses (6–24mth apart)
14y old	Tetanus, diphtheria, and polio Meningococcal ACWY	Td/IPV MenACWY

* If contraindicated, inactivated vaccine is given to at-risk groups.

Revised September 2018 📖 https://www.gov.uk/government/publications/the-complete-routine-immunisation-schedule.

Antimicrobial resistance (AMR) and stewardship (ASP)

AMR is a global threat to human health and hence is a major priority of the WHO. Rates of developing AMR are linked to antibiotic use in animals and the health care industry (especially primary care):

- Up to 40% of hospitalized children in Europe receive antibiotics.
- Up to 50% of antibiotic use in hospitals is inappropriate/unnecessary.
- AMR has a huge cost implication due to ↑ risk of complications, longer hospital stays, and use of more expensive drugs.

Inappropriate use of antibiotics is the result of multiple factors, including patient expectations, lack of rapid diagnostic tests (especially in children), and lack of awareness of appropriate antimicrobial use in health care professionals. ASPs are designed to combat AMR and improve antimicrobial use by using strategies such as:

- Initiation of appropriate antibiotics, based on local guidelines.
- Sending diagnostic samples before commencing antibiotics.
- Clear documentation of indication for treatment and choice.
- System in place for review at 48–72h in order to de-escalate or decide treatment duration, based on culture results/sensitivities.
- Monitoring of antimicrobial use and surveillance of AMR.
- Providing feedback to prescribers.

Table 16.3 provides empirical suggestions for common infections.

Table 16.3 Empirical suggestions for some common infections*

Infection	Antibiotic choice	Minimum duration
Bacterial sore throat	Phenoxymethylpenicillin Clarithromycin (if penicillin allergy)	5–10 days
Peritonsillar abscess	Ceftriaxone + metronidazole PO switch 48h after drainage (co-amoxiclav)	10 days
Otitis media	Amoxicillin Co-amoxiclav (if not improving)	5–7 days
Lower UTI (age >3mth)	Trimethoprim/nitrofurantoin Amoxicillin, cefalexin	3 days
Pyelonephritis	Cefalexin/co-amoxiclav IV ceftriaxone/co-amoxiclav (if severe)	7–10 days
Sinusitis	Phenoxymethylpenicillin Co-amoxiclav (severe disease)	5 days
Pneumonia	Amoxicillin (mild to moderate) Co-amoxiclav (severe) Clarithromycin (>4y, likely atypical, allergy to penicillin)	Mild—3 days Severe—7 days Complicated 2–4wk

* Adapted from NICE antimicrobial prescribing guidelines and McMullan et al ℜ http://dx.doi.org/10.1016/.

Further reading

Fever and sepsis

National Institute for Health and Care Excellence. (2013). *Fever in under 5s: assessment and initial management*. Clinical guideline [CG160]. Available at: ℘ https://www.nice.org.uk/guidance/cg160.

National Institute for Health and Care Excellence. (2014). *Fever in under 5s*. Quality standard [QS64]. Available at: ℘ https://www.nice.org.uk/guidance/qs64.

National Institute for Health and Care Excellence. (2016). *Sepsis: recognition, diagnosis and early management*. NICE guideline [NG51]. Available at: ℘ https://www.nice.org.uk/guidance/ng51.

Meningitis

National Institute for Health and Care Excellence. (2010). *Meningitis (bacterial) and meningococcal septicaemia in under 16s: recognition, diagnosis and management*. Clinical guideline [CG102]. Available at: ℘ https://www.nice.org.uk/guidance/cg102.

TB

National Institute for Health and Care Excellence. (2016). *Tuberculosis*. NICE guideline [NG33]. Available at: ℘ https://www.nice.org.uk/guidance/ng33.

Tropical disease

TravelHealthPro. Tropical disease and country-specific malaria prophylaxis. Available at: ℘ https://travelhealthpro.org.uk.

AMR and ASP

National Institute for Health and Care Excellence. (2015). *Antimicrobial stewardship: prescribing antibiotics*. Key therapeutic topic [KTT9]. Available at: ℘ https://www.nice.org.uk/advice/ktt9.

Public Health England. (2011). *Antimicrobial stewardship: Start smart – then focus*. Available at: ℘ https://www.gov.uk/government/publications/antimicrobial-stewardship-start-smart-then-focus.

World Health Organization. (2015). *Global action plan on antimicrobial resistance*. Available at: ℘ https://www.who.int/antimicrobial-resistance/publications/global-action-plan/en/.

Immunization

Public Health England. (2013). *Immunisation against infectious disease: the green book*. Available at: ℘ https://www.gov.uk/government/publications/immunisation-against-infectious-disease-the-green-book-front-cover-and-contents-page.

Public Health England. (2014). *Complete routine immunisation schedule*. Available at: ℘ https://www.gov.uk/government/publications/the-complete-routine-immunisation-schedule.

HIV

Children's HIV Association. Paediatric HIV guidelines. Available at: ℘ https://www.chiva.org.uk/guidelines/.

Chapter 17

Rheumatology

General assessment of limb pain or stiffness

Background

The prevalence of pain in the paediatric population is high, increasing with age, and pain, in itself, is not a sensitive marker of disease. Musculoskeletal (MSK) pain, especially of the knees, back, shoulders, and feet, is particularly common, with 6–13% of consultations in paediatric primary care for such assessment. Of note:

- The site to which the pain can be attributed is often vague and all tissues need to be assessed, including joints (disease of synovium, cartilage, or bone), entheses, tendons, and muscles, or more frequently a combination of structures.
- The level of distress from pain does not correlate well with the severity of the underlying or causative pathology. All should be believed and all thoroughly assessed, guided by age:
  - Some children complain little of pain but 'silently' lose function of a limb due to inflammation of a joint, muscle, or bone.
  - Other children, perhaps fuelled by concern or lack of concern of a parent, are distressed with an essentially normal examination.
- The duration of pain is not a sensitive marker of disease and chronic severe pain (>3mth and affecting quality of life) is common, with a prevalence of up to 16% in secondary school-aged girls.
- The majority of causes (>80%) of MSK pain are self-limiting and have little impact on quality of life. In this respect, pain is not a sensitive marker of disease, yet it is still important to provide reassurance to avoid symptom amplification and prolonged disability.
- MSK pain can be a presenting feature of conditions not to be missed or long-term conditions that result in tissue damage, followed by reduced participation in activities and quality of life.
- The challenge is to understand pain in the context of other symptoms and signs. Many diagnoses are made without investigations.

Key features

To facilitate diagnosis, patterns of pain/disease are subclassified into:

- Features/conditions not to be missed (see ➔ Conditions 'not to be missed', p. 659).
- Normal variants (see ➔ Normal musculoskeletal variants, p. 666).
- Inflammatory arthritis (see ➔ The acutely swollen or painful joint, p. 669).
- Non-inflammatory MSK pain (see ➔ Non-inflammatory MSK conditions, pp. 674–5).

Conditions 'not to be missed'

Conditions not to be missed include cancer, infection, and NAI. Complex regional pain syndrome (CRPS) is also on this list since early intervention is essential to avoid high levels of distress and incapacitation. Alerts to these conditions are:

- *Unexplained focal pain and bony tenderness* lasting >2wk in children is a 'red flag' for suspicion of bone cancer. ('Focal' means able to clearly point to site of bone pain or tenderness and cannot be explained by osteochondroses, trauma, or infection.)
- *Systemic features* such as fever, malaise, anorexia, weight loss, rash, and raised acute phase response may point to:
  - Septic arthritis or osteomyelitis (high fever, hot and tender joint, or limb pain).
  - Leukaemia, lymphoma, neuroblastoma, lupus, or vasculitis (persistent low-grade fever >2wk, typically associated with rash).
  - KD (high spiking fever in <6y olds with limb pains).
  - Macrophage activation syndrome (MAS) and multisystem inflammatory disorders.
  - Reactive arthritis.
- *Incongruence between the level of pain and disability reported and the objective findings* on examination may indicate NAI when symptoms are dismissed or CRPS when symptoms are amplified.

Other key features which should trigger referral for further assessment

- Limp (see also ⊃ Limp and hip disorders, p. 680).
- Joint restriction or persistent joint swelling.
- Impaired functional ability.
- School absence or teacher concern.
- Morning symptoms unexplained by previous day activities and tiredness after disturbed sleep.
- Widespread pain.
- Worrying thoughts or anxiety of the patient or parent.
- Report of loss of milestones.
- Loss of peer or social contact or significant reduction in physical activity.

History taking: keynotes by age

The non- or minimally verbal child

- Parents may volunteer impairments of sleep or activities such as movement of a leg when nappy changing.
- Precise localization of the pain/tenderness is difficult. Palpation or resistance to joint movement may elicit change in facial expression.
- Babies and toddlers are better examined on a parent's lap.

The toddler and school-aged child

- Young children may not understand the word 'pain', but parents may help in choice of language. Use of a picture or cuddly toy may help to localize the site of pain.
- Much information is gained from watching the child at play while history taking, and thereafter all children and toddlers are best approached with confidence and ease.

Teenagers

- Whenever possible, teenagers should be offered to be seen on their own, with parents included fully in the consultation thereafter. This is now considered best practice.
- By speaking directly to the young person, an accurate picture will be acquired and will optimize examination and future appointments.
- Supplemental information from parents may be helpful, as may any discordance between histories.
- Identify problems with sleep. Early morning wakening with pain may be associated with inflammatory or malignant conditions, whereas difficulty with sleep initiation or maintenance may be associated with chronic pain.
- Frequent associations with chronic pain include bowel, bladder, and psychological disturbances.

History: specific and system enquiries

Infectious features

- Preceding coryza or rash may indicate viral reactive arthritis (other viral features are 'slapped cheek' of parvovirus B19, widespread and facial macular rash of rubella, and sore throat of mumps).
- Vaccinations may be associated with arthralgia and myalgia but are not associated with juvenile idiopathic arthritis (JIA).
- Reactive arthritis typically lasts 3–6wk, although, when associated with HLA-B27, may last longer. The latter may be associated with conjunctivitis, urethritis, and psoriasiform rash and preceded by a history of diarrhoea.
- If there is bloody diarrhoea and fever, check stool cultures for *Shigella*, *Yersinia*, *Campylobacter*, and *Salmonella*. *Escherichia coli* and *Clostridium difficile* are also known to trigger reactive arthritis.
- Post-streptococcal arthritis is associated with sore throat, no cough, and painful, marginally swollen, and often flitting polyarthritis. Scarlet fever is associated with typical rash and strawberry tongue.
- Consider acute rheumatic fever (ARF) (see ➔ Rheumatic fever, pp. 214–15) when there are additional clinical features, e.g. erythema marginatum, skin nodules, pericardial rub or new murmur (prolonged PR interval), and chorea (see ➔ Chorea, p. 400).
- Routine enquiry should also include contact with infectious diseases, including TB, animal contact, and tick bites (see ➔ Infections characterized by rash, p. 625; ➔ Tuberculosis: presentation and diagnosis, pp. 639–40; ➔ Tropical infections, pp. 644–5; ➔ Travel history and infectious contacts, p. 663).

Character of bone and joint symptoms

- Arthritis is commonly associated with persistent and prolonged morning stiffness and joint restriction. Pain is not a major feature, and any report of joint swelling unreliable.
- Intense, often spasmodic, long bone or vertebral pain with tenderness raises suspicion of neoplasia.
- Entheseal pain, including the heel, patella, ASIS, and plantar fascia, is often disproportionate to the observed findings, may be associated with a restless quality, and can be difficult to distinguish from a pain processing problem such as CRPS.

History of trauma

- Trauma is common and often the event that draws attention to an already swollen joint.
- Attributing pain to non-specific trauma/sprain or internal disruption of a joint can be reassessed after 2–3wk to see if it has resolved.
- Haemarthrosis from internal joint disruption or periarticular swelling from quadriceps contusion or tear occurs within 2h of trauma.
- Trauma includes penetrating injury with FB punctum.

- A mechanism of injury incongruous with examination findings may raise suspicion of NAI (see ➔ Physical abuse, pp. 914–15) or CRPS (see ➔ Complex regional pain syndrome, pp. 676–7).
- An amplified response to minor trauma is also found with juvenile fibromyalgia and sensory integration–autistic spectrum and anxiety disorders, leading to high levels of disability from altered pain processing. There can be complete school absence and grossly abnormal sleep routines attributed to pain.

Systems enquiry and past medical history

- Weight falling across centiles or unexplained weight loss of >5% in an adolescent needs detailed assessment.
- Systems enquiry may indicate features of coeliac disease or IBD or raise concern for multisystem disorders (e.g. SLE or vasculitis).
- Other conditions associated with ↑ risk of arthritis include CF, coeliac disease, Down's syndrome, and other genetic conditions.

Family history

- Enquire about arthritides, including ankylosing spondylitis and related conditions such as IBD, psoriasis, and previous iritis.
- Patients may volunteer haemophilia, familial Mediterranean fever, SLE, and other autoimmune diseases.
- A good family history explores parental or patient concerns and perceptions about arthritis or joint pains, as witnessed in an older family member with RA or osteoarthritis, fibromyalgia, or other conditions.

Travel history and infectious contacts

- History of contact with TB, *Salmonella*, and other enteric organisms should be sought and, depending on the area visited, may also include leishmaniasis and brucellosis with consumption of unpasteurized milk products.
- Insect bites and contact with ticks, including travel to endemic rural areas, may lead to consideration of Lyme disease (see ➔ Infections characterized by rash, p. 625) and other conditions.
- Cat scratches with lymphadenitis or lymphangina are suggestive of *Bartonella* infection.

Clinical examination

Routine examination includes height and weight and a paediatric Gait Arms Legs Spine (pGALS) assessment. Some key pointers to a successful examination include:

- Be attentive of, and reassuring about, painful movements.
- Assess general muscle conditioning and posture, including spinal contour, noting any loss of, or ↑, lordosis.
- Screen for rashes, mouth ulcers, nail and nail bed changes, and organomegaly. Assessment of reactive arthritis includes cardiac auscultation.
- Ocular examination may reveal a red eye or changes of the iris.
- Muscle weakness, muscle fatigue, numbness, focal pain, and delayed development may also indicate neuromuscular disease, including muscular dystrophies, congenital and metabolic myopathies, and neuropathies.
- Widespread pain or a pain processing problem is associated with an essentially normal, although hesitant, examination and often with multiple trigger points (characteristic points of tenderness).
- Hypermobility does not indicate the cause of the pain. Care must be taken when using the term 'hypermobility', as it can be perceived as disabling with a poor outcome. The cause of pain is often complex, but with effective communication and a range of integrated strategies that include focus on self-management and resilience, the outcome will be excellent with full participation and normal quality of life.
- Functional weakness, not attributable to fear of movement from pain, may be indicated by walking on tiptoes and difficulties climbing stairs and putting on T-shirts or jumpers.

Regional MSK examination

Assessment specifically looks for asymmetry, muscle wasting, scars, deformity, tenosynovitis, enthesitis, and spinal and hip disease. Key features to also consider are:

- Normal fat pads, especially in toddlers, may appear as swelling and should be distinguished from subcutaneous oedema, lymphoedema, cellulitis, haematoma, or swelling of tendons or joints.
- *Clicking* is common and normal, unless associated with a jarring or locking movement.
- *Pain at end of range of joint movement* typically indicates intra-articular pathology.
- *Muscle wasting*, a clear sign of chronicity, typically affects the vastus medialis with knee involvement and the calf with ankle involvement. Upper limb muscle wasting is usually less prominent.

- *Tenosynovitis* is more commonly seen around the ankle and may be mechanical in origin, rather than inflammatory. Involvement of the tendons of the hand may result in trigger finger.
- *Tenderness* at the insertion of Achilles tendon, patellar tendon, or plantar fascia, or at the attachment of quads and hamstrings to pelvis suggests enthesitis, as in the specific form of JIA called enthesitis-related arthritis (ERA).
- *Examination of the spine* includes forward flexion for scoliosis, the Schöber's test of lumbar spinal drift, and palpation and distraction of the sacroiliac joints (with the four quadrant test).

pGALS

The pGALS is a quick, excellent screening tool for joint restriction, often key to finding multiple joint involvement when just one or two joints were initially suspected. A full demonstration of pGALS can be found at ℬ https://www.versusarthritis.org/media/3080/student-handbook-11-2.pdf. Of note:
- It is a valuable and playful way of engaging a younger child in examination without touching the child and avoiding distress.
- It includes examination of gait.
- It should be demonstrated by the doctor facing the patient and encouraging them to copy.
- Limbs should be adequately exposed.
- Even subtle differences in range of motion may signify synovial thickening.
- Range of motion and asymmetry of jaw opening is checked.
- Particular attention should also be paid to flexion at all finger joints, extension of the elbow, and inversion and eversion of the foot, checking subtalar and midfoot joints.
- Any doubt about the presence of synovitis can be addressed with US (or MRI, as directed).

Characteristic rashes

In joint conditions, include:
- Psoriasis and associated nail pits (see ➲ Psoriasis, p. 788).
- Palmar pustulosis and acne of synovitis, acne, pustulosis, hyperostosis, and osteitis (SAPHO).
- HSP (see ➲ Henoch–Schönlein purpura, pp. 701–2).
- Erythema chronicum migrans of Lyme disease.
- Erythema marginatum.
- Erythema nodosum of vasculitis and sarcoid.
- Lipodystrophy and/or skin thickening with pink halo in scleroderma.
- Other vasculitic rashes, especially involving the palm or fingertips.
- Nail bed capillary changes of SLE, juvenile dermatomyositis (JDM), scleroderma, and autoimmune overlap conditions.

Normal musculoskeletal variants

Effective reassurance that a child has a normal variant avoids unnecessary referral, investigation, and intervention. Table 17.1 describes common normal variants of MSK development and indicates when referral to orthopaedics, rheumatology, or neurology may be considered.

Table 17.1 Normal MSK variations

Variant	Prevalence	Notes
Genu varum (bow legs)	Very common in <2y olds	If progressive: consider Blount disease, rickets, and skeletal dysplasia. Abnormal when mechanical axis deviates into/beyond medial quadrant
Genu valgum (knock knees)	Physiological, 4–7y, and mild is common thereafter	Refer if intermalleolar distance >8cm, unilateral, modified gait, deteriorating or new onset in adulthood
In-toeing/ out-toeing	Common in <5y olds	Usually resolves by 9y. Causes are metatarsus adductus, femoral anteversion, and tibial torsion. Refer after 9y if affecting gait
Toe walking	7–24% of children (especially in autistic spectrum disorder)	Resolves by 3y. If obligate, new, progressive, or unilateral, consider neuromuscular and orthopaedic disorders
Femoral anteversion	Common 4–7y	Presents as in-toeing and occasionally limb pain. Rarely requires surgery
Hypermobile hands	Common in <5y; at 13y, 30% boys, 46% girls	No association with pain. May be associated with development/ coordination delay, needing writing support
Hypermobile knees	Common <5y; 8–11% at 13y	May be associated with patellofemoral pain and biomechanical imbalances
Flat feet (pes planus)	All initially; >40% at 3–6y; 1 in 7 adults	Longitudinal arch at 3–5y. Shoe inserts stabilize but do not correct the foot. Exercises address biomechanical pain. Rigid flat foot indicates bone/neural problem
High arch (pes cavus)	10% of population	Assess neuromuscular status (especially if progressive) and biomechanics. Consider spinal tumour if unilateral
Benign nocturnal limb pain of childhood	Common in 3–12y. Peak age 6y. Up to 40% under 5y	Further assessment if disability, focal tenderness, fever, weight loss, weakness, swelling, erythema, prolonged morning stiffness

Imaging investigations

Imaging should be discussed with a radiologist, whenever possible, with the aim of minimizing procedure time and radiation exposure. Tests that are considered include:

- *Radiographs* which are the investigation of choice if considering periosteal lesions, traumatic or stress fractures, mineralization defects (e.g. rickets or periarticular osteopenia), loose bodies of osteochondritis, or major structural conditions like skeletal dysplasia.
- *US* can be helpful when examination findings are equivocal, but there is a high false −ve rate in routine clinical situations, especially for feet, ankles, and small joints of the hand.
  - Consider US if there is likelihood of joint/tendon synovitis, an osteochondral lesion, or a ligament, enthesis, or tendon lesion.
- *MRI* shows chondral changes and bone and entheseal oedema and is the investigation of choice for pelvic and spinal assessment. Gadolinium enhancement reduces the false +ve rate.
  - Whole-body MRI is used when malignancy, infection, or non-bacterial osteomyelitis, including chronic recurrent multifocal osteomyelitis (CRMO) and SAPHO, are suspected.
- DEXA scanning grades bone mineral density (BMD) against the average expected, but data need adjustment for bone growth and pubertal changes.

Laboratory tests and samples

Blood tests

Key points to consider when ordering blood tests include:

- There are no absolutely diagnostic laboratory tests (including ANA) for JIA, and ESR and FBC may be normal.
- *RF +ve polyarticular JIA* occurs in <5% of JIA and has a characteristic symmetrical appearance. RF should not be considered a routine test and is often misinterpreted.
- *Autoimmune serology* is helpful in multisystem inflammatory disorders. Weakly +ve results may need repeating.
- *ANA:* associated with uveitis, but it can occur when ANA –ve.
- *Thrombocytosis:* is common in most inflammatory conditions, particularly in systemic-onset JIA (SoJIA), when associated with neutrophilia. Low platelet and lymphocyte counts occur in SLE and antiphospholipid antibody syndrome (APS).
- *Low platelet and neutrophil count:* in the presence of raised inflammatory markers and arthritis may indicate malignancy.
- *Fall in cell count and ESR with rise in ALT/AST:* may indicate MAS and needs correlating with clinical condition and ferritin level.
- *Unexplained ESR:* >15mm/h has a differential diagnosis similar to that of fever or pyrexia of unknown origin (PUO):
  - Persistent increase (over 6–12wk) in platelets and CRP raises the likelihood of inflammatory disease being found.
  - Biopsy of a suspected lesion can be helpful, and whole-body MRI can be used to screen for malignancy or to locate inflammation.
  - Other causes are renal disease, especially when there is azotaemia, multiple myeloma, and anaemia of chronic disease.
- Interpretation of *ASOT* is difficult. The most reliable feature of streptococcal infection is sore throat without cough. Serial ASOT, anti-streptococcal DNAse B, and streptozyme may be helpful.
- *Lyme serology:* should be requested, in keeping with Lyme disease diagnostic guidelines (see ➲ Box 16.1).
- In suspected TB, IGRA, CXR, and Mantoux tests are important if synovial aspiration is not done (see ➲ Tuberculosis: presentation and diagnosis, pp. 639–40).

Joint aspiration and synovial biopsy

These may need GA or inhalational agents. Synovial biopsy is helpful when considering pigmented villonodular synovitis (PVNS), sarcoid, chronic in-fections, and malignancy. Arthroscopy has higher yield than needle biopsy. When aspirating synovial fluid, consider:

- Joint aspiration for Gram stain and culture when investigating septic arthritis or when considering TB synovitis.
- Bloody taps are common, but haemarthrosis is considered when blood runs through the whole sample and may be attributable to trauma, bleeding diathesis, PVNS, or haemangioma.
- Crystal arthropathy is very rare in children and adolescents.

The acutely swollen or painful joint

To help in the assessment of an acute swollen or painful joint, categorization is by age, systemic features, and joint number, using a threshold of three joints to define multi-articular involvement. The conventional approach in JIA (see ➔ Juvenile idiopathic arthritis, pp. 692–3) does not help with improved diagnosis, treatment, or prognosis. Assessment of conditions not to be missed can be found in ➔ Conditions 'not to be missed', p. 659 (see Table 17.2):

- Mono-/oligoarticular arthritis in children (1–2 joints).
- Multi-articular arthritis in children (≥3 joints).

Table 17.2 Differential of a swollen or painful joint

Condition	Examples	Investigations
Monoarticular disease	Septic arthritis TB PVNS FB synovitis Sickle-cell/haemophilia Leukaemia Non-bacterial osteomyelitis/CRMO Lyme disease and cat-scratch fever Travel-associated brucellosis and leishmaniasis	Blood cultures and synovial fluid aspirate, Mantoux, IGRA, USS, MRI, synovial biopsy, blood film, genetics, coagulation, factor assays
Post-infectious arthritis	Viral-associated arthritis Post-enteric arthritis Post-streptococcal arthritis Rheumatic fever	Viral serology, ASOT, anti-DNAse B, throat swab, echocardiography
Juvenile arthritis and spondyloarthropathies	HLA-B27-associated reactive arthritis, IBD-associated arthritis, enthesitis	Faecal calprotectin, MRI
Multisystem disorders	(See Table 17.8) Differential of fever, rash, and arthritis	
Non-inflammatory conditions	(See Table 17.5)	X-ray, MRI
Pain conditions	CRPS CWP (including hypermobility)	Diagnosis based on history and examination

Septic arthritis and osteomyelitis

Septic arthritis and osteomyelitis are less common than juvenile arthritis but require urgent orthopaedic assessment and intervention with antibiotics to avoid complications.

- 50% of *septic arthritis* presents in the first 2y, with 75% affecting lower limb joints. Shoulder involvement is also common.
- 50% of *osteomyelitis* occurs at <5y of age, often with preceding trauma. Organisms may not be isolated from culture or biopsy.

Causes

The commonest pathogen is *Staphylococcus aureus*. Others include:

- By age: neonates—*E. coli*, GBS; 2mth to 5y—GAS, *Streptococcus pneumoniae*, and *Haemophilus* in non-vaccinated; and adolescents— *Neisseria gonorrhoeae*.
- *Mycobacterium tuberculosis* is increasingly recognized.
- Viral-induced transient synovitis is an important differential when there is hip involvement.
- For travel-associated pathogens and zoonoses, see travel history (see ➲ Travel history and infectious conditions, p. 663) and laboratory tests (see ➲ Laboratory tests and samples, p. 668).

Presentation

Depends on organism and host immunity. Infants may have few signs and may appear well with no fever, although they resist limb movement. Toddlers may become unable to weight-bear. In osteomyelitis, there is usually a history of trauma, typically of a long bone metaphysis, and there may be haematogenous spread from infections of the lung, skin, ear, nose, or throat. There are acute, subacute (2–3wk delay), chronic (rare in children), and non-bacterial (e.g. CRMO or SAPHO) forms of osteomyelitis.

Examination

Examination of a septic joint shows a hot, swollen, and often tense joint, with complete or partial limitation of movement. Bony involvement includes marked tenderness, swelling, and overlying erythema. *Kocher's prediction algorithm* for differentiating septic arthritis from transient synovitis includes:

- Fever >38.5°C.
- Non-weight-bearing or pain with passive motion of the joint.
- ESR >40mm/h.
- WCC >12 × 10⁹/L.

Investigations

The yield from joint/bone aspirate and biopsy is poor.

Management of septic arthritis

IV antibiotics and analgesia will depend on local policies, but as a guide, according to age, see Tables 17.3 and 17.4. The following are recommended:
- <3mth old: IV cefotaxime and amoxicillin.
- 3mth to 5y: IV cefuroxime.
- >5y: IV flucloxacillin.

Table 17.3 Summary of antibiotics by age group

Neonate (<3mth)	Benzylpenicillin and gentamicin Or cefotaxime Add amoxicillin if *Listeria* is suspected PO: switch to co-amoxiclav
3mth to 5y	Cefuroxime PO: switch to cefalexin or co-amoxiclav
>5y	Flucloxacillin or clindamycin If *Pseudomonas* suspected: ceftazidime or ciprofloxacin PO: switch to co-amoxiclav or flucloxacillin or clindamycin

Reproduced with permission from Sukhtankar P, Clark J, Faust S. (2013–10). Bone and joint infections in children. In *Oxford Textbook of Rheumatology*. Oxford, UK: Oxford University Press, Table 99.3.

Table 17.4 Post-immediate management of septic arthritis in children

Diagnostic status	Management
Diagnosis not confirmed and clinically improved	Splint and continue IV antibiotic 1–2wk Then switch to PO co-amoxiclav for a total treatment duration of 4–6wk, according to clinical condition
Confirmed diagnosis (pus ± 50 000 WBC ± pathogen in blood or synovial fluid)	Splint and continue IV antibiotic 1–2wk and adjust, based on culture/susceptibility Then switch to PO co-amoxiclav for a total treatment duration of 4–6wk, according to clinical condition and pathogen Weekly clinical and laboratory follow-up
Diagnosis not confirmed Clinically not improved	Review antibiotics Obtain paediatric infectious diseases advice Further evaluation to consider other types of non-infectious arthritis

Malignant bone tumours

(See also ➲ Bone tumors, pp. 600–1; ➲ Benign bone tumours, p. 686.)

Malignant bone tumours are rare (annual incidence of 6 per 1 million children), of which 55% are osteosarcoma and 35% are Ewing's sarcoma. Malignancy should be suspected, particularly in an adolescent, if there is *persistent pain* of long bones or vertebrae of >2wk with associated:

- Point tenderness.
- Night awakening.
- Pain out of proportion to clinical findings, or
- Other features, including: bony swelling or enlargement, weight loss, malaise, pathological fracture (5–10%), and rarely lung involvement.

Other malignancies

Many other childhood malignancies also have MSK features at presentation, in particular ALL, lymphoma, and neuroblastoma.

NB: isolated hip or back involvement in a young child raises the suspicion of leukaemia in the absence of sepsis.

Joint pains with systemic features

Our approach to instances of presentation with joint pains and systemic features include the following steps. (See ➔ Conditions 'not to be missed', p. 659.)

History

Address travel, infectious contacts, and social and family histories.
- Screening questions about each organ system may point to a diagnosis of multisystem inflammatory disorders.
- Characterizing the fever, including fluctuation throughout the day, periodicity, and duration, may indicate KD or specific periodic fevers (see ➔ Kawasaki disease, pp. 630–1; ➔ Multisystem inflammatory disorders, pp. 700–2). A 'quotidian' fever occurring once or twice a day with return to baseline is characteristic of SoJIA.
- *Inflammatory arthritis* has key features, including:
  - Consistent morning stiffness lasting >30min.
  - Swelling with joint restriction.
  - Associated muscle atrophy.
  - Involvement of >1–2 joints (see Table 17.2).
- *Post-infectious arthritis* causes an acute painful and swollen joint (for symptom enquiry, see Table 17.2). Causes include Lyme disease, *Brucella*, cat scratch/*Bartonella*, and leischmaniasis.

Examination

In addition to the general examination already outlined in ➔ Clinical examination, pp. 664–5:
- *Characterize any rash* as it may facilitate diagnoses of SoJIA, lupus, dermatomyositis, periodic fevers, and vasculitis. Other important rashes are those of pyoderma and neutrophilic dermatoses, scleroderma, and Behçet's disease.
- *Ocular features* may include red eye, pain, double vision, photophobia, and blurring.
- *ENT features* may include sinusitis, crusting, bloody discharge, tinnitus, hearing loss, facial weakness, oral ulceration, sore throat, parotitis, and dry mouth.

Non-inflammatory MSK conditions

Biomechanical and non-inflammatory pain is very common in healthy children and adolescents and is by far the commonest cause of MSK pain. Hypermobility in the normal population is also common, and care should be taken before ascribing focal or widespread MSK pain to hypermobility syndrome or type III Ehlers–Danlos syndrome (EDS). Inappropriate or overzealous use of this diagnostic label can reflect a misunderstanding of the multifactorial nature of MSK pain and project a 'disabling', rather than 'enabling', formulation onto patients → parental confusion → lack of flexibility over treatment → excess disability.

History

Non-participation in physical education, extracurricular sport, or other physical activity may indicate a significant impact of a condition, general deconditioning, or cycles of behavioural response to pain.

- Features suggesting a *functional disorder* include IBS, dizziness, paraesthesiae, headaches, and bladder dysfunction.
- *Family history* may indicate other painful conditions, but these are very unlikely to be genetically related other than through body type and patterns of movement and behaviour.
- *Skeletal dysplasias* may also present with limb pain and deformity but usually present with a family history and disproportionate short stature or, in the case of osteogenesis imperfecta (OI), fractures.
- *Biomechanical pain* typically increases with activity and occurs in the evening or following morning. It may be associated with stiffness at these times or with minor swelling and tenderness, and may occur with inflammatory or other conditions. It commonly occurs with chronic arthritis because of muscle and joint inhibition from active inflammation and subsequent MSK imbalance.

Factors contributing to chronic non-inflammatory MSK pains may be identified in the history, e.g.:

- MSK imbalance from tight and/or weak musculature or ligaments.
- General deconditioning, whether through overall lack of effective background physical activity, excess sedentary behaviour, or avoidance of activity due to pain. Strength may also be suboptimal for the range of joint movement.
- Repetitive physical activity with suboptimal muscular control.
- Subchondral or other bony stress.
- Delayed gross motor development (including proprioception), which continues through to puberty and requires myelination and neuromuscular imprinting, so practice will not improve rate of change.
- Adverse gait maturation/efficiency or other patterns of movement (e.g. tracking of patella), which continue until after skeletal maturity.

- A 'boom and bust' approach to physical activity.
- Loss of confidence in specific movements.
- Difficulty in pain self-appraisal and sensitization of pain pathways.
- Ruminating or attentive behaviours.
- Reinforcing parental or other family member responses.
- Social and environmental factors, including those at school.

Assessment

A therapist's assessment of 'engagement' will provide an understanding of the patient's cooperation with home exercise and this can be correlated with examination findings (e.g. persistence of tight musculature or specific areas of deconditioning). Also, be aware of other causes that may be evident on examination (see Table 17.5):

- *Focal bone pain* occurs with osteochondroses and osteoid osteoma, and although very rare, osteosarcomas should be considered in the absence of typical features of osteochondrosis.
- *Neuromuscular conditions* manifest by weakness and may present with (often initially focal) pain.

Table 17.5 Typical non-inflammatory MSK disorders

Painful conditions from focal lesions
- Patellofemoral syndrome and other biomechanical imbalances.
- Tendinopathy and enthesitis.
- Perthe's disease.
- SUFE.
- Osteochondroses and osteochondritis dessicans.
- Stress fracture.
- Tarsal coalition.
- Osteoid osteoma and neoplasia.
- PVNS.
- Haemophilia.
- CRPS.
- Trauma and NAI.

Conditions that may be associated with widespread MSK pain
- Juvenile fibromyalgia.
- NAI.
- Skeletal dysplasias.
- MFS and EDS.
- OI (focal or multiple fractures).
- Muscular dystrophies and other neuromuscular conditions.
- Rickets (pain rare if no muscular weakness/X-ray changes).
- Vitamin C deficiency (scurvy).
- Hyperparathyroidism.
- X-linked hypophosphataemic rickets (fractures/bone pain).

Complex regional pain syndrome

The characteristic finding of CRPS is a level of pain, tenderness, and disability disproportionate to the mechanism of injury or signs apparent from examination and/or persistence of these symptoms beyond the time of normal healing. This condition is illustrated by the presence of excess pain and dysesthesia in up to a half of distal forearm fractures in adults, despite allowance for normal healing and irrespective of the mechanism or extent of injury or the level of intervention.

• Trauma (e.g. fracture, burn, surgery, etc.) is the commonest triggering event. The event may be trivial.
• Often no cause is identified.
• CRPS may also occur in response to chronic inflammatory or other MSK conditions.

Suspicion and early intervention are key. This approach avoids a cycle of clinical decline and excessive investigation with inadvertent iatrogenesis from medical reinforcement of further pain and threat. The cycle of decline includes:

• Failure of effective pain appraisal.
• Increasing fear and avoidance of pain and pain sensitization.
• Deteriorating physical function, and sequelae such as loss of sleep and ↑ anxiety.

The pathogenesis of CRPS is not fully known but involves peripheral and central sensitization of pain processing and secondary imbalances of autonomic function leading to colour change and late signs of sweating dysfunction, hair loss, and deteriorating skin integrity. CRPS has been sub-characterized by the presence (type 2) or absence (type 1) of injury to a specific peripheral nerve, although the value of this distinction is unclear and a determined search for evidence of neural tissue damage can undermine management strategies.

CRPS in children and adolescents differs from that in adults in that the lower limb or multiple limbs are more commonly involved and dystrophic changes and long-term disability are less common. Hence:

• More commonly seen involving the distal part of a limb.
• There are similar disorders of the back, chest, abdomen, and scalp, and disruption of internal pain perception also occurs where it may be related to organ dysfunction (e.g. gut and headache).
• Other features of threat arising from sleep dysfunction, anxiety, family disruption, and parental behaviours contribute to the pain experience and should be fully assessed and included in management.

Clinical features of pain

Patients may become 'depersonalized' from their affected limb, with a feeling that it no longer belongs to them. Particular characteristics of the pain include:

- Descriptions of 'burning' and paraesthesiae or numbness.
- *Allodynia*— an otherwise innocuous stimulus that produces pain.
- *Hyperalgesia*—↑ pain perception to a given stimulus.
- *Hyperpathia*—delayed over-reaction, often after repetitive cutaneous stimulus.

Investigations

Frequently over-interpreted and prevent a diagnosis of CRPS from being made. There are few corroborative tests, and radiological investigations may show sequelae such as bone oedema (MRI), osteopenia, and disturbance of regional blood flow on bone scintigraphy. Abnormalities of ESR, CRP, and FBC do not rule out CRPS.

Management

Staging of CRPS may have some prognostic benefit but is not considered particularly useful clinically, although it is for research purposes. Success in treating CRPS relies on:

- Early and accurate diagnosis.
- Early treatment in order to prevent chronicity (once persisting beyond 6–8mth, it is difficult to reverse).
- Effective explanation: 25–35% of children and adolescents with CRPS are resistant to routine practice and will benefit from more intense programmes of care, as described in ⊃ Chronic pain in children, pp. 718–21.
- Graded exercise programme supervised by a therapist experienced in chronic pain management and frequent desensitization. Working on the four pillars of care (education, pain relief, physical rehabilitation, and psychological intervention) improves resilience and most patients respond within 4–6 therapy sessions. Patients can expect to be pain-free and return to all activities.
  - Attention to anxiety, psychosocial stressors, pain behaviour, and sleep disturbance is important.
  - Desensitization of the affected region can help to normalize the sensations of hyperalgesia and allodynia. This is achieved by applying different textures to the affected area, concentrating particularly on the interface between normal/abnormal sensations.
  - The value of early IV pamidronate in relieving pain, especially if there are bony changes on imaging, and short courses of glucocorticoids is debatable.
  - Tricyclic antidepressants can help correct sleep disturbance and increase pain threshold. However, like gabapentin or pregabalin, their direct role in pain management is unproven in adolescents.

Normal gait

Normal gait is a complex automatic process that requires the development of muscles, bones, joints, and ligaments effectively coordinated by the nervous system. Imbalances will lead to problems and delay may still be within normal development. A simple view of normal gait includes:
* *A stance phase* starting with the heel strike, progressing through plantar flexion, to toe-off. Assessment also looks at base width and single limb support time.
* *A swing phase,* from toe-off to heel strike, with forward rotation and tilting of the pelvis and a stable lumbar spine and abdomen. Assessment also includes cadence and stride length.

In general, do not ascribe hypermobility or hypotonia to delay of normal gait. Slower development may be perceived as a problem but is not a medical disorder, as catch-up and fine adjustments to gait may take up to age 8–10y. (See ➔ Identifying abnormal gait, pp. 678–9 for abnormal gait.)

Identifying abnormal gait

Assessment by age group

Toddlers and preschool children
Observe the gait closely and compare with normal development and variants (see ➔ Normal gait, p. 678; ➔ Normal musculoskeletal variants, p. 666):
* Note any preceding illness; take care not to ascribe limp to trauma.
* Avoid simple focus on the hip; observe foot position and knee straightening when walking; examine the back, abdomen, and groin.
* Morning stiffness is typical of JIA.
* Any incongruence in the history may suggest NAI.
* Trivial injury may be unwitnessed, and fractures missed on X-ray.
* Weakness and loss of motor milestones occur in neuromuscular conditions.

School-aged children and adolescents
An insidious onset of limp is typical of Perthes disease and JIA, the latter having associated stiffness after prolonged rest.
* Also consider other osteochondroses, SUFE, or bone tumour.
* Association with exercise and evening predominance is typical of biomechanical conditions.
* Consider sports-related injuries and overuse syndromes.
* Hip restriction or pain at the limits of passive rotation requires further investigation.

Further assessment/examination
* *Watch:* neurology; measure and compare leg lengths; observe walk, run, hop, and coordination; assess strength.
* *Look at the shoes* and wear patterns.
* *Assess skin:* the whole body, including soles of feet and nails.
* *Evaluate muscle:* any pain or weakness, including difficulties climbing stairs, getting up from the floor, and dressing.

- Weakness is assessed using Gower's sign, rising out of a chair without use of upper limbs, sustained neck flexor strength, and winging of scapulae when pushing against a wall.
- Benign myositis of childhood is a transient illness that presents with calf pain in a 4–10y old, 3 days after fever and high CK.
- G-BS affects distal muscles and is associated with gradual progression, marked weakness, sensory symptoms, and normal CK.
- Chronic myositis (e.g. JDM, SLE, pyomyositis) is associated with rash, low-grade fever, muscle tenderness, and high CK.
- Muscular dystrophies and atrophies, upper motor neuron lesions, including spinal cord compression, neuropathies, and metabolic muscle disease, are not associated with pain.
- Muscle weakness and Trendelenberg gait are seen in gross deconditioning from sedentary behaviour and chronic pain conditions. Symptomatic deterioration occurs in the evening.

Predictive patterns of gait abnormality

- *Antalgic:* pain / stiffness from trauma / inflammation → shorter stance phase.
- *Trendelenburg limp:* weak hip abduction, causing a body sway in the stance phase and a droop in the hip in the swing phase; may be due to neuromuscular disorders or hip joint disorders.
- *Waddling:* attributable to neuromuscular or articular stiffness around the pelvis.
- *Stiff-legged (peg-leg):* results from loss of knee flexion and circumduction, with pelvic elevation on the affected side. Causes include hemiplegia or leg length discrepancy from chronic knee synovitis.
- *Toe walking:* habitual, typically resolving at 3y, or due to muscle contractures or spasticity from upper motor neuron lesion, especially if unilateral or a heal strike cannot be encouraged. When unilateral, may indicate a lower extremity length inequality or a wound to the heel.
- *High stepping:* from difficulties with foot dorsiflexion, usually associated with peroneal neuropathies, lower motor neuron disease (e.g. spina bifida, polio), and peripheral neuropathies (e.g. Charcot–Marie–Tooth).
- *Stooped:* might indicate abdominal pathology.
- *Clumsy:* often described, but rarely seen in formal assessment. Partly the result of inattention and may be from subtle developmental delay (often associated with handwriting difficulty and learning disability). May include frank neurodevelopmental or metabolic disorders.
- *Ataxic:* wide-based, unsteady, and staggering and appears 'not ordered'.

Limp and hip disorders

Most cases of acute limp (asymmetric gait pattern) are seen in accident and emergency (A&E). Infection and malignancy are considered if there are systemic features, or *Perthes disease* and *slipped upper femoral epiphysis* (SUFE) otherwise. Most cases of an acute limp, however, have a preceding illness and are diagnosed as *transient tenosynovitis* or irritable hip.

Perthes disease

An insidious onset of limp and pain in the groin or referred to the knee/thigh that is relieved by rest:

- There may be limitation of hip internal rotation and abduction (due to adductor spasm).
- Leg length inequality suggests femoral head collapse. There may be spontaneous resolution, especially in younger patients, in whom conservative management is indicated.
- Early surgical review is required.

Slipped upper femoral epiphysis

A pathological translation of the head of the femur in relation to the femoral neck in a backward direction through the epiphysis.

- It affects teens and pre-teens (boys > girls) who are still growing and causes pain, stiffness, and instability in the affected hip.
- It usually develops gradually over time, but there may be a sudden presentation. It may be missed when assessment suggests rectus femoris tear in athletic individuals.
- It requires early recognition and surgery to stop the femoral head from slipping further. This will avoid the need for more involved surgery and the potential for early-onset degenerative change.

Developmental dysplasia of the hip

Previously called 'congenital dislocation of the hip'. Developmental dysplasia of the hip (DDH) includes hip instability/subluxation/dislocation acetabular dysplasia.

- Incidence: 1:500 (1:50 newborn hips are unstable; 90% spontaneously stabilize by 9wks).
- Risk factors: family history, female > male (5:1), breech birth, large birth weight (>5kg).
- Aetiology: capsular laxity (type III collagen, maternal oestrogens), intrauterine volume (breech position, first born, oligohydramnios).
- Associations: other 'packaging' disorders: torticollis (20%), metatarsus adductus (10%), talipes calcaneovalgus, Down's syndrome.
- Teratologic dislocation: hip dislocation before birth associated with neuromuscular syndromes (e.g. myelodysplasia, lumbosacral agenesis, chromosomal abnormalities).

Examination

Screen all newborns for DDH at newborn examination (NIPE) and then again at 6wks. High-risk infants are selected for additional ultrasound screening.

In the neonate:
- Is hip dislocated? If so, is it reducible? Ortolani's test (O for out). Gently elevate (anteriorly) and abduct the dislocated hip to reduce it (clunk of reduction).
- If not dislocated, can I dislocate it (i.e. dislocatable)? Barlow's test. Gently adduct and depress (posteriorly) femur; vulnerable hip dislocates.

These 2 provocation manoeuvres become unreliable after age 6–8wks.

Treatment

Depends on age of child. A Pavlik harness (holds hips in abduction during first few months of life) avoids surgical intervention in >90% of cases. If teratogenic or late diagnosis (after 8 wks), surgery usually required. Urgent referral to a paediatric orthopaedic surgeon whenever DDH is detected.

Regional musculoskeletal diagnoses

Wrist and hand pain

Isolated MSK lesions in the wrist and hands of children are rare:
- Small swellings may be ganglia that resolve spontaneously in 50%.
- Congenital trigger thumb or finger affects 1 in 300 children. Spontaneous resolution in 60% within 2y.
- Persistent swelling in wrists and fingers may denote JIA. USS is a relatively easy and acceptable way to confirm.
- Wrist pain is presenting feature of skeletal dysplasia or rickets.

Thoracic back/chest pain

Chest pain is a common presentation to primary care and A&E in patients aged 10–21y. It is often alarming to parents and patients, but rarely caused by a serious condition:
- Chest pain is classified into MSK, respiratory, GI, cardiac, and other conditions. Acute chest pain is cardiac in origin in <6%.
- One-third of adolescents with chest pains who present to outpatients have a history of stressful events and typically associated with other somatic complaints and sleep disturbance.

Pelvic, groin, and thigh pain

(See also ⮕ Developmental dysplasia of hip, p. 681; ⮕ Limp and hip disorders, p. 680.) Ask the patient to point to the site of pain. Intra-articular hip pain localizes to the groin. Lateral hip and pelvic pain are usually biomechanical in origin.

Knee pain and lower limb development

Assess the knee, foot, and ankle to exclude developmental variants (see Table 17.1), then:
- *Growing pains* are common and often seen in <6y olds. There is nighttime predominance, hence the term '*benign nocturnal pain of childhood*'. Knees, thighs, shins, and feet are key sites.
- *Osteochondroses* of knee structures are common in the growing skeleton (see Table 17.6).
- *Osteochondritis* affects the articular cartilage and when a fragment separates, it is 'dissecans'.
- *Patellofemoral syndrome*, the commonest cause of anterior knee pain in adolescents, is attributable to an underlying biomechanical imbalance, including muscle tightness, that leads to abnormal loading of the knee and patella maltracking.
- *Patella instability* varies from a mild dynamic imbalance to recurrent patella dislocation.
- Other causes of anterior knee pain in active children include *insertional enthesitis*, local *bursitis*, and *fat pad syndrome*.
- The knee is a common presenting site for JIA, PVNS, TB/septic arthritis, and haemarthrosis (trauma).

Evaluation of back pain

Back pain in children and adolescents is common, with a lifetime prevalence of up to 70–80% by 20y. Low back pain (LBP) in childhood or adolescence is a significant risk factor for LBP in adulthood. Unless <5y of age, most cases of back pain are non-specific and self-limiting. Of those that present to doctors or physiotherapists, the likelihood of finding an underlying pathology remains low. However, concern arises when dealing with:

- A young child.
- Refusal to walk, irritability, loss or delayed acquisition of developmental milestones, or early development of hand preference.
- Neurological symptoms.
- Intractable pain or night pain.
- Systemic features.

History

A full history, and also find out about:

- Trauma, especially twisting (sudden or repetitive), which may aggravate/cause a *pars defect* (spondylolysis) → spondylolisthesis.
- Inflammatory, mechanical, systemic, and neurological symptoms.
- Previous use of systemic corticosteroid treatment, which may suggest osteoporosis as a cause.
- Assess night sweats and relevant TB contact risk.
- Back pain: LBP is especially common in athletic young people. Back pain is commoner at times of rapid growth, particularly in girls and those with high and low levels of activity.
- Social history, including stresses and loss of sleep.

Examination

A full examination, but also focus on:

- Disproportionate disability (including school absence), compared to examination, which may indicate pain amplification.
- Assessment of focal bony tenderness, neurology, gait, and posture.
- Survey the skin for possible bruising, hairy patches overlying the spine, and café-au-lait or axillary freckling (NF).
- Neurological examination.
- Modified Schober's test for lumbo-sacral spine mobility is useful in JIA.
- Reduced hamstring flexibility (determined by popliteal angle) and tight hip flexors (Thomas' test) are commonly associated with back pain.

Osteochondroses and osteochondritis dissecans

The cause of these benign, but disruptive, conditions is site-dependent and not clearly understood. An avascular theory has been proposed for Perthes disease of the hip, whereas at other sites, traction apophysitis results in disturbance of endochondral ossification. The eponyms of different sites can be found in Table 17.6.

Diagnosis

Based on tenderness of the anatomical sites:
• X-rays are rarely necessary, other than in atypical cases when bone tumour may be considered.
• X-ray may show epiphyseal or apophyseal disruption or fragmentation.

Management

Includes patient and family education, correction of biomechanical imbalance, and NSAIDs. Aggravating sporting activity may need to be reduced.

Surgical review

Required for Blount and Perthes disease:
• Osteochondritis dissecans is thought to result from microtrauma from biomechanical stress. If it causes persistent locking, giving way, or sharp pain, surgical review is required.
• Plain radiographs will show a well-circumscribed, sclerotic lesion, but in young patients before skeletal maturity, there is a good chance of dissecans healing.

Table 17.6 Osteochondroses

Scheuermann's disease	Vertebral epiphyseal osteochondritis in adolescence results in painless dorsal kyphosis with compensatory lumbar lordosis. Lateral spine X-ray shows vertebral end-plate irregularity, anterior vertebral wedging, and kyphosis
Legg–Calvé–Perthes disease	Perthes disease is osteonecrosis of the femoral epiphysis and occurs in the age range of 3–8y, most frequently in boys (ratio 4:1). Perthes disease is bilateral in 10–20% of cases
Osgood–Schlatter's disease	This osteochondrosis is probably due to repetitive trauma at the site of patellar tendon insertion into the tibial tubercle. It typically occurs in athletic adolescents, especially young ♂ aged 14–16y. Pain is usually on exercise and eases with rest
Sinding–Larsen–Johansson's disease	Overloading of the patella at its secondary centre of ossification, producing traction apophysitis at the patella lower pole. Although not exclusive to the group, it is a typical sports-related injury in adolescent athletes who jump, e.g. high-jump, basketball
Köhler's disease	This osteochondrosis is essentially an osteonecrosis lesion of the tarsal navicular. Changes may represent a developmental variation in ossification and it presents with a painful limp. Weight-bearing is more comfortable on the outside of the foot and the navicular is tender
Freiberg's disease	An osteonecrosis of the metatarsal (usually the second) head, following trauma. It is commonest in adolescent ♀. Pain is localized and worse on weight-bearing, with swelling sometimes detectable
Elbow capitellum	In the elbow, the capitellum and radius touch to absorb forces from the wrist—usually in sports such as gymnastics or involving heavy lifting. This sometimes causes injury to bone and cartilage

Fractures

Up to 42% of boys and 27% of girls experience a fracture by 16y of age and many experience up to three fractures:

- The rate of fracture increases with age, being highest at 14y of age, largely due to sport, fights, and road traffic accident.
- Fractures in infants should always raise suspicion of NAI.
- Low-impact insufficiency fractures may raise suspicion of OI, which, in the absence of short stature, is generally the classical or type 1 form. This may be associated with blue sclerae, hypermobile joints, and adverse dentition.
- It is always important to understand the mechanism and force involved in all instances, not only to identify NAI and insufficiency fractures of OI, but also to help identify strategies to avoid future fractures.

Management

- X-rays help to elicit the involvement of growth plates.
- Interpretation of radiographs needs to take account of the child's age and whether findings are due to age-related normal variants.
- The rate of complication depends on the type of fracture, physis involvement, and remaining growth capacity. Of note:
  - Distal femur and proximal tibia are the most susceptible to physeal involvement.
  - Fractures in children are at risk of greater deformity.

Benign bone tumours

(See also ⊃ Bone tumours, pp. 600–1; ⊃ Malignant bone tumours, p. 672.)
These tumours are often initially identified on X-ray and include:

- *Osteoid osteoma:* small, painful radiolucent nidus affecting lower limb long bones.
- *Osteoblastoma:* which causes pain and swelling from within the bone.
- *Osteochondroma, endochondroma and chondroblastoma:* cartilaginous tumours which typically cause painful masses and have a low potential for malignant transformation.
- Other benign tumours: include *fibrodysplasia* which produces a ground-glass matrix.

Vitamin D deficiency and rickets

Rickets results from defective bone and cartilage mineralization before closure of the epiphyses. Although debated, levels of 25-hydroxyvitamin D (25-OHD) in the UK are considered:
• Replete: when >50nmol/L.
• Deficient: when <30nmol/L.

Causes of rickets

• *Vitamin D deficiency:* low sunlight exposure, dietary lack, or suboptimal metabolism.
  • Both vitamin D_2 (ergocalciferol) from dietary vegetables and D_3 (colecalciferol) from animal tissues and *de novo* synthesis in skin are metabolized to active 1,25-OHD2 and D3, respectively.
  • PTH is raised due to vitamin D-associated Ca^{2+} lack. High PTH can increase bone turnover and bone loss.
• *Resistance to vitamin D* (see ➜ Vitamin D, p. 426).
• *Non-PTH-related defect in renal handling of phosphate.*

Examination findings

Children with rickets may have:
• *General:* hypotonia, apathy, growth retardation, and delayed walking.
• *Bones and skeleton:* on weight-bearing, long bones become bowed. Typically, you may see:
  • Wrist: irregularity of the metaphyseal–epiphyseal junction associated with pain and bony enlargement.
  • Costochondral junctions/ribs: rachitic rosary; softened ribs and indentation along diaphragm attachments (Harrison's groove).
  • Skull: rapid growth of softened skull leads to craniotabes, parietal bone flattening, and frontal bossing. Dentition is delayed and poor.
• *Peripheral and CNS:* paraesthesiae and tetany, seizures, psychosis.
• *Heart:* cardiac dysrhythmia.
• *GI:* underlying intestinal disorders with fat malabsorption that is the cause of vitamin D deficiency.

Management

Of note, bony deformities may persist despite treatment and may require surgery. Specific treatment includes:
• *25-OHD replacement:* normalizes secondary hyperparathyroidism and symptom control. Bone pain and muscle weakness respond quickly. However:
  • Type I vitamin D-dependent rickets: rare AR disease → low 1,25-OHD → rickets before 2y and failure to respond to normal vitamin D replacement. Treatment is with *calcitriol*.
  • Type II vitamin D-dependent rickets: AR disease involving vitamin D receptor; 70% of patients have alopecia.
• *Co-treatment with Ca^{2+} supplements:* not necessary in all cases.

Generalized skeletal disorders

Osteogenesis imperfecta

OI is a set of brittle bone disorders caused by mutations in the *COL1A1* or *COL1A2* genes, which are responsible for the production of collagen type I. It affects 1 in 20 000 live births. The *differential diagnoses* of OI include NAI, idiopathic juvenile osteoporosis, Cushing's, and homocystinuria. There are four main types of OI (and at least 17 distinct genotypes), the commonest being type 1. Type 2 is fatal in infancy, and types 3 and 4 are severe variants associated with short stature and bone deformity. Of note:

Fractures
- OI exhibits considerable interfamilial variability in the number of fractures and degree of disability.
- Fracture tendency is constant from childhood to puberty, decreases thereafter, and often increases after menopause or >60y in men.
- Fractures are treated with standard orthopaedic procedures and heal rapidly with good callus formation and usually without deformity.

Other features
- Blue sclerae, ligament laxity, easy bruising, poor dentition, and hearing deficit in 50%, beginning in the late teens.

Bisphosphonate treatment
Used in children/adults with type 1 OI:
- Associated with BMD gains and reduced fracture risk. Greatest gains are probably in the first 2–4y of treatment.
- Long-term skeletal effects of anti-resorption therapy are unknown.

Conditions with joint hypermobility

There are a number of childhood conditions associated with joint hypermobility, including:
- OI.
- EDS, e.g. classical, vascular.
- MFS.
- Loeys–Dietz syndrome.
- Stickler syndrome.
- Trichorhinophalangeal syndrome.
- Meier–Gorlin syndrome.

Marfan's syndrome and related disorders

(See ➔ Marfan's syndrome, p. 876.) MFS is an AD condition characterized by tall stature, long extremities, fingers, and feet, lens dislocations, and cardiac defects.

Diagnosis

Based on the Ghent criteria (a scoring system; see ⚘ https://www.marfan.org), and a mutation is often found in the fibrillin 1 (*FBN1*) gene on chromosome 15. MSK features should raise suspicion but alone are non-diagnostic:
- *Height:* compared to non-MFS children, height is a discriminant criterion for MFS when >3.3 SDs above the mean. Other measurements show a span:height ratio of >1.05 and an upper segment:lower segment ratio of <0.89.
- *Cardiac:* 35% of affected persons have mitral valve prolapse or aortic root enlargement, or both, on echocardiography, recommending ECHO, CT, or MRI in all patients. Aortic aneurysm and dissection later in life are associated with ↑ mortality.
- *Others:* include chest wall deformity, scoliosis, joint laxity, myopia, high-arched palate, mandibular hypoplasia, striae distensae, pulmonary blebs (which predispose to spontaneous pneumothorax), and spinal arachnoid cysts or diverticula.

MFS has overlapping features with Loeys–Dietz syndrome (craniosynostosis, cleft palate, hypertelorism, vascular lesions, and translucent and hyperelastic skin) and Beals syndrome (congenital contractural arachnodactyly).

Ehlers–Danlos syndrome

(See also ➲ Ehlers-Danlos syndrome, p. 882.) An umbrella term for a set of conditions that variably have skin fragility, ligament laxity, short stature, spinal deformity, vascular fragility, and (rarely) retinal detachment.

Diagnosis

Increasingly through genotyping, although many gene variants can be of un-certain significance:

- *Classical EDS (cEDS):* hyperextensible skin, easily torn, and poor repair and wound healing; herniae; hypermobile joints with subluxations, dislocations, and early-onset arthritis; difficulties in pregnancy.
- *Vascular EDS (vEDS):* in the absence of family history, typically diagnosed after arterial vascular event (aneurysm, dissection, or rupture); shortened median lifespan (men 49y, women 53y).
- *Hypermobility-type EDS* (or benign joint hypermobility syndrome, *EDS 3*): controversial diagnosis and errant use may inculcate a view of body insufficiency or failure in the child/parent → overmedicalization. There are no genetic defects or validated diagnostic criteria. However, irrespective of the diagnosis, effective management strategies exist for all children and adolescents with chronic widespread pain and biomechanical imbalances.

Relationship of hypermobility and chronic MSK pain

(See ➲ Chronic pain in children, pp. 718–21.) A theoretical basis for prob-lems with hypermobility is that individuals with hypermobility require greater muscular control to avoid stress and possible damage of the joint capsule or associated ligaments. As a result, it is inferred that hypermobility may be a risk factor for chronic MSK pain. However, although there is some, if inconsistent, evidence that hypermobility in children and adolescents is associated with an ↑ risk of MSK pain, the true value of a diagnostic label of *hypermobility spectrum disorders* (HSD) as the cause of pain is unclear and may even be harmful in asserting a life-long condition when this is un-proven. That said:

- It is recognized that hypermobility is present at high levels in the normal paediatric population and especially in preschool children.
- In teenage girls and boys (mean 14y), a large UK study found generalized joint laxity in 28% and 11%, respectively, using a cut-off of four hypermobile joints.
- Hyperextensibility at the little finger has been found in >40% girls. One explanation of this is that hypermobility may be normal in a teenage population.

Therefore, in a child with chronic pain where there is some evidence for hypermobility, rehabilitation and functional restoration are best achieved by a 'needs', rather than a 'diagnostic', focus.

Juvenile idiopathic arthritis

JIA is a chronic inflammatory arthritis which causes stiffness, swelling, joint restriction, and damage and is one of the commonest causes of disability in childhood. JIA is an umbrella term for several forms of arthritis (see ➔ JIA subtypes, pp. 694–5). Of note:
- JIA affects 1 in 1000 children and young people <16y of age.
- Annual incidence of 1/10 000 children and young people.

Diagnosing arthritis in children

There are no diagnostic tests for JIA and so diagnosis requires a thorough history and examination to distinguish JIA from other causes of joint pain or swelling. (For a differential diagnosis for JIA, see ➔ Tables 17.2, 17.7, and 17.8.) JIA should be considered if:
- Joint swelling from presumed trauma (including knee and ankle) persists beyond 2wk; involvement of several joints.
- Prolonged morning stiffness (>20min).
- Joint restriction in the absence of an orthopaedic course.
- Aseptic tap from a swollen joint.

Examination

To confirm swelling, identify joint restriction (using pGALS; see ➔ pGALS, p. 665 and Table 17.7) and any secondary effects such as:
- Muscle atrophy, synovial cysts.
- Leg length discrepancy from limb overgrowth or growth restriction.
- Other joint-specific features identified in paediatric MSK matters (paediatric regional examination of the musculoskeletal system (pREMS)] assessment (see ♫ http://www.pmmonline.org).

Table 17.7 Regional examination in JIA

Wrist	Ventral displacement, grip strength, handwriting
Fingers	Dactylitis, nail pitting, nodules, handwriting
Elbow	Flexion deformity, inability to touch shoulder
Shoulder	Winging of scapulae and scapula instability, dressing
Neck	Lordosis, rotation
Back	Lordosis, Schöber's test, midline or sacral bony tenderness, pelvic and lower limb muscle length
Hips	Apparent leg length, Trendelenberg gait, loss of hip swing, pain at end of range of rotation, FABER test, Thomas' test
Knees	Leg length, flexion deformity, synovial cyst, vastus medialis atrophy
Ankles	Gait—heel strike and foot position, foot inversion, calf muscle length, bulk and power, midfoot rigidity
Jaw	Restricted or asymmetric jaw opening, crepitus

Initial investigations in JIA

Bloods

- ESR and CRP may be normal and do not correlate well with the extent or severity of arthritis.
- Low Hb may indicate anaemia of chronic disease, rather than iron deficiency.
- Falling ESR and Hb, with climbing liver transaminases, may indicate MAS (see ⊃ Systemic-onset JIA, p. 695), as may ferritin >10 000ng/mL.
- ANA positivity is not diagnostic or predictive of outcome but is associated with ↑ risk of eye disease. RF positivity is rare in JIA and often difficult to interpret.

Imaging

- USS is usually the radiological investigation of choice to corroborate arthritis and evaluate tenosynovitis and joint damage. Its false −ve rate is higher in foot and ankle disease than for other joints.

Arthroscopy

Should be avoided unless a biopsy or culture is required.

Ophthalmology clinic

Since there is a strong association between JIA and uveitis, all patients should be seen within 6wk of diagnosis.

JIA subtypes

Oligoarticular JIA

Acounts for 30–40% of JIA and is characterized by ↑ risk of uveitis. It predominantly affects ♀, with ages of onset between 2 and 4y, and 7–13y.

- *50% are monoarticular in presentation*, with the commonest joints involved being the elbow, knee, and ankle; if early hip involvement, especially in <7y olds, search for other causes (e.g. irritable hip, septic arthritis, leukaemia, and IBD).
- If ≥5 joints become involved after 6mth of disease, the condition is reclassified as extended oligoarticular JIA and, pragmatically, like polyarticular arthritis (see → Polyarticular JIA, p. 694).
- >80% have little or no disability/damage after 15y of follow-up.

Polyarticular JIA

Accounts for 20–30% of JIA and is subdivided by the presence/absence of RF.

- Diagnosed when ≥5 joints involved within the first 6mth of disease activity (excluding psoriatic arthritis, IBD-associated arthritis, and ERA).
- RF +ve JIA occurs in <5% of JIA and in girls >12y, and is an aggressive, symmetric polyarthropathy.
- Often incomplete control of arthritis despite treatment; associated with higher levels of disability, especially during flares.
- Joint restriction indicates disease activity, so-called 'dry synovitis', and is associated with muscle atrophy, disability, and joint damage.
- Jaw involvement is often insidious. If left undertreated, it may result in micrognathia and dental malocclusion.
- Neck involvement can cause marked irritability and is disabling in the classroom; requires occupational therapy assessment.

Juvenile psoriatic arthritis (JPsA)

Considered in the presence of psoriasis in the patient or a first-degree relative, nail pitting, dactylitis, acute panuveitis, and spondyloarthropathy. It overlaps with oligoarticular and polyarticular disease but is frequently resistant to conventional treatment for these conditions, including steroid resistance.

Enthesitis-related arthritis/juvenile ankylosing spondylitis (JAS)

Are considered in patients >6y, especially ♂, with asymmetric large joint involvement. Enthesitis is inflammation at sites of bony insertion of tendons and capsule. It is commonly very painful, which may appear disproportionate to examination findings. HLA-B27 is found in 30–50% of ERA cases and is associated with an ↑ risk of spondyloarthropathy. ERA is generally associated with a low-grade, grumbling disease persisting into adulthood.

Systemic-onset JIA

An arthritis presenting with fever and rash is rare (5–8% of the JIA population). It is best considered as an umbrella term that covers several auto-inflammatory disorders (see ❥ Periodic fevers and autoinflammatory syndromes (AIS), pp. 716–17) and polyarticular JIA presenting with a viral infection.

- *Still's disease* is a redundant/confusing term for paediatric disease.
- Characteristic fever, rash, polyarthritis, lymphadenopathy, and hepatosplenomegaly overlap with *conditions that should not be missed* (see ❥ Conditions 'not to be missed', p. 659 and Table 17.8) that should be assessed by the paediatric rheumatology service.
- A full travel history and contact with infectious diseases, animals, or ticks should be assessed.
- There are no diagnostic tests, and arthritis may present late.
- Fever, of up to 39°C, is typically quotidian—occurring once or twice per day in a diurnal distribution, with return to normal baseline between fever spikes.
- Typical blood results include high ESR and CRP, neutrophilia (of the order of 20×10^9/L), thrombocytopenia (often $>600 \times 10^9$/L), and anaemia of chronic inflammation (often <80g/L).

Table 17.8 Differential diagnoses of fever, rash, and arthritis

Condition	Investigation
ALL	Blood film, bone marrow aspirate, whole-body MRI [short T1 inversion recovery (STIR)]
Neuroblastoma	Urine or blood metadrenalines (see local policy)
Lymphoma	CXR, abdominal USS, whole-body MRI
Sepsis or TB	Blood cultures, serology, PCR, MRI, Mantoux, IGRA, joint aspiration
SLE or APS	Coagulation, complement, autoantibodies, urinalysis
JDM	Thigh MRI, CK, LDH
Reactive arthritis and rheumatic fever	Lyme, *Bartonella*, and *Brucella* serology, ASOT and throat swab, echocardiogram
Vasculitides	Echocardiogram/ECG, urinalysis, detailed history, angiography, biopsy
Viruses and zoonoses	EBV, CMV, parvovirus, rubella, Lyme
Travel-associated pathogens	Tests according to suspicion
Periodic fevers	Genetic tests, IgD, mevalonic aciduria
IBD	Faecal calprotectin, endoscopy, barium swallow (see ❥ Inflammatory bowel disease, pp. 300–1)

General management of JIA

There is a window of opportunity in the first few months of arthritis to gain optimal control and avoid a spiral of decline, albeit slow, with joint damage causing further inflammation. Rapid control is also used to minimize the adverse effects of treatment and support the general physical and mental health of the patient. A patient-centred, holistic approach requires an MDT with dedicated experience in JIA. Overall, management focuses on:

• Treatment of the acutely swollen joint (see ➜ The acutely swollen joint, p. 669).
• Long-term control of arthritis and its sequelae (see ➜ Long-term management of JIA, p. 668).
• Uveitis screening and treatment (see ➜ Uveitis screening and treatment, pp. 698–9).
• Specific treatment for the rare complication of MAS (see ➜ Macrophage activation syndrome, pp. 714–15).

Treatment of the acutely swollen joint

Although rare, consider infection/sepsis and treat if present. Then the approach is:

• *NSAIDs* (e.g. ibuprofen, naproxen, diclofenac): 2wk to see anti-inflammatory effect, while awaiting paediatric rheumatology review.
• *Intra-articular steroids* (IAS) for limp, disability, and joint restriction; persistent marked joint swelling; or as a bridge while awaiting long-term medication to become effective.
• *PO/IV steroids*: used if many joints involved, or IAS not immediately available, or the effect of IAS is only short-lived.

Long-term management of JIA

Requires collaboration between members of the MDT and the regional network, as well as *shared care*. Medication is only one part of management.

Principles of shared care

• *Promotion of physical activity*: corrects muscular imbalances that result in pain, injury, loss of joint protection, and deconditioning.
• *Provision of information and education*: for parents and patients is critical for participation in joint decision-making and adherence to agreed treatment plans and helps dissipate lingering anxiety.
• *Pain management*: using strategies other than medication.
• *Vaccination advice*: when possible, give live vaccines (MMR, flu, and chickenpox) before starting disease-modifying antirheumatic drugs (DMARDs). Live vaccines are given while on DMARDs because benefits far outweigh risks. Give routine non-live vaccines.
• *Liaison*: between school, primary care, and community services.
• *Effective transition*: to adolescent and adult care that includes age-appropriate services for young people from puberty onwards.
• *Healthy diet*: avoids some of the problems of growth restriction or delay and inappropriate weight gain from reduced physical activity or steroid use.

Long-term medication

Aims to reduce the frequency and impact of flares of arthritis or uveitis. These treatments take a few weeks to become effective and may require bridging with steroids (IAS, PO, or IV). Long-term medication or DMARDs are used for:

- Persistent or extension of arthritis to other joints or uveitis.
- Presence of chronic complications or tissue damage.
- Effects on wrist and hand function, the hip, or jaw mobility.

Given the extensive support and experience required, these drugs are best instituted by a specialist service or within a clinical network.

DMARDs

- *Methotrexate:* is the standard drug for JIA and uveitis. National registries show long-term use is safe. The SC form is preferred to PO, especially in the very young:
  - *Dose:* 10–20mg/m².
  - *Side effects:* nausea which may be avoided with prophylactic ondansetron. The benefit of folic acid is debatable.
  - *Monitor:* FBC, LFTs, and ESR/CRP monthly for first 6mth; then follow as per local guidelines. Most rises in aminotransferases and falls in neutrophils are attributable to other causes (e.g. viral infection), but follow local guidelines about withholding.
- *Alternative monotherapy:* includes leflunomide, sulfasalazine, and hydroxychloroquine. Azathioprine and ciclosporin may have a role in both arthritis and uveitis, whereas MMF and tacrolimus are considered to have a specific role in uveitis.
- *Combination therapy:* not well studied in JIA, but used with good effect in some, and are associated with more adverse effects.

Biologic therapies

Used when JIA, uveitis, or other inflammatory condition is refractory to, or the patient is intolerant of, methotrexate or other DMARDs. There is NICE approval for the use of abatacept, adalimumab, etanercept, and tocilizumab in patients with JIA.

Supplementary medications

Include those for pain, gastritis, and nausea and those used to optimize bone density and strength in the presence of steroids or reduced physical activity. Treatment of arthritis with fever and rash may differ slightly and includes:

- NSAIDs: initial trial of high dose for 2wk to allow investigation.
- PO/IV steroids: limited course commonly used to treat SoJIA and temporize pain, fatigue, and disability, and as rescue if MAS present.
- IVIG: also effective for MAS and other systemic inflammatory conditions.

Uveitis screening and treatment

Uveitis affects 10–20% of JIA patients and accounts for silent and irreversible visual loss in ~25% of untreated JIA. It may occur after only a few weeks of uncontrolled inflammation.

- Uveitis is present in 40% of patients on the first eye screen; it is not predictable and is unrelated to the severity of arthritis.
- Other causes of uveitis are:
  - *Infectious:* Toxoplasma, varicella, HSV, CMV, TB, Lyme, *Bartonella*, *Toxocara*, *Ascaris*, histoplasmosis, fungal, syphilis.
  - *Non-infectious:* trauma (sympathetic ophthalmia); IBD, sarcoidosis, and Blau syndrome; periodic fevers and Behçet's; tubulointerstitial nephritis–uveitis, Vogt–Koyanagi–Harada, MS, vasculitis, and KD.
- Complications, especially cataract, occur in up to 40%. Other major concerns include glaucoma, macular oedema, retinal detachment, band keratopathy, and hypotony.
- Poor outcome from uveitis is associated with: ocular damage at presentation, uveitis preceding arthritis, delay in onset of intervention, and failure to achieve early remission.

Surveillance

Since it is difficult to detect uveitis, screening is undertaken by experienced ophthalmology teams. In the absence of uveitis, eye screening ends at 12y of age when a patient can self-report floaters and pain (Table 17.9). If there has been uveitis, screening is annual after the age of 12y.

Table 17.9 Frequency of eye screening slit-lamp examination summarized from the Royal College of Ophthalmology guidelines

Condition	Age of onset of JIA	ANA status	Frequency
So-JIA	Any		Yearly
Oligoarticular JIA Polyarticular JIA; RF–ve	<7y old	ANA +ve	2-monthly for 6mth, 3-monthly for 3.5y, 6-monthly for 3y or until aged 12y
		ANA –ve	6-monthly for 7y or until aged 12y
	>7y old		6-monthly for 4y

Management of uveitis
- *First-line treatment:* steroid eye drops (dexamethasone, e.g. Maxidex® or prednisolone, e.g. Predsol®) given up to hourly. There is a dose-dependent increase in risk of cataract formation from using steroid eye drops.
- *Other topical agents:* mydriatics (cyclopentolate) to reduce the risk of the iris sticking to the lens (posterior synechiae); glaucoma agents.

Macrophage activation syndrome
(See also → Macrophage activation syndrome, pp. 714–15.) MAS is a life-threatening complication of SoJIA and other paediatric autoimmune diseases, and management should be undertaken by a specialist centre. A high level of suspicion is needed in JIA, particularly when:
- ↑ irritability or disconnect between clinical findings and blood tests.
- Very high levels of ferritin (>10 000ng/mL).
- Climbing liver transaminases, hyperbilirubinaemia.
- Rapidly falling ESR.

Outcome of JIA
Even though control of inflammation is often incomplete, outcome is usually favourable due to current treatment strategies. Joint replacement is now rarely required. Outcomes by type are:
- *Oligoarticular:* 50–75% of patients with persistent oligoarticular JIA achieve remission by early teens but may still experience flares in adulthood.
- *Polyarticular:* 20–30% of patients with polyarticular JIA achieve drug-free long-term remission.

  Poorer prognosis is associated with:
- Delayed referral.
- Suboptimal control, including from inadequate engagement of family and patient.
- Disease-specific factors such as ocular damage at presentation, persistently active SoJIA by 6mth, psoriatic arthritis, hip involvement, and early X-ray changes.

Multisystem inflammatory disorders

Primary vasculitides

In children are rare, but life-threatening, multisystem conditions with perivascular inflammation.

The commonest conditions are acute, usually self-limiting:
- HSP (see ➍ Henoch–Schönlein purpura, pp. 701–2).
- KD (see ➍ Kawasaki disease, pp. 630–1).

Rare chronic vasculitides include:
- Polyarteritis nodosa (PAN) (see ➍ Polyarteritis nodosa, p. 704).
- Takayasu arteritis (TA) (see ➍ Takayasu arteritis, p. 704).
- ANCA-associated vasculitis (see ➍ ANCA-associated vasculitides, p. 704).
- Leukocytoclastic (hypersensitivity vasculitis; HSP is a form).
- CNS vasculitis (see ➍ Primary angiitis of the CNS, p. 705).
- Behçet's (see ➍ Behçet's disease, p. 705).

Vasculitis may also occur with other conditions such as malignancies, lupus, and drug reactions.

Diagnosis

Suspicion typically arises in the presence of fever (often low grade), weight loss, and a multisystem presentation with a rash.
- A careful history (including infections, immunizations, drug exposure, and detailed family history) and clinical examination are key.
- Several classification criteria for chronic vasculitis exist, each with their own sensitivity and specificity of diagnostic accuracy.

Kawasaki disease

Kawasaki is a condition that requires a multidisciplinary care team, including a rheumatologist, infectious disease specialist, and cardiologist. In this book, text on KD is consolidated in Chapter 16 (see ➍ Kawasaki disease, pp. 630–1), mainly so that the section on KD and the section on the recently described association between COVID-19 and a KD-like, post-infectious inflammatory condition are next to each other (see ➍ Coronavirus and COVID-19, pp. 632–3).

Henoch–Schönlein purpura

HSP is a small-vessel, non-granulomatous IgA *leukocytoclastic vasculitis* of unknown aetiology that occurs between the ages of 2 and 11y (75%), and rarely in infants and young children. Its characteristic purpuric rash on the back of legs, buttocks, and arms needs to be distinguished from menin-gococcal septicaemia, acute haemorrhagic oedema of infancy, immune thrombocytopenic purpura, acute post-streptococcal glomerulonephritis, and HUS.

Presenting symptoms
By system, include:
- Skin (95%): purpura (legs, buttocks, arms), urticaria, angio-oedema, and a bruising or necrotic appearance.
- GI (72%): abdominal pain (often precedes rash by up to 2wk), vomiting, haematemesis, and melaena. Severe complications include intussusception, appendicitis, cholecystitis, pancreatitis, ulceration, infarction, or perforation.
- MSK (47%): self-limiting arthralgia or arthritis of knees and ankles.
- Renal (>25%): nephritis in 25–60% of patients [NB: HSP nephritis accounts for 1.6–3% of all childhood cases of end-stage renal failure (ESRF) in the UK].
- GU (rare): orchitis.
- CNS (rare): cerebral vasculitis.
- Respiratory (rare): pulmonary haemorrhage.

Clinical course
HSP is generally a benign, self-limiting disease, with most patients experien-cing full resolution within 8wk, and overall <5% experience chronic symp-toms. However:
- Recurrences occur in 50% within 6wk.
- One-third have symptoms for up to a fortnight and another third for up to 1mth, and recurrence of symptoms within 4mth of resolution in one-third.

Clinical monitoring
Weekly for the first month; alternate weeks for 1mth, and then monthly. Increase the frequency if *renal involvement* because:
- 97% of renal disease occur within 3mth of disease onset, but screening with monthly urinalysis is recommended for up to 6mth.
- Although <10% require referral for consideration of renal biopsy, usually in the presence of nephrosis and persisting haematuria, 20% of patients with nephrotic syndrome progress to ESRF. However, there is no clear effective treatment to avoid ESRF (see ➲ Management of CKD, p. 358–9).
- Predictors of serious nephropathy include a persisting rash and bloody stools. Prognosis is better in children aged <7y.

Treatment
- There is no treatment that shortens the duration of HSP or improves long-term renal outcome. So treatment is primarily symptomatic with rest, analgesia, and hydration. Hospital admission is for management of:
  - GI: severe abdominal pain or GI haemorrhage.
  - GU: acute scrotum or renal failure.
  - MSK: disabling arthritis.
- *Steroids:* prednisolone, often at a dose of 1mg/kg/day (PO for 5–7 days), is used for symptomatic improvement to enable discharge from hospital.
- Avoid excess steroid use; the dose is adjusted according to response, and methylprednisolone use is guided by a tertiary specialist centre.
- Often used (without evidence) for persisting nephrosis and 50% crescents on renal biopsy. (See ➔ Chapter 8 for other treatments of severe renal disease, e.g. immunosuppression, antiproteinuric and antihypertensive agents.)

Other leukocytoclastic or hypersensitivity vasculitis

These common cutaneous and small-vessel forms of vasculitis may be secondary to medication (including herbal remedies), food additives, underlying infection, multisystem autoimmunity (e.g. lupus and IBD; 10–15% of cases), and malignancy (4%). In 50%, the disorder is idiopathic, and 10% have a chronic or recurrent condition.

Presentation
Palpable purpura, often associated with urticaria, vesicles, bullae, and pustules. Itch, pain, or burning is uncommon. Organ system involvement may include joints, gut, and kidneys.

Investigations
Directed to identifying the underlying cause (see list below), but biopsy may be needed if there is multisystem involvement:
- Infection: GAS, viral hepatitis, HIV.
- Autoimmunity.
- Malignancy.
- Urticarial vasculitis and cryoglobulins: send haemolytic complement (CH50 or CH100), C3, C4, and anti-C1q antibodies.

Chronic multisystem vasculitis

Polyarteritis nodosa

PAN is a condition that is usually idiopathic in origin but may be secondary to viral hepatitis. Mortality is now 4%, and relapses occur in 35–50%. The diagnosis is based on the presence of malaise, fever, >5% weight loss, myalgia, and arthropathy *plus*:

- Vasculitic rash.
- Mono- or polyneuropathy.
- Testicular tenderness or pain.
- Muscle tenderness or focal weakness.

Cutaneous polyarteritis nodosa (cPAN) is a benign medium-vessel vasculitis, predominantly of the skin, with arthralgia, myalgia, and neuralgia, but *no organ damage*.

Complications

Include CNS morbidity (stroke, encephalopathy, myelopathy, and neuropathy), cardiac morbidity (pericarditis, aneurysms, and ischaemia), GI bleeding and infarction, and renal failure.

Treatment

Is led by a tertiary centre, often using steroids, along with MMF, methotrexate, azathioprine, or cyclophosphamide.

Takayasu arteritis

TA is a large-vessel vasculitis affecting the aorta and its major branches. Clinical sequelae of panarteritis is luminal narrowing or occlusion, with bruits, claudication, or diminished/absent pulses. ESR may be normal. Systemic arterial hypertension is a common feature (70–80%) and raises suspicion of vasculitis.

ANCA-associated vasculitides

These conditions include:

- Granulomatosis with polyangiitis (GPA): formerly known as Wegener's granulomatosis; typified by upper airways, lung, renal, and skin involvement.
- Microscopic polyangiitis (MPA): renal and GI involvement commoner than in GPA.
- Eosinophilic granulomatosis with polyangiitis (eGPA): formerly known as Churg–Strauss syndrome.

Tissue diagnosis with biopsy of renal, skin, or nasal mucosa is important for therapeutic decision-making. There is considerable disease-related morbidity and significant mortality.

Primary angiitis of the CNS

Primary CNS vasculitis is an increasingly recognized inflammatory brain disease. The clinical presentation is with:
- *Non-focal* symptoms (50%): headaches and altered mental state.
- *Localizing* symptoms: lateralized weakness (30%), aphasia (15%), ataxia (15%), visual (15%), seizures (15%), and myelitis (10%).

Behçet's disease

A very rare multisystem disorder often considered when there is recurrent oral and genital ulceration, although diagnosis requires specific criteria in the UK and the support of the national centre. Vasculitis can affect large or small vessels and thrombophlebitis may raise suspicion.

Treatment
Includes:
- Colchicine: the mainstay.
- Anti-TNF therapy: used for refractory or severe disease.

Juvenile SLE

Juvenile SLE (J-SLE) is often a more severe phenotype, accruing more organ damage and a twofold higher mortality rate than the condition in adults. The overall incidence of J-SLE is 0.4–0.6/100 000 (higher in ♀, and Afro-Caribbean and Asian populations), and 20% present before 18y of age, commonly 12–14y.

Diagnostic classification

Is in accordance with the *Systemic Lupus International Collaborating Clinics* (SLICC) or the *American College of Rheumatology* (ACR) criteria. The SLICC criteria are preferred and include characterizing 18 features (see ♪ https://qxmd.com/calculate/calculator_274/slicc-sle-criteria) such as:

- Acute, subacute, and chronic cutaneous lupus: malar rash (30%).
- Non-scarring alopecia.
- Oral or nasal ulcers.
- Joint disease.
- Serositis.
- Renal (up to 80%): abnormal urine findings (proteinuria or RBC casts); biopsy-proven lupus nephritis.
- Neurologic involvement: neuropsychiatric (40%).
- Blood: haemolytic anaemia; leucopenia or lymphopenia; thrombocytopenia, low complement (C3, C4, or CH50).
- Antibodies: ANA, anti-dsDNA (60%), anti-Sm nuclear antigen, antiphospholipid, DCT.

Prognosis

Is often determined by the severity of renal disease. Other risk factors for poor outcome include severe flares, infection, and neuropsychiatric manifestations.

Management

Early and aggressive therapy is paramount to improving outcome and preventing organ damage. Also, provide advice about sun avoidance and use of sunblock (SPF 50) to reduce flares and photosensitive rashes.

Induction therapy

- *IV methylprednisolone* (for three daily doses): typically used, followed by a weaning regime of PO prednisolone (from 1–2mg/kg/day) plus a disease-modifying agent.
- *IV cyclophosphamide:* its role in induction is unclear, and MMF is typically preferred in lupus nephritis. Cyclophosphamide is still used in neurological disease, systemic vasculitis, and refractory lupus nephritis.

Treatment by disease condition/features
- *Mild to moderate disease* is treated with corticosteroids, MMF, or azathioprine.
- *Disease with predominance of arthritis/cutaneous manifestations* is treated with methotrexate.
- *Refractory J-SLE* is treated with rituximab.

Other treatments
- *Heparin and/or warfarin:* prescribe in coexisting thromboses from antiphosholipid syndrome.
- *Aspirin:* use in cases of +ve lupus anticoagulant or anticardiolipin antibodies.
- *ACE inhibitors:* use in cases of hypertension and proteinuria to aggressively manage and prevent further renal damage.

Juvenile idiopathic inflammatory myositis

The group of conditions categorized as juvenile idiopathic inflammatory myositis are heterogenous inflammatory conditions in young people aged <17y, characterized by proximal myopathy, classical rashes, and other organ involvement. They are classified into groups that share similar clinical features, laboratory changes, treatment response, and prognosis and include:

- JDM (80%).
- Juvenile polymyositis (JPM) (5%).
- Overlap myositis (10%) (associated with scleroderma, arthritis, or lupus).
- Rare forms: macrophagic myofasciitis, focal myositis, and graft-versus-host myositis.
- Inclusion body myositis (including critical illness myopathy seen on PICU) and cancer-associated myositis are generally considered confined to adults.

Differential diagnosis of muscle weakness

- *Viral myositis.*
- *Benign acute childhood myositis*: a self-limiting condition that presents with calf pain, walking difficulty, and very high CK levels.
- *JDM or JPM.*
- *Musculodystrophy and congenital myopathy* (see ➔ Muscular disorders, pp. 390–1).
- *Multisystem inflammatory diseases*: mixed connective tissue disease (MCTD), SLE, vasculitides.
- *Juvenile fibromyalgia.*
- *Skeletal dysplasias* (see ➔ Skeletal dysplasias, p. 887).
- *Electrolyte imbalances*: K^+ and Ca^{2+}.
- *Drug-induced myopathy.*
- *Critical illness myopathy.*

Juvenile dermatomyositis

The incidence is 2–4 per million (United States and the UK), with a median age of onset of 7y. Unlike in adults, JDM is not typically associated with neoplasia and as such, investigations are not required.

Diagnosis

Classically based on Bohan and Peter criteria and requires:

- *Rash:* the facial rash is often photosensitive in a malar distribution with nasolabial sparing like in SLE. However, the classic heliotrope (dusky, purple-red hue to the upper eyelids) and Gottron's papules (shiny red marks on knuckles, elbows, knees, and ankles) are distinguishing features.
- *Symmetrical proximal muscle weakness:* determined by examination. It manifests as difficulty getting upstairs or out of bed, difficulty with putting on a jumper or T-shirt, or tiring more quickly than usual during sport.
- *Elevated serum skeletal muscle enzymes:* include CK, aldolase, glutamate oxaloacetate and pyruvate transaminases, and LDH.
- *Electromyographic (EMG) triad:* short, small, polyphasic motor unit potentials; fibrillations, +ve sharp waves, and insertional irritability; and bizarre, high-frequency repetitive discharges.
- *Muscle biopsy:* abnormalities of degeneration, regeneration, necrosis, phagocytosis, and interstitial mononuclear infiltrate.

NB: raised CK and MRI evidence of myositis is now preferred for diagnosis over EMG and biopsy (reserved for atypical or subtle cases).

Other features include low-grade fever, weight loss, arthralgia, abdominal pain, melaena, change in character of the voice, and difficulty swallowing. Interstitial lung disease and dilated cardiomyopathy may also occur in chronic disease.

Modern ACR criteria include the following categories:

- *Amyopathic JDM:* with the characteristic rash, but no obvious muscle disease, although muscle inflammation and weakness may be subclinical. Calcinosis or interstitial lung disease are rare.
- *Overlap myositis:* occurring with scleroderma, SLE, JIA, Sjögren's, and IDDM and is often associated with Raynaud's and interstitial lung disease, resulting in higher mortality.
- *JPM:* which presents as a very rare and more clinically apparent proximal and distal muscle weakness in adolescents. Also, very high CK levels, little skin involvement, but often cardiac effects.

Clinical course
Falls into different patterns:
- *Monocyclic* (25–40%): lasting up to 3y.
- *Polycyclic* (50–60%): periods of remission and relapse, or chronic, and can be lifelong.
- *Ulcerative* (10–20%).

Treatment
Requires a multidisciplinary approach to optimize muscle strength, function, and quality of life, while controlling inflammation of the skin, to avoid calcinosis, muscle, gut, and other organs. Calcinosis cutis (occurring in up to one-third of JDM) can be a major cause of morbidity because of pain, cosmetic problems, and tethering of skin, muscles, and nerves, and as a nidus for infection. Hence, early aggressive treatment to rapidly and completely control inflammation is essential to fully restore muscle function and avoid damage and calcinosis.

Corticosteroids are the mainstay of treatment and universally supplemented with DMARDs (methotrexate, hydroxychloroquine, ciclosporin, and IVIG). The consensus guidelines on treatment are:
- *Induction*: IV methylprednisolone 30mg/kg (maximum 1g) for 3 days and then weekly in severe cases.
- *Weaning regime*: prednisolone from 1–2mg/kg/day, aiming to be off by 12mth.

Other therapies, as determined by the specialist centre for refractory disease, include:
- Methotrexate: 15mg/m².
- IVIG: 2g/kg every 2wk for three doses and then monthly.
- Cyclophosphamide: typically used for ulcerative cases, severe muscle disease, including dysphonia, and interstitial lung disease.
- MMF, rituximab, and TNF inhibitors.

Juvenile scleroderma

Scleroderma is a spectrum of autoimmune diseases with chronic inflammation → excess collagen deposition, fibrosis, and skin thickening.

Localized scleroderma (LS)

Has an incidence of 3.4 per million children per year. Survival normal, but permanent sequelae in 40–90%—may improve with new treatments. *Cutaneous* features include:

• *Plaque morphoea* (26%): a benign, round, circumscribed single patch or multiple lesions, often erythematous at the start, then becoming indurated and woody, and with halo or altered skin pigmentation.
• *Generalized morphoea* (7%): ≥4 large plaques involving ≥2 areas.
• *Linear morphoea* (65%): affects limbs.
• *En coup de sabre (Parry–Romberg or progressive hemifacial atrophy):* linear lesion on face and scalp, with loss of hair over affected area. Extent of inflammatory involvement determined by response to steroids. Intracranial brain lesions are rare, but possible.
• *Other* (3%): bullous morphoea, deep morphoea, guttate morphoea, nodular morphoea.

Extra-cutaneous features include: articular (19%), CNS (4%), Raynaud's, ocular, GI (2%), respiratory, renal, and cardiac (<1%).

Juvenile systemic sclerosis (jSSC)

Very rare (0.27 per million children per year) and often refractory to treatment. Mortality is up to 12%, which is similar to adult-onset disease. *Cutaneous* features include:

• *Generalized* diffuse, waxy skin thickening, starting with the face and hands. Raynaud's phenomenon in up to 76%.
• *Limited cutaneous systemic sclerosis* (lcSSc).
• *Skin changes confined to distal* arms, legs, head, and neck.
• *Overlap syndromes:* more commonly than in adults, children often present common features with J-SLE and JDM, with milder outcome.

Extra-cutaneous features include: Raynaud's, GI (30%), respiratory (29%), articular, renal, and cardiac.

Examination, investigations, and treatment

Examination
Perform a general examination, but focus on:
- Growth.
- Skin.
- MSK: gait, any limb length discrepancy, joint contractures.

Investigations
Focus on extra-cutaneous involvement:
- CVS: BP, echocardiography.
- Respiratory system: lung function test/transfer factor, chest CT.
- GI: barium swallow if symptoms.
- Urinalysis.

  LS is often associated with:
- *Inflammatory markers:* normal and ANA is not diagnostic or helpful in prognosis.
- *Skin:* biopsy is useful if any diagnostic uncertainty. Monitoring is with serial photographs, thermography, and capillaroscopy.
- *Imaging:* MRI helps define the depth and extent of disease.

Treatment
Prednisolone and methotrexate, as for JDM.
  jSSC requires cardiopulmonary follow-up and:
- Prognostic autoantibodies: Scl-70 (34%) and anti-centomere (7%).

Macrophage activation syndrome

MAS is a rare and life-threatening (mortality is 8–22%) condition attributable to overstimulation of the immune system by infection, autoimmune conditions (including KD), and neoplasia. A key histological feature is engulfment of haematopoietic cells by macrophages, i.e. *secondary HLH*. Primary HLH is usually seen in children <2y old with consanguinous parents (see ➲ Haemophagocytic lymphohistiocytosis, p. 607). There may be a history of death of a young family member with unexplained fever and a primary CNS presentation.

Diagnostic suspicion

Should arise when you see:
- An already unwell child.
- Unremitting fever and high levels of inflammation despite broad-spectrum antibiotics.
- Unexpected fall in ESR associated with new-onset cytopenia and hyperferritinaemia.

Table 17.10 summarizes the clinical and laboratory features of MAS.

Table 17.10 Summary of clinical and laboratory features of MAS

Clinical signs	Laboratory findings
High, persistent, unremitting fever or change in pattern of fever	Low/falling ESR in the context of active inflammatory disease or high CRP
New-onset hepatosplenomegaly	Low/rapidly falling WBC, Hb, or platelet count
CNS features, including irritability	
Lymphadenopathy	Low/falling or unexpectedly normal platelet count
New-onset heart, lung, or kidney failure	Low/falling or unexpected normal fibrinogen
Petechiae or haemorrhages	Rising AST, ALT, GGT, bilirubin, triglycerides, and LDH
	Ferritin higher than would be expected for patient's diagnosis

Haemophagocytosis in the bone marrow aspirate is present in 40–60% of MAS cases and is a relatively late sign. Absence of haemophagocytosis does not rule out MAS.

Treatment

Treatment started promptly potentially avoids a poor prognosis and includes:

- *Broad-spectrum antibiotics:* used empirically.
- *Steroids:* if conditions not to be missed (see ➲ Conditions 'not to be missed', p. 659) have been excluded, IV steroids are used as first-line treatment, then PO; steroid therapy is effective in over 50%. Use methylprednisolone 30mg/kg/day (maximum 1g) for 3 days, followed by tapering PO prednisolone 1mg/kg/day.
- *IVIG:* used in refractory MAS at 1–2g/kg.
- *Ciclosporin:* and biologic therapy are also used at specialist centres.
- *IL-1 inhibition* (e.g. anakinra): dramatic effect in MAS (and increases survival rate versus placebo in adult sepsis with features of MAS).
- *Other options:*
  - Anti-IL-6 receptor (tocilizumab).
  - Anti-TNFα.
  - Etoposide.
  - Rituximab (anti-CD20+ B-cell therapy) for EBV-driven MAS.
  - Cyclophosphamide in SLE-associated MAS (see ➲ Juvenile SLE, pp. 706–7).

Periodic fevers and autoinflammatory syndromes (AIS)

These conditions are rare monogenic immune-mediated disorders that typically present in childhood with recurrent bouts of fever, high inflammatory markers, and systemic involvement, between which the patient is entirely well, hence the term *periodic fever*.

The term *autoinflammatory syndrome* (AIS) arises from the understanding that a gene mutation results in the switching on of uncontrolled innate immune activity that has a secondary effect on adaptive immunity. This differs from autoimmunity in which failure of recognition between self and non-self is stimulated by self-reactive T-cells, involves MHC class II molecules, and leads to circulating antibodies.

Since the discovery of *MEVK*, the gene for familial Mediterranean fever, the genes of other AIS have been identified and collectively have proven valuable in understanding inflammatory pathways. Although AIS are not, in general, life-threatening, an early diagnosis may avoid high levels of morbidity, years of hospital visits, unnecessary investigations and treatment, reduced quality of life, and severe complications from systemic amyloid A (AA) amyloidosis.

Familial Mediterranean fever is the quintessential and commonest form of AIS (carrier frequency in Middle Eastern populations is 1 in 3 to 1 in 5). Other periodic fevers (AIS) include:

- TNF receptor-associated periodic syndrome (*TRAPS*).
- Cryopyrin-associated periodic syndrome (*CAPS*).
- HyperIgD syndrome (*HIDS*).

Diagnosis

Based on clinical suspicion, especially if recurrent fevers or multisystem inflammation of unknown aetiology begin in infancy. The approach includes:

- *Exclude:* infection, neoplasia, and autoimmune diseases.
- *Review family history:* important clues include ethnicity and any sibling/infant deaths.
- *Fever:* age of onset; characterization of fever (duration and periodicity), which also helps to understand the burden of disease on quality of life; also note whether there was prolonged fever with immunization.
- *Assess rash or concomitant manifestations of AIS:*
  - *Urticarial eruptions:* typical in CAPS, but often indistinguishable from chronic urticaria.
  - *Urticarial vasculitis:* fixed in shape for >24h, also in CAPS.
  - Multiple *sterile abscesses:* seen in *PAPA* syndrome (Pyoderma gangrenosum, cystic Acne and Pyogenic sterile Arthritis); *SAPHO*; *Majeed syndrome* (chronic recurrent multifocal osteomyelitis and congenital dyserythropoietic anaemia); *DIRA* (deficiency of the IL-1 receptor antagonist); early-onset IBD; and several other AIS.
  - *Psoriasiform rashes:* seen in congenital forms of psoriasis, e.g. CARD-14-mediated pustular psoriasis (*CAMPS*) and *SAPHO*.
  - *Ichthyosiform rash:* tan-coloured and scaly, seen in ~90% of patients with Blau syndrome.

- Organ systems review:
  - GI: any diarrhoea, which may be present in 75% of HIDS.
  - Special senses: uveitis and SN hearing loss in CAPS.

Investigations

Include:
- *Blood:* high inflammatory markers (ESR/CRP) and neutrophilia that normalize between febrile episodes.
- *Genetic testing:* good for confirmation of AIS, but up to 50% of AIS patients have −ve results.
- *Urine screen:* needed to assess any proteinuria, which raises the possibility of secondary AA amyloidosis.

Chronic pain in children

NB: for *chronic fatigue syndrome (CFS)/myalgic encephalomyelitis*, see NICE guidelines (available at: ℞ (https://www.nice.org.uk/guidance/cg53).

In childhood and adolescence, pain is a ubiquitous experience, affecting >80% of individuals in the preceding 3–6mth. This threat or danger sensation is associated with a neuroendocrine, MSK, and inflammatory response and provokes threat appraisal and behavioural adaptation that may be attentive or avoidant. The prevalence of chronic (recurrent or persistent) pain in children and adolescents is also high (11–38%), with 5% experiencing significant pain-related dysfunction. It affects most body sites (e.g. head, abdomen, back, generalized), with a prevalence that increases with age.

Of note, in primary care, over 10% of all contacts with adolescents are attributable to MSK pain. Although the international criterion for chronicity is 3mth (constant or intermittent), which is taken from the definition in adults, a diagnosis can often be made sooner. For example:

- Careful enquiry of site, character, and severity of pain and any loss of function is often incongruous with the mechanism of any injury or background disease (JIA, SCD, IBD, etc.)—a finding that will override the relevance of duration.
- Most chronic MSK pain can be attributed to biomechanical imbalances and stresses that result from tissue tightness and changes in patterns of muscle use with normal growth and development.

Key considerations in the assessment of chronic pain

Framing of consultation

- Patients are likely to have seen other professionals, so start by asking patient and parent about expectations from the consultation.
- Local, regional, and widespread pain occurs; this includes the terms CRPS (see ➲ Complex regional pain syndrome, pp. 676–7) and juvenile fibromyalgia, both pain processing or neuromatrix problems. So use such terms guardedly because prognosis is far better in children and adolescents than in adults and your words may have unintended interpretations.
- Parenting behaviours often maintain the child's pain by *pain bias* when interpreting ambiguous emotional expressions. If a parent also has chronic pain, the child is at risk of worse health outcomes, ↑ anxiety and depression, and ↑ family dysfunction.

Context of diagnostic appraisal

- Thinking of chronic pain as a diagnosis made by exclusion will undermine any assessment, since it may raise suspicion in the patient or parent that not all investigations have ruled out other causes of pain.
- If ordering investigations, the purpose should be explained and should be framed in the context of a +ve diagnosis.
- The levels of disability and distress for both localized and widespread chronic pain are usually well in excess of the clinical findings from history and examination but should not be dismissed.
- The commonest cause of regional and widespread chronic pain is biomechanical—typically associated with growth and development and includes *benign nocturnal limb pains* of childhood.

Therapeutic strategy
- Chronic pain may appear mysterious and unexplained to other professionals, and inconsistent assessment and explanation may agitate the family.
- The needs of chronic pain patients should be clearly identified to help direct effective management that often requires a multidisciplinary approach (physiotherapy, occupational therapy, and psychology).
- The role of medication is unclear. If used, monitor any benefit or side effect. Medication is more effective when used to support engagement with physical and psychological therapies.

Chronic localized pain

Is usually of biomechanical origin, related to inappropriate patterns of muscle use, which may derive from previous injury, repetitive sport or dance activities, or commonly deconditioning due to sedentary behaviour. Other localized pain, such as *CRPS*, is associated with an episode of minor trauma in circumstances that may be challenging or alarming (e.g. unanticipated somersault on a trampoline, unexpected fall, or presence of exhaustion from lack of sleep or heat stroke).

Chronic widespread pain (CWP)

Is usually insidious, with gradual effect on quality of life. CWP is preferred to juvenile fibromyalgia, joint hypermobility syndrome (see ⮕ Relationship of hypermobility and chronic MSK pain, p. 691), or other labels that intimate poorly established causes, have overlapping diagnostic criteria and heterogeneity, and may unnecessarily trap patients into a story of lifelong disability.
- *Triggers or coexistence with disorder* (5–20%): seen in organic disorders (e.g. SCD, IBD, JIA, CHD, or cancer).
- *Enigmatic symptoms* (50%): dizziness, fatigue, blurring of vision, 'blackouts', and tachycardia attributable to variations in threat signalling and deconditioning, and may be exacerbated by anxiety.
- *Unhelpful labels*: 'post-orthostatic tachycardia syndrome' (POTS), 'autonomic dysfunction', or 'chronic Lyme disease' are usually unhelpful and most of the clinical symptoms resolve with effective explanation and engagement in a rehabilitative programme.
- *Other common associations* with chronic pain and pain amplification include obesity, reduced sleep, lower socio-economic status, parental catastrophizing, risk aversion, thought/attention problems, anxiety, low mood, rule-breaking, aggressive behaviour, and hypermobile joints, but the extent to which these factors are contributory in childhood varies.

Management of chronic pain

Irrespective of the medical setting, there is always a potential to positively intervene:
- *Begin with recognition* of a primary pain disorder and making time for the patient to explain their history, the impact, and their understanding. The therapeutic consultation acknowledges the pain and explains the role of pain as a threat signal.

- *Further explanations* about pain processing and understanding promote engagement in treatment and reduces a sense of helplessness.
- *Understanding disruptions to the four 'S'*: sleep, sports, social life, and school—explanation on how to return to normal routines will improve resilience and quality of life, reduce the psychological impact of pain, and enhance biofeedback to counteract pain signals.

Programmes of care

Effective programmes target the level of resource to meet the level of need. This often requires integration across a network of services, including community and schools. The focus of care is a return to normal function first, and an incident decrease in pain following. Core features of a programme include a range of interventions.

Pain workshops promote a shared experience through peer support, educate in an engaging way, dispel myths, and create a narrative to increase participation despite minimal changes in levels of pain.

Physical therapies, including PT and OT are most effective when goal-oriented.

- PT: reduces the fear of movement and supports the patient back into physical and other activities. ↑ participation promotes resilience, normal patterns of muscle use, strength, stamina, and balance and reduces muscle tightness.
- OT: provides a diverse range of strategies and supports graded return to many activities, including school and social life, improved sleep, and management of bullying.

Psychological intervention uses an array of strategies, in addition to CBT. Effective programmes reduce barriers to engagement, focus on resilience and coping strategies, and enhance patient strengths. A 2014 Cochrane review showed that psychological treatments reduce pain intensity and disability in various forms of chronic pain and these benefits are maintained. Evidence for the effects of psychological therapies on mood is limited, as it is for effects on disability in children with headache.

Active mind–body techniques are useful in promoting self-management, including breathing strategies (square, diaphragmatic, and slow-exhale breathing), mindfulness, yoga or pilates, and progressive muscle relaxation. This is not an exclusive list and benefit varies between patients.

Parent coaching by keyworkers help to manage the considerable emotional, and often financial, toll on family life. Pain-related disability is more consistently related to poor family functioning than to pain intensity.

- *Normalizing parental protectiveness* reduces guilt and defensiveness and refocuses parents' attention on healthy and adaptive behaviours. Parents are taught how to calm themselves and use skills to distract and avoid emotional escalations or other faulty pain behaviours. Focus is maintained on their child's function and participation.
- *Address parental pain experiences* and discuss openly with the child and their parent(s) and clearly point out that the patient's pain is different from the parent's disability and pain, with an expectation that the child can become pain-free.
- *Teach parents how to optimize their teenager's independence* and encourage self-management skills.

Pharmacotherapy for primary pain disorders

There is little evidence to support the sole use of medication as a treatment strategy without the measures discussed in ➲ Key considerations in the assessment of chronic pain, pp. 718–19. However, medications are associated with a strong placebo effect in chronic pain, and in multiple randomized controlled trials (RCTs) for migraine, an effective placebo response is seen over 50%. Placebo also decreases headache frequency from 5.6 to 2.9 headaches per month. Hence, medications may have a role in the integrated management plan and include using:

- *Simple analgesics:* no RCTs showing benefit of *paracetamol*, but limited evidence for *ibuprofen* exists, although both are associated with potential long-term side effects, including overuse headaches.
- *Opioids:* avoid because of poor safety and side effect profiles associated with worse outcomes. Care should be taken with opioid use when IBD or SCD is associated with a primary pain disorder. *Codeine* has been withdrawn from the World Health Organization (WHO) pain ladder for children.
- *Adjuvant therapies:* include low-dose *TCAs, gabapentinoids, selective serotonin reuptake inhibitors* (SSRIs), and *melatonin*—may be helpful. There are no RCTs to support the use of *gabapentin* in paediatric pain and its use may result in cognitive impairment and reduced resilience. However, the anxiolytic effects of this drug, TCAs, and SSRIs may help to improve engagement and resilience from improved sleep.

Further reading

Fatigue

National Institute for Health and Care Excellence. (2007). *Chronic fatigue syndrome/myalgic encephalomyelitis (or encephalopathy): diagnosis and management.* Clinical guideline [CG53]. Available at: ℰ https://www.nice.org.uk/guidance/cg53.

Arthritis

Arthritis and Musculoskeletal Alliance (ARMA). (2010). *Standards of Care for children and young people with juvenile idiopathic arthritis.* Available at: ℰ http://arma.uk.net/wp-content/uploads/pdfs/Juvenile%20Idiopathic%20Arthritis.pdf.
British Society for Paediatric and Adolescent Rheumatology. Available at: ℰ http://www.bspar.org.uk.
British Society for Paediatric and Adolescent Rheumatology (BSPAR). BSPAR guidelines. Available at: ℰ http://www.bspar.org.uk/clinical-guidelines.
NHS England. (2013). *NHS standard contract. Paediatric medicine: rheumatology (E03/S/b).* Available at: ℰ http://www.england.nhs.uk/commissioning/spec-services/npc-crg/group-e/e03/.
NHS England. *Specialised services quality dashboards.* Available at: ℰ http://www.england.nhs.uk/commissioning/spec-services/npc-crg/spec-dashboards/.

Child development

Managing and living with disability

(See also ➜ Special educational needs, p. 898; ➜ Children with disabilities, p. 899.) Diagnosis of a child with disability is invariably devastating for the family. Parents will react in different ways and their needs and support will vary. Health professionals should provide clear, practical information and be open, realistic, and honest in approach. Do not withhold information.

Multidisciplinary team

The MDT involved in the coordination and provision of care for the child and their family includes:

- Specialist paediatricians.
- Physiotherapists.
- Occupational therapists.
- Language therapists.
- Specialist nurses (e.g. community paediatric, epilepsy, learning disability).
- Key worker who takes responsibility for coordinating appointments and information.
- Social care.
- Education.

Ongoing evaluation

Ongoing evaluation of long-term needs in a child with disability requires attention. Each of the following is as important as the child's medical needs:

- Mobility problems.
- Hearing and vision difficulties.
- Communication difficulties.
- Self-care and continence issues.
- Educational provision: special schooling, statements of special educational needs.
- Feeding difficulties.
- Sleeping difficulties.
- Behaviour problems.

Social considerations

These are often able to provide support and advice for the family. A child with a disability is a 'child in need', according to the Children Act, and there-fore is entitled to an assessment, which can include:

- Provision of temporary respite care for parents.
- Provision of suitable accommodation (e.g. wheelchair access, bathroom access).
- Financial support (e.g. disability living allowances).

Transition to adult services must be carefully coordinated.

Normal development

(See also ➔ Visual development and UK screening, pp. 966–7.) Early child development is best divided into four functional areas:

- Gross motor (see ➔ Gross motor development, p. 726).
- Fine motor (see ➔ Fine motor development, p. 727).
- Speech (language and hearing) (see ➔ Speech and language development, p. 728).
- Social (emotional and behavioural) (see ➔ Social, emotional and behavioural development, p. 729).

Cognitive development refers to higher intellectual function and develops as the child gets older. Development is the result of a combination of hereditary and environmental factors. The environment must meet the child's physical and psychological needs. Developmental progress is about the acquisition of functional skills. There is remarkable consistency in the pattern of skills acquisition, although there is a wide normal range.

Gross motor development

Key motor developmental milestones

Head control

- *Newborn:* head lag on pulling to sit; head extension in ventral suspension.
- *6wk:* lifts head on lying prone and moves it from side to side.
- *3mth:* infant holds head upright when held sitting.

Primitive reflexes

'Primitive' reflexes disappear by 4–6mth (see Box 18.1).

Box 18.1 Primitive reflexes

- *Moro reflex:* sudden head extension causes symmetrical extension of the limbs, followed by flexion.
- *Grasp reflex:* fingers/toes grasp an object placed on the palm/sole.
- *Rooting reflex:* head turns to tactile stimulus placed near the mouth.
- *Stepping reflex:* infant held vertically, will step on a surface when foot is placed on it, followed by an up-step by the other foot.
- *Asymmetric neck reflex:* lying supine, if head turned, a 'fencing posture' is adopted—outstretched arm on the side, the head is turned.

Sitting

By 6–8mth, without support. relies on two reflexes:

- Propping or parachute reflex in response to falling.
- Righting reflex to position head and body back to the vertical on tilting.

Children not sitting by 9mth should be referred for evaluation.

Locomotor skills

An infant initially becomes mobile usually by crawling, but some will bottom-shuffle and others will commando-crawl (creep).

- By 10mth, infants pull to stand and cruise round furniture.
- By 12mth, 50% of infants walk independently.

Children not walking by 18mth must be referred for evaluation.

Further development of motor skills

- *Age 3y:* can jump from a step, stand on one leg, and pedal a tricycle.
- *Age 4y:* can balance on one leg for a few seconds, go up and down stairs one leg at a time, and pedal a bicycle with stabilizers.
- *Age 5y:* can skip on both feet.

Fine motor development

Fine motor development and vision

Fine motor skills are usually assessed alongside visual development.

Early visual alertness
- A *newborn infant* will fix and follow a near face in the field of view.
- By *6wk*, infant will turn the head through 90° to follow an object.
- By *3–4mth*, a baby will spend a lot of time watching their hands.

NB: Squints beyond the 8wk check must be referred to an ophthalmologist.

Early fine motor skills

As the grasp reflex decreases, infants will start to reach for objects.
- At 6mth:
  - Grip is usually with the whole palm (palmar grasp).
  - Holds objects with both hands and will bang them together.
  - Transfers objects between hands.
- By *10mth*, infant is developing a pincer grip (thumb and first finger).
- By *12mth*, infant will use index finger to point to objects.

Preschool fine motor development

Fine motor skills assessment is shown in Table 18.1.

Table 18.1 Fine motor skill developmental milestones

Age	Pencil skills	Brick building
18mth	Scribbles	
2y		Builds 6-brick tower
2.5y	Copies a circle	Builds 8-brick tower or train with four carriages
3y	Draws a circle	Copies/makes bridge
4y	Draws a cross	Copies/makes steps
4.5y	Draws a square	
5y	Draws a triangle	

Speech and language development

Speech is assessed in conjunction with hearing (see ⊃ Hearing assessment, pp. 854–5). Impaired hearing will affect language development. Age of acquisition of language is very varied.

Early signs of normal hearing and vocalization

- *Newborn* will quieten to voices and startle to loud noises.
- *By 6wk:* responds to mother's voice.
- *By 12wk:*
  - Will vocalize alone or when spoken to.
  - Begins to coo and laugh.

Early language development

- *At 6mth*, will use consonant monosyllables, e.g. 'ba' or 'da'.
- *By 8mth*, will use non-specific two-syllable babble, e.g. 'mama' or 'dada'.
- *By 13mth*, two-syllable words become appropriate, and develops understanding of other single words (e.g. 'drink' or 'no').
- *By 18mth:*
  - Vocabulary of ten words.
  - Demonstrates six parts of the body.

Phrase and conversation development

Conversation becomes increasingly complex, with sentence development in the second year.

- *By 24mth*, begin to combine two words together, progressing to 3-word phrases by the age of 2y (e.g. 'Give me toy' or 'Get me drink').
- *By 3y*, knows age, name, and several colours.

Social, emotional, and behavioural development

Early social development

- *At 6wk:*
  - Starts smiling.
  - Becomes increasingly responsive socially.
- *At 10mth*, shows separation anxiety when separated from parent and ↑ wariness of strangers.
- *By 10mth*, begins to wave 'goodbye'.

Social and self-help skills development

- *At 8mth*, begins to start to feed self using fingers.
- *At 12mth*, will drink from a cup.
- *At 18mth*, uses spoon to feed self.
- *By 2y*, removes some clothes and will soon start to try to dress self.

Bladder and bowel training

Very variable. Some children are potty-trained by 2y, but others can be much older when they develop this behaviour. Night-time dryness always takes longer; 10% of 5y olds still wet the bed at night.

Symbolic play

- *By 24mth*, children start to copy actions and activities that they see around them (e.g. feeding a doll, making tea, dusting, and cleaning).
- *They progress in the second year* to play on their own or alongside peers in parallel play.
- *From 3y*, they start to have interactive play, taking turns and following simple rules.

Cognitive function

Cognition refers to higher mental function.

- *Preschool children:*
  - Thought processes are called preoperational; children are at the centre of their world.
  - 'Magical' thinking and play with toys as if they were alive.
- *Junior school age:* thoughts become operational and thought processes are more practical and orderly.
- *Teenage years:* formal operational thought has developed, including abstract thought and complex reasoning.

Developmental assessment

The Denver Developmental Screening test (see Box 18.2) is used as a relatively quick test of children's abilities and as an assessment of whether they have achieved their age-appropriate developmental milestones (see Fig. 18.1).

Developmental assessment should always consider developmental progress over time within each area of skill. The pattern and rate of attainment of developmental milestones may also vary.

> **Box 18.2 How to use the Denver Developmental Screening Test**
> - A vertical line is drawn at the child's chronological age.
> - If premature, subtract the months of prematurity from the chronological age (up until the age of 2y).

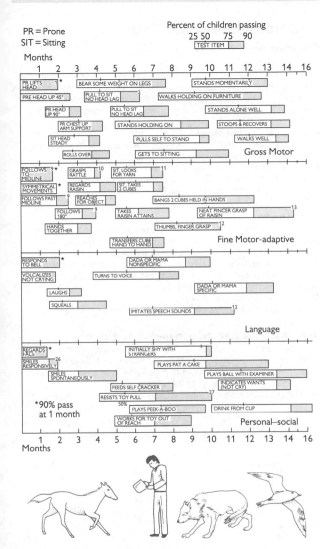

Fig. 18.1 Denver developmental screening.

Reproduced from Frankenburg WK, Dodds JB. The Denver developmental screening test. *J Pediatr.* 1967;71(2):181–91, with permission from Elsevier.

Neurodevelopmental delay

Common presentations

Delayed walking

Children may show early delay in the acquisition of motor milestones, with failure to crawl or sit unsupported at the appropriate age. A child who is not walking at the age of 18mth should be referred for a further opinion and may need to see a physiotherapist or a specialist paediatrician. It is important to exclude the following conditions:

- CP (see ➲ Cerebral palsy, pp. 392–3).
- DMD or other muscular disorders (see ➲ Neuromuscular disorders, pp. 384–7; ➲ Muscular disorders, pp. 390–1).
- Global neurodevelopmental delay as part of a syndrome or other unidentified cause (see ➲ Developmental delay, p. 502; ➲ Global neurodevelopmental delay, p. 733; ➲ Genetic testing in cognitive impairment, pp. 878–9).

Delayed speech

Delayed speech may be an isolated finding, either in the production of actual sounds or in the use of language. Language is divided into receptive language (language comprehension) and expressive language (speech to communicate). A speech and language therapist should assess language delay. A hearing test should be considered, especially if the child has not had their hearing screened as a neonate or there are other concerns (see ➲ Hearing assessment, pp. 854–5).

The causes of delayed speech development are shown in Box 18.3.

> **Box 18.3 Causes of delayed speech development**
> - *Familial:* a family history of language delay where parents have been late in developing language skills or have had speech therapy.
> - *Hearing impairment:* chronic otitis media (glue ear) is a common cause for delayed or poor clarity of speech in preschool age.
> - *Environmental:* poor social interaction/deprivation.
> - *Neuropsychological:*
>   - GDD.
>   - Autistic spectrum disorder.

Global neurodevelopmental delay

(See ➔ Chapter 25.)

Global developmental delay (GDD) indicates delay in all skill areas. Often it is more pronounced in fine motor, speech, and social skills. The degree of gross motor deficit is variable. There are many causes of developmental delay (see Box 18.4), although in some cases, the cause will remain unknown. If the delay is severe or profound, then it is more likely that a cause will be found.

> **Box 18.4 Causes of global neurodevelopmental delay**
>
> *Genetic*
> - Chromosomal disorders, e.g. Down's syndrome, fragile X.
> - DMD.
> - Metabolic syndromes, e.g. PKU.
>
> *Congenital brain anomalies*
> - For example, hydrocephalus or microcephaly.
>
> *Prenatal insult*
> - Teratogens, e.g. alcohol and drugs.
> - Congenital infections, e.g. rubella, CMV, or toxoplasmosis.
> - Hypothyroidism.
>
> *Perinatal insult*
> - Complication of extreme prematurity, e.g. IVH, periventricular leucomalacia.
> - Birth asphyxia.
> - Metabolic disorder, e.g. hypoglycaemia or hyperbilirubinaemia.
>
> *Postnatal events*
> - Brain injury: trauma; anoxia, e.g. suffocation or drowning.
> - CNS infection: e.g. encephalitis/meningitis.
> - Metabolic: e.g. hypoglycaemia.

Learning difficulties/disabilities

Learning difficulty is categorized as mild, moderate, severe, or profound.

Cognitive function can be assessed by an IQ test (see Table 18.2), but it may be difficult to assess all skill areas, especially in preschool age groups—assessment can be significantly affected by language problems and motor skills.

Table 18.2 Cognitive function assessment using an IQ test

Assessment	IQ
Normal	70
Mild learning difficulty	50–69
Moderate learning difficulty	35–49
Severe learning difficulty	20–34
Profound learning difficulty	<20

Mild learning disability may only be detected once a child is in school. A child with moderate learning difficulty will need significant support in their education. One with severe difficulties will learn basic personal care and develop simple speech, but will always need supervision. A child with profound difficulty is unlikely to develop speech and will always be dependent.

Developmental coordination disorder (DCD)

See also ➔ Developmental coordination disorder, p. 900. Previously known as *dyspraxia* or *clumsy child syndrome*.

Communication difficulties

Children may have an isolated language disorder and difficulty with social skills. However, when these two developmental problems are present on a background of other difficulties (limited play, obsessions, and lack of social awareness), autism must be considered (see ➔ Autism spectrum disorders, p. 757).

Child and family psychiatry

Classification, categories, and dimensions

Diagnosis is used in child and adolescent psychiatry to:
• Collect and organize information collected at assessment.
• Guide treatment planning.
• Inform about prognosis.

Classification systems assist with the standardization of the diagnostic process, and the use of a reliable and effective classificatory system can serve several important functions:
1. Their use results in greater precision in planning treatment at both the individual and population levels.
2. They are a prerequisite for the conduct of many types of clinical research and facilitate the communication of research findings.
3. They allow for the collection of epidemiological data, a process which is central to health care planning.

The two most influential diagnostic systems are the WHO's *International Classification of Diseases* (ICD) and the American Psychiatric Association's *Diagnostic and Statistical Manual of Mental Disorders* (DSM) system. Current versions are ICD-10 (ICD-11 released in June 2018, with plan for ICD-11 to be used for reporting from 2022) and DSM-V (updated in 2017). Both are categorical systems. They both include sections describing disorders first diagnosed in childhood and adolescence, but also allow children and adolescents to meet criteria for most 'adult' mental health disorders. A key requirement of both systems is that they insist that both symptoms and associated impairments be present in order for a diagnosis to be made.

Assessment

A thorough assessment and understanding of the presenting difficulties form the basis for any treatment interventions offered for children, young people, and their families or carers. As mental health problems rarely occur in isolation, with comorbidity the norm, it is essential that any assessment is sufficiently comprehensive to ensure that a clear and complete formulation of the presenting problems has been made. An assessment will usually have four major components:

- Identification of problems, history, signs, and symptoms.
- Information gathering stages.
- Evaluation/synthesis.
- Care/treatment planning.

Psychiatric history and examination

Psychiatric history and examination of child and adolescent mental health problems bears many similarities to that of adults. However, there are several differences in detail and emphasis. The assessment will usually be conducted as part of a joint interview with parents and the child/young person and will often require more than one visit.

Interview with parent(s)/carers

Clarify the presenting complaints with a systematic evaluation of psychopathological symptoms and a description of how problems developed over time.

- *Developmental history:*
  - Pre- and postnatal factors.
  - Early developmental history (e.g. milestones, language, attachment, sleep, feeding problems, early temperament).
- *Medical history:* especially tics and epilepsy, and psychosis for adolescents.
- *Medication:* e.g. anticonvulsants, antihistamines, sympathomimetics, and steroids.
- *Family history:* functioning, problem-coping styles, warmth and hostility, social networks, and other resources.

Interview with the child/young person

- *Functioning:* in the family, the school, and the peer group.
- *Emotional problems* and self-esteem.
- *Self-report rating scales:* may be useful as supplement, especially for emotional symptoms in those ≥9y.
- *Behavioural observation:* during clinical examination, can be very useful when problems are seen. Observe for social disinhibition and evidence of language disorder.
- *Systematic screening:* for psychiatric symptoms/disorders.
- *Physical examination.*

Notes on history taking

Why have multiple informants?

Neither parents nor their children may be aware of, or see, the whole picture. They may also withhold information from you, e.g. the teenage girl with anorexia nervosa who wants to avoid admission may exaggerate the amount she is eating and minimize her level of exercise.

Whom to get information from?

This is a balance between 'the more sources, the better' and the demands of confidentiality and time.

- A good starting point is the *referral details* and information from both the young person and members of the family.
- Information from the *school* should also be sought, though this may not be practicable in an emergency situation.
- Where relevant, *others* should be approached, e.g. social services, child and adolescent mental health services, youth offending teams.

Interviewing the family

To an extent, the family interview is an efficient way of gathering information and hearing the views of the patient, siblings, and parents all in one go. However, to see it this way is missing the point. It is an opportunity to learn so much more:

- Are there obvious tensions or conflicts?
- Is tension between the parents diffused by the child's behaviour?
- Are the children allowed appropriate autonomy, or do they 'rule the roost'?
- Is one parent a 'switchboard' through which all communication is routed?
- Are family members able to listen to each other's views?
- Is disagreement tolerated?
- Is there a family 'story' that informs how they interact around the presenting problem? Examples include 'no one listens to us', 'we have tried our best and can't do any more', 'it is all this child's fault', and 'he/she cannot be helped, but at the same time someone has to do something about her/him'. This sort of mixed message around a scapegoated child can often be very difficult to work with.

Family structures are variable. Often the interview is with one parent. Sometimes it can be illuminating if grandparents are also present. Are there coalitions across generations (e.g. grandparent and child), in effect combining forces to undermine one of the parents?

A further area to note is how the family responds to you. Are you treated as a threat, a hope, a parent/grandparent, or just a doctor? Do you feel pulled to take sides in a dispute?

Communicating

Tips for communicating with children

- Children's anxiety is often ↓ if first interviewed with an adult they trust.
- Assume children do not fully understand why they are being seen.
  - Often children assume they are 'in trouble'.
  - Often children equate doctors with physical illness, often with painful procedures such as injections.
- Be prepared to see a child several times to gain trust and rapport.
- Learn and/or practise child-appropriate communication, i.e. drawing, colouring, storytelling, pretending, building, making, exploring, appreciating tall tales, talking about current TV, and technology. Do not take 'over play'; remember to retain sensible adult behaviour.
- Practise age-appropriate language.
- Avoid undermining the parents' efforts by appearing too competent.

Tips for communicating with adolescents

(See also ➲ Chapter 20.)

- Don't assume they have chosen to be there.
- Understand they may be ambivalent about recognizing they have a problem dealing with, or denying, it. They may see you as a source of help or as a threat—or both.
- Discuss the context of your conversation—why are you meeting?
- Discuss what you will do with what she/he tells you (confidentiality and its limits may be crucial).
- It may be helpful to ask about neutral areas first.
- Be prepared to ask closed questions, accepting a 'yes' or 'no' answer.
- Speak naturally: avoid talking like an adult pretending to be a teenager.
- Convey your desire to understand by checking whether you are getting it right. 'I am hearing that unless something changes pretty quick, you are not going to be able to go to school anymore. Have I got it right?'
- Do ask the adolescent what she/he would like to happen, but accept they may have mixed feelings.
- Be patient—unless it is an acute situation, consider continuing your assessment over more than one session.
- Do see the adolescent alone, as well as with his/her parents.

Asking the difficult questions

About sexual abuse

(See also ➲ Sexual abuse, p. 916.) Sexual and other forms of abuse are common specific and non-specific vulnerability factors for poor mental health and must be excluded as aetiological factors. The clinician's task is to find an approach to asking about abuse that they are comfortable with and the child to be comfortable with. One approach is a hierarchical set of questions.

- *Introductory comment:* 'I ask these questions to all children I see.'
- *Ask the child to respond* to a broad, non-leading statement: 'Some children tell me something has happened to them that they wish had never happened.' The child's response may be verbal or non-verbal affirmation, denial, or looking perplexed; they may not understand the question at all.
- *Ask more specific questions:* 'Some things are done by other people . . . ' or ' . . . are touched in places they wished they had not been touched.'
- *Ask very specific questions:* 'Some people are touched in places like their private parts/vagina/penis (language depends on age, may also point or draw picture). Has this happened to you?'

Partial affirmation or non-verbal cues suggesting possible abuse should be followed up later. One caveat is differences between a forensic and a clinical interview. In both settings, open, non-leading questions are preferable. Local protocols will guide assessments. Consider completing a *child sexual exploitation* (CSE) questionnaire.

About suicidal ideation and intent

Clinicians must ask about suicidal thinking, especially in adolescents with any depressive features. Asking does not create or promote suicidal thinking. Again, a hierarchical approach is used effectively by many clinicians.

- *Introductory comment:* 'I ask these questions to everyone I see.'
- *Ask adolescent to respond to a broad statement:* 'Some young people tell me they feel life is not worth living anymore.' Again, note verbal responses or any non-verbal affirmation or denial.
- *Ask more specific questions:* 'Have you considered what it would be like to not be alive?' or 'Some people think it would be better to be dead.'
- *Ask very specifically to clarify risk and extent of planning:* 'Have you thought of killing yourself?'; 'Have you ever made a plan to kill yourself?'; 'Have you ever lost control and started your plan?'

As above, partial affirmation or non-verbal cues that suggest possible abuse should be followed up during later appointments.

Depression

Prevalence

~10% of 10y olds are reported by parents and teachers, and 20% of 14y olds report themselves to be often miserable. The rate of diagnosable depressive disorder in a community sample of 11–16y olds is closer to 3%. The discrepancy is due to those who suffer low moods but do not meet full diagnostic criteria.

Aetiology

Genes increase both the risk of developing depression and of experiencing −ve life events. Post-pubertal ♀ are twice as likely as ♂ to become depressed, and possible links to oestrogen levels, either *in utero* or post-puberty, have been suggested. ♀ may also be more influenced by lack of +ve relationships, close friendships, or a supportive peer network.

- *Environmental factors* include early adversity and attachment difficulties, −ve or traumatic life events or abuse, death of a parent, drug and alcohol abuse, and bullying.
- *Psychosocial factors* include social isolation and −ve interpersonal relationships, poor academic achievement, unstable family environment, and parental drug and alcohol abuse.

Clinical features

Diagnosis of depressive disorder requires that mood is persistently lowered and accompanied by a loss of interest and enjoyment and/or ↑ fatiguability for >2wk, with a significant effect on functioning. There should also be at least two of the following symptoms:
- Reduced concentration and attention.
- Reduced self-esteem and self-confidence.
- Ideas of guilt and unworthiness.
- Bleak and pessimistic views of the future.
- Ideas or acts of self-harm.
- Diminished appetite.
- Disturbed sleep.

Amongst those referred to child psychiatric clinics, comorbidity is common, e.g. conduct disorder (CDD), OCD.

Depressive disorders are frequently recurrent, so it is always important to ask about past episodes.

Dysthymia is a chronic enduring depressed state lasting for >1y, but without the intensity of a depressive episode.

Management

Initial assessment should identify:
- Significant risk of self-harm or suicide.
- Significant lack of self-care or neglect.
- Symptoms of manic episode or psychotic disorder.
- Comorbid psychiatric disorder.
- *Previous history of moderate or severe depressive episodes.* When these are present, referral to a specialist child and adolescent mental health service is appropriate.

Treatment

Mild depressive disorder with symptoms <4wk

Supportive therapy and *psychoeducation* about depressive disorders are effective first-line interventions in 30% of children and adolescents with recent onset of mild to moderate depressive symptoms:
- Give advice on sleep hygiene, nutrition, activity, and exercise.
- If no response to supportive management after 2–3mth, young people should be referred to Tier 2/3 Child and Adolescent Mental Health Services (CAMHS) for more intensive psychological therapy.

Moderate to severe depressive disorders

Psychological therapies are recommended as first-line treatments for treating child and adolescent depressive disorders. Recommended practice is that a block of psychological therapy should be undertaken before considering antidepressant medication. Approaches are:
- CBT and interpersonal therapy. Brief family therapy may be effective in some cases.
- Response to treatment should be reviewed after 12wk.
  - If good response to treatment, the course of therapy should be completed and follow-up provided for 12mth after remission of symptoms.
  - If poor response to treatment after 12wk, the assessment, formulation, and treatment plan should be reviewed (see ➔ Assessment, pp. 740–1).

If a diagnosis of depression remains, consider alternative psychological therapy and/or antidepressant medication. The most commonly used medications are SSRI antidepressants.

Prognosis

While recovery from a depressive disorder is likely, this may take months or, in some cases, years. Prognosis is worsened by increasing severity of disorder and by the presence of comorbid oppositional defiant disorder (ODD). Even in those who have made good recovery, further depressive episodes are not uncommon. Prolonged follow-up is therefore wise.

Suicide and non-fatal deliberate self-harm

Suicide is very rare in pre-pubertal children, but incidence rises through the teenage years. It is the fourth commonest cause of death in the 15–19y age group (UK: 4–8/100 000), with a ♂:♀ ratio of 4:1. Non-fatal deliberate self-harm is far commoner, with some 7% of those aged 15–16y having engaged in an act of deliberate self-harm in the previous year and 10% in an act of deliberate self-harm in their lifetime. It is commoner in ♀ (♀:♂ ratio 4:1).

Predisposing characteristics to completed suicide include:
- *Psychiatric disorder:* e.g. CDD, depression, substance misuse, ADHD, and psychosis.
- *Social isolation.*
- *Physical illness.*
- *Low self-esteem.*

Relevant family factors include a family history of abuse and neglect or of psychiatric illness and suicide, and family dysfunction.

Methods of self-harm

Those who kill themselves use a range of methods. The majority of non-fatal deliberate self-harm is through overdosing, generally with analgesics or prescribed drugs. Cutting is very common, particularly amongst adolescent girls. Unless the cutting is deep and over the site of major blood vessels, it should not be seen as necessarily linked to suicide or attempted suicide. Those who cut describe it as easing a build-up of bad feelings and resolving emotional numbness, or sometimes as a form of self-punishment.

Assessment

Careful assessment should happen soon after the self-harm. It should include the young person, the family, and information from other sources such as the family doctor or social services. Initial assessment should identify:
- Injuries from self-harm.
- Likely/potential effects of ingestion of substance.
- The child/young person's capacity to consent to, or refuse, treatment.
- Presence or absence of mental illness.
- Risk of further episode of self-harm.

Appropriate medical treatment should be provided. A further separate interview should be conducted with the child once the acute situation is stable. Take a general history and address the following.

- *History of act of self-harm:*
  - Circumstances leading up to self-harming behaviour.
  - Degree of suicidal intent at time of deliberate self-harm.
  - Intensity, frequency, and duration of self-harm thoughts.
  - Behaviour at time of overdose/self-harm.
  - Impulsivity or planned nature of the self-harm episode.
  - Help-seeking or help-avoiding behaviour.
  - Ongoing plans for further self-harm or suicide.
  - Previous history of self-harming behaviours.
- *A full mental state assessment* (see ➔ Assessment, pp. 740–1).
- *A clinical interview with the parents should include:*
  - A corroborative history of events surrounding the self-harm episode.
  - An exploration of parental response to the episode of self-harm.
  - An assessment of family functioning and support for the child.
  - Identification of symptoms suggesting a psychiatric disorder.

Management

Treat the physical effects of the self-harm episode and arrange mental health assessment. Following risk assessment, ensure appropriate levels of supervision are in place. Consider access to medication and other means of self-harm. If there are significant concerns about ongoing suicide risk, consider admission to an inpatient unit. If there are concerns about child protection, a referral should be made to social services. Treat any comorbid psychiatric disorder.

Management options for deliberate self-harm

Aims of intervention
- Address self-esteem issues.
- Improve interpersonal skills and address relationship difficulties.
- Improve communication skills.
- Learn more helpful ways to communicate emotions.

Family work
Family support and counselling with more structured and intensive family therapy may be appropriate.

School-based interventions
- Entire school programmes focusing on self-esteem issues and addressing peer relationships.
- Peer support programmes.
- Development and implementation of anti-bullying policies in school.

Prognosis

Ten per cent of those who self-harm will repeat within a year. A significant proportion will kill themselves within 5y—4% of girls and 11% of boys.

Anxiety disorders

Diagnostic criteria

One disorder is specific to children and adolescence: separation anxiety disorder (SAD). Other anxiety disorders that may occur in children and adolescents include: generalized anxiety disorder (GAD), panic disorder (with and without agoraphobia), simple and social phobias, and post-traumatic stress disorder (PTSD). Specific physical and cognitive symptoms are described for each disorder. Developmental principles apply.

- *Very young children* experience 'stranger danger', later simple phobias, and SAD with the beginning of the school years.
- *Middle childhood* presentations include fears of animals, the dark, burglars, and anxiety-related abdominal pain. A recrudescence or first presentation of SAD may occur at the onset of secondary schooling.
- *Adolescents* may experience social phobia, and panic with or without agoraphobia.

Post-traumatic stress disorder

Diagnostic criteria

A range of psychopathology may be experienced following an emotionally traumatic event, dependent on pre-existing vulnerabilities, event exposure, and related loss and grief. PTSD occurs as a response to an exceptionally threatening or catastrophic event. This leads to:

- *Re-experiencing phenomena*: e.g. nightmares, flashbacks, and intrusive memories.
- *Persistent avoidance of reminders of the trauma*.
- And either:
  - *Inability to recall,* either partially or completely, some important aspects of the period of exposure to the stressor; or
  - *Persistent symptoms of* ↑ *psychological sensitivity and arousal*: e.g. difficulty falling or staying asleep, irritability or outbursts of anger, difficulty concentrating, hypervigilance, exaggerated startle response. Emotional numbing and detachment are also often reported.

Age-specific symptoms

- *Younger children*: regression, altered sleep and feeding routines; exhibiting clingy, anxious, or aggressive behaviour; or engaging in post-traumatic play.
- *Young children*: cannot report emotional numbing or detachment; parents report these symptoms as a 'personality change'.

Differential diagnosis

Other anxiety disorders include event-related phobias, GAD, OCD, or, if of lesser severity, an adjustment disorder. Comorbidity with depression is common. If trauma is repetitive, expect disruptive behaviours in boys and early evidence of personality dysfunction in teenagers.

Treatment

If severe, treatment can be complex and take time.

Interventions include: *cognitive strategies* such as identifying and modifying dysfunctional schema; *behavioural strategies*, including prolonged re-exposure and skills acquisition such as relaxation techniques; *supportive therapy*; and *family interventions* to monitor for secondary impairment and altered family functioning.

- Eye movement desensitization and reprocessing (EMDR) has a role.
- Psychopharmacology may provide some symptomatic relief.

Prognosis

Long-term problems include: symptom chronicity, generalization of fears, and generalized impairment. A history of chronic, repetitive trauma, such as sexual abuse, is overrepresented in other mental health presentations, including drug/alcohol abuse and bulimia.

Obsessive–compulsive disorder

Diagnostic criteria

- *Obsessions*: recurrent, persistent thoughts, images, or impulses that are distressing, time-consuming, and functionally impairing. Young people recognize these thoughts as their own and perceive them as unhelpful and at times senseless.
- *Compulsions*: mental or physical behaviours, completed in an attempt to neutralize anxiety caused by the obsessional thoughts or images.
- *Rituals and habits*: present in two-thirds of preschool children. They are similar in form and content to compulsions in OCD, but:
  - Are less frequent and intense.
  - Do not impact on functioning.
  - Do not cause distress.

A diagnosis of OCD requires symptoms to be present on most days for at least 2 successive weeks and be a source of distress or interference with activities. Children are not required to have insight into the nature of their thoughts to meet the criteria for a diagnosis of OCD.

Prevalence

In children/adolescents, prevalence is ~0.5%. Up to 50% of adults with OCD will have had symptoms since age <18y. Onset is commoner in pre-pubertal boys and post-pubertal girls.

Treatment

Age- and developmentally appropriate psycho-education and guided self-help regarding both the psychological and biological perspectives of OCD are essential components of treatment for all children and young people. CBT and pharmacotherapy are effective and often required for more severe cases.

Prognosis

The course of OCD may be acute or chronic. Longitudinal studies of adults with a diagnosis of OCD suggest that prognosis is variable; most people fall into one of three patterns:
1. 40% recover and experience only mild symptoms.
2. 40% experience a fluctuating illness course, with symptoms remitting and relapsing.
3. 20% develop a chronic illness pattern.

Schizophrenia

Schizophrenia is characterized by disorders of thought, perception, mood, and sometimes posture. Peak onset is in young adult life. Prevalence in mid teens is ~70%, with equal numbers of ♂ and ♀. A +ve family history is common.

Clinical features

Onset may be insidious or acute. Core features of schizophrenia include the following:

- *Thought disorder:* thoughts inserted or removed from one's head or broadcast to others, often with abnormal speech patterns.
- *Auditory hallucinations:* external voices discussing the patient or commenting on his/her behaviour.
- *Delusions:* fixed beliefs that are false, not open to reason, and not in keeping with the patient's developmental or cultural context.
- *Disorders of posture:* holding abnormal postures.

Differential diagnosis

Important differential diagnoses include: affective psychosis (bipolar disorder/psychotic depression), drug-induced psychoses, and psychoses secondary to other organic conditions (e.g. N-methyl-D-aspartate-receptor encephalitis), temporal lobe epilepsy, autism spectrum disorder.

Assessment

As a schizophrenia-type psychosis can be caused by organic conditions, it is essential that signs of these be sought. Include full neurological examination, and check for thyroid, adrenal, or pituitary dysfunction and drug screen.

Management

Children and adolescents require a combination of:

- Specific therapies, aimed at reducing the core symptoms.
- General therapies, relating to the psychological, social, and educational needs of the child/young person and their family.

Traditional psychotherapies have little effect, but learning-based therapies and those that increase family support can improve functioning and decrease relapse rates. *Antipsychotic medication,* most commonly the newer atypical antipsychotics with preferable side effect profiles, is often effective. Relapses are fewer when families are supportive.

The acute phase can progress to a chronic state with poor motivation and inactivity.

Prognosis

Relatively good for a single acute episode in a previously well-functioning teenager. It is worse for insidiously developing illness, particularly if pre-existing developmental difficulties.

Somatoform disorders and typical consultation–liaison presentations

This is a poorly defined area with a whole host of overlapping terms and confusions between descriptive terms and implied aetiology. Some of the terms in common usage are:

- *Psychosomatic*: a very general and rather unhelpful term that can include both illnesses brought on by stress (e.g. tension headache) and physical symptoms secondary to psychiatric illness (e.g. hypothermia secondary to malnutrition in anorexia nervosa).
- *Somatoform disorders*: physical symptoms with no organic basis. These are subdivided into:
  - Conversion disorders.
  - CFS (see ➲ Chronic fatigue syndrome, pp. 902–3).
  - Pain syndromes (see ➲ Chronic pain in children, pp. 718–21), hypochondriasis.
  - Somatization disorder.

While many of these terms are entrenched, and so unlikely to disappear, the concept of somatoform disorders has been much criticized on the following grounds:

- It implies a cause that is not demonstrable and often intuitively does not appear to be correct.
- It is often unacceptable to patients and parents and is therefore an obstacle to forming a collaborative relationship.
- Its use may result in missing psychiatric or physical diagnoses.
- There seems little relationship between this term and other diagnoses commonly applied to the same patients in non-mental health settings, e.g. IBD, chronic fatigue.

Conversion disorder

(See also ➲ Conversion or 'psychologically mediated' disorders, p. 401.) Conversion disorder is characterized by the presence of physical symptoms (e.g. paralysis, seizures, and sensory deficits) or mental symptoms (e.g. amnesia), but without any evidence of physical cause. Previously called hysteria. The proposed underlying mechanism is transformation of emotional conflict into mental or physical symptoms. The postulated splitting off of mental processes from each other is referred to as dissociation. There may be secondary gain (e.g. when the child who is being bullied at school develops paralysis), which keeps them at home. Conversion disorders are rare in childhood, particularly under 8y.

Treatment

Principles of treatment include attempts to resolve any apparent emotional difficulties, avoidance of unnecessary physical investigation, removal of secondary gain, and help in returning to normal life.

Prognosis

Generally favourable.

Anorexia nervosa

Diagnostic criteria

- *Dietary restriction* (may be accompanied by vomiting, exercise, laxative abuse, or other weight control methods), leading to significant and unhealthy self-induced weight loss (e.g. to <85% of expected body weight for height or age, or a BMI <17.5kg/m^2).
- *Intense fear of gaining weight*, even when severely underweight.
- *Body image distortion* with dread of fatness.
- *Amenorrhoea* (may be primary or secondary).

Risk factors

A genetic predisposition, a perfectionist personality, and low self-esteem seem to be implicated.

Epidemiology

While varying with age, a sex ratio of 9:1 (girls:boys) is fairly typical. Pre-pubertal cases are rare but do occur.

Treatment

(See MARSIPAN guidance in ⮕ Further reading, p. 758.) The evidence base for treatment is small. An MDT approach is used. The key to success in individual treatment is engagement with the therapist, rather than the type of therapy provided.

Treatment is likely to be lengthy and to involve attention to anorexic behaviours, to recognizing and not acting on anorexic thoughts and feelings, and to returning to aspects of normal function such as school and home life. At times, compulsory treatment (requires use of the Mental Health Act) may be needed. Clearly, correction of dangerous weight loss or its secondary complications may be urgent. Patients who are unable or un-willing to manage adequate oral nutrition may need NGT feeding. In any rapid refeeding plan, the risks of refeeding syndrome (see ⮕ Method, p. 291) should be remembered.

Prognosis

Anorexia nervosa carries a significant risk of death and morbidity. Many children will carry the diagnosis into adult life. The risks to long-term physical health are greater without early attention to malnutrition and include:

- Growth retardation, delayed or arrested puberty.
- Reduced bone density.
- Higher likelihood of LBW baby.

Risk factors for poorer outcome include:

- Late onset.
- Vomiting and purging as part of the clinical picture.
- Poor social adjustment or poor parental relationships.
- Being ♂.

Bulimia nervosa

Epidemiology

Bulimia nervosa is rare at <13y of age, and it is unusual for a person to present for help before their early twenties. In teenagers, bulimia may occur alongside other externalizing teenage behaviours (i.e. sexual promiscuity, drug-taking, drinking, and self-harming). ≥90% are ♀. Bulimia is associated with westernized lifestyle, with a lower prevalence in developing countries and rural areas. There may or may not be a preceding history of anorexia nervosa.

Causes

Similar factors contribute to the aetiology of bulimia nervosa, as are found for anorexia nervosa. In contrast to anorexia nervosa, bulimia is associated with high expression of emotions, impulsivity, and a chaotic lifestyle.

Additional risk factors include:
- Adverse family life events.
- Family history of obesity.
- Parental substance misuse.
- Family history of affective disorder.
- Poor social network.
- Critical parents.

Diagnostic features

- *Persistent preoccupation with eating*: craving for food, with recurrent episodes of binge eating, associated with feeling out of control.
- *Regular use of mechanisms to reduce weight gain* from bingeing (e.g. vomit induction, laxatives, diuretics, appetite suppressants, excessive exercise).
- *Morbid fear of fatness*.
- *Body weight higher than required* for the diagnosis of anorexia.
- *Repeated vomiting and/or laxative abuse*: may result in serious electrolyte disturbance, seizures, tetany, haematemesis, or stomach rupture.

Management

Usually best managed by an MDT and including the family from the start. CBT, including educational input about healthy eating, starvation, and binging. Motivational interviewing and family therapy can also be helpful. Pharmacotherapy (e.g. fluoxetine) is rarely used but may reduce food craving.

Prognosis

Full recovery occurs in up to 50% of cases. Between 66% and 75% show at least partial recovery at 10y follow-up. Bone density follow-up shows no osteopenia or osteoporosis in recovered bulimic patients.

Oppositional defiant and conduct disorders

ODD and CDD are related disruptive behaviour disorders, typified by defiance, disobedience, and violation of social rules and the rights of others.

Epidemiology

Prevalence varies greatly, depending on the age of the sample and the diagnostic criteria used.

- Both CDD and ODD are commoner in ♂.
- ODD is commoner in younger children (<10y); ODD prevalence in 5–10y olds is ~5% in boys and ~2% in girls.
- CDD prevalence increases with age: ~1% in children and 4% in adolescents.

Causes

Many patients are likely to have an underlying genetic vulnerability and an association with various pre- and perinatal risk factors.

Subsequent exposure to coercive parenting (intrusive parenting and subsequent reinforcement of child counterattack and parent withdrawal) early in life has also been implicated. Later involvement of vulnerable individuals with a deviant peer group predicts a CDD pathway, as does a variety of psychosocial risk factors (e.g. low socio-economic status, peer relationship difficulties, parental mental illness, and child maltreatment, neglect, and abuse).

Clinical features

- ODD is highly descriptive (i.e. hostile, negativistic, and defiant), particularly to the parents. The defiant behaviour pattern must last ≥6mth and cause impairment across a variety of domains.
- CDD is defined by more serious aggressive behaviour and rule violations, property damage, theft, arson, truancy, and running away, which again must have been present for ≥6mth and result in functional difficulties.

Management

Early intervention with ODD in very young children use universal parenting programmes, targeting coercive parenting and parental abuse. If ODD and CDD are established, programmes with intensive interventions that involve children, parents, and other participants in the child's social ecology have proved effective. Multisystemic therapy is an example of such an intervention. Remedial education is likely to be needed and can also be helpful as self-esteem rises.

Attention-deficit/hyperactivity disorder

ADHD is a complex neurodevelopmental disorder.

Prevalence

Prevalence of ADHD in children is 6.5%, and in adolescents 2.7%. ADHD is 2–3 times commoner in boys.

Causes

ADHD displays considerable heterogeneity at the genetic, pathophysiological, cognitive, and behavioural levels of analysis. While the exact cause of ADHD is unknown, considerable research supports a strong genetic component (heritability of 0.7), with non-shared environmental factors contributing most of the residual variance.

Diagnostic criteria

- *Inattention:* e.g. failure to attend to detail, difficulty sustaining attention, does not follow through, difficulty organizing tasks, easily distracted.
- *Hyperactivity:* e.g. often fidgets, leaves seat in classroom, runs and climbs excessively, acts as if driven by a motor.
- *Impulsivity:* e.g. often blurts out an answer before the question has finished, has difficulty waiting turn, interrupts and butts in.

Symptoms must be present for ≥6mth, be present before 7y, and result in impairment in two or more functional domains or settings. Common comorbidities include:

- Disruptive behaviour disorders (ODD and CDD).
- Anxiety (22–37%).
- Depression (12–17%).
- Learning, speech, and language disorders are also overrepresented.

Treatment

- *Psychopharmacology:* drug therapies include psychostimulants (methylphenidate, dexamfetamine) and the non-stimulant atomoxetine.
- *Behavioural interventions:* integrated home–school behaviour management, token economies, and parent effectiveness training. The effectiveness of family interventions is inconclusive.

Prognosis

Seventy to 80% continue to display symptoms and impairments as adolescents, and 50–65% as adults. Only 10–20% reach adulthood without any psychiatric diagnosis, functioning well, and without symptoms of their disorder. Pharmacological treatments may be continued into adulthood.

Autism spectrum disorders

Autism spectrum disorders include:
- Autism (prevalence ~1/1000).
- Rett's syndrome (prevalence 1/15 000).
- Asperger's disorder (prevalence 3–4/1000).

Aetiology

It is likely that autism spectrum disorders are heterogenous in aetiology. Most believe there are underlying complex genetic vulnerabilities, with subsequent environmental influences and factors that trigger gene expression.

Clinical features

Usually identified in preschool years but may be found later in individuals with above-average IQ.
- *Problems with social interactions:* include appearing aloof, impaired non-verbal behaviours, difficulty establishing friendships, and poor or absent emotional reciprocity.
- *Language problems:* include marked delay or lack of speech, inability to converse, and abnormal speech, including stereotypical speech.
- *Behaviour problems:* include preoccupied and stereotypical behaviours (e.g. hand flapping). In adolescence, aggressiveness, mood variability, and sexually inappropriate behaviour can be problematic.

Mental retardation, language delay, ADHD, and medical complications, such as epilepsy, often coexist with an autism spectrum diagnosis.

Management

Psychosocial interventions, often with an emphasis on behaviour management and parent involvement, can often lead to ↑ child skills and high parent satisfaction.

Prognosis

- 70% remain with severe disability.
- 50% develop useful speech.
- Only 5% will lead independent adult lives.

Individual psychotherapy

There are a wide range of individual therapies, including the following.

Behaviour therapy

This treatment is brief and directed at encouraging desired behaviours and eliminating problem behaviours. Problems are dealt within a behavioural framework, rather than through focusing on underlying thoughts, feelings, or past causes.

Cognitive behavioural therapy

As above, but with a wider focus on thoughts and attribution of meaning, as well as behaviour. This is one of the better researched therapies. CBT involves keeping of diaries and homework carried out between sessions.

Psychodynamic psychotherapy

Longer-term treatment directed at underlying problems and the presenting symptom. Central to treatment are theories of the unconscious mind. The patient is encouraged to use their relationship with the therapist to explore dysfunctional patterns of behaviour. The therapist is able to comment on these and help the patient to understand new ways of relating.

Family therapy

These treatments share the idea that problems are affected by communication between family members and such communication can serve to maintain or to ameliorate their difficulties.

Family therapy based on *systems theory* might identify recurring dysfunctional patterns of interaction and typically might hypothesize that the presenting problem in one family member is a manifestation of this. An example of such an approach is the school-refusing child who is being kept home to act as a buffer between parents who are in conflict. The child's presence may prevent dangerous escalation but may also interfere with the parents' ability to resolve their differences. Therapy in this case might focus on helping the parents to address their difficulties without involvement of the child, and for the child to trust his/her parents to do this and to get on with being a child, e.g. going to school.

Further reading

Anorexia nervosa

Royal Colleges of Psychiatrists, Physicians, and Pathologists. (2014). *MARSIPAN: Management of Really Sick Patients with Anorexia Nervosa*, second edition. Available at: ℛ https://www.rcpsych. ac.uk/docs/default-source/improving-care/better-mh-policy/college-reports/college-report-cr189.pdf?sfvrsn=6c2e7ada_2.

Other

See reference list in: Royal College of Psychiatrists. (2017). ADHD and hyperkinetic disorder: for parents and carers. Available at: ℛ https://www.rcpsych.ac.uk/mental-health/parents-and-young-people/information-for-parents-and-carers/attention-deficit-hyperactivity-disorder-and-hyperkinetic-disorder-information-for-parents-carers-and-anyone-working-with-young-people.

National Institute for Health and Care Excellence. (2018). *Attention deficit hyperactivity disorder: diagnosis and management*. NICE guideline [NG87]. Available at: ℛ https://www.nice.org.uk/guidance/NG87.

Volkmar FR, Lord C, Bailey A, *et al.* Autism and pervasive developmental disorders. *J Child Psychol Psychiat* 2004; **45**: 135–70.

Chapter 20

Adolescent health and well-being

Adolescence: an overview

Adolescence is the developmental phase that defines the shift from dependent childhood to autonomous adulthood. It involves major changes in physical maturity and brain structure and function, as well as puberty. Though experienced by all humans, an individual's adolescence is as unique as they are.

Terminology is important and can be confusing. *Adolescence* describes the time period, but the group living it prefer the term 'young person' to 'adolescent'. 'Young person' and 'adolescent' will be used interchangeably in this chapter. 'Teen' or 'teenager' are not accurate in regard to brain development in adolescence, since it continues well into an individual's twenties.

Traditionally, the most commonly used age is 10–19y, based on the WHO definition. However, expert opinion now suggests it is reasonable to consider young people as those between the age of 10y and 24y, which takes account of a global shift towards earlier puberty and the later acquisition of traditional adult statuses such as marriage and parenthood. The legal and health service configurations in each country place artificial boundaries at different ages in the 10–24y period.

Psychological development

Adolescence marks the beginning of the development of more complex thinking processes. These include:
- Ability for abstract thinking (thinking about possibilities).
- Ability to reason from known principles (form own new ideas or questions).
- Ability to consider many points of view according to different criteria (i.e. compare or debate ideas or opinions).
- Ability to think about the process of thinking.

These developments go in parallel with a significant shift in brain structure and function, with massive synaptic pruning in the grey matter. This pruning follows a predictable pattern in which the limbic system (i.e. the areas of the brain associated with reward and risk-taking) matures faster than the prefrontal cortex, with its vital role in regulating behaviour. This pattern has been likened to a car gaining a more powerful accelerator before any work improving its brakes.

Social development

Adolescence marks the period during which there is a gradual shift from dependence on parents, through dependence on friends and peers, before gaining a position of relative independence. The value of friends' and peers' opinions is of utmost importance and the presence of others significantly increases risk-taking, particularly around driving behaviour.

Physical development

Adolescence also describes the period in which the human body undergoes some of its most dramatic physical changes, with both a large and final growth spurt and also the development of secondary sexual changes that result in a mature reproductive system. During this time of physical change, the body is vulnerable to diseases occurring at the same time as the creation of self-identity. This magnifies the impact of disease, e.g. a skin complaint like acne can have a huge impact on self-esteem and well-being.

Key areas to consider in management

- *Communication:* adopt non-judgemental, open communication style.
- *Physical examination:*
  - Ensure privacy and personal integrity.
  - Perform pubertal assessment (with another health care professional as chaperone) when indicated.
- *Psychosocial issues:*
  - Personal identity.
  - Concordance with treatment.
  - Provision of opportunistic health promotion.
- *Ethical and legal issues:* consent, competence, and confidentiality.
- *Service configuration issues:*
  - Ensure meaningful engagement and co-design.
  - Use quality standards (i.e. UK's Department of Health benchmark 'You're Welcome'—see ℘ http://www.doh.gov.uk).
  - Consider clinic times that fit the lives of young people.

Communication and consultations

Getting communication with young people right is vital. It is the surest way to ensure relevant information is shared and understood and that prescribed or suggested treatments are understood and followed. The adolescent consultation can be challenging, but enormously rewarding.

Top tips

- Introduce yourself with 'Hello, my name is'.
- Give an overview of the structure of the consultation.
- See young people by themselves, as well as with their parents.
- Remind the young person about confidentiality and its limits.
- Place the young person at the centre of the consultation, even when their parents are present.
- Use an open, empathetic, non-judgemental approach.
- Avoid medical jargon.
- Use gender-neutral terminology whenever possible.
- Explore the young person's hopes and fears to include them in all decisions about their health and treatment.
- Summarize the key 'take home messages'.

Each consultation offers an opportunity to give opportunistic health screening, particularly in emergency settings where the young person may have experienced an adverse outcome from their behaviour and be amenable to the 'teachable moment.' HEEADSSS (see Box 20.1) is a psychosocial history toolkit designed for adolescent health-related consultations and can be completed in 5min. While asking some of these questions can feel awkward at first, such an approach improves the satisfaction of the young person with the consultation. Before undertaking such screening, it is important to familiarize yourself with locally available support services, should an issue be highlighted.

Box 20.1 The HEEADSSS protocol[1]

H—Home, including relationship with parents.
E—Education or employment, including financial issues.
E—Eating, including diet, exercise, and body image.
A—Activities, including online/social media life.
D—Drug use, including cigarettes and alcohol.
S—Sex, including sexuality, relationships, and contraception.
S—Suicide, including general mood and potential self-harm.
S—Safety, including accident and violence prevention.

1. Goldenring JM, Rosen DS. Getting into adolescent heads: an essential up-date. *Contemp Pediatr*. 2004;**21**(1):64–90.

Adolescent health issues

While the majority of young people live healthy and happy lives, there is a sizeable minority for whom this is not the case.

Adolescent mortality

Adolescence and young adulthood are traditionally seen as the healthiest time of life, free from potentially fatal infectious diseases of childhood and not yet affected by long-term non-communicable conditions of adulthood. Sadly, it is no longer the case, with rates of death in the UK now almost three times higher in 15–19y olds, compared with 5–9y olds. Sadly, the rapid improvements seen in infant and child mortality over the last century are not mirrored in young people.

Most deaths in resource-rich countries sadly occur due to external causes (see Table 20.1). These are not random events, but often predictable or preventable with public health and psychosocial interventions.

Adolescent health problems

The pattern of adolescent illness is distinct and reflects the transitional nature of this period of life (see Box 20.2). With improvements in the survival of premature neonates and those with profound disabilities, many such children live into and beyond adolescence. Many long-term physical and mental health conditions begin in adolescence and their management in this time often sets trends that last well into adult life.

There are also the more specific issues related to adolescence, whether it is a physical issue with growth or pubertal development or the direct impacts of psychosocial issues such as substance misuse or sexually transmitted infections (STIs). Finally, there are a small, but often resource-intensive, group of young people with CFS and medically unexplained physical symptoms (see ➋ Chronic fatigue syndrome, pp. 902–3) who require expert multidisciplinary care in order to reach their maximum potential into adulthood.

Table 20.1 Leading causes of adolescent mortality

	UK	Worldwide
1	Suicide	Road traffic accidents
2	Road traffic accidents	LRTIs
3	Homicide	Self-harm
4	Cancer	Diarrhoeal diseases
5	Neurological	Drowning

Adolescent service use

Adolescents form an often under-appreciated group in primary and secondary health care settings since they are spread over a wide number of clinical teams and locations. In the UK, there is higher service use by those aged 10–19y than those aged 1–9y. *Task: look around your institution. Do you know how many young people you treat and what for?*

> **Box 20.2 Common adolescent-related health issues**
> * Acne.
> * Cancer.
> * Long-term physical health conditions:
>   * IDDM.
>   * Asthma.
>   * Epilepsy.
>   * Arthritis.
>   * HIV.
> * CFS and chronic pain (see ➋ Chronic fatigue syndrome, pp. 902–3; ➋ Chronic pain in children, pp. 718–21).
> * Medically unexplained physical symptoms.
> * Constitutional delay in growth and puberty.
> * Acute deliberate self-harm.
> * Substance abuse:
>   * Alcohol.
>   * Tobacco.
>   * Illegal drugs.
> * Long-term mental health conditions:
>   * ADHD.
>   * Anxiety disorders.
>   * Conduct/behaviour disorders.
>   * Depression.
>   * Eating disorders—anorexia nervosa, bulimia nervosa.
> * Gynaecological disorders:
>   * Oligomenorrhoea/dysmenorrhoea.
>   * PCOS.
> * Sexual health issues:
>   * Teen pregnancy.
>   * STIs.
> * Obesity.
> * Sports-related injuries.
> * Trauma.

Substance misuse

The use of alcohol, tobacco, and other recreational drugs has long been a common part of adolescence, but for a minority, this can cause significant problems acutely and longer-term issues of dependence. Alcohol and tobacco are traditionally the most commonly used substances due to ease of access and social acceptability. Most young people who use alcohol or tobacco do not progress to using illicit substances. However, most users of illicit drugs will have used alcohol and tobacco.

- *Alcohol:* reducing in the UK; 44% of 11–15y olds have tried alcohol. Most drink <1 time/wk, though issues with binge drinking persist.
- *Smoking:* reducing in the UK and Western Europe, but concerning rise in tobacco use in resource-poor settings. In the UK, 3% of 11–15y olds smoke regularly. Use of e-cigarettes is increasing.
- *Illegal drugs:* use of traditional recreational drugs is declining in the UK. Cannabis remains the most commonly used substance in teenagers in most developed countries, with 8% of 11–15y olds in the UK having used it at least once (it is higher in North America). There have been worrying rises in use of novel psychoactive substances (formally known as 'legal highs') and nitrous oxide, though a number of governments have recently tightened legislation.

Dealing with acute drug intoxication can be challenging. Resources such as TOXBASE® (℠ https://www.toxbase.org/) and FRANK (℠ http://www.talktofrank.com) are vital in ascertaining drug taken and any treatments required. The list below of *vulnerabilities and concerning behaviours* not only applies to substance misuse, but also to other areas of concern such as grooming, gang recruitment, and radicalization.

Vulnerabilities
- *History of abuse or neglect*
- *Looked-after child/care leaver*
- *Young carers*
- *Parental drug/alcohol dependence*
- *Low self-esteem/self-confidence*
- *Homelessness*
- *Truancy*
- *Refugee or unaccompanied asylum seeker/trafficked*
- *Poor mental health*
- *Learning difficulties and disabilities*

Concerning behaviours
- Unexplained changes in behaviour
- Inappropriate sexual behaviour
- Disengagement from family or friends
- Disengagement from school/truancy
- Unexplained gifts
- Multiple mobile phones
- Repeated STIs/pregnancies
- Involvement in crime

Sexual health

Sexual health is a hugely important area for young people. Developing good sexual health is about more than simply avoiding unwanted pregnancy and infections. It includes development of emotional maturity, relationship skills, and healthy body image.

The median age of first sexual intercourse in the UK remains 16y, with younger age associated with ↑ risky behaviour. The exponential growth of Internet use (via smartphones and tablets) has seen pornography use rise and *sexting* (sharing sexually explicit images/videos) becoming common practice. Age of consent varies by country, as do social and cultural expectations around sex and sexuality, but there are some areas that should always cause concern (see Box 20.3).

> ## Box 20.3 Sexual health red flags
> - Age <13y.
> - Age or power imbalance in relationships.
> - Evidence of excessive secrecy or of bribery and coercion, as often seen in the latter stages of grooming/CSE.
> - Any reports of aggression or sexual violence.
> - Association with substance misuse.

LGBTQ

~4% of 16–24y olds in the UK identify as lesbian, gay, bisexual, transgender, or questioning (LGBTQ). There has been a welcome shift in public acceptance of these sexualities and of the fluidity of gender. It is vital to use gender-neutral language and not to assume sexuality.

Pregnancy

There has been a significant reduction in under-18y old conception rate in the UK, with 2016 showing the lowest rate since records began, at 18.9/1000 women, due to better sex and relationship education, improved educational expectations for young women, and improved access to long-acting reversible contraception. This rate is still higher than other northern European countries, with most unwanted teenage pregnancies in the context of poverty, low educational achievement, and adverse social factors (e.g. mental health problems, sexual abuse, and crime). Infants of teenage mothers are at ↑ risk of being born LBW or suffering abuse and neglect.

Sexually transmitted infections

Adolescence is the commonest time to be diagnosed with an STI, with the rate twice as high in 15–24y olds, compared with 25–59y olds. Chlamydia remains the most frequently diagnosed condition. Gonorrhoea has reduced a little, but there are deeply concerning trends in antibiotic resistance. There has been a marked reduction in diagnoses of first genital warts in both girls and boys, reflecting the uptake of the human papillomavirus (HPV) vaccine.

Long-term conditions and transition

A long-term issue is a condition for which there is currently no cure, and is managed with medications and other treatments. Twenty-three per cent of young people have a long-term condition or disability in the UK, with the incidence of asthma and IDDM still increasing.

Impact on the adolescent

Young people with a long-term condition often face additional challenges, compared with their healthy peers. Their illness can impact physical, psychological, emotional, and social development and well-being. For example:

Physical
- Constitutional delay in growth/pubertal development (see ➲ Constitutional delay in growth and puberty, pp. 442–3).
- Medication side effects, e.g. moon facies with steroid use.

Psychological
- Poor self-esteem.
- –ve body self-image.
- Sense of alienation.
- Depression.
- Anxiety.
- Behavioural problems.

Social and educational
- Poor school performance.
- Social isolation/integration.
- Difficulties in attending social events or participating in sport.

Impact on the family

Chronic illness can adversely impact on the young person's family. Parents have to provide additional time for care and support of the young person with a chronic illness, often with financial consequences. Parents may experience guilt, frustration, and anxiety, and the frequency of mental health problems is ↑. Siblings can also be affected, often missing out on parental time and attention. The support of specific charities and sometimes child and adolescent psychology services is often required and may be helpful.

Impact on health professional relationships

Young people are usually more concerned about the 'here and now' issues of adolescence, and less interested in the long-term consequences of their treatment and their behaviour towards it. This often leads to a conflict of priorities between health professionals (and parents) and the adolescent and may lead to problems with compliance.

Treatment

Improving compliance may be helped by the following.

Treatment discussions
- Should be developmentally and cognitively appropriate.
- Should be alone and in confidence.

- Adopt a non-judgemental approach.
- Explore understanding of illness and treatment. Correct any misunderstanding and educate.
- Identify potential barriers to concordance.
- Avoid medical jargon.
- Encourage treatment 'routine'.

Treatment goals
- Should be relevant to (current) adolescent issues, e.g. appearance, socializing, recreational opportunities.
- Include the adolescent in negotiations.
- Keep goals short term (weeks to months).
- Use the simplest regimen possible.
- Tailor to the adolescent's daily routine.

Treatment application
- Give written instructions.
- Suggest simple reminder strategies, e.g. calendar, alarms, phone apps.
- Enlist support and help from parents, family, peers, MDT, and groups.

Transition to adult health services

Adolescents requiring ongoing specialist care will eventually need transfer to 'adult' health care services. This transition requires more than a 'simple' transfer of medical records from one service to another. The key principles of successful transition are:
- Start early, at least by 13–14y old.
- Involve families.
- Ensure good documentation—proformas are great.
- Regularly review confidence and independence.
- Facilitate familiarity with the adult service; shared clinics can work really well.

As much as is possible in our often inflexible health care models, final transfer of the young person should occur at a time when they are ready, to ensure that there is no breakdown in treatment with potential acute exacerbations or flares of their condition.

Further reading

FRANK. Drug use information for patients. Available at: ℜ http://www.talktofrank.com.

Northumbria Healthcare NHS Foundation Trust. (2017). *Making healthcare work for young people. A toolkit to support delivery of 'Developmentally Appropriate Healthcare' in the NHS.* Available at: ℜ https://www.northumbria.nhs.uk/wp-content/uploads/2017/04/nhs-making-healthcare-work-web-02.pdf.

TOXBASE®. Available at: ℜ https://www.toxbase.org/.

Royal College of Paediatrics and Child Health, National Children's Bureau, British Association for Child and Adolescent Public Health. (2014). *Why children die: deaths in infants, children and young people in the UK.* Part A. Royal College of Paediatrics and Child Health, London.

World Health Organization. (2017). *Global Accelerated Action for the Health of Adolescents (AA-HA!): guidance to support country implementation.* World Health Organization, Geneva.

Dermatology

Assessment of a rash

Red flag signs/symptoms in dermatology
- Skin pain.
- Mucous membrane involvement.
- Unwell child.

History

It is worth seeing adolescent patients separately from their parents for history (especially if sexual or drug history is appropriate).
- When and where did the rash start? Is it itchy, painful, or asymptomatic? Is the rash fixed or does it move about (evanescence)?
- Any mucous membrane involvement? Any exacerbating or relieving factors? Any contacts with patients with the same rash?
- Medication history (new and any ceased in the last 3mth).
- Immunization status and past medical history.
- Family history (especially of psoriasis or atopy; consanguinity).
- Any recent foreign travel?
- What treatments have been tried (how much and how long? Did they help or not? Were they creams (white) or ointments (clear)?

Examination

Undress the child (ideally with parents), leaving underwear, and inspect all the skin. Check the hair, scalp, nails, and mucous membranes. Palpate the skin. Check for tenderness and temperature, and feel (e.g. hard, firm, or soft). Ask about genital involvement. In order to generate a differential diagnosis, define rash morphology.

Step one: define the primary lesion
Is it flat or raised? Is it symmetrical? Is the size <5mm or >5mm?
- *Macule:* flat, symmetrical lesion; <5mm.
- *Patch:* flat; >5mm (may be symmetrical or asymmetric).
- *Papule:* raised, palpable, round lesion; <5mm.
- *Nodule:* raised, palpable, round lesion; >5mm.
- *Plaque:* raised; >5mm; may be asymmetric.
- *Vesicle:* fluid-filled papule.
- *Bulla:* blister containing clear fluid; >0.5cm in diameter.
- *Pustule:* pus-filled papule.
- *Purpura:* non-blanching red-purple skin discoloration due to RBC extravasation; macular or papular (palpable purpura = vasculitis).
- *Petechia:* purpuric macule; <2mm in diameter.
- *Erosion:* superficial loss of epidermis.
- *Ulcer:* loss of epidermis and/or dermis (dermis or fat at base).
- *Telangiectasia:* visible small blood vessel.
- *Wheal:* raised, itchy, white papule surrounded by red flare.

Step two: describe secondary changes
- *Scale:* thickened stratum corneum/excess keratin.
- *Crust:* dried serum, pus, blood, and other debris.
- *Lichenification:* skin thickening with prominent skin markings.
- *Excoriation:* small punctate erosions caused by picking.
- *Atrophy:* thinning (epidermal, fine wrinkles; dermal/fat, depression).
- *Induration:* subtle thickening of the skin.
- *Maceration:* occurs when skin is moist—appears white.

Step three: define the colour of the rash
- *Erythematous:* red.
- *Hypopigmented:* reduced pigment, compared with normal skin.
- *Depigmented:* absence of pigment, e.g. vitiligo.
- *Hyperpigmented:* ↑ pigment, compared with normal skin.
- *Violaceous:* violet (lichenoid, inflamed dermoepidermal junction).

Step four: describe the way the rash is arranged (configuration)
- *Agminate:* in a group or cluster.
- *Annular:* a ring shape.
- *Arcuate:* arch-like.
- *Discoid or nummular:* coin-shaped.
- *Digitate:* like fingers placed on the skin.
- *Guttate:* dew drop-sized.
- *Gyrate:* spiral-shaped.
- *Linear:* in a line.
- *Mammillated:* breast-like projections.
- *Reticular:* net-like.
- *Serpiginous:* like a snake.
- *Stellate:* star-shaped.
- *Target lesion:* a bullseye (three zones).
- *Umbilicated:* with a central dimple.
- *Verrucous:* wart-like.

Step five: define the distribution of the rash
- *Generalized:* all over.
- *Flexural:* flexural surfaces.
- *Extensor:* extensor surfaces (eg elbows, knees).
- *Intertiginous:* areas where skin is apposed (e.g. axillae, groin).
- *Palmoplantar:* palms and soles.
- *Blaschkoid:* along epidermal cell migration lines.
- *Dermatomal/zosteriform:* following dermatomes.
- *Periorificial:* affecting skin around the mouth, eyes, or perianal.
- *Periungual:* around the nails.
- *Photodistributed:* in photo-exposed sites (spares the submental area, in contrast to rashes caused by airborne exposure).

Rash morphology and diagnoses (1)

While there are some straightforward diagnoses in dermatology, more commonly, a differential diagnosis is based on rash morphology and history. If diagnosis is uncertain, then investigate, including: swabs (MC&S for virus and bacteria), tissue biopsy (histopathology, immunofluorescence, and culture), or sometimes imaging. Since biopsies (see ➲ Skin procedures on children, p. 803) are difficult in young children, early involvement of a dermatologist is prudent.

Erythematous macular eruptions (synonym: toxic erythema)

- Cellulitis, erysipelas, intertrigo.
- KD.
- Acute cutaneous lupus.
- Sunburn/phototoxic reactions.
- Capillary vascular malformations (port wine stains; see Plate 1).
- Mastocytosis.

Hyperpigmented macular eruptions

- Post-inflammatory hyperpigmentation.
- Pigmentary mosaicism.
- Café-au-lait macules: *if* >6—work-up for genodermatoses (NF commonest, but can see multiple macules in legius syndrome and NS, amongst others).
- Lentigines.
- Congenital and acquired melanocytic naevi.
- Mongolian blue spots (dermal melanocytosis).

Hyperpigmented plaques

- Acanthosis nigricans.
- Congenital melanocytic naevi.
- Dermal melanocytosis (Mongolian blue spots).
- Sebaceous naevi.
- Connective tissue naevi.
- Lichen amyloidosis.
- Morphoea.
- Scars (keloid scars).

Hypopigmented macular eruptions

- Vitiligo (absolutely depigmented).
- Post-inflammatory hypopigmentation.
- Ash leaf macules and confetti-like macules seen in TS.
- Pigmentary mosaicism.
- Lichen sclerosus et atrophicus.
- Guttate hypomelanosis.
- Pityriasis alba (slightly scaly).

Maculopapular eruptions (i.e. morbilliform eruptions, exanthematous eruptions)

- Viral exanthema (see Plate 2).
- Drug rashes (type IV hypersensitivity).
- Connective tissue disease.
- Erythema marginatum.

Papular eruptions

- Insect bite reactions.
- 'id' eruptions (auto-eczematization can be secondary to intense inflammation at a primary site: bacterid, dermatophytid, eczematid).
- Gianotti Crosti (papulovesicular acrodermatitis).
- Keratosis pilaris.
- Scabies.
- Papular eczema.
- Miliaria rubra.
- Molluscum contagiosum (umbilicated papules; see Plate 3).
- Plane warts.
- Lichen planus.
- Lymphomatoid papulosis.
- Pityriasis lichenoides et varioliformis acuta (PLEVA).
- Rosacea (including granulomatous rosacea and demodicosis).
- Atypical infection (e.g. atypical mycobacterial and fungal infections).
- Dermal infiltrates may present with papules, e.g. granuloma annulare, sarcoidosis, histiocytosis, xanthomas).
- Juvenile xanthogranulomas can present as multiple/isolated papules.

Vesicular eruptions

- Herpes simplex.
- Varicella-zoster.
- Hand, foot, and mouth disease (enteroviruses).
- Gianotti Crosti (papulovesicular acrodermatitis).
- Acute contact dermatitis.
- Phytophotodermatitis.
- Toxic epidermal necrolysis (TEN).
- Erythema multiforme (see Plate 4).
- Miliaria crystalline.
- Vesicular stage of incontentia pigmenti.
- Epidermolysis bullosa (see Plate 5).
- Dermatitis herpetiformis.
- Polymorphic light eruption, juvenile spring eruptions.
- Actinic prurigo.
- Porphyrias.
- Prurigo pigmentosa.

Rash morphology and diagnoses (2)

Bullous eruptions

- Bullous impetigo.
- Staphylococcal scalded skin: superficial bullae → break → eroded areas.
- Bullous dermatophyte.
- Chronic bullous disease of childhood.
- Burns.
- Friction blisters.
- Bullous insect bite reactions.
- Fixed drug eruptions.
- Erythema multiforme (see Plate 4).
- TEN.
- Staphylococcal scalded skin.
- Pemphigus: flaccid bullae that quickly deroof, leaving erosions.
- Bullous pemphigoid.
- Epidermolysis bullosa (see Plate 5).
- Bullous lupus.
- Mastocytosis or solitary mastocytoma.

Pustular eruptions

- Folliculitis (bacterial, pityrosporum).
- Impetigo.
- Scabies.
- Acne (comedones should always be present).
- Periorificial dermatitis (pustules without comedones).
- Rosacea.
- Acute generalized exanthematous pustulosis.
- Pustular psoriasis.
- Any vesicular eruption → secondary infection, e.g. chickenpox.
- Candidiasis.
- Miliaria pustulosa.
- Atypical infections (mycobacterial, fungal, *Nocardia*).
- Tinea incognito: dermatophyte and topical steroids → pustular.
- Hidradenitis suppurativa.

Nodular eruptions

- Nodular prurigo.
- Metastases.
- Pityriasis lichenoides acuta.
- Insect bite reactions.
- Erythema nodosum.
- Actinic prurigo.
- Lymphomatoid papulosis.
- Lymphoma.
- Pseudolymphoma.
- Histiocytosis.

Epidermal plaques (with scale)
- Atopic dermatitis (ill-defined borders).
- Psoriasis (see Plate 6).
- Seborrhoeic dermatitis.
- Tinea.
- Pityriasis rubra pilaris.
- Pityriasis versicolor.
- Pityriasis rosea.
- Pityriasis lichenoides chronica.
- Cutaneous T-cell lymphoma.
- Sarcoidosis.
- Discoid lupus.
- Lichen planus.
- Atypical infections (TB, atypical fungal infections).
- Syphilis.
- Skin cancers.

Dermal plaques (no scale)
- Urticaria (evanescent; see Plate 7).
- Erythema multiforme.
- Subacute lupus, tumid lupus.
- Sweet syndrome.
- Granuloma annulare, actinic granuloma.
- Vascular tumours, e.g. infantile haemangiomas.
- Naevi, e.g. congenital melanocytic naevi.
- Histiocytosis.
- Morphoea.
- Lichen sclerosus.
- Urticaria pigmentosa.
- Other infiltrates: atypical infections, lymphoma, other neoplasias.

Ulcerative conditions
- Ulcerated infantile haemangiomas.
- Pyoderma gangrenosum.
- Infections.
- Cutaneous Crohn's.
- Hidradenitis suppurativa.
- Aplasia cutis.
- Trauma or factitial disease.
- Severe napkin dermatitis (Jacquet's irritant dermatitis).
- Erythema induratum.

Rash morphology and diagnoses (3)

Petechiae and purpura

- Capillaritis.
- Leucocytoclastic vasculitis (including HSP and haemorrhagic oedema of infancy).
- Medium-vessel vasculitis.
- Thrombophilias.
- Thrombocytopenia.
- DIC (including purpura fulminans).
- Septic emboli.
- Warfarin necrosis.
- Leukaemia cutis.
- Trauma, including NAI and dermatitis artefacta.
- Drug reactions.
- Vasomotor straining, e.g. strenuous coughing or isometric exercise.

Photosensitive conditions

- Photosensitivity secondary to medications (e.g. tetracyclines, retinoids, thiazide diuretics, voriconazole).
- Phytophotodermatitis.
- Connective tissue disease (e.g. dermatomyositis, cutaneous lupus).
- Polymorphic light eruption.
- Juvenile spring eruption.
- Actinic prurigo.
- Porphyrias.
- Inherited defects in DNA repair (e.g. xeroderma pigmentosum).
- Photo-exacerbated dermatoses (e.g. photo-exacerbated eczema, psoriasis, etc.).

Poikiloderma (telangiectasia, hyperpigmentation, and atrophy of the skin)

- Sun damage (seen in xeroderma pigmentosum in children).
- Connective tissue disease (e.g. lupus and dermatomyositis and other photosensitive disorders).

Reticular eruptions

- Livedo reticularis: primary (symmetrical, associated with cold weather, disappears on warming; similar to cutis marmorata); secondary to vasculitis, thrombophilia, or other condition.
- Livedo racemosa (more broken rings/branch-like; similar differential to livedo reticularis; APS is a major cause).
- Erythema ab igne (heat injury).
- Livedoid vasculopathy.
- Parvovirus B19.

Periorificial and acral dermatitis

Flaky paint dermatitis with erosions around the mouth, nose, and anus. Often associated when severe with loss of hair and secondary infections):
- Zinc deficiency (acquired or inherited).
- Protein or amino acid deficiency.
- Essential fatty acid deficiency.
- Holocarboxylase or biotinase deficiency.
- Nutritional deficiency may be secondary to systemic disease (e.g. malabsorption), ↑ needs (e.g. cancer and infections).

Telangiectasia (permanently dilated small vessels)

- Fair-skinned individuals.
- Associated with photoageing (seen in adults and children with photosensitive disorders and DNA mismatch repair defects).
- Spider naevi.
- Multiple telangiectasias (>5) may be seen in:
  - Hereditary haemorrhagic telangiectasia (AD genetic disorder with telangiectasia on the lips, tongue, and nasal epithelium, risk of recurrent epistaxis ± GI haemorrhage).
  - Ataxia telangiectasia (see ◑ Box 16.5).
  - Hereditary benign telangiectasia.

Alopecia (hair loss)

- Localized areas:
  - Alopecia areata.
  - Tinea capitis.
  - Trichotillomania.
  - Trauma.
  - Congenital: aplasia cutis (often hair collar sign); naevi (sebaceous naevi or organoid naevi).
- Diffuse:
  - Nutritional: iron deficiency, zinc deficiency, protein deficiency.
  - Thyroid disease, IDDM.
  - Syphilis.
  - Connective tissue disease.
  - Diffuse variant of alopecia areata.
  - Medication-related.
  - Congenital hypotrichosis.

Rash morphology and diagnoses (4)

Blistering rash on a neonate (with vesicles or erosions)

- Infection: HSV; HZV; hand, foot, and mouth; bullous impetigo; staphylococcal scalded skin; congenital syphilis; atypical infections.
- Bullous congenital ichthyosiform erythroderma.
- Ichthyosis bullosa of Siemens.
- Epidermolysis bullosa (may be simplex, junctional, or dystrophic).
- Incontinentia pigmenti.
- Immunobullous conditions: bullous pemphigoid, pemphigus, linear IgA, epidermolysis bullosa acquisita, SLE (all transplacental).
- Aplasia cutis (presents with absence of skin).
- Congenital erosive dermatosis with reticulate and supple scarring.
- SJS (see Plate 8)/TEN.
- Bullous mastocytosis.
- Friction blisters (at site of vacuum or forceps) and sucking blisters are more localized and easily recognized.
- Nutritional deficiency: zinc, protein/amino acids, essential fatty acids, biotinase.
- Congenital porphyria.
- Some rare genodermatoses can rarely present with erosions.

Blueberry muffin baby (blue nodules and plaques in the skin often representing extramedullary haematopoiesis, purpura, or metastases)

- Blood disorders: e.g. haemolytic disease of the newborn, HS, twin–twin transfusion syndrome.
- Infections: TORCH [toxoplasmosis, other (syphilis, hepatitis B, Coxsackie virus, varicella, parvovirus B19), rubella, CMV, HSV].
- Tumours: e.g. leukaemia cutis, RMS, neuroblastoma, LCH.

Erythrodermic baby (>80% of body surface area with rash)

- Atopic dermatitis (see Plate 9).
- Inherited ichthyosis: e.g. non-bullous ichthyosiform erythroderma.
- Netherton's syndrome.
- Conradi–Hünermann syndrome.
- Infection: staphylococcal scalded skin, toxic shock, candidiasis.
- Immunodeficiency: Omenn syndrome (SCID), GVHD.
- Metabolic: essential fatty acid deficiency, biotinase deficiency.
- Holocarboxylase synthetase deficiency.
- Medications: vancomycin and ceftriaxone reported.
- Mastocytosis.
- Rarely psoriasis, pityriasis rubra pilaris, and seborrhoeic dermatitis.

Collodion baby (baby born in casing of thick skin)

- 25% self-healing ichthyosis.
- AR congenital ichthyoses (lamellar ichthyosis, congenital ichthyosiform erythroderma, Harlequin baby—a severe subtype).
- Bullous congenital ichthyosiform erythroderma.
- Gaucher disease.
- Sjögren–Larsson syndrome.
- Neutral lipid storage disease.
- Trichothiodystrophy.
- Loricrin keratoderma.
- X-linked hypohidrotic ectodermal dysplasia.

Atopic eczema

(See also ➲ Eczema, p. 530.) Atopic eczema and atopic dermatitis are terms used interchangeably.
- Prevalence of 5–15% in developed countries.
- Age of onset <6mth in 75%.
- Fundamental cause is epidermal barrier defect.

Water is lost more easily → dry skin that may itch. Irritants, allergens, and microbes penetrate the skin more easily, often causing flares. This is the reason for the atopic march (eczema → hayfever → asthma), as sensitization first occurs through the skin.

Presentation

(See Plate 9.)

Acute eczema may be erythematous and weeping. Chronic eczema may be lichenified and dry. There are often changes of excoriation, post-inflammatory hypo-/hyperpigmentation, and infection.
- *Infant:* often cheeks, elbows, and knees with crawling.
- *Childhood:* often flexural; also wrists and ankles.
- *Adolescent and adult:* also flexural, but may affect head and neck, nipples, palms, and soles.

Approach to treatment

Explain the diagnosis and provide education for the family and patient. Focus on treating flares and then on maintaining skin integrity.

General measures
- Soap avoidance, including soap-free wash and no bubble bath.
- Short showers and baths, not too hot.
- Avoidance of irritants:
  - Rinse after exposure to chlorine and salt water.
  - Don't overdress.
  - Minimize skin contact with sand grass and carpet.
  - Avoid fragranced products.
  - Minimize skin exposure to synthetic material and rough fabrics.
  - Keep fingernails short.
- Moisturize:
  - *Avoid lotions.*
  - *Creams* are good moisturizers but sting on open excoriated skin.
  - *Ointments* do not sting, but to limit coating clothes and impairing sweating, apply to wet skin and then pat the child dry.

Specific measures
- *Treat itch and inflammation* with topical corticosteroids daily until the eczema is clear (the skin feels normal); then taper off on alternate days for 1wk and stop. If eczema returns, resume once-daily application until clear and then recommence taper.
- *Treat infection* if appropriate:
  - Topical antiseptics such as bleach baths can reduce itch and bacterial load without leading to resistance or gut microbiome disruption. In severe cases, PO or topical antibiotics may be required.
  - Punched-out erosions should be swabbed for viral infection.

Additional ways to break the itch–scratch cycle
- Wet dressings (apply steroid ointment and then a wet, warm material for 5–10min).
- Occlusion (with zinc-impregnated bandages or dressings).
- Sedative antihistamines at night.
- Hospital admission.

  In some patients who do not respond to treatment, consider:
- Compliance issues.
- Diagnosis is not eczema: beware zinc and protein deficiency masquerading as eczema.
- Allergic contact dermatitis: refer for patch testing.
- Secondary infection.

Some patients will require hospital admission and treatment with immuno-suppression (locally with phototherapy or systemically). Try to avoid using PO prednisolone in eczema—patients who need this therapy should be referred to tertiary services. A major reason for treatment failure is concerns about steroid use and prescription of topical steroids that are too weak.

Steroids for atopic eczema

Address concerns about steroid use and discuss side effects and clinical endpoint (skin feels normal, not just redness gone). Explain steroids have different potencies and skin has different thickness in different areas, hence different topicals on different sites (see Table 21.1).

Mild eczema

Using a mild-potency topical corticosteroid ointment, e.g. 1% hydrocortisone, is appropriate daily for anywhere on the body.

Mild to moderate eczema

Using a moderate-potency topical corticosteroid ointment, e.g. clobetasone butyrate 0.05%, is appropriate and safe for daily use on the face and body, but *not the groin*.

Moderate to severe eczema

Using a potent topical corticosteroid ointment, e.g. mometasone furoate, is appropriate daily for the body, but *not the face or groin*. Patients should treat until the skin feels normal but be warned not to treat post-inflammatory hypo- or hyperpigmentation with topical steroids and to re-present if things are not clearing within 4wk.

Eczematous eruption

If not responding to adequate-potency topical steroids (and compliance is good), consider nutritional deficiency (zinc, amino acids, essential fatty acids, or biotin), tinea, and contact allergy.

Table 21.1 Potency ranking of topical corticosteroids

Class	Drug	Concentration
Class I: mild	Hydrocortisone	0.5–1.0%
	Hydrocortisone acetate	0.5–1.0%
Class II: moderate	Clobetasone butyrate	0.05%
	Hydrocortisone butyrate	0.1%
	Betamethasone valerate	0.02%
	Betamethasone valerate	0.05%
	Triamcinolone acetonide	0.02%
	Triamcinolone acetonide	0.05%
	Methylprednisolone aceponate	0.1%
Class III: potent	Betamethasone dipropionate	0.05%
	Betamethasone valerate	0.05–0.1%
	Mometasone furoate	0.1%
Class IV: very potent	Betamethasone dipropionate	0.05%
	Clobetasol propionate	0.05%

Complications of atopic eczema

- Sleep disturbance.
- Family dysfunction.
- Eczema herpeticum (HSV), eczema coxsackium (enterovirus), punched-out erosions, and failure to clear with usual treatment.
- *Staphylococcus aureus* infection.
- Growth delay.
- Atopic cataracts.

Prognosis

The natural history tends towards resolution with age. Predicting this is difficult; however, early-onset severe disease with associated atopy (hayfever and asthma) and elevated IgE may be associated with a worse prognosis.

Irritant and allergic contact dermatitis

Napkin dermatitis

(See also → Nappy rash, p. 178.) In children, irritant contact dermatitis due to urine, faeces, and friction in the napkin area is common. It spares the folds and favours convexities and there may be associated *Candida* infection (often signalled by micropapules or satellite lesions; see Plate 10). Frequent nappy changes, drying after bathing, and using barrier cream may prevent dermatitis. Hydrocortisone ointment, in combination with an antifungal barrier cream, is the treatment of choice. Failure to clear or respond should prompt review, as rarely another cause will be found (e.g. psoriasis, zinc deficiency, LCH). *LCH* is thought of in infants with petechiae in intertriginous areas and excoriated papules on the abdomen and scalp. A biopsy is needed.

Pruritus ani

Localized peri-anal itching.

Causes
- Contact dermatitis due to faecal soiling, sweat, and chronic diarrhoea.
- Allergic contact dermatitis, e.g. toilet paper, haemorrhoid cream.
- Threadworms.
- Anal disease (e.g. anal fissure, haemorrhoids, CD).
- Localized skin disease (e.g. candidiasis, peri-anal streptococcal dermatitis, psoriasis).

Investigations
Threadworms may be seen during anal inspection (especially in the night) or their eggs seen on microscopy of 'Sellotape' applied to the anus. Swabs of peri-anal skin for MC&S.

Treatment
- Treat underlying disease.
- Improve peri-anal hygiene.
- Mild topical steroid ointment and white soft paraffin or zinc oxide containing barrier creams may relieve symptoms once infective cause is excluded.

Pruritus vulvae

Localized perivulval itching.

Causes
- Irritant contact dermatitis due to skin contact with urine and faeces.
- Infection (e.g. candidiasis).
- Diabetes mellitus.
- Threadworm.
- Contact dermatitis.
- Localized skin disease (lichen sclerosus, psoriasis).

Management
Examine to make sure no evidence of lichen sclerosus. Rule out infection and diabetes, and treat for pin worms.
• For the commonest cause (*irritant dermatitis*), it is very important that children take time to toilet (don't rush) and visit the toilet regularly, so as to avoid incontinence. Double voiding (void and then count to 10) can help. Any damp underwear should be changed. Girls need to be taught to wipe from front to back and to adequately wipe the area to clear faeces.
• In acute inflammation, use of a topical steroid bd (e.g. 1% hydrocortisone ointment or methylprednisolone aceponate) until redness settles and then white soft paraffin-based emollient bd for 2wk to act as a soothing barrier cream as the skin heals.

Allergic contact dermatitis

Allergic contact dermatitis (delayed type IV hypersensitivity) is less common but often occurs in older children. Strong reactions often cause an acute blistering and weeping eczema.
• *Common allergens:* include nickel (earrings), colophony (sticking plasters), methylchloroisothialinozone (preservative), topical medicaments (topical neomycin and preservatives), some henna tattoos, plants (e.g. poison ivy), and rubber.
• *Diagnosis:* patch testing (patches on for 48h, then removed and marked, and final reading on days 5–7. Repeat open application testing is an alternative. The proposed cause is applied to a spot on the forearm bd for 7–14 days. If eczema occurs at the site, then an allergy to a part of the cream is likely.
• *Treatment:* allergen withdrawal and potent topical steroids.

Perioral eczema and lip lick dermatitis

Eczema around the mouth is common in winter in mouth breathers. This needs a different treatment:
• *General measures:* as usual for eczema.
• *Frequent lip balms.*
• *Topical steroid ointment:* bd to tds (1% hydrocortisone ointment or methylprednisolone aceponate) and reduction of irritant foods for 2–3wk (as the barrier reforms) to avoid irritancy exacerbating the condition.
• *Irritant foods:* include citrus and other acidic fruits, tomato-based sauces, vinegar, and salty food.

Psoriasis

(See Plate 6.) Psoriasis affects 1–2% of the population. One-third develops the disease before 20y. It is an immune-mediated disorder of T cells. There is a strong genetic component in childhood psoriasis; however, environmental factors such as infection (streptococcal and HIV), stress, smoking (pustular psoriasis), and drugs (beta blockers, calcium channel blockers, thiazides, lithium, interferon, and antimalarials) also play a role.

Presentation

- Red, well-demarcated plaques with overlying silvery scale.
- Classically affects elbows, knees, and scalp.
- However, facial (40%) and napkin (25%) psoriasis is a common presentation in children.
- The clinical appearance may be site-modified in the scalp (concretions), genital area (glazed), palms, and sole (pustules).
- Variant presentations include guttate (small plaque), annular (ring-like), pustular, and erythrodermic (>90% skin affected).
- Common nail signs include pitting, onycholysis (separation of the nail plate from the nail bed), and subungual hyperkeratosis (distal thickening).
- Psoriatic arthropathy may develop (see ➔ Juvenile psoriatic arthritis, p. 694).

Treatment

General measures
- Soap avoidance.
- Moisturize immediately after bath/shower.
- Provide emotional support (very important).
- Remove any precipitating triggers.

Specific measures
- Topical steroids.
- Topical tar and salicylic acid creams.
- Topical calcipotriol (vitamin D derivative).
- Refer patients not responding to topical therapy and general measures. Dermatologist may use phototherapy and systemic agents (acitretin, ciclosporin, methotrexate, and biologics).

Prognosis
May be life-long or spontaneously remit.

Stevens–Johnson syndrome/toxic epidermal necrolysis

Severe and overlapping condition with erythema multiforme, except usually drug-induced, with viral infection rarely implicated.
- SJS: <10% BSA involved.
- SJS/TEN overlap: 10–30% BSA involvement is overlap syndrome.
- TEN: >30% BSA involved.

Presentation

(See Plate 8.)
- Widespread blisters/bullae over erythematous, purple macular or haemorrhagic skin. Rubbing causes skin separation at epidermo-dermal junction (= +ve Nikolsky sign).
- *Skin pain.*
- Mucous membranes often affected with haemorrhagic crusting.
- Possible fever, arthralgia, myalgia, prostration, renal failure, pneumonitis, conjunctivitis, genital and oesophageal ulceration.

Management

Supportive, as for severe burns (e.g. hydration, airway protection). So manage in burns unit in severe cases. These cases often need long-term IV access as soon as possible. Identify the causative antigen and remove/treat. In addition:
- *Fluids:* monitoring with in-dwelling catheter.
- *Biochemistry:* monitor and treat serum K^+, Mg^{2+}, and PO_4^-.
- *Skin:* non-adhesive dressings, frequent emollients; frequent eye, oral, and genital cleansing with saline/lubricating eye drops; do not debride the skin.
- *Ophthalmology:* review and input.
- *Pain:* adequate analgesia.
- *Infection:* monitor for secondary infection.
- *Nutrition:* high-protein diet, often with NG feeding.
- *Other:* consider these treatments if condition progressing (but evidence is based on small uncontrolled studies), e.g. IVIG, systemic corticosteroids, ciclosporin, TNF blockers, G-CSF.

Prognosis

Can be life-threatening. Recovery usually occurs in 3–4wk. Commonest long-term sequela is dry eyes. If severe, eye involvement can have scarring and blindness. Genital fusion can occur. Post-inflammatory hypo- and hyperpigmentation can be severe and take months to years to settle in darker skin types.

Chronic urticaria

(See ➲ Acute urticaria, p. 536.) Urticaria (hives) is caused by mast cell degranulation of histamine and vasoactive mediators that cause localized vasodilatation and ↑ capillary permeability. It is characterized by wheal or urticarial plaque.

- Acute urticaria: lasts <6wk.
- Acute intermittent urticaria: recurrent episodes lasting <6wk.
- Chronic urticaria: daily symptoms >3mth that usually regress after 2–3y. Chronic spontaneous urticaria has a good prognosis with 95% of children symptom-free in 7y.

Causes

Up to 50% of cases of chronic urticaria are idiopathic. Other causes include:
- Chronic infections, e.g. parasites, *Candida*.
- Foods.
- Physical urticaria: e.g. dermographism, delayed pressure, cholinergic, cold, etc.
- Autoantibody-stimulating mast cells.

Presentation

(See Plate 7.)

Rapidly developing erythematous eruption with central white wheals. May have angio-oedema. May have annular and arcuate-shaped plaques. Any part of the body can be affected and often itchy. Lesions last 4–24h and may have associated fever and arthralgia (serum sickness).

Investigations

Apart from a good history, investigation is usually not necessary. SPT is rarely helpful, but consider a food and symptom diary, stool studies (threadworms, oocytes and parasites), and the list in Table 21.2.

Table 21.2 Chronic urticaria investigations

Baseline investigations	Additional investigations
FBC	Infection screen
TFTs	Autoimmune screen (ANA)
LFTs	Skin biopsy
Inflammatory markers	SPT/sIgE if identifiable allergen
Coeliac screen	

Treatment

Avoid medications that cause mast cell degranulation (NSAIDs, codeine/opioids, muscle relaxants, contrast, and some food dyes). With dermatologist use:
- First-line treatment is high-dose second-generation antihistamine, e.g. cetirizine up to 40mg/day.
- Leukotriene receptor antagonist can be used as additional therapy.
- Severe cases add short-course PO prednisolone 0.5mg/kg/day, weaning over 3wk.
- Anti-IgE therapy (omalizumab) is also effective in severe cases.

Angio-oedema

Variant of urticaria with significant swelling of subcutaneous tissues—often involves lips, eyelids, genitalia, tongue, or larynx. If severe, may cause acute upper or lower respiratory tract obstruction and may be life-threatening.

Causes

As for urticaria. Hereditary angio-oedema is a rare AD condition caused by active C1-esterase inhibitor deficiency (see ➲ Hereditary angio-oedema, p. 537).

Investigations and management

As for urticaria (see ➲ Chronic urticaria, p. 790). If hereditary angio-oedema is suspected, then measure serum C4 complement level initially.

Treatment for severe angio-oedema

(See ➲ Anaphylaxis, pp. 524–5; ➲ Anaphylaxis, p. 52; ➲ Hereditary angio-oedema, p. 537.)
- Give facial O_2.
- IM 0.1mL/kg adrenaline 1:10 000.
- IM/IV hydrocortisone 12-hourly.
- Nebulized salbutamol.

Prophylaxis

In severe and recurring cases of hereditary angio-oedema, tranexamic acid or anabolic steroids (e.g. danazol boosts liver production of C1-esterase inhibitor) are effective, but the latter is rarely used in childhood due to its androgenic effects.

Exanthematous eruptions

(See also ➔ Infections characterized by rash, p. 625.) These blanching, symmetrical maculopapular eruptions (also called morbilliform) are commonly triggered by infections and drugs. In non-immunized children, consider infections that rarely present in the immunized population (measles, mumps, rubella, and hepatitis), and returned travellers have an additional set of potential causes.

Most children with viral eruptions are quite well. Reduced feeding, reduced wet nappies, and ↓ LOC are *red flags*. Also differentiate the following from exanthems, since treatment differs:

- Severe bacterial infections.
- Gianotti Crosti syndrome (lasts 6–12wk).
- Pityriasis rosea (lasts 6–12wk).
- Erythema multiforme.
- SJS.

Erythema multiforme

Cause

Immunologically mediated syndrome. Usually precipitated by infection (e.g. *Mycoplasma*, HSV, other viruses) or, more rarely, drugs (e.g. sulfonamides, penicillin).

Presentation

(See Plate 4.) Crops of characteristic symmetrical, fixed urticarial plaques develop with a pallid/purple centre surrounded by an erythematous ring. Target lesions (three zones) are pathognomonic. Lesions also:

- Are haemorrhagic, red macules, or large bullae.
- Present for 2–3wk.
- Are distributed favouring the extremities—hands, feet, elbows, knees, ears, and face, but can be widespread.
- Tender, burning sensation (not itchy).
- Typically, mucous membrane ulcers (buccal, eye, genitalia).

Treatment

If precipitating infection recurs, treat early as tends to cause rash again, e.g. PO aciclovir for recurrent HSV. Otherwise:

- Fluid maintenance.
- Analgesic mouthwashes.
- Lip emollient ointment.
- PO antihistamines.
- PO corticosteroids: use in severe cases (e.g. prednisolone equivalent 0.5mg/kg, weaning over a 3wk period).

Prognosis

Complete recovery, but may recur. Post-inflammatory pigment change is common but resolves with time.

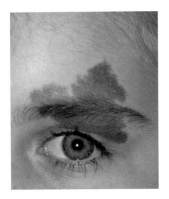

Plate 1 Capillary vascular malformation (port wine stain).

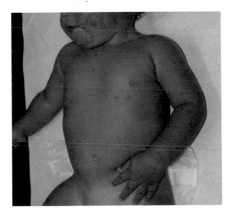

Plate 2 Viral exanthema.

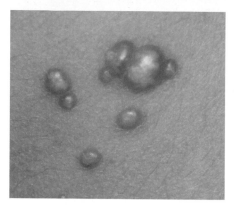

Plate 3 Molluscum contagiosum.

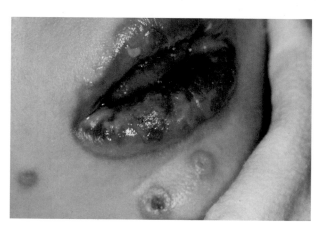

Plate 4 Erythema multiforme.

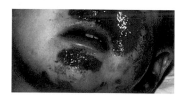

Plate 5 Epidermolysis bullosa.

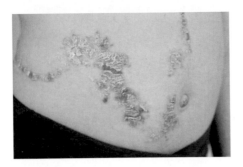

Plate 6 Psoriasis.

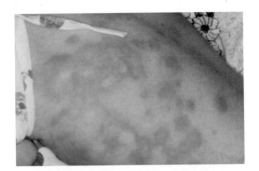

Plate 7 Urticaria.

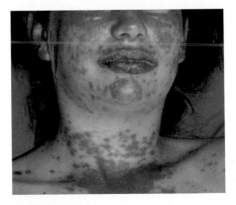

Plate 8 Stevens–Johnson syndrome.

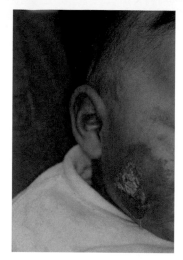

Plate 9 Atopic dermatitis.

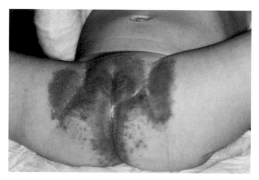

Plate 10 Irritant napkin dermatitis with candidiasis.

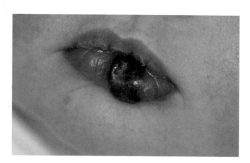

Plate 11 Superficial haemangioma.

Viral skin infections

Warts

Very common. Caused by infection with HPV. Affect any age, but mainly school-aged children. Warts exist as painless, firm papules with a rough hyperkeratotic surface. Capillary ends can usually be seen superficially. Typically affect hands, knees, face, and feet. Usually resolve spontaneously within 3y.

- *Plantar warts* (verrucae): may be painful due to pressure-induced ingrowing.
- *Genital or peri-anal warts* (condyloma acuminata): may occur in sexual abuse, which should be considered in the differential.

Treatment

Not usually needed. All treatments try to encourage immune recognition of the virus, so none are 100% effective. If painful or embarrassing, consider:
- Destructive techniques:
  - Keratolytic agent (e.g. salicylic acid, lactic acid).
  - Liquid nitrogen cryotherapy.
  - Cover (duct tape, etc.).
  - Podophyllotoxin.
  - Rarely intralesional bleomycin.
  - Surgical removal.
- Immune-based techniques: HPV vaccination, immunotherapy.

Molluscum contagiosum

Common pox virus infection affecting infants and young children (see Plate 3).

Presentation

Pink, umbilicated (central dimple) papules. Usually affects moist areas but can occur anywhere. Exacerbated by active eczema and picking.

Treatment

None if uncomplicated, as usually spontaneously resolves within a year. If problematic, consider:
- Treating any associated eczema (topical steroids).
- Covering to prevent spread and auto-inoculation.
- Pinch forceps liquid nitrogen cryotherapy (with local analgesic cream).
- Lesion curettage (after application of numbing cream).
- Cantharidin.
- Application of mild irritant daily, e.g. benzoyl peroxide 5%, salicylic acid 10–20%.

Fungal skin infections

Diagnostic fungal studies

To do a fungal scraping, make sure no cream has been applied to the area for 72h to maximize yield. A glass slide is scraped across the skin surface and then any scale tapped into a sterile container, and the slide sent to the laboratory (even if you cannot see much macroscopically) will often yield results. The microscopy takes a week to come back, and culture often takes 2–6wk.

Dermatophyte infection

Tinea corporis (ringworm)

Appearance of annular, scaly lesion with central clearing and sharp edge on trunk, face, or limbs.
- *Investigation:* skin scrapings for microscopy and culture.
- *Treatment:* topical antifungals, e.g. imidazole or terbinafine cream.

Tinea capitus (scalp ringworm)

Appearance of red, scaling scalp lesions with hair loss and short hair stumps. May present as tender, erythematous patch with pustules (kerion).
- *Investigation:* skin scrapings and hair pull for microscopy/culture.
- *Treatment:* topical antifungal shampoo for 1wk; PO griseofulvin 20mg/kg/day for 6–8wk (plus PO steroids if kerion). Terbinafine or itraconazole, depending on dermatophyte species cultured.

Tinea pedis (athlete's foot)

Appearance of itchy, irritable skin between the toes ± sole of foot.
- *Treatment:* careful drying between toes, topical antifungal (e.g. terbinafine cream). Dispose of shoes worn without socks or try antifungal powder to decontaminate.

Tinea unguium (onychomycosis)

Appearance of nail infection causes discoloured, friable, and deformed nails.
- *Investigation:* microscopy and culture of nail clippings.
- *Treatment:* PO antifungal for 3mth (e.g. terbinafine).

Candida albicans infection

Predisposing factors
- Moist body folds.
- Nappies.
- Treatment with broad-spectrum antibiotics.
- Immunosuppression.
- Diabetes mellitus.

Variants include the following:
- *Cutaneous candidiasis* (e.g. napkin rash; see Plate 10). Macular erythema, slight scaling, small outlying 'satellite' lesions in body folds.
- *Chronic paronychia.*
- *Chronic mucocutaneous candidiasis* (a congenital immunodeficiency disorder).

Investigations
Skin scrapings or swabs for microscopy and culture.

Treatment
Topical ± anti-candidal drugs, e.g. nystatin, fluconazole, clotrimazole.

Pityriasis versicolor (tinea versicolor)

Malassezia infection in post-pubertal children. Asymptomatic or itchy, scaly plaques that may be hypo-/hyperpigmented on trunk/upper limbs. After acute infection, post-inflammatory hypopigmentation may persist for months. This takes time to settle and does not need to be treated with antifungal agents.

- *Treatment*: topical imidazole foaming lotion for three consecutive nights. An antifungal shampoo (2% econazole, selenium sulfide, or zinc pyrithione) may be used intermittently as a wash to prevent recurrence.

Bacterial skin infections

Impetigo

Highly contagious *S. aureus* or β-haemolytic streptococcal superficial skin infection. May complicate other skin disease (e.g. HSV infection, eczema, scabies). Risk factors include overcrowding and poor hygiene.

Presentation

Superficial, rapidly spreading, initially clear blisters that rapidly develop into straw-coloured, 'dirty'-looking lesions with yellow crusting. Often starts around the nose and face; neonates may develop bullous impetigo. Risk of staphylococcal scalded skin syndrome or acute GN (streptococcal).

Investigations

Skin swabs for bacterial culture and sensitivity. Swabs from distant blisters will not grow bacteria. Need to swab primary site of impetigo (e.g. around nose, eyes, etc.).

Management

Rapidly resolves if:

- *Bathe crusts* off using antiseptics (contain infectious bacteria).
- *Antibiotics* (e.g. topical mupirocin 2% ointment or PO cefalexin or flucloxacillin).
- Treat any *predisposing condition*.
- Treat any *other affected family* members.
- In recurrent cases: nasal swabs and decolonization of patient and family with intranasal mupirocin bd for a week; hot washing of all clothes, sheets, and towels; antiseptic washes.

Staphylococcal scalded skin syndrome

(See also ➔ Scalded skin syndrome , p. 628.) Exotoxin-mediated epiderm-olysis to *S. aureus* infection (which may be trivial). Occurs in children <5y.

Presentation

Extensive tender erythema with flaccid superficial blisters/bullae ('scalded appearance'). Erosions and +ve Nikolsky sign. Crusting around the eyes and mouth; fever.

Treatment

Supportive treatment and analgesia. Anti-staphylococcal antibiotics (PO or IV). Gentle skin care, emollient ointments.

Prognosis

Rapid recovery without scarring.

Parasitic skin infections

Scabies

Caused by *Sarcoptes scabiei* mite. Common at all ages.

Diagnosis

Diagnosis is not easy, so look closely for clues. Classically, it causes an itchy papular rash, with visible burrows affecting the finger and toe webs, palms, soles, wrists, groin, axillary folds, and buttocks (truncal in infants). Excoriation, eczematization, urticaria, or impetigo may develop. Papules on shaft of penis are highly suspicious. Diagnosis is confirmed by microscopy of mite removed from burrow (rarely needed).

Treatment

Treat whole household and close contacts simultaneously with 12h topical application below the head (in children <2y old all body, except face) with permethrin cream (5%) or 24h of malathion liquid (0.5%) washed off and then repeated the next day. Simultaneously, launder bed linen and under-wear in a hot wash. Antihistamines or calamine lotion for itch, which may last for 10 days.

Apply weak topical corticosteroid if scabies nodules are present.

Lice

Infestation with *Pediculus capitis* (scalp 'nits'), *Pediculus corporis* (body), or *Phthirus pubis* (pubic area 'crabs').

Pediculosis capitis

Common in all ages. Localized pruritus, secondary impetigo, or regional lymphadenopathy. Lice are difficult to see, but small white eggs (nits) are easily seen attached to hair shafts. Treatment includes:
- Daily thorough combing with fine-toothed comb, combined with single shampoo with lotions of malathion (0.5%), permethrin (1%), and ivermectin (0.5%). Resistance to permethrin has been reported in some areas. Combing with conditioner can be helpful but needs to be repeated daily for 1–2wk.
- Shaving the head can be effective, but extreme.
- PO co-trimoxazole and ivermectin for recalcitrant cases.

Other insects

Many biting insects (e.g. fleas, midges, bedbugs, mosquitoes) may cause erythematous macular lesions with a central punctum or papular urticaria. Treatment includes:
- Avoiding bites, e.g. treat infested pets, long clothes, and repellant.
- PO antihistamines.
- Topical steroids under occlusion for bites.
- Antibiotics if there is secondary bacterial infection.

Acne vulgaris

Acne affects 90–100% of teenagers. However, acne may occur in:
- Neonates: spontaneous improvement without treatment.
- Infant: often requires treatment and may imply severe acne in later years.
- Adults: often women older >25y.

Cause

Hormones (GH, sex and stress hormones, as well as insulin) result in excess *sebum production* → *comedone formation* (open comedones are known as blackheads, closed comedones as whiteheads) → bacterial proliferation → inflammation and *inflammatory acne* (papules, pimples, cysts). There may be post-inflammatory erythema and *scarring* in the resolution phase. Hyperandrogenism should be suspected if acne is severe, sudden, and of early onset and if there are other signs of hyperandrogenism, including irregular periods, hirsuitism, ♂ or ♀ pattern hair loss, and deepening of the voice in women.

Treatment

General measures
- Twice-daily facial cleansing.
- Use oil-free and non-comedogenic make-up and sunscreens.
- Eat a low-glycaemic index, low-dairy diet.
- Regular exercise (with face washing within 30min of exercise).

Specific measures
- To target the comedones:
  - *Topical retinoids* for comedonal acne (e.g. adapalene, tretinoin). These often need to be weaned on and patients with sensitive skin may better tolerate a cream, rather than a gel base.
  - *Oral contraceptive pill* containing an anti-androgen progestogen (e.g. drospirenone or cyproterone acetate) for girls who have had 12–18mth of regular periods. Care to discuss potential side effects and review contraindications (family history of venous thromboembolism, breast cancer, personal history of migraines), and discuss contraceptive activity of the oral contraceptive pill.
  - *PO isotretinoin* if severe scarring or failure or intolerance of other options. This should be prescribed by a specialist. Careful counselling regarding teratogenicity needed. Main side effects are photosensitivity, dry skin and mucous membranes, and reduced wound healing. Rarely headaches and liver dysfunction. Avoid in familial hypertriglyceridaemia. Important to discuss controversial link to depression.
- To target the inflammatory acne:
  - Topical antiseptics, e.g. benzoyl peroxide 2.5–5%.
  - Topical antibiotics, e.g. clindamycin, dapsone.
  - PO antibiotics, e.g. erythromycin, tetracyclines, co-trimoxazole.
- If scarring is present: PO isotretinoin is first-line agent.

Prognosis

Resolves but may persist for years in some cases. Psychological support is important. Post-inflammatory erythema may persist for 6–12mth, even once acne is controlled. Scarring can be treated, but acne needs to be quiescent. Various lasers (mainly ablative fractionated lasers) are effective for acne scarring.

Periorificial dermatitis

This is a misnomer, as it is an *acneiform condition* caused by overgrowth of skin commensals (why swabs are not useful). Topical steroids suppress the disease but do not cure it. The condition is slightly itchy and consists of tiny pustules that can coalesce into plaques.

Treatment

General measures

Avoid occlusive moisturizers, sunscreens, and topical steroids. Cleanse the face twice daily with a gentle cleanser. Clean the nasofacial groove and alar crease carefully. Some mild cases will resolve with these measures alone.

Specific measures

Topical antibiotics and antiseptics can be helpful but often sting, making the condition worse. Patients must be warned that the condition will get worse before it gets better if topical steroids have been used. PO antibiotics are used for longer than for other infections (4–12wk) and include:
- *Children <10y:* PO erythromycin or roxithromycin.
- *Older children:* PO doxycycline or minocycline.

Vascular malformations and tumours

Vascular malformations

Consider referral for all cosmetically sensitive capillary vascular malformations (as soon as possible), as intervention with the pulse dye laser works best in the first 2y of life. Segmental and multiple port wine stains should also be referred, as these may form part of a syndrome (e.g. Sturge–Weber syndrome, capillary malformation macrocephaly syndrome, etc.). There are new and evolving treatments for lymphatic and venous malformations available at specialist centres (e.g. sclerotherapy, surgery, and topical and PO rapamycin therapy). Conditions include:

- *Capillary malformations:*
  - Port wine stains (see Plate 1): may be solitary or associated with various syndromes.
  - Salmon patches: naevus simplex.
  - Telangiectasia.
  - Cutis marmorata telangiectatica congenita.
- *Lymphatic malformations (LMs):*
  - Common: microcystic, macrocystic, mixed.
  - Generalized lymphatic anomaly.
  - LM in Gorham–Stout disease.
  - Channel-type LM.
  - Primary lymphoedema.
- *Venous malformations (VMs):*
  - Common.
  - Familial.
  - Blue rubber bleb naevus syndrome.
  - Glomuvenous malformation.
  - Cerebral cavernous malformation.
- AVM.
- Arteriovenous fistulae.
- *Combined malformations* and syndromes with vascular malformations and other anomalies also exist (e.g. Klippel–Trenaunay syndrome).

Vascular tumours

- Infantile haemangiomas: commonest, *Glut-1* +ve.
- Congenital haemangiomas: rapidly involuting, partially involuting, and non-involuting.
- Tufted angiomas.
- Kaposiform haemangioendothelioma.
- Pyogenic granulomas.
- Angiosarcoma.
- Some malignant tumours may have a vascular appearance.

Infantile haemangiomas (capillary, 'strawberry' haemangiomas)

(See Plate 11.)

These conditions occur in 10% of infants. They often present in the first few weeks of life and are commoner in ♀, first-born children, premature infants, and Caucasian children. They may be superficial (red colour), deep (blue colour), or mixed. They often undergo a rapid proliferative phase that persists until 3–18mth of age and then the haemangioma slowly involutes over several years (most completely involuted by 7y old). Some small telangiectatic vessels and fibrofatty residual may occur.

Complications

Include ulceration, bleeding, infection, and compromise of vision.

Referral

Haemangiomas that should be referred for PO or topical β-blocker and/or pulse dye laser:
- Ulcerated.
- Cosmetically sensitive.
- Blocking vision, mouth, nose, neck/beard area, and genital area.
- >5 (need USS of head and liver, possibly TFTs).
- Overlying spine in midline (spinal dysraphism).
- Segmental over face and perineum.
- PHACES (posterior fossa abnormalities, haemangioma, arterial anomalies, cardiac anomalies, eye abnormalities, sternal cleft or supra-umbilical raphe) syndrome.
- PELVIS (perineal haemangioma, external genital anomalies, lipomyelomeningocele, vesicorenal abnormalities, imperforate anus, and skin tags) syndrome.

Infantile haemangiomas have no risk of Kasabach–Merritt syndrome (comprises thrombocytopenia and consumptive coagulopathy; only occurs in tufted angiomas and kaposiform haemangioendotheliomas).

Treatment

Reassurance and monitoring in most cases are all that is required. However, those in critical or cosmetically sensitive sites may now be treated with PO propranolol by a dermatologist.
- *Referral is urgent*, as propranolol works to stop the proliferative phase.
- Pulse dye laser is a useful treatment for ulceration and residual telangiectasia after involution.
- Surgical correction may be required to remove fibrofatty residual after involution of large haemangiomas.

Congenital naevi (birthmarks)

A *naevus* refers to a benign collection of cells. A melanocytic naevus is a benign collection of melanocytes. Congenital melanocytic naevi behave slightly differently to acquired naevi in childhood. They are divided into small (<1cm), medium (1–20cm), and giant (>20cm):

* There is an ↑ risk of melanoma in children with giant congenital melanocytic naevi in the first 10y and they should be monitored by a dermatologist.
* If children have >2 congenital melanocytic naevi, they should be reviewed by a dermatologist as they have an ↑ risk of neurocutaneous melanocytosis.

Other birthmarks (e.g. sebaceous naevi and connective tissue naevi) may be associated with certain genodermatoses or underlying syndromes, so if in doubt, referral to dermatology is suggested.

Skin procedures on children

- *Don't perform painful procedures* on children. If unavoidable, do procedures early in the day and:
  - Use topical LA (e.g. EMLA) before cannulation, skin biopsy, and blood tests.
  - Apply LA creams 60–120min before, and use occlusion (with plastic wrap or specialized dressings).
- *Cover children's eyes*, so they do not see what you are doing works (special goggles).
- *Prepare the room in advance.*
- *Have adequate staff.*
- *Ensure parents' consent* before the procedure (anticipation makes the child more anxious).
- *Punch biopsies* are quick and keep the tissue intact.

Further reading

Use of steroids

Australasian College of Dermatologists. (2015). *Adverse effects of topical corticosteroids in paediatric eczema: Australasian consensus statement*. Available at: ℘ http://www.sedermstafford.com.au/wp-content/uploads/2017/12/Steroidsconsensus.pdf.

Australasian College of Dermatologists. (2017). *The Australasian College of Dermatologists Consensus Statement: topical corticosteroids in paediatric eczema*. Available at: ℘ https://www.dermcoll.edu.au/wp-content/uploads/ACD-Consensus-Statement-Topical-Corticosteroids-and-Eczema-Feb-2017.pdf.

Classification of vascular anomalies

International Society for the Study of Vascular Anomalies. (2018). *International Society for the Study of Vascular Anomalies classification of vascular anomalies*. Available at: ℘ https://www.issva.org/UserFiles/file/ISSVA-Classification-2018.pdf.

Paediatric surgery

Symptoms and signs that should cause concern

Neonates and infants

As a paediatrician, it is important to recognize important symptoms and signs that indicate a surgical emergency.

Neonatal intestinal obstruction

- Bile-stained vomiting: the cardinal sign of an intestinal obstruction.
- Emergency assessment: check vital signs; commence fluid resuscitation, and pass an NGT.
- X-ray: all children with bile-stained vomiting should have AXR.

Radiology

- Dilated bowel loops on the AXR suggest intestinal obstruction.
- Look for free air to indicate a perforation. In the supine film, this will outline the falciform ligament (umbilical vein).
- Be aware of the radiological appearance of a midgut volvulus (see → Midgut volvulus, p. 820): prompt diagnosis is essential for bowel salvage.

Clinical assessment

- Anus: make sure the baby has an anal opening.
- Meconium: most babies pass meconium within 48h of birth. Delayed passage of meconium in a baby with abdominal distension could mean Hirschsprung's disease (HSD) (see → Hirschsprung's disease, p. 832).
- Rectal examination: do not perform a rectal examination, insert a suppository, or perform a rectal washout without seeking advice first, because some surgeons use lower GI contrast studies for diagnosis and this may obscure the signs of HSD.

Oesophageal atresia (OA)

- The combination of polyhydramnios and a mucousy baby is suspicious of OA (see → Oesophageal atresia and tracheo-oesophageal fistula, pp. 810–11).
- Pass an NGT before attempting feeds.
- Babies with OA and distal TOF who are ventilated are a surgical emergency because of risk of gastric distension and gastric perforation.

Congenital diaphragmatic hernia

Most CDHs are now diagnosed antenatally. Delivery should be in a neonatal surgical centre. At delivery, secure IV access so that the baby can be sedated, paralysed, and then intubated (see also → Congenital diaphragmatic hernia, p. 814).

- Avoid bag–mask ventilation because this distends the stomach.
- If the diagnosis is not made prenatally, suspect CDH in a baby with respiratory distress and apparent dextrocardia.

Intussusception in infants
Suspect intussusception in any infant who is inconsolable, vomits bile, or has blood in the stool (see also ➋ Intussusception, p. 822).

Assessment
- Resuscitation: these patients often require large volumes of fluid to restore the circulation. NGT and broad-spectrum antibiotics.
- Confirm diagnosis by USS.
- Do not consider radiological reduction unless you have a surgeon and an anaesthetist who are able to operate on the child in the event of perforation or failure.

Incarcerated inguinal hernia
An irreducible hard swelling in the groin in a baby who is vomiting is probably an incarcerated inguinal hernia (see also ➋ Incarcerated hernia, p. 830).
- Resuscitate the baby.
- *Give analgesia (may require opiates).*
- Transfer to a paediatric surgeon; do not wait overnight.

Older children
Acute appendicitis
Be wary of children with abdominal pain who are taking antibiotics for a presumed sore throat or UTI. The diagnosis may be appendicitis, but the history and abdominal signs may be atypical (see also ➋ Acute appendicitis, p. 826).
- Observe: admit the child for observation.
- USS: request if there is clinical doubt, history of >5 days suggesting appendix mass/abscess, or possibility of ovarian pathology.

Acute scrotal pain
Any boy with acute scrotal pain has a testicular torsion until proven otherwise (see also ➋ Testicular torsion, p. 838).
- Refer all these children urgently to a urologist/surgeon.
- The medicolegal consequences (and the patient's, of course) of missing a torsion are substantial.

Congenital abnormalities: upper airway

Choanal atresia (CA)

Congenital obstruction of the posterior choana of the nose—may be unilateral or bilateral. Babies are obligate nose breathers and bilateral obstruction presents with asphyxia during feeding and sleep. Unilateral obstruction may pass unnoticed. CA may be a presenting feature of the CHARGE association, which is:

- *Coloboma*.
- *Heart* defects.
- *Atresia* of the choanae.
- *Retardation* of growth and development.
- *Genitourinary* abnormalities.
- *Ear* abnormalities and hearing loss.

Diagnosis
- NGT: diagnosis excluded if passage of an NGT via each nostril.
- CT scan: to determine whether obstruction is membranous or bony.

Treatment
- Emergency treatment: comprises an oropharyngeal airway and an orogastric tube for feeding.
- Surgery: performed transnasally, restores patency of the choanae.

Cleft lip and palate

(See also ➔ Orofacial cleft, p. 173.) ~1 baby per 1000 is born with a cleft lip and palate. This may occur sporadically or there may be a family history. A cleft lip is immediately apparent. An isolated cleft palate may not be noticed immediately but will present with feeding difficulties, particularly nasal regurgitation of milk. A cleft palate will interfere with breastfeeding as it precludes the generation of suction. Bottle-feeding may also be difficult unless a squeezable bottle, rather than a rigid bottle, is used.

Management
- Lip repair: at around 3mth of age.
- Palate repair: at around 6mth of age.
- Follow-up: long-term because of problems with speech, dentistry, and hearing.

Pierre–Robin sequence

The Pierre–Robin sequence (see Fig. 22.1) is characterized by three features:
- Micrognathia.
- Glossoptosis.
- Cleft palate.

Management
- The large tongue has a tendency to obstruct the airway, causing apnoea, particularly during sleep.
- Prone positioning may help, allowing the tongue to fall forward, but occasionally tracheostomy is necessary.
- ETT intubation is often difficult.
- Tube feeding may be necessary.
- The palate is generally repaired between 9 and 18mth of age.
- The airway problems invariably improve with growth.

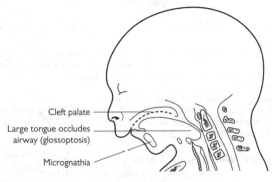

Cleft palate

Large tongue occludes airway (glossoptosis)

Micrognathia

Fig. 22.1 Pierre–Robin sequence.

Congenital abnormalities: tracheo-oesophageal

Oesophageal atresia and tracheo-oesophageal fistula

(See also ➜ Oesophageal atresia, p. 806.) The incidence of OA and TOF (see Fig. 22.2) is 1/3500 live births. There are five anatomical subtypes (see Table 22.1).

Table 22.1 Gross classification of OA types

Type	Description	Frequency (%)
A	OA alone	6
B	OA with proximal TOF	5
C	OA with distal TOF	84
D	OA with proximal and distal TOF	1
E	H-type fistula	4

Antenatally, polyhydramnios is common, with other signs including small or absent gastric bubble. However, antenatal USS has only 42% sensitivity and most cases are still diagnosed postnatally. Babies present at birth with:
- Excessive salivation.
- Choking and cyanosis on attempted feeds.
- 50% associated malformations, usually VACTERL (vertebral anomalies, anal atresia, cardiac malformations, tracheo-oesophageal fistula, renal and limb anomalies) (see Box 22.1).

> **Box 22.1 VACTERL association**
> - Vertebral anomalies (fused vertebrae, hemivertebrae).
> - Anorectal anomalies (imperforate anus).
> - Cardiac anomalies (all types).
> - TOF.
> - Renal abnormalities (all types).
> - Limb abnormalities (radial ray anomalies, e.g. hypoplastic thumbs).

Diagnosis
- Inability to pass NGT >10cm from the mouth.
- CXR: NGT stops in the upper thorax. Air in the stomach indicates a fistula between the trachea and distal oesophagus (TOF).

Acute management
- *Minimize risk of aspiration pneumonia:* aspirate upper oesophageal pouch with low pressure (preferably via a Replogle tube).
- Standard IV fluids started.
- Preoperative antibiotics.
- Babies who require mechanical ventilation must be referred for urgent surgery because gas will produce progressive gastric distension → impaired ventilation → gastric perforation.

Surgery
- Disconnection of the TOF and anastomosis of upper and lower oesophagus through a right thoracotomy or thoracoscopically.
- Long-gap OA may require a feeding gastrostomy in the neonatal period, followed by oesophageal replacement during infancy.
- High-risk babies may have a staged procedure—the TOF is ligated and then the OA repaired a few days later.
- Complications include anastomotic leak, anastomotic stricture, GOR, and recurrent fistula.

Follow-up
- Respiratory morbidity in the early years after OA/TOF repair is relatively high, particularly in winter. Consider admitting these children during respiratory infections.
- Tracheomalacia can be life-threatening and warrant aortopexy.
- Obstruction of the oesophagus by food bolus is common. Refer for urgent endoscopic removal.

Isolated tracheo-oesophageal fistula (H type)

TOF is usually associated with OA. However, isolated TOF present with:
- Choking or coughing during feeding; or recurrent pneumonia.
- Abdominal distension.

Tube oesophagram (contrast) and bronchoscopy are the investigation of choice. Treatment is surgical ligation of the TOF via neck incision.

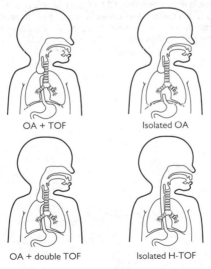

OA + TOF   Isolated OA

OA + double TOF   Isolated H-TOF

Fig. 22.2 Types of OA/TOF.

Congenital abnormalities: lung

Congenital pulmonary airway malformation (CPAM)

CPAM is a congenital multicystic lung mass due to proliferation of terminal bronchioles at the expense of alveolar tissues. The majority of CPAMs are now diagnosed prenatally by USS, and high-risk cases will be associated with hydrops. Symptomatic CPAMs should be resected:

- Large CPAMs present at birth with respiratory distress that is managed along conventional lines.
- Small CPAMs will be asymptomatic at birth but may present in early childhood with pulmonary sepsis.

Sequestration

Bronchopulmonary sequestrations are cystic masses of non-functioning lung parenchyma that lack connection to the tracheo-bronchial tree, with an anomalous blood supply from the aorta. The majority are detected antenatally. Management, though debatable in asymptomatic cases, is resection.

- Large sequestrations will present at birth with respiratory distress or heart failure from high flow through the feeding vessel.
- Sequestrations may present in infancy or childhood with pulmonary sepsis.

Congenital lobar emphysema (CLE)

CLE is an unusual lung bud anomaly characterized by massive air trapping in the emphysematous lobe. This compresses the surrounding normal lung and may result in mediastinal shift. CLE presenting with progressive respiratory distress within the first few weeks or months of life nearly always requires lobectomy. In the acute phase, +ve pressure ventilation may produce rapid worsening of emphysema.

Congenital abnormalities: chest

Congenital diaphragmatic hernia

(See ➲ Congenital diaphragmatic hernia, p. 806; ➲ Fig. 4.6.) The incidence of CDH is 1/3000 live births. The main problem is not the diaphragmatic hernia, but rather the associated pulmonary hypoplasia and pulmonary hypertension that are often severe and determine prognosis. The commonest type of diaphragmatic defect is posterolateral (Bochdalek) and left-sided, occurring in 90% (see Figs. 22.3 and 22.4).

- *Antenatal screening:* most CDHs are identified on antenatal USS, but prognosis for these fetuses is poor (i.e. 20% survive).
- *Birth:* if the diagnosis is not made antenatally and the baby presents at birth, clinical findings may include respiratory distress, scaphoid abdomen, and apparent dextrocardia. Prognosis for survival is 60%—worst with associated anomalies.
- *Coincidental:* 10% are discovered during early childhood, including most anterior (Morgagni) defects. Prognosis is excellent.

Neonatal management

An emergency:

- Initial management consists of sedation, paralysis, ETT intubation, and MV with FiO_2 1.0.
- NGT placement and avoid bag–mask–valve ventilation.
- If oxygenation is good and pulmonary hypoplasia is not severe, repair of the diaphragmatic defect is undertaken after a few days either by primary suture or insertion of a prosthetic patch.

Hiatus hernia (HIH)

HIH refers to herniation of the stomach into the chest through the oesophageal hiatus in the diaphragm. The LOS also moves and becomes incompetent. Most HIHs present with GOR. The two types of HIH (see Fig. 23.5) are:

- Sliding (common).
- Rolling or para-oesophageal (rare).

Management

- Diagnosis is made radiologically by barium meal.
- Treatment comprises management of GOR, initially medically.
- Surgery is reserved for children who fail to respond to medication, complicated reflux (e.g. peptic strictures), and para-oesophageal hernias (because of the risk of incarceration and infarction of the herniated stomach). Surgery involves repair of the hiatus hernia and fundoplication to prevent GOR.

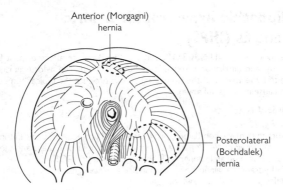

Fig. 22.3 Types of diaphragmatic hernia.

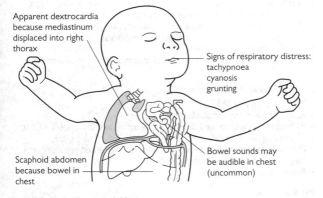

Fig. 22.4 Clinical features of CDH.

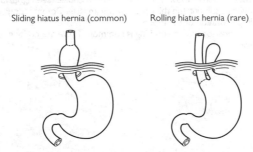

Fig. 22.5 Types of hiatus hernia.

Idiopathic hypertrophic pyloric stenosis (IHPS)

The incidence of IHPS is 3/1000 live births. Boys are affected most frequently, and familial occurrence is well documented. The pylorus enlarges due to hypertrophy of the circular muscle to produce the typical 'tumour'. The cause remains unknown.

Clinical features

(See Fig. 22.6.)

- Vomiting: milky, non-bilious, progressive, and projectile; starting in the fourth week of life. Vomiting occurs within an hour of feeding and the baby is immediately hungry. Often misdiagnosed as GOR.
- Dehydration, malnutrition, and jaundice are late signs.
- IHPS is rare beyond 12wk of age.

Diagnosis

- Test feed: the examiner palpates the baby's abdomen during a feed. Visible waves of gastric peristalsis may be seen passing across the upper abdomen, and a thickened pylorus is palpable as a firm, olive-shaped mass, just above and to the right of the umbilicus.
- USS: if a mass cannot be felt.
- Biochemistry: hypochloraemic, hypokalaemic metabolic alkalosis (see Fig. 22.7).

Preoperative management

- Nil by mouth and NGT.
- Rehydrate and correct alkalosis before surgery.
- IV fluids: maintenance of NS with 5% dextrose and 20mmol/L KCl at 150mL/kg/day; use NS replacement of NG losses mL for mL.
- Electrolytes and capillary blood pH: should be checked regularly until they return to normal (usually 24–48h).
- Blood glucose monitoring.

Surgery

- Ramstedt's pyloromyotomy: the treatment of choice (see Fig. 22.8). This involves splitting the thickened pyloric muscle. Complications include perforation of the mucosa.
- Transient post-operative vomiting is common. There are no long-term sequelae.

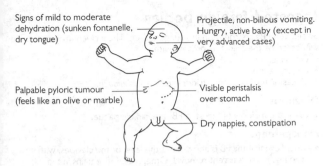

Signs of mild to moderate dehydration (sunken fontanelle, dry tongue)

Projectile, non-bilious vomiting. Hungry, active baby (except in very advanced cases)

Palpable pyloric tumour (feels like an olive or marble)

Visible peristalsis over stomach

Dry nappies, constipation

Fig. 22.6 Clinical signs of pyloric stenosis.

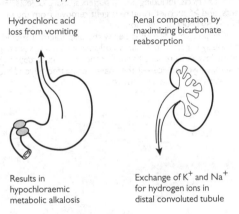

Hydrochloric acid loss from vomiting

Renal compensation by maximizing bicarbonate reabsorption

Results in hypochloraemic metabolic alkalosis

Exchange of K^+ and Na^+ for hydrogen ions in distal convoluted tubule

Fig. 22.7 Biochemical abnormalities in pyloric stenosis.

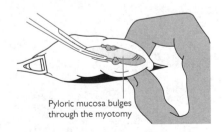

Pyloric mucosa bulges through the myotomy

Fig. 22.8 Ramstedt's operation.

Ingested foreign bodies

Swallowed FBs are common in young children. The incident may have been witnessed or the child may present with:
- Drooling.
- Regurgitation.
- Occasionally cough and stridor—*consider inhalation*.

Diagnosis
- CXR: the majority of ingested FBs are radio-opaque.

Management
- *Oesophageal:* if the FB is above or at the level of the clavicles, with drooling, it needs urgent removal. Otherwise if it remains in the oesophagus, it should be removed within 24h by endoscopy.
  - *Hazardous objects*, including *button batteries*, sharp objects, very large objects, and >1 magnet, require urgent removal from the oesophagus within a few hours of ingestion.
- *Below the diaphragm:* if the FB is below the diaphragm, it should pass spontaneously per rectum. Colicky abdominal pain and vomiting warrant review and a repeat X-ray. For the above *hazardous objects*, always seek surgical advice—if they have not passed beyond the pylorus at 12h, endoscopic retrieval is advised.

Midgut malrotation and volvulus

(See Fig. 22.9 and ➔ Neonatal intestinal obstruction, p. 806.) During the first trimester, the fetal midgut rotates to bring the caecum to lie in the right iliac fossa and the duodenojejunal flexure (DJF) to lie to the left of the midline. Malrotation is failure of this normal rotation that leaves the caecum high in the right upper quadrant and the DJF to the right of the midline. The result is a narrow base for the midgut mesentery through which the superior mesenteric artery runs, which is prone to volvulus.

Midgut malrotation

Midgut malrotation predisposes to midgut volvulus. To prevent this complication, surgical correction of a malrotation is advised using Ladd's procedure, with an incidental appendicectomy.

Midgut volvulus

A time-sensitive surgical emergency with catastrophic consequences
The immediate effect is high intestinal obstruction at the duodenal level that is rapidly followed by necrosis of the entire midgut.

Symptoms and signs
• Bile-stained vomiting: *beware a grass-green vomit can be the only sign in an otherwise clinically well baby.*
• Scaphoid tender abdomen.
• Bloody stools.
• Circulatory collapse.

Diagnosis
• AXR (see Fig. 22.10): may see 'double bubble' and a paucity of gas elsewhere in the abdomen. *Beware this may be confused with duodenal atresia or may look normal.*
• The diagnosis is confirmed by an urgent (even in middle of the night) upper GI contrast study.

Surgical treatment
• Immediate laparotomy to untwist the volvulus.
• If the bowel is healthy, a Ladd's procedure is performed.
• If bowel viability is doubtful, a second-look laparotomy may be necessary after 24h. The risk is massive intestinal necrosis not compatible with life or short gut requiring long-term parenteral nutrition and consideration for transplant.

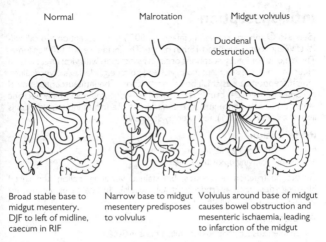

Normal

Malrotation

Midgut volvulus

Duodenal obstruction

Broad stable base to midgut mesentery. DJF to left of midline, caecum in RIF

Narrow base to midgut mesentery predisposes to volvulus

Volvulus around base of midgut causes bowel obstruction and mesenteric ischaemia, leading to infarction of the midgut

Fig. 22.9 Intestinal rotation and volvulus. RIF, right iliac fossa; DJF, duodenojejunal flexure.

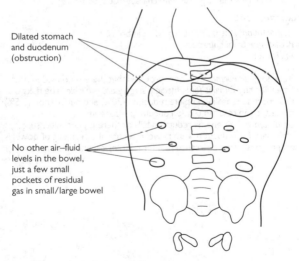

Dilated stomach and duodenum (obstruction)

No other air–fluid levels in the bowel, just a few small pockets of residual gas in small/large bowel

Fig. 22.10 Features of volvulus on AXR.

Intussusception

(See also ➲ Intussusception in infants, p. 807.) Intussusception typically affects infants between 6 and 18mth of age. The incidence is 1/500 children.
The majority of intussusceptions occur in association with viral infections. In
older children, consider a pathological lead point, e.g. Meckel's diverticulum.
Intussusception causes small bowel obstruction. The intussuscepted bowel
becomes ischaemic → causes rectal bleeding → becomes eventually necrotic
→ perforation → peritonitis. The commonest site for an intussusception is
ileocolic (see Fig. 22.11), followed by ileo-ileal.

Presentation

- Intermittent colicky abdominal pain.
- Episodic drawing up of the knees.

As the obstruction progresses, bile-stained vomiting, pallor, and rectal
bleeding (described as 'redcurrant jelly stools'). In late cases, circulatory
shock or peritonitis will be present.

Assessment

- Palpable sausage-shaped abdominal mass in 30%.
- Blood may be noted on rectal examination.
- AXR: small bowel obstruction and paucity of gas in the RIF.
- USS: confirms the diagnosis with characteristic 'target sign'.

Management

- *Resuscitation:* at least 20mL/kg NS fluid bolus.
- Broad-spectrum *antibiotics*.
- *Analgesia*.
- *NGT*.
- Radiology *air enema* reduction: provided that there is no evidence of
  peritonitis and facilities for immediate surgery are available. The risks of
  this procedure are incomplete reduction (30%) and perforation (2.5%);
  the latter can result in tension pneumoperitoneum.
- *Laparotomy:* if air enema reduction fails or there is peritonitis, surgery is
  necessary for reduction, with bowel resection if a segment of bowel is
  gangrenous; 10% recurrence rate for radiological and surgical treatment.

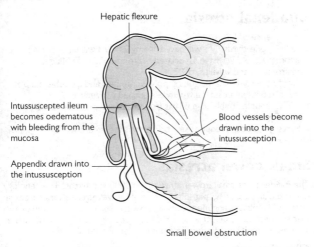

Fig. 22.11 Ileocolic intussusception.

Duodenal atresia

The incidence of DA is 1/5000 live births.
- Rule of one-thirds: 1/3 will have trisomy 21; 1/3 will have cardiac anomalies; 1/3 will have associated malrotation (see ➲ Midgut malrotation and volvulus, p. 820).
- Commonly antenatal diagnosis: polyhydramnios and a double bubble, but can present postnatally with bile-stained vomiting.
- AXR: 'double bubble' sign of gas in stomach and proximal duodenum (see Fig. 22.12).
- Surgery: duodenoduodenostomy; prognosis is excellent.

Small bowel atresias

The incidence of small bowel atresia is 1/3000 live births. The aetiology is a vascular insult. The pathology of small bowel atresias varies from an intraluminal obstructing membrane to a widely separated atresia with a V-shaped mesenteric defect and loss of gut (see Fig. 22.13). About 10% of atresias are multiple (consider immunodeficiency, familial, and CF).

Clinical aspects

- *Bile-stained vomiting*: babies present shortly after birth with bile-stained vomiting and abdominal distension.
- AXR shows a few dilated loops (see Fig. 22.14).
- *Laparotomy*: end-to-end anastomosis. Prognosis depends on the length of the remaining small bowel.

Meconium ileus (MCI)

The incidence is 1/2500 live births. *Ninety-five per cent of neonates presenting with MCI will have CF.* Lack of pancreatic enzymes results in meconium that is thick and viscous, causing an intraluminal obstruction in the terminal ileum. Occasionally, the distended obstructed bowel will perforate or result in volvulus *in utero*, so-called 'complicated' MCI. Babies present at birth with intestinal obstruction.

Management

Treatment of MCI involves relieving the intestinal obstruction.
- *Gastrografin® enema*: 'simple' MCI is successfully relieved by hypertonic contrast in two-thirds of cases. *Fluid resuscitation required.*
- *Laparotomy*: for unsuccessful enema or complicated MCI.
- Further management will be for CF.

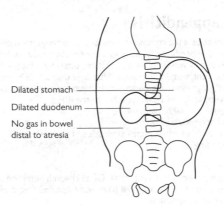

Fig. 22.12 Features of duodenal atresia on AXR.

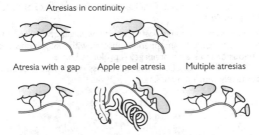

Fig. 22.13 Types of small bowel atresia.

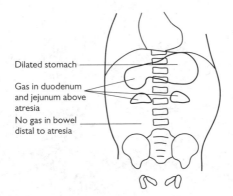

Fig. 22.14 Features of jejunal atresia on AXR.

Acute appendicitis

Acute appendicitis is the commonest abdominal emergency in children (see also ➲ Acute appendicitis, p. 807; ➲ Perioperative care, p. 846). Acute appendicitis begins with luminal obstruction, often by a faecolith, and this causes vague central abdominal pain. After a further 24–36h, the appendix will become gangrenous and perforate. Irritation of the peritoneum results in more severe abdominal pain localized to the RIF.

• Pain is aggravated by movement.
• Fever and anorexia are common.
• Localized RIF involuntary spasm in muscles of the abdominal wall—'guarding'.

Diagnosis

The diagnosis of appendicitis is clinical. Of all children admitted to hospital with abdominal pain, only ~30% will have acute appendicitis; if there is any doubt, admit for observation.

• *Urinalysis*: abnormal in 30% of children with acute appendicitis. Don't assume a diagnosis of UTI unless the urine culture is +ve.
• USS: investigation of choice if clinical doubt, particularly to exclude ovarian pathology.

Late presentations can mimic gastroenteritis with diarrhoea and minimal abdominal signs. Exclude an appendix abscess with USS, as this requires percutaneous or transrectal drainage. A prolonged history of >5 days also warrants an USS to rule out an appendix mass which would be managed non-operatively with antibiotics.

Mesenteric adenitis

Mimics acute appendicitis. It is usually the result of an intercurrent viral infection. Children with mesenteric adenitis typically present with a high fever (>39°C) and abdominal pain in the *absence of peritonism*.

Diagnosis

After a period of observation, analgesia, and hydration, the symptoms remain static or improve, rather than progress, as would be expected with appendicitis.

Meckel's diverticulum

- Persistence of the embryonic vitello-intestinal duct.
- Present in 2% of the population and the majority are asymptomatic.

Symptoms

- GI bleeding, obstruction, inflammation, and umbilical discharge.
- Rectal bleeding is painless and fresh—*consider as a strong differential of rectal bleeding when there is an acute drop in Hb*.

Management

- ^{99m}Tc-pertechnetate isotope scan: 2% have ectopic gastric mucosa.
- *Surgical excision (laparotomy or laparoscopic-assisted) for symptomatic cases.*

Gastroschisis

The incidence of gastroschisis is 1/3000 live births, and the incidence is increasing. Majority antenatally diagnosed, and delivery arranged in a regional neonatal surgical centre. The abnormality is immediately apparent at birth as a defect in the abdominal wall to the right of the umbilicus (see Fig. 22.15). The bowel is eviscerated and not covered by a sac. As a result of contact with amniotic fluid, the bowel is thickened and matted. Associated malformations are uncommon, except intestinal atresias (10%).

Management

- Immediate: cover the exposed bowel with cling film.
- Keep the baby warm
- Fluid resuscitation, broad-spectrum antibiotics, and NGT.
- Surgery: either primary closure of the defect or if there are concerns about abdominal compartment syndrome, a silo is used. The silo is reduced serially over a period of days, followed by closure of the defect.
- Nutrition: TPN is often required for at least a month, as intestinal function is slow to commence. The majority have an excellent outcome, with 96% survival rates; however, complex cases have short gut syndrome.

Exomphalos (omphalocele)

The incidence of exomphalos is 1/7000 live births (see Fig. 23.15). It is characterized by:
- Herniated bowel into the base of the umbilical cord, covered by a sac (amnion).
- Exomphalos major: defect >4cm and/or sac containing the liver.
- Exomphalos minor: defect <4cm.

Majority diagnosed antenatally, with <10% of antenatal diagnostic workload reaching operative repair. Pulmonary hypoplasia can be severe. Associated malformations are found in 50% of cases:
- Chromosomal defects: trisomies 18, 13, and 21 and Turner's syndrome.
- Cardiac defects.
- Syndromes: BWS.

Surgical treatment
- Closure of the defect in one or more stages.
- Conservative approach with topical agents to promote epithelialization for giant omphalocele.
- Prognosis depends on associated malformations.

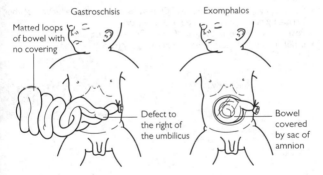

Fig. 22.15 Anterior abdominal wall defects.

Inguinal hernias

Groin hernias in children are almost invariably *indirect inguinal hernias* caused by failure of the processus vaginalis (PV) to obliterate after testicular descent through the inguinal canal.

- Commoner in boys and prematurity.
- 15% of hernias are bilateral.

Clinical care

- A reducible swelling in the groin, often extending into the scrotum (see Fig. 22.16).
- Surgical herniotomy. Infants should be repaired within a few weeks of diagnosis because the risk of incarceration is high. The risk of incarceration lessens after the age of 1y.

Incarcerated hernia

Incarceration (irreducible) results in intestinal obstruction and then strangulation.

- *In ♂*: risk of testicular infarction due to cord compression.
- *In ♀*: the ovary can herniate and become trapped, risking infarction if not reduced.

Treatment

- Resuscitation, analgesia such as PO morphine, and then reduction of the hernia by gentle and sustained pressure (*taxis*).
- Post-reduction herniotomy performed 24–48h later.
- If hernia not reducible → emergency surgery (rarely needed).

Hydroceles

Common. Same aetiology as hernias, smaller PV. There is no history of an intermittent groin swelling suggestive of hernia.

- *Clinical signs:* soft swelling around the testis that transilluminates and above which the examiner can get (see Fig. 22.16).
- Most resolve by the second year: persistent hydroceles are offered a cosmetic repair.

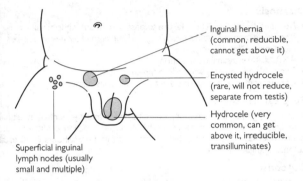

Inguinal hernia (common, reducible, cannot get above it)

Encysted hydrocele (rare, will not reduce, separate from testis)

Hydrocele (very common, can get above it, irreducible, transilluminates)

Superficial inguinal lymph nodes (usually small and multiple)

Fig. 22.16 Groin swellings.

Hirschsprung's disease

The incidence of HSD is 1/5000 live births; 95% of cases sporadic. Associated with trisomy 21.
- Caused by failure of ganglion cells to migrate into the hindgut.
- Defect → functional intestinal obstruction at the junction ('transition zone') between normal bowel and distal aganglionic bowel.
- Variable bowel length affected: 75% of cases rectosigmoid, 5% total colonic aganglionosis.

Diagnosis

- *Neonatal bowel obstruction:* failure to pass meconium, abdominal distension, and bile-stained vomiting; *99% of normal term newborns pass meconium within 48h of delivery.*
- AXR: distal intestinal obstruction.
- Rectal biopsy: no ganglion cells in the submucosa.
- Can present later in childhood with chronic constipation.

Surgical treatment

A single-stage pull-through in infancy, after initial management of intestinal obstruction with home rectal washouts. A staged procedure with an initial stoma needed for failure to decompress with rectal washouts or in total colonic aganglionosis.

Outcome

- *Long-term outcome good:* 75% of children acquire normal bowel control, smaller numbers with chronic constipation and soiling.
- *Beware HD enterocolitis:* a dramatic illness characterized by fever, abdominal distension, diarrhoea, septicaemia, and risk of mortality.
- Urgent resuscitation, IV antibiotics, and transfer to surgical centre.

Rectal prolapse

Rectal prolapse refers to mucosal or full-thickness herniation of the rectum through the anal canal. Most commonly seen in constipated toddlers and *self-limiting*. Rarely associated with CF—*arrange sweat test*.

Management

- Often the prolapse reduces spontaneously after defecation. If not, gentle digital reduction should be performed.
- Treat constipation and toilet step to avoid straining.
- Recurrent prolapse may be managed with injection sclerotherapy.
- More complicated surgical procedures are rarely necessary.

Anorectal malformations

The incidence of anorectal malformation is 1/5000 live births. Anorectal malformations comprise part of the VACTERL association (see Box 22.1). The abnormality should be identified at birth by:

- Failure to pass meconium.
- Abdominal distension.
- Bile-stained vomiting.
- Absent or abnormally sited anal opening.

In boys, the commonest anomaly is an imperforate anus with a recto-urethral fistula (see Fig. 22.17). Meconium can be seen passing from the urethra into the urine. Another common anomaly is a perineal fistula where a small-calibre rectal fistula emerges in an ectopic position.

In girls, the commonest anomaly is the recto-vestibular fistula (see Fig. 22.18). The rectum opens into the back of the introitus, so there is the appearance of an imperforate anus, with meconium seen to emerge from the introitus.

Surgical treatment

A defunctioning colostomy within the first 48h of birth, reconstruction at a few months of age (most commonly involving a posterior sagittal anorectoplasty performed through a midline perineal incision), and then closure of the colostomy.

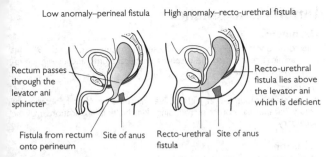

Low anomaly–perineal fistula

High anomaly–recto-urethral fistula

Rectum passes through the levator ani sphincter

Recto-urethral fistula lies above the levator ani which is deficient

Fistula from rectum onto perineum

Site of anus

Recto-urethral fistula

Site of anus

Fig. 22.17 ♂ anorectal malformations.

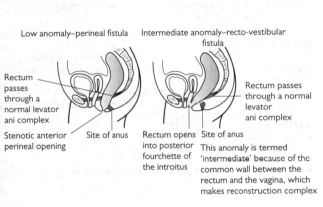

Low anomaly–perineal fistula

Intermediate anomaly–recto-vestibular fistula

Rectum passes through a normal levator ani complex

Rectum passes through a normal levator ani complex

Stenotic anterior perineal opening

Site of anus

Rectum opens into posterior fourchette of the introitus

Site of anus

This anomaly is termed 'intermediate' because of the common wall between the rectum and the vagina, which makes reconstruction complex

Fig. 22.18 ♀ anorectal malformations.

Umbilical anomalies

Granuloma

The commonest umbilical abnormality seen in infants (see Fig. 22.19). This is a harmless reaction to the resolving umbilical stump and usually disappears by the third week.

Treatment

If persistent, cauterization with a silver nitrate stick after application of yellow paraffin to protect surrounding skin. Multiple applications may be necessary.

> ### Caution
> A persistent 'granuloma' discharging faeculant material signifies a patent vitello-intestinal duct (see Fig. 22.19). Treatment involves surgical exploration of the umbilicus and excision of the duct with a small segment of the ileum. The diagnosis is clinical.

Urachal remnants

These are uncommon anomalies. The urachus is an embryonic tubular connection between the bladder and the allantois that normally obliterates before birth.

- Main symptom: persistent discharge of urine from the umbilicus.
- Bladder outlet obstruction (PUVs) should be excluded by micturating cystography. Treatment is surgical closure.
- Umbilical hernias (see Fig. 22.19).
- Common, particularly in Afro-Caribbean children.
- Most will close spontaneously.
- Complications are rare.
- Cosmetic repair offered if persistent defect at 4y of age.

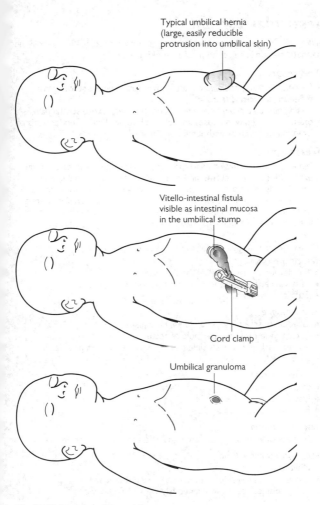

Typical umbilical hernia (large, easily reducible protrusion into umbilical skin)

Vitello-intestinal fistula visible as intestinal mucosa in the umbilical stump

Cord clamp

Umbilical granuloma

Fig. 22.19 Disorders of the umbilicus.

Testicular torsion

A time-sensitive emergency. The age distribution is bimodal—first peak in the neonatal period and second peak around puberty.

Presentation

- *Perinatal testicular torsion:* neonate with a hard, painless scrotal mass, reflecting a necrotic testis.
- *Torsion outside the perinatal period:* sudden-onset, severe scrotal pain, often associated with nausea and lower abdominal pain. Tender testis on examination, with or without abnormal lie.

Treatment

- *Perinatal testicular torsion:* warrants surgical referral for possible scrotal exploration, orchidectomy, and contralateral fixation. Variable practice.
- *Torsion outside the perinatal period:* urgent surgical referral for immediate scrotal *exploration is mandatory* to salvage the testis, which should then be fixed to prevent recurrence. The contralateral testis should also be fixed, as torsion is due to a bilateral anomaly.

Differential diagnosis of acute scrotal pain

Testicular torsion
- Sudden-onset pain, swelling, and nausea.
- Testis is very tender and may lie transversely in scrotum.
- Scrotal skin may be red.

Torted hydatid
- Gradual onset of less severe pain; no nausea.
- Focal tenderness at upper pole of testis.
- Torted hydatid may be visible through scrotal skin as a pea-sized, blue/black swelling.

Epididymo-orchitis
- Insidious onset of dysuria and fever.
- Usually associated with UTI.
- Red, tender scrotum.

Testicular trauma
- History obvious and there are signs of trauma/haematocele.

Idiopathic scrotal oedema
- Child is well.
- Scrotal skin is cellulitic, but the testes are not tender.
- The condition settles spontaneously within a few days.

Epididymo-orchitis

- *Symptoms:* fever, urinary symptoms, and scrotal pain
- Can have associated UTI: *exclude renal tract anomaly by USS in recurrent cases.*
- *Management:* antibiotics once urine has been sent for MC&S. Adolescents should be screened for STI (see ⊃ Sexually transmitted infection, p. 767).

Undescended testes (cryptorchidism)

Undescended testes result from incomplete descent to the scrotum (see Fig. 22.20). Affects 3% of full-term boys. Spontaneous descent may occur in first 6mth, but not later. Commoner in premature infants.

Clinical aspects

Undescended testes are subdivided into the following.
- *Palpable* undescended testes (80%): usually at the external inguinal ring. *Treatment:* groin orchidopexy.
- *Impalpable* testes (20%): intra-abdominal, inside the inguinal canal, or absent. There is risk of malignant degeneration in an intra-abdominal testis (1 in 70, compared with 1 in 5000 for normal testis).

Treatment

Diagnostic laparoscopy since imaging is unreliable. If the vas and vessels enter the deep inguinal ring (30%) → groin orchidopexy. If the vas and vessels end blindly at the deep ring (30%), then testis torted *in utero* and resorbed. No further action necessary. If a testis is intra-abdominal, then remove or bring down as two-stage orchidopexy.

> ### When should boys be referred to a surgeon?
> - Impalpable testis at any age.
> - Undescended palpable testis beyond age 3mth, aiming for orchidopexy at age 6–12mth or at point of detection in older child.

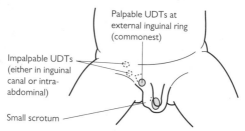

Palpable UDTs at external inguinal ring (commonest)

Impalpable UDTs (either in inguinal canal or intra-abdominal)

Small scrotum

Fig. 22.20 Undescended testes (UDTs).

Retractile testes

The cremasteric muscle is overactive and the testes retract into the groin. The scrotum is well developed, and the parents may notice that the testes are in place when the child is in a warm bath. The testes can be manipulated into the scrotum. Surgery is not necessary.

Hypospadias

Hypospadias affects 1 in 350 ♂ births. Characterized by an abnormal position of the urethral meatus and is classified according to the location of the meatus (penis down to the scrotum; see Fig. 22.21). Severe forms of hypospadias may be associated with chordee—ventral curvature of the penis. The consequences of hypospadias are difficulty urinating while standing and an abnormal cosmetic appearance. Sexual function is not affected unless chordee is present, which may cause painful erections.

> **Hypospadias advice**
> - Make sure you document the diagnosis in the notes.
> - Tell the parents not to circumcise the child.
> - Give the parents a letter stating this advice.
> - Refer the child to a paediatric urologist.

Surgery

Correction involves straightening of any chordee and reconstruction of the urethra to the glans. This may involve tubularizing skin from the prepuce, so circumcision is contraindicated. The correction can be completed in one or more operations during early childhood.

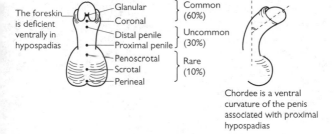

The foreskin is deficient ventrally in hypospadias

Glanular ⎫
Coronal ⎬ Common (60%)

Distal penile ⎫
Proximal penile ⎬ Uncommon (30%)

Penoscrotal ⎫
Scrotal ⎬ Rare (10%)
Perineal

Chordee is a ventral curvature of the penis associated with proximal hypospadias

Fig. 22.21 Classification of hypospadias.

Phimosis and paraphimosis

The foreskin is normally non-retractable in early childhood. It is common for boys to complain of intermittent redness and discomfort from the prepuce. Rarely the result of infection, but simply a chemical irritation from urine under the foreskin. As foreskin maturation occurs, the foreskin balloons out on micturition. These symptoms are self-limiting and resolve during childhood without circumcision.

Circumcision

The medical indications for circumcision are:

- *Balanitis xerotica obliterans* (BXO) (or lichen sclerosis), which is an uncommon, progressive scarring dermatitis. Thickened white appearance of a non-retractile foreskin. Very rare in those aged <5y.
- Paraphimosis: the prepuce retracts as the boy gets an erection and becomes stuck behind the glans which becomes oedematous. Paraphimosis should be reduced under GA, and circumcision scheduled a few weeks later to prevent recurrence.
- Recurrent balanitis: this is rare.
- PUVs.

Balanitis/balanoposthitis

Balanoposthitis is acute inflammation of the glans and foreskin associated with a purulent discharge from the preputial orifice.
• Treatment: 5-day course of PO co-amoxiclav is appropriate. Topical antibacterials or antifungals are of no value.

Priapism

Priapism is a prolonged penile erection lasting >4h and is rare in childhood. It is a urological emergency, as ischaemic priapism can cause permanent cavernosal damage and erectile dysfunction. The commonest cause of priapism in children is SCD (see ➲ Sickle crises and problems, p. 820). Other causes are trauma, idiopathic, and pharmacologically induced. Occasionally, priapism is a presenting symptom of acute leukaemia.

Miscellaneous conditions

Labial adhesions

Common in ♀ toddlers. Nappy rash and exposure to urine causes chronic labial irritation, which adhere. There is invariably a small anterior opening through which urine escapes. Labial adhesions are asymptomatic and usually separate without treatment, but they are a major source of anxiety to parents. Treatment is best deferred until the child is out of nappies. Topical oestrogen cream for 2wk will result in separation of most adhesions, but occasionally gentle separation under GA may be necessary.

Ankyloglossia (tongue-tie)

A common congenital oral anomaly in 4% of children, characterized by ↓ mobility of the tongue tip caused by a short, thick lingual frenulum. Tongue-tie can affect the ability of newborns to breastfeed, and division of the lingual frenulum in the newborn period can improve this. Bottle-feeding is not affected. Other indications for division include future speech development, although this remains controversial.

Dermoid cysts

Common in children (see Fig. 22.22). Dermoids are non-tender, mobile subcutaneous cysts filled with keratin, hair follicles, and sebaceous glands. They should be excised to prevent infection. Dermoid cysts occur most frequently along the lines of embryological fusion, e.g. lateral corner of the eyebrows (external angular dermoid), neck midline, over the nasal bridge, and suprasternal notch.

Thyroglossal duct cysts (TDCs)

Present with midline neck swelling, just below the hyoid. The swelling rises with tongue protrusion and swallowing. TDCs develop from epithelial remnants left after descent of the developing thyroid from the foramen caecum at the base of the tongue. TDCs gradually enlarge and eventually become infected, which makes excision more difficult. Treat by surgical removal of the central portion of the hyoid, along with the cyst and track.

Branchial remnants

Persist from branchial clefts during embryogenesis of the head and neck. Anomalies of the second branchial cleft are by far the commonest.
- *Branchial sinuses*: present as small cutaneous openings along the anterior lower-third border of the sternocleidomastoid muscle that discharge mucus (see Fig. 23.23). They can communicate with the tonsillar fossa (branchial fistula). Manage by excision to prevent infection.
- *Branchial cysts*: uncommon neck swellings along the anterior border of the sternocleidomastoid. Manage by surgical excision.

Cystic hygroma (CH)

A congenital malformation of the lymphatic system that presents in early childhood as a soft multilocular cystic swelling, appearing either antenatally (chromosomal anomalies) or postnatally. CHs are more often found in the neck and axillae, although they can occur anywhere, including inside the abdomen or thorax. Large cervical CHs may present at birth with airway obstruction. Small CHs require no treatment. Large lesions infiltrate the surrounding tissues, making complete surgical excision impossible. Intra-lesional sclerotherapy injection is an alternative to surgery.

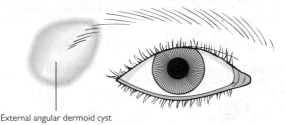

External angular dermoid cyst

Fig. 22.22 External angular dermoid cyst.

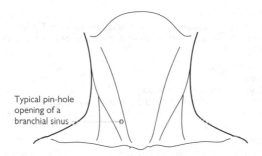

Typical pin-hole opening of a branchial sinus

Fig. 22.23 Branchial sinus.

Perioperative care

Elective children

Take a history and carry out an examination:
- The presenting complaint should be documented and confirmed.
- Record previous medical history, medication, and allergies.
- Brief clinical examination should be performed. In the case of undescended testes, hydroceles, and inguinal hernias, a mark should be made on the child's thigh to document the side for operation.
- If the child is unwell with intercurrent illness, discuss with the anaesthetist who may decide that the child is unfit for anaesthesia.
- Blood tests: including preoperative cross-match; will vary according to diagnosis and the type of surgery.
- Fasting prior to elective surgery (see Box 22.2).

> **Box 22.2 Minimum fasting times before elective surgery (Association of Paediatric Anaesthetists recommendations)**
> - Solid food: 6h.
> - Formula milk: 6h.
> - Breast milk: 4h.
> - Clear fluids (dextrose solution, water): 2h.

Newborns

Preoperative resuscitation and preparation are essential for best surgical outcomes. Newborns with congenital malformations will be admitted to NICU.

Routine preparation
- IM vitamin K.
- FBC to determine Hb concentration.
- Cross-matching blood. Many laboratories require a sample of maternal blood for typing and this should accompany the baby if the mother is unable or unfit to travel.

Echocardiography
OA, duodenal atresia, exomphalos, and anorectal malformations, for example, have possible associated cardiac defects.

Renal imaging
Provided the baby passes urine (indicative of functioning nephrons), renal imaging can be arranged electively. Anuria necessitates renal USS to exclude renal agenesis.

Intestinal obstruction
- IV fluid: resuscitation, normal maintenance, and replacement of losses.
- NG decompression: a wide-bore 8Fr NGT is necessary to empty the stomach.
- Biochemistry and acid–base balance: necessary in babies with prolonged vomiting (e.g. pyloric stenosis).

Consent for surgery

(See also ⊃ Assent and consent, pp. 956–7.)

Consent for surgery: clinical practice

The best person to obtain consent is the surgeon performing the operation.

Children

- Whenever possible, the procedure should be explained to the child in language that he/she can understand.
- Children aged <16y can give consent if Fraser-competent, but if they refuse, the law allows a person with parental responsibility to consent in their place.

Parents

Informed consent must include:

- An explanation of the diagnosis and proposed operation, along with alternative treatments, risks and benefits, and likely outcomes.
- It is prudent to discuss potential complications and provide an estimate of risk. The risk of adverse reactions to GA in fit, healthy children is between 1 in 10 000 and 1 in 100 000, which is comparable with the risk of injury crossing a road.

Emergency

- In an emergency, it is justifiable to treat without parental consent.
- It must, however, be documented clearly that the child's life is in danger and that attempts have been made to contact the parents.
- Ensure that entries in the records are signed, timed, and dated.
- Verbal consent from the parents is acceptable in an emergency and this should be recorded on the consent form.

Post-operative care: fluids

Major surgery

After major surgery, children will return to the ward or NICU/PICU. The operation notes should include specific instructions regarding antibiotics, catheters, IV fluids, etc.

- *Post-operative IV fluids:* will depend on the nature of the surgery. NS with 5% dextrose is often used with 20mmol/L KCl added to fluids after the first day. The rate of infusion should be adjusted according to the weight of the child.
- *NG aspirates:* it is easy to underestimate 'third space losses' (i.e. fluid translocating into the peritoneum, bowel, or chest) after major surgery. Remember to replace losses (e.g. NG aspirates).
- *Biochemistry:* children who remain on IV fluids, e.g. those with post-operative ileus or high stoma losses, should have daily U&E monitoring. Frequent adjustments to the electrolyte content and rate of infusion may be necessary to avoid hyponatraemia.
- *Nutrition:* following abdominal surgery if prolonged IV fluid therapy is necessary (>5 days), consideration should be given to parenteral nutrition.

Newborns and infants

Newborns and infants <44wk post-conception should be transferred to NICU or a special care baby unit post-operatively. The risk of post-operative apnoea after GA is relatively high.

Post-operative care: analgesia

(See also ➲ Pain management, p. 932.)

Analgesia for day cases

In many cases, LA blocks or wound infiltration will provide complete analgesia for several hours. After this, simple analgesia, such as paracetamol or ibuprofen, are usually all that is required.

Analgesia for major surgery

After major surgery, stronger analgesia is required for a longer period. This applies to neonates, as well as to older children.

Continuous epidural infusions of local anaesthetics

There are many advantages to local or regional analgesia, and continuous epidural infusions of LA (e.g. bupivacaine) work particularly well after major abdominal or thoracic surgery. These are rarely used on a general paediatric ward in a district general hospital.

- Epidural infusions are not without risk. It is essential that close nursing supervision is maintained (i.e. vital signs and level of the epidural block).
- In many hospitals, there is a *'paediatric pain team'* who supervise the epidural. If not available, close liaison with the anaesthetist responsible.
- If analgesia is inadequate, advice should be sought before either removing the epidural catheter or starting opiates.

Continuous IV infusion of morphine

Infusion of morphine or other opiates is another very effective method of post-operative analgesia. For older children, this may be in the form of a patient-controlled analgesia (PCA) pump with a button the child can press to obtain an increment of analgesic. Contact the local pain team for advice and setting up a patient-controlled device.

Further reading

Paediatric surgery textbooks

Holcomb III GW, Murphy PJ, Ostlie DJ. *Ashcraft's Pediatric Surgery*, sixth edition. Elsevier Saunders, New York, NY; 2014.

Hutson JM, O'Brien M, Beasley SW, Teague WJ, King SK (eds). *Jones' Clinical Paediatric Surgery*, seventh edition. Wiley Blackwell, Chichester; 2015.

Paediatric urology textbooks

Wilcox D, Godbole P, Cooper C. *Pediatric Urology Book*. Available at: ℻ http://www.pediatricurologybook.com/index.htm.

eLearning module in paediatric surgery emergencies

Royal College of Surgeons. *Paediatric surgical emergencies* (eLearning). Available at: ℻ https://www.rcseng.ac.uk/education-and-exams/courses/postgraduate-certificate-in-surgery/paediatric-surgery-emergencies/.

Audiology

Ear: pain and discharge

Ear discharge (otorrhoea)

May be due to drainage of blood, ear wax, pus, or fluid from the external or middle ear, e.g.:

- Otitis externa.
- Eczema and other skin irritations.
- Foreign object impaction.
- Otitis media.
- Mastoiditis.
- Perforated eardrum.
- Head injury—CSF leak.

Earache (otalgia)

Can be a symptom of the conditions noted above. However, it may be the result of pain referred from pathology at another location (referred otalgia), e.g.:

- Parotitis.
- Teeth and jaw (impacted molars, dental caries).
- Acute tonsillitis.
- Oropharyngeal tumours.

Hearing assessment

A fetus will respond to sound in the latter part of pregnancy (from third trimester). At birth, the baby will react to noise, with a marked preference for voices.

Hearing screening

(See also ➲ Delayed speech, p. 732.)

Early detection of hearing loss is important. Hearing loss impairs speech and language development, cognitive development, and socialization. A baby who does not startle when parents come into view may not have heard them approach due to deafness. These children need *urgent* audiological assessment, along with children who show absence of appropriate vocalization by age (see bullet points below). Specific screening questions can be asked when evaluating hearing:

Birth
- Does baby startle to loud noise?

12wk
- Does baby quieten to mother's voice, even when mother cannot be seen?
- Does baby quieten to prolonged loud noise?
- Does baby settle to a musical toy?

5mth
- Does baby smile to familiar voice?
- Does he/she take turns to vocalize when spoken to?

7mth
- Does baby turn to look towards a new sound?
- Does he/she make tuneful vocalization?

9mth
- Does baby recognize own name?
- Does baby recognize and react to familiar tunes and music?

11mth
- Will baby react to calling from out of sight?

Hearing tests

All health authority areas in the UK have a universal newborn hearing screening (UNHS) programme. UNHS involves otoacoustic emission testing in the first 48h after birth. In the test, a small earpiece is inserted into the ear canal. This delivers a sound that evokes an emission from the inner ear hair cells if the cochlea is normal.

Current hearing screening programmes

There is currently some regional variation in the type of tests used. A general summary of hearing screening is described below.

- *Within a few weeks of birth:* this is known as newborn hearing screening and it is often carried out before the baby leaves hospital after birth. This test is routine for all children and even those having a home birth will be invited to come to hospital. *Tests include:* otoacoustic emission, auditory brainstem-evoked potential, and auditory response cradle test.
- *8mth to 1y old:* a follow-up to the newborn hearing screening may be required at this time for some children. The *distraction test* (see
  ⊃ The distraction test, p. 855) would be employed in the first instance.
- *From 8mth to 2.5y of age:* parents may be asked if they have any concerns about their child's hearing, as part of a review of the child's health and development, and hearing tests can be arranged if necessary. *Tests include:* pure tone audiometry (from 3y), speech discrimination test, and impedance audiometry.
- *4 or 5y old:* most children will have a hearing test when they start school; it may be conducted at school or in an audiology department. *Test includes:* pure tone audiometry.

The distraction test

Based on the principle that a normal response is observed when sound is presented to an infant and the infant turns his/her head to locate the source of the sound. Two testers are required—one presents the sound out of the infant's line of vision, while the other holds the infant's attention in a forward direction. The test involves delivering a frequency-specific stimulus presented at quiet levels (35dB) to the side and slightly behind an infant who is seated on a parent's knee.

Distraction testing requires a behavioural response and is therefore a direct test of hearing sensitivity. The major disadvantages of this test are that an infant must be mature enough to sit erect and to head turn, and it is subject to all the common biases found in behavioural testing of hearing. It is therefore unsuitable for neonates, which makes identification of hearing loss at <6mth of age very difficult.

Childhood deafness

Hearing loss or deafness may be congenital or acquired and can be divided into SN or conductive loss. Hearing loss of up to 20dB tends not to affect development, but a loss of over 40dB will affect speech and language development.

Sensorineural

Inherited/genetic
- *Non-syndromic.*
- *Syndromic:*
- Usher syndrome (see Table 23.1).
- Waardenburg syndrome (see Table 23.1).

Acquired
- *Perinatal:*
- Birth asphyxia.
- Hyperbilirubinaemia.
- Congenital infection (rubella, CMV, syphilis).
- *Postnatal:*
- Drugs (aminoglycosides).
- Meningitis.
- Head injury.
- Labyrinthitis.
- Acoustic neuroma.

Conductive
- *External ear abnormalities.*
- *Ear canal atresia/stenosis.*
- *Middle ear abnormalities:*
- Acute otitis media.
- Chronic otitis media (tympanic perforation, cholesteatoma).
- Secretory otitis media.

Table 23.1 Syndromes associated with childhood deafness

Syndrome	Characteristics
Waardenburg	SN deafness and pigmentation anomalies (white forelock)
Klippel–Feil sequence	Deafness (SN or conductive) and short neck with low hairline
Treacher Collins	Conductive deafness and midface hypoplasia
Pierre–Robin sequence	Conductive deafness and mandibular hypoplasia, with cleft soft palate
Alport	SN deafness, pyelonephritis, haematuria, and renal failure
Pendred	SN deafness and hypothyroidism
Usher	SN deafness and RP
Jervell–Lange–Nielsen	SN deafness and long QT interval on ECG

Disorders of the ear

Otitis media

(See also ➔ Table 16.3, p. 655.) Infection of the middle ear is associated with pain, fever, and irritability. *Examination* reveals a red and bulging tympanic membrane, with loss of normal light reflex. Occasionally, there is acute perforation of the tympanic membrane. Causative organisms include:

• Viruses.
• *Pneumococcus.*
• Group A β-haemolytic *Streptococcus.*
• *Haemophilus influenzae.*

Treatment is with broad-spectrum antibiotics (e.g. PO amoxicillin or co-amoxiclav) and analgesia. Decongestants may also help. Complicating mastoiditis (see ➔ Acute mastoiditis, p. 859) or meningitis are rare. Recurrent ear infections can lead to secretory otitis media.

Secretory otitis media

This is a middle ear effusion without the symptoms and signs of acute otitis media. It is often the result of recurrent episodes of acute otitis media. Duration often last months (chronic secretory otitis media) and the effusions may be serous (thin), mucoid (thick), or purulent. Children, although asymptomatic, may be noticeably inattentive or complain of hearing loss.

Examination shows the eardrum is retracted and does not move easily. Fluid effusion may be visible behind the tympanic membrane, which appears opaque. Chronic (>3mth) secretory otitis media, particularly when associated with suspected hearing loss, needs referral to the audiology and otolaryngology (ENT) teams for further evaluation and possible *treatment* with myringotomy and insertion of ventilation tubes ('grommets').

Otitis externa

Itching of the external ear canal is common in swimmers and after minor trauma. There may be progressive pain and discharge.

Examination reveals an inflamed ear canal that may be oedematous.

Treatment is with suction clearance under the microscope and a combined antibiotic (hydrocortisone 1% plus gentamicin 0.3%) and steroid preparation applied topically.

Cholesteatoma

An erosive condition affecting the middle ear and mastoid. Consists of squamous epithelium that is trapped within the skull base and that can erode and destroy important structures within the temporal bone. It may lead to life-threatening intracranial infection. Signs include:

• Recurrent painless ear discharge and offensive discharge.
• Conductive hearing loss.
• Vertigo.
• Rarely facial nerve palsy.

Urgent referral to the ENT team is required for surgery and antibiotics.

Acute mastoiditis

Is uncommon but may follow an episode of acute otitis media. In the early stage, symptoms are indistinguishable from those of acute otitis media but may evolve to include intense pain, swelling, or tenderness over the mastoid process. The latter is due to acute mastoid osteitis and occurs when infection and destruction of the mastoid bony trabeculae have occurred.

Examination may also reveal outward and downward displacement of the pinna and swelling of the posterior–superior wall of the external ear canal. Purulent discharge may also be present. Diagnosis is largely clinical, although CT scan is helpful. Urgent referral to ENT for IV antibiotics and sometimes mastoidectomy is indicated.

Foreign body impaction

Parents may observe a child putting an object in the ear canal, which otherwise may take several days to come to notice.

Examination with an auroscope—objects that are easily visible (and with a cooperative child) may be extracted using a hook. Use of forceps should be avoided, as they tend to push the object further down the ear canal and may damage the tympanic membrane unless the FB is paper or cotton bud that can be grabbed. Refer to ENT.

Ear malformations

Abnormal shape, orientation, or position of the ears should raise suspicion of a congenital, inherited disorder or syndrome. Problems with hearing should also be suspected and evaluated.

Referral to clinical genetics is required. The following conditions are associated with ear malformations.

Low-set ear position
- Turner's syndrome (see ➜ Turner's syndrome, p. 884).
- NS (see ➜ Noonan's syndrome, p. 877).
- Rubenstein–Taybi syndrome.
- Treacher Collins syndrome (see ➜ Table 23.1 and Table 24.1).

Malformed auricles
- CHARGE association (see ➜ Choanal atresia, p. 808).
- EDS (see ➜ Ehlers–Danlos syndrome, p. 882).
- di George syndrome (see ➜ Deletion 22q11 syndrome/ velocardiofacial syndrome/ di George syndrome, p. 876).
- Down's syndrome (see ➜ Down's syndrome, pp. 872–3).

Clinical genetics

Clinical genetics and counselling

Genetic counselling

This is 'the process by which individuals or relatives at risk for a disorder that may be hereditary are advised of the consequences of the disorder, the probability of transmitting it and the ways in which this may be prevented, avoided or ameliorated'.[1]

It is axiomatic that this aim will be most satisfactorily achieved when a secure diagnosis has been established. Accordingly, the primary purpose of clinical genetics in practice is the recognition and objective confirmation of the specific disease entity.

Role of the clinical geneticist

Clinical geneticists are doctors with wide training in medicine and its sub-specialties whose expertise is the identification and diagnosis of inherited disorders. These skills lend themselves to the assessment of the child with multiple birth defects, but clinical geneticists see patients of all ages and comprising all manner of clinical presentations. When families come to the genetics clinic, they usually have a number of questions, which may be summarized as follows:

• What is the diagnosis?
• Why did it happen?
• Will it happen again?
• If so, what can be done to ameliorate or prevent it?

The main role of the clinical geneticist is to establish an accurate genetic diagnosis, which is essential in order to:

• Gain an understanding of the condition and possible prognosis.
• Guide optimal management for the child.
• Identify other systems that need surveillance, e.g. hearing or vision.
• Address concerns about events during pregnancy or delivery.
• Enable accurate genetic advice for parents and other family members about the risk of recurrence in future pregnancies.
• Establish a secure predictive test for other family members.

A basic principle of genetic counselling is that advice is non-directive.

When to refer to clinical genetics

A majority of underlying chronic disorders in children either are clearly genetic or have a genetic susceptibility. It is important for paediatricians to recognize genetic disorders and to know when to refer to a clinical geneticist.

Useful definitions
- Dysmorphic features: physical features, particularly unusual facial features, that are not usually found in a child of the same age or ethnic background.
- Abnormal growth parameters: height or weight or OFC >98th centile or <2nd centile.

Indications for referral to clinical genetics
- *Congenital anomalies:*
  - Multiple congenital anomalies.
  - Isolated congenital anomaly in conjunction with dysmorphic features/ developmental delay/abnormal growth parameters/family history.
- *Dysmorphic features:*
  - Especially in conjunction with developmental delay, learning disability, congenital anomaly, and abnormal growth.
- Family history suggestive of a recurrent abnormality.
- Developmental delay or learning disability:
  - Unexplained severe developmental delay or learning disability.
  - Developmental delay or learning disability in conjunction with dysmorphic features, congenital anomaly, abnormal growth parameters, and family history.
- *Multiple problems and no diagnosis:*
  - Child with multiple problems and under the care of many specialists, with no unifying diagnosis.
- *New diagnosis of a genetic disorder:*
  - Enables explanation of the genetic basis of the condition.
  - Essential if the diagnosis may have implications for other relatives.
  - Important if parents would like advice regarding future pregnancies.
- *Teenager with a genetic disorder:*
  - If a genetic diagnosis was made in infancy or early childhood, refer patient back to clinical genetics in mid teens, so that the young adult understands the genetic basis of their condition and the risks to their own offspring.

Taking a family history

One of the key skills in clinical genetics is taking a family history and drawing a family tree with all relevant symbols (see Fig. 24.1). The approach described here is intended for routine use in a general paediatric setting. A more detailed approach is indicated when assessing a patient with a known or possible genetic disorder.

Drawing a basic family tree

- *Start with your patient:* draw ♂ symbol for a male, and ♀ symbol for a female.
- Add symbols for your *patient's parents and siblings*. Record basic information only, e.g. age, whether they are in good health, and whether there are any concerns regarding development. If an individual has died, note age and cause of death and annotate the family tree with an oblique stroke through the symbol.
- Ask whether there is any *inherited disorder running in the family*.
- Ask whether your patient's parents are related (*consanguinity* increases the chance of an AR disorder). Consanguinity is indicated by drawing a double line on the family tree.
- Ask the key question '*Has anybody else in your family had a similar problem to the patient?*' Be aware that some conditions have variable expression, e.g. del 22q11 may present with cleft palate in one member of the family and CHD in another.
- *Extend the family tree upwards* to include grandparents, and sideways to include aunts, uncles, and cousins. If you have not revealed a familial problem by this stage, do not go further as you are unlikely to have missed an important familial disease with onset in childhood. In suspected X-linked disorder, extend the family tree further on the maternal side (ask a clinical geneticist to help you with this).
- Shade those people in the family tree *affected by the disorder*. This will help determine whether there is a genetic problem, and, if there is, it will help to suggest the pattern of inheritance.
- For an example of drawing a family tree, see Fig. 24.2.

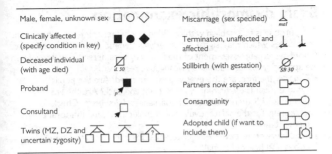

Male, female, unknown sex □ ○ ◇

Clinically affected (specify condition in key) ■ ● ◆

Deceased individual (with age died) d. 50

Proband P

Consultand

Twins (MZ, DZ and uncertain zygosity)

Miscarriage (sex specified) mal

Termination, unaffected and affected

Stillbirth (with gestation) SB 30

Partners now separated □—○

Consanguinity □═○

Adopted child (if want to include them) □─○ [○]

Fig. 24.1 Basic family tree symbols.

Reproduced from Firth HV, Hurst JA, Hall JG (2005). *Oxford Desk Reference of Clinical Genetics.* With permission of Oxford University Press.

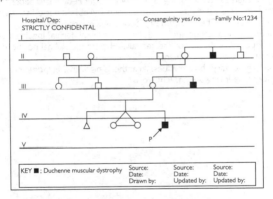

Fig. 24.2 Example of a family tree.

Firth HV, Hurst JA, Hall JG (2005). *Oxford Desk Reference of Clinical Genetics.* With permission of Oxford University Press.

Basic dysmorphic examination

The purpose is to establish with confidence whether there are clinical signs or features which may signal an underlying genetic disease or syndrome. A brief systematic assessment of the following parameters will often inform the appropriate diagnostic and investigative response.

- *Consider the face:* are the eyes widely separated? Are the pupils symmetrical? Is the hairline normal, front and back? Are the lips prominent? Is there evidence of coarseness? Hirsuitism? Check intraorally for the palate, uvula, and frenulum. Lip pits? Intraoral or lip pigmentation?
- *Ears:* low-set? Rotated? Associated pits? External ear canals patent? Lobes and helices normal?
- *Limbs:* asymmetrical? Normal length? Normal proportion between the segments? Nails present? Additional creases or absent creases? Evidence of joint restriction or laxity? Evidence of extra digits (scars/nubbins)? Broad thumbs? Overlapping digits? Trident sign? Fetal finger pads?
- *Neck and chest:* skin pits or sinuses? Goitre? Webbed neck? Sternal malformation? Chest asymmetry? Scoliosis? Gynaecomastia?
- *Abdomen:* umbilical position and shape? Umbilical hernia? Inguinal hernia? Micropenis? Ambiguity of the genitalia? Hypospadias? Anal position? Sacral pit? Caudal appendage?
- *Skin:* pigmentary abnormalities? Acanthosis nigricans? Hypopigmented lesions? Haemangiomata? Ichthyosis?

Genetic testing

Appropriate situations for genetic testing in a child

- Diagnostic testing in a child who has features of a genetic disorder, e.g. chromosome analysis in a child with suspected Down's syndrome.
- The child is asymptomatic but at risk of a genetic condition for which preventive or other therapeutic measures are available, e.g. testing to determine if a child of an affected parent with retinoblastoma (with a known mutation) requires screening by frequent periodic examination under anaesthesia. This is predictive testing and should involve a clinical geneticist.
- The child is at risk of a genetic condition with paediatric onset for which preventive therapeutic measures are not available, e.g. SMA type 1.

Involve a clinical geneticist in these situations. The decision to undertake a genetic test requires careful balancing of benefit/harm; each case is assessed on its individual merits. Generally, testing is done at parental discretion after careful discussion.

As a general rule of good practice, it is unwise for the paediatrician to embark upon specialist investigation which will require specialist knowledge for test interpretation.

Inappropriate situations for genetic testing in a child

- An asymptomatic child is at risk of a genetic condition that usually has onset in adult life for which preventive or effective therapeutic measures are not available, e.g. Huntington's disease.
- Testing for carrier status, e.g. siblings of a child with CF. Practice does vary, but it is usually considered that testing be deferred until the child is old enough to seek testing in their own right or at least to take part in the discussion about testing. Parents sometimes request testing of young children without having necessarily thought through the difficulties this may lead to later on. We suggest referral to clinical genetics if parents remain keen to perform carrier test.
- Genetic testing of children for the benefit of another family member should not be performed unless testing is necessary to prevent substantial harm to the family member.

Chromosome tests

Karyotype analysis

A standard chromosome analysis involves a G-banded karyotype viewed by a cytogeneticist using a light microscope. Using this approach, the maximum resolution is 75–10Mb. One of the major advantages of chromosome analysis is that it is a genomic survey, i.e. it looks in outline at the whole genome. The normal ♂ karyotype is 46, XY. The normal ♀ karyotype is 46, XX.

This is a highly labour-intensive process which has been supplanted by microarray analysis in clinical practice. It will be extremely uncommon for a paediatrician to require a karyotype nowadays.

Fluorescence *in situ* hybridization

Targeted studies are possible at higher resolution using specific FISH probes. Using FISH, it is possible to see submicroscopic deletions responsible for WS (7q) and Angelman syndrome (AS) (15q), but only if the clinician requests this. Microarray has displaced FISH, which is now used as a specialist examination by clinical geneticists.

Molecular kayotyping using microarrays

This is a newly established technology which enables much higher-resolution DNA analysis than is possible with light microscopy. It has recently been especially valuable in identifying patients with chromosomal abnormalities previously not diagnosable by standard techniques.

Genome-wide arrays

These give coverage at varying degrees of resolution, ranging from 1Mb to 100kb, i.e. 10–100 times greater than light microscopy. It is important to appreciate that at high levels of resolution, there is considerable normal variation in the human genome. Copy number variation is routinely identified both in pathological states and as normal family variants. Differentiating between pathological and non-pathological variation requires a specialist. In requesting microarrays, be aware that ~25–30% of such tests will need parental sample analysis to facilitate interpretation of the array report.

It is important to understand arrays and how they differ from karyotypes, apart from the higher sensitivity. Arrays measure the ratio between patient DNA and a standard population norm. They are sensitive to microdeletion and microduplication conditions, trisomy, monosomy, and triploidy. They do NOT detect intragenic mutations, balanced chromosome rearrangements such as translocation, and fragile X syndrome. Array testing is warranted in dysmorphic children, developmentally delayed children, and multiple congenital anomaly presentations and by way of confirming a suspected chromosomal diagnosis.

Molecular genetic analysis

The human genome contains 73 000 000 000 DNA base pairs and 725 000 genes. In genetic disorders, the pathology may range from a whole extra chromosome (e.g. Down's syndrome) to a single DNA base pair alteration (e.g. achondroplasia). Molecular genetic tests are highly specific tests that only reveal information about one very specific gene analysis, generally selected because of a strong clinical diagnosis (e.g. achondroplasia).

If there is a commonly occurring mutation, analysis is simple and comparatively inexpensive (e.g. CF where the CF29 kit tests for the 29 commonest mutations in the Caucasian population, and achondroplasia in which two common mutations (G1138A and G1138C in the *FGFR3* gene) account for ~98% of mutations in children with achondroplasia.

If the mutation in a family is known, analysis is straightforward and takes ~2–4wk for most tests. Such tests, based on information obtained from other family members, should involve a clinical geneticist.

If the mutation is unknown, but a specific clinical condition is suspected, an entire gene may have to be sequenced. Genetic testing in this situation can be laborious and expensive, and only a small proportion may be available as diagnostic tests. In the UK, reporting times are being reduced for these tests and now routinely take about 6–8wk, even for a very large challenging gene, e.g. *FBN1* in MFS and *TSC1* and *TSC2* in TS. Consult a clinical geneticist about whether genetic testing is appropriate in these circumstances.

Panel testing refers to a situation where the specific diagnosis is not known, but there is a likelihood of a disorder which has multiple genetic causes. MFS represents a good example. True cases have a mutation of the *FBN1* gene, but there are several lookalike syndromes (Loeys–Dietz syndrome and homocysteinuria included) which are clinically inseparable from MFS. In that instance, the laboratory will test a 'panel' of genes known to be associated with a Marfan-like clinical presentation. The clinician needs to be aware of which genes were tested and early referral to a clinical geneticist is advised.

Whole exome sequencing (WES) is a specialist tool used in situations when there is no apparent clinical diagnosis, to attempt to identify a possible causal genetic disorder. Multiple sequence variations are certain to be found and careful back confirmation to the clinical situation is necessary if 'cause and effect' is to be confidently ascribed to the genetic variation seen on WES. It is immensely powerful but has the scope to be diagnostically misleading. A specialist tool only.

Practical issues in genetic testing

Counselling the family before testing

Think carefully about the potential impact of the diagnosis you may make with a genetic test. Some genetic conditions are relentlessly progressive and life-limiting (e.g. DMD). Others imply lifelong impairment of a child's ability to learn and communicate (e.g. AS, fragile X syndrome). If you make a genetic diagnosis, it is likely to remain a permanent aspect of that child's life. There may be some treatable elements to the condition, but it is unlikely to be transient or curable. The diagnosis may have implications for other family members. The family should preferably be counselled by a clinical geneticist, before a genetic test is performed. Ensure that the parents understand what you are testing for and why. Explain how long it may take to obtain a result and make careful arrangements for communicating the result.

Predictive testing

The circumstances in which this may be appropriate can be complex and can vary for different disorders. This should be arranged through a clinical geneticist. Predictive testing is inappropriate in a paediatric setting.

Down's syndrome

Incidence ~1/600–700 live births (incidence increases with advancing maternal age).

Cause

The great majority (~95%) of babies with Down's syndrome have trisomy 21, usually due to non-disjunction during maternal oogenesis.
- 72%—the result of a Robertsonian translocation.
- 72% mosaic, with normal cell line, as well as trisomy 21 cell line.

Clinical features

Usually presents at birth with:
- *Generalized hypotonia* and marked head lag.
- *Facial features:* small, low-set ears, up-slanting eyes, prominent epicanthic folds, a flat facial profile, protruding tongue. Later Brushfield's spots apparent in the iris (whitish spots).
- *Flat occiput* (brachycephaly) and short neck.
- *Typical limb features:* short, broad hands (brachydactyly); short, incurved little fingers (clinodactyly); single transverse palmar crease; and a wide 'sandal' gap between the first and second toes.
- *Mildly short stature.*
- *Intellectual impairment* becomes apparent; IQ range 25–70.
- *Social skills:* often exceed other intellectual skills.

Associated conditions

- CHD (~40–50%): most commonly AVSD, ASD, VSD, ToF.
- GI problems include: duodenal atresia, anal atresia, and HSD.
- Risk of infection.
- Developmental hip dysplasia.
- Eczema.
- Deafness: both SN and conductive.
- Cataracts.
- Leukaemia (1%). (See also ➔ Leukaemia and Down's syndrome, p. 593.)
- Acquired hypothyroidism.

Diagnosis

If there is clinical suspicion of Down's syndrome, a senior paediatrician should discuss their concerns with the parents. The diagnosis is confirmed by chromosome analysis showing an additional chromosome 21. Most cytogenetics laboratories are able to offer a rapid analysis, usually by microarray.

Management

- *Specialist referrals:* detailed cardiac assessment, hip USS, and audiology and ophthalmology (1- to 2-yearly).
- *Genetic counselling* by a clinical geneticist should be offered. It is not necessary to undertake parental chromosome analysis if the cause is non-disjunctional trisomy 21 or mosaic trisomy 21, but this is very important if the karyotype shows a translocation. Remember that an array will NOT distinguish between a translocation and a non-disjunctional trisomy.
- Putting the parents in contact with a support organization, such as the *Down's Syndrome Association*, is often helpful (ℛ http://www.downs-syndrome.org.uk and ℛ http://www.ndss.org).
- *Long-term follow-up* should be by an MDT led by a paediatrician with special expertise in child development. Physiotherapy to improve tone and posture is often required.
- Test *TFTs annually.*
- Almost all children with Down's syndrome are now educated in mainstream schools, with appropriate educational support.

Prognosis

If deaths from CHD are excluded, life expectancy is well into adult life, although somewhat shortened as almost all develop Alzheimer's disease by age 40y. The majority of adults can live semi-independently with supervision.

Common chromosomal disorders

Down's syndrome

(See → Down's syndrome, pp. 872–3.)

Klinefelter's syndrome (47, XXY)

- Affects ~1/600 to 1/800 boys; majority caused by non-disjunction during maternal oogenesis.
- *Diagnosis* by chromosome analysis.
- Boys with Klinefelter's syndrome:
  - Enter puberty normally, but by mid puberty, the testes begin to involute and the boys develop hypergonadotrophic hypogonadism with ↓ testosterone production (often tall and may develop feminine body build).
  - Testes are small in adult life and men with Klinefelter's syndrome are generally infertile (azoospermia).
  - Gynaecomastia develops at puberty in ≥50%.
  - IQ ~15 points lower than their siblings.
- Many boys with Klinefelter's syndrome remain undiagnosed throughout childhood, with the diagnosis only coming to light during investigation of infertility.

Patau syndrome (trisomy 13)

- Incidence is ~1/12 500 live births; ~75% caused by non-disjunction during maternal oogenesis; ~20% Robertsonian translocation; ~5% result from mosaicism.
- *Diagnosis* confirmed by chromosome analysis (additional chromosome 13). Most cytogenetics laboratories are able to offer a rapid analysis. This is usually by microarray. Antenatal USS needed, since the majority of affected babies have multiple anomalies.
- Typical malformations include:
  - Holoprosencephaly.
  - SGA.
  - Microcephaly.
  - Microphthalmia.
  - Cleft lip/palate.
  - CHD (e.g. ASD or VSD).
  - Renal anomalies (e.g. fused kidneys).
  - Post-axial polydactyly.
  - IQ: severe/profound mental retardation.
- If there is clinical suspicion of trisomy 13, a senior paediatrician should discuss their concerns with the parents. Median survival is 8.5 days, based on UK data. However, there are occasional exceptions, who may survive many years.

Edwards' syndrome (trisomy 18)
- Incidence is ~1/8000 births, caused by non-disjunction during maternal oogenesis.
- *Diagnosis* confirmed by chromosome analysis, and beware that array analysis will not detect translocation-associated cases.
- Babies usually:
  - SGA (mean birthweight 2240g), with an OFC <3rd centile.
  - Other common features include: CHD (usually VSD ± valve dysplasia), short sternum, overriding fingers, and 'rocker-bottom' feet.
  - Strong ♀ excess.
- Median life expectancy is 74 days, although some affected babies live for several months.
- If there is clinical suspicion of trisomy 18, a senior paediatrician should discuss their concerns with the parents.

Turner's syndrome (45, X)
(See ➲ Turner's syndrome, p. 884.)

Genetic disorders with cardiac features

Many chromosomal disorders and genetic syndromes are characterized by CHD.

Deletion 22q11 syndrome/velocardiofacial syndrome/di George syndrome

- Incidence is ~1/4000.
- Caused by a microdeletion on chromosome 22q11.2. Most children have a *de novo* microdeletion, but in ~15%, the condition is inherited from an affected parent.
- Apart from cardiac defects, usually involving the aortic arch, features include subtle dysmorphism (wide and prominent nasal bridge, down-slanting eyes, small mouth), parathyroid aplasia/hypoplasia (hypocalcaemia), and thymus aplasia (T-cell deficiency). Short stature is common.
- Consider this condition in all children diagnosed with ToF or aortic arch abnormalities, e.g. interrupted aortic arch (~20% will have del(22q11)).
- Also consider in any child with CHD, e.g. VSD, who has hypernasal speech, cleft palate, including submucous cleft palate (may present as nasal regurgitation of milk), hypocalcaemia, asymmetric crying facies, recurrent infections, or learning difficulties, especially speech and language delay.
- Diagnosis will be missed on routine chromosome analysis; it requires FISH study. It is best identified by microarray analysis.

Marfan's syndrome

(See also → Marfan's syndrome and related disorders, p. 690.)
- Incidence ~1/5000 births.
- Variable AD multisystem disorder caused by mutation in the *FBN1* gene on chromosome 15q. There is high new mutation rate (~30%).
- *Features include:* tall and slim body build with long limbs, pectus malformation of the sternum, scoliosis, high narrow palate, long fingers (arachnodactyly), and joint laxity. Most affected children are myopic and some may develop lens dislocation (a major diagnostic feature).
- *Cardiac features:* initially, there may be a floppy mitral valve. With time, dilatation of the aortic root (another major diagnostic feature) may occur, leading eventually to ascending aortic aneurysm and aortic dissection. Treatment with losartan has greatly improved the outlook in terms of stabilizing aortic aneurysms.
- If genetic confirmation of the diagnosis is required, this may be possible (in conjunction with a clinical geneticist) by mutation analysis of the *FBN1* gene.

Noonan's syndrome

- Incidence ~1/2500 births.
- *AD disorder:* NS is genetically heterogenous, with ~50% caused by mutation in the *PTPN11* gene on chromosome 12q. Mutation in several other genes in the RAS/MAP kinase pathway have been reported in other NS cases and in clinically overlapping disorders of cardio-facio-cutaneous syndrome and Costello syndrome.
- *Features:* short stature, typical facial features (hypertelorism, ptosis, ear abnormalities), broad neck, CHD (especially pulmonary stenosis), cardiomyopathy, chest malformation with pectus carinatum superiorly and pectus excavatum inferiorly, mild developmental delay, and undescended testes.
- Genetic confirmation of diagnosis is possible (in conjunction with a clinical geneticist) for some children by mutation analysis of the *PTPN11* gene. In practice, most laboratories will offer molecular analysis of a panel of NS-related genes. Parental clinical assessment and counselling are for a clinical genetics setting.

Williams syndrome

- Incidence is 1/7500 live births.
- Caused by a microdeletion on chromosome 7q11 that encompasses the elastin gene.
- Associated cardiac defect is supravalvular aortic stenosis, often with peripheral pulmonary branch stenosis.
- Facial features include: periorbital fullness, full cheeks, anteverted nares, wide mouth with full lips, and small and widely spaced teeth. Most have mild mental retardation, with strengths in language, but poor visuospatial skills.
- The typical behavioural phenotype is that of overfriendliness, short attention span, and anxiety.
- ~15% of infants have hypercalcaemia.
- Diagnosis is by microarray which will establish the characteristic microdeletion of 7q11.
- For further information, including growth charts, see: ♫ http://www.williams-syndrome.org/.

Genetic testing in cognitive impairment

Amongst children with severe mental retardation, a high proportion will have a genetic cause. In the absence of a family history, *de novo* chromosomal events or, indeed, new mutations within specific genes will account for most cases. These investigations and the interpretation of the resulting data are highly specialized and open to misinterpretation. Accordingly, such investigation is best undertaken in a clinical genetics environment. Referral to clinical genetics should be considered for all children with unexplained severe GDD/mental retardation. The referring paediatrician may undertake some basic diagnostic genetic testing, including the following:

- *Microarray analysis:* whereas ~10% of all cases of mental retardation are due to a gross chromosomal abnormality, arrays have shown that a chromosomal basis can be demonstrated in an additional 10–15% of cases.
- *Fragile X analysis:* this is the commonest cause of inherited learning disability but remains a rare disorder. As it is often difficult to diagnose on clinical grounds, genetic testing should be offered to all children with developmental delay. This requires a specific molecular analysis not covered by microarray or WES.
- *CK in boys:* DMD may present with speech delay and delayed motor milestones and/or global delay.
- *TFTs:* children born in the UK should have been tested for congenital hypothyroidism on the newborn blood spot screen. If this result was normal (needs confirmation), repeat investigation is not required, unless there are clinical signs suggestive of hypothyroidism.
- *Amino and organic acids:* IEM are individually rare but may present with non-specific features, e.g. developmental delay and/or FTT. Plasma and urine samples should be arranged if there are developmental regression, episodic decompensation, parental consanguinity, family history, or physical examination findings consistent with a metabolic disorder (e.g. microcephaly, macrocephaly, hepatosplenomegaly). 'Non-specific' abnormalities are commoner than true diagnoses.
- *Urine glycosaminoglycans* (MPS): consider if developmental regression, glue ear, coarse features, and macrocephaly.
- *Ophthalmological opinion:* especially if there is concern regarding vision, eye signs (e.g. nystagmus), neurological signs, and microcephaly.
- *Audiology assessment:* especially if there is speech delay or concern regarding hearing.
- *Consider congenital infection:* in children with IUGR, microcephaly, and eye/hearing signs. Requires comparison of maternal booking and current maternal serology. Useful for children up to ~18mth of age.

Angelman syndrome

- Incidence ~1/40 000.
- AS is caused by impaired or absent function of the maternally imprinted *UBE3A* gene on chromosome 15q11.13.
- Severe developmental delay, speech impairment, ataxic and wide-based gait, and specific behavioural phenotype (excitable personality, hand-flapping, and inappropriately happy affect). Seizures common.
- The genetics of AS are complex. Refer to a clinical geneticist.

Fragile X syndrome (FRAXA)

- Incidence ~1/5500 ♂; commonest inherited cause of mental retardation.
- Caused by a full expansion (>200 repeats) in the (CGG)n triplet repeat in the *FRAXA* gene on chromosome Xq27.3.
- Boys with FRAXA typically have GDD, often with gaze avoidance, stereotyped repetitive behaviours such as hand-flapping, and resistance to change of routines.
- Up to 50% of girls with full FRAXA expansion have learning/behavioural difficulties similar to affected boys, but less severe.
- Genetic counselling is complex and there will be genetic implications for relatives. Referral to a clinical geneticist is recommended.

Prader–Willi syndrome

(See ⊃ Prader–Willi syndrome, p. 885.)

Rett's syndrome

- Affects ~1/10 000 ♀ births.
- Caused by mutation in the *MECP2* gene on Xq28. Girls with Rett's syndrome appear normal in the first 6mth of life.
- Severe neurodevelopmental disorder. Almost exclusively girls. Presents >1y, usually with developmental regression and loss of purposeful hand movements. May develop seizures, scoliosis, erratic breathing with episodes of breath-holding and hyperventilation, and stereotypic hand-wringing.

Smith–Magenis syndrome

- Affects at least 1/25 000 children.
- Usually caused by *de novo* microdeletion on chromosome 17p11.2.
- Features: broad face, mid-face hypoplasia, brachydactyly, obesity, and developmental delay/learning disability with behavioural disturbance, especially of sleep (night-time waking, daytime somnolence).
- Most cases identified by microarray. However, cases due to an intragenic mutation within the *RAI1* gene wikll require molecular analysis of the gene to confirm (undertaken by clinical genetics).

Williams syndrome

(See ⊃ Williams syndrome, p. 877.)

Genetic disorders with neuromuscular features

The majority of severe neuromuscular disorders affecting infants and children have a genetic basis. In addition to accurate assessment and examination of the child, a detailed family history and examination of the parents may sometimes be very helpful in establishing the diagnosis.

Congenital myotonic dystrophy

(See ➲ Muscular dystrophy, p. 390.)

- Caused by a triplet repeat expansion (CTG)n in the *myotonin* gene on chromosome 19q. Congenitally affected infants usually have a huge expansion of the triplet repeat with >1000 repeats.
- Occurs in affected babies born to women who also have myotonic dystrophy (an AD disorder with onset usually in adult life), even when mild or undiagnosed.
- Typically, there is polyhydramnios and at delivery the baby is floppy and may require prolonged ventilatory support.
- Diagnosis is usually possible by careful examination of the mother (percussion myotonia) (also enquire if the mother sleeps with the eyes open) and analysis of a DNA sample from the infant.
- Useful to establish if there has been early onset of cataracts—common in patients with myotonic dystrophy in their 20s and 30s and extraordinarily unusual in the general population <50y.
- Neonatal mortality is ~20%. Survivors have static or slowly progressive weakness. Most have associated intellectual impairment.

Duchenne muscular dystrophy

(See ➲ Duchenne muscular dystrophy, p. 390.)

- Affects ~1/3500 ♂ births—DMD is the commonest and most severe form of childhood muscular dystrophy.
- Caused by mutations (deletions, duplications, and point mutations) in the *dystrophin* gene on chromosome Xq28.
- Presents with developmental delay, especially late walking and speech delay. In the early phase of the disease, boys have difficulty rising from the floor (Gower's manoeuvre sign where the child climbs up his thighs with his hands to get up off the floor). Later there is early loss of ambulation (mean age ~9y). Affected boys develop progressive cardiomyopathy. ~30% of boys with DMD have mild learning disability that is not progressive.
- Serum CK is grossly elevated, usually >10 times normal levels. Diagnosis is usually possible by genetic testing, avoiding the need for muscle biopsy.
- DMD follows X-linked recessive inheritance and expert genetic counselling is an essential part of management. One-third of cases represent new mutation.
- Death from cardiorespiratory failure or infection usually occurs in the late teens or early 20s.

Spinal muscular atrophy

(See ➔ Spinal muscular atrophies, p. 385.)

- An AR disorder caused by bi-allelic mutation in the *SMN* gene on 5q13. ~95% of infants with SMA type 1 are homozygously deleted for exon 7 of the *SMN1* gene.
- In severe cases, babies usually feed normally for the first few weeks, with the earliest sign often being of a tiring infant who does not finish his feed. Clinical examination may show fasciculations of the tongue, an important clinical indicator.
- Develop symmetrical proximal muscle weakness as a consequence of degeneration of the anterior horn cells of the spinal cord. Intelligence is unaffected.
- Several types:
  - SMA type 1 (severe)—onset in first few months of life. Never able to sit or walk. Historically, usually die from respiratory failure by age 6–12mth.
  - SMA type 2 (intermediate)—onset before age 18mth. Able to sit, but not to walk unaided. Survival into adult life is usual.
  - SMA type 3 (mild)—onset of proximal muscle weakness after age 2y. Ability to walk independently initially; survival into adult life.
- Diagnosis can be made by molecular genetic testing.

Genetic disorders with dermatological features

Sometimes it is the cutaneous features that are the key to diagnosis of a genetic disorder (see also ➲ Chapter 21).

Ehlers–Danlos syndrome

(See ➲ Ehlers–Danlos syndrome, p. 691.)
- Incidence ~1/5000 births.
- There are several types of EDS. Classical EDS is AD and caused by mutation in the *COL5A1* and *COL5A2* genes.
- All forms of EDS characterized by skin fragility, unsightly bruising and scarring, musculoskeletal discomfort, and susceptibility to osteoarthritis. The skin is soft and hyperextensible, with easy bruising and thin, atrophic 'cigarette paper' scars, joint hypermobility, varicose veins, and a risk of premature delivery in affected fetuses.
- Hypermobile EDS: common and usually mild AD disorder characterized by soft skin with hypermobility of large and small joints.

Neurofibromatosis type 1

(See ➲ Neurofibromatosis, p. 383; ➲ Neurofibromatosis, p. 423.)
- NF1 has a prevalence of ~1/4000.
- AD condition caused by mutation in the *NF1* gene on 17q11.2.
- Clinical diagnosis: the patient should have ≥2 of the following:
  - ≥6 café-au-lait spots (≥0.5cm in children).
  - ≥2 neurofibromata of any type (dermal neurofibromata are small lumps in the skin that appear in adolescence) or one or more plexiform neurofibromata.
  - Freckling in the axilla, neck, or groin.
  - Optic glioma (tumour in the optic pathway).
  - ≥2 Lisch nodules (benign iris hamartomas).
  - A distinctive bony lesion, e.g. sphenoid wing dysplasia or dysplasia or thinning of the long bone cortex (e.g. pseudoarthrosis).
  - A first-degree relative with NF1.
- NF1 is a highly variable disorder, with a small risk of serious complications (e.g. scoliosis), pressure effects of tumours or malignant change (e.g. neural crest tumours), and hypertension (due to renal artery stenosis or phaeochromocytoma). Regular surveillance (e.g. annual review) is recommended to try and detect these early and facilitate early intervention.

X-linked hypohidrotic ectodermal dysplasia

The condition follows X-linked recessive inheritance and is caused by mutation in the *EDA-1* gene. Boys have reduced/absent sweating that may cause dangerous hyperpyrexia in infancy. Carrier ♀ may be mildly affected. Absent eyebrows are an easy clue in affected boys.

Tuberous sclerosis complex

(See also ➔ Tuberous sclerosis complex, p. 382.)

- Affects ~1/10 000 individuals.
- A highly variable AD multisystem disorder caused by mutation in the *TSC1* gene on 9q or the *TSC2* gene on 16p.
- Characterized by hamartomas in the brain, skin, and other organs.
- Commonly presents with infantile spasms. Seizures and mental retardation are often associated.
- Hypomelanotic macules ('ash-leaf' spots) occur in ~95% of affected individuals by the age of 5y. Wood's light (ultraviolet) may be needed to visualize these. Angiofibromata occur in later childhood in a butterfly distribution over the nose and cheeks. Other cutaneous features include forehead fibrous plaque, shagreen patches, ungual fibromata, and dental pits.
- 50% of individuals with TSC have normal intelligence, but children who develop infantile spasms and severe epilepsy in the first year of life often have learning disability.
- Thorough clinical evaluation, e.g. cranial MRI, eye exam, renal USS, is indicated to make the diagnosis prior to genetic testing.
- Expert genetic advice, with careful evaluation of the parents, is important. ~60% of cases arise as a result of new mutations.
- Genetic testing is possible by mutation analysis of *TSC1* and *TSC2*, but it is helpful to establish a clear clinical diagnosis before embarking on genetic testing.
- Useful to be aware that the *TSC2* gene is adjacent to *PKD1* (polycystic kidney disease on chromosome 16) and there are patients who have features of both disorders.

Incontinentia pigmenti

- Rare X-linked dominant disorder caused by mutation in the *NEMO* gene on Xq28 (~80% carry a common deletion).
- Affected ♂ pregnancies almost invariably miscarry. Girls present in the neonatal period with blistering lesions, cropping circumferentially on the trunk and in a linear distribution on the limbs. Ultimately, lesions regress by late childhood/adult life to leave atrophic streaky areas of pigmentation or hypopigmentation (often most noticeable on the back of the calves). The child remains well and continues to feed. There is often marked eosinophilia in the blood.
- ~50% have associated abnormalities of the dentition, eye (cataracts), or CNS (seizures, microcephaly).
- Genetic testing is possible; ~80% of affected individuals carry a large deletion in the *NEMO* gene.
- No specific treatment available.

Genetic disorders of growth

Assessment of growth plays an important role in deciding whether a child may have an underlying genetic disorder. Measurements <0.4th centile or >99.6th centile nearly always merit further assessment, unless there is a clear explanation. Measurements between the 0.4th and 2nd centiles or 98th and 99.6th centiles need to be interpreted in context and may be clinically significant. If in doubt, discuss with a senior colleague.

Intrauterine growth retardation

Silver–Russell syndrome

- Incidence is unclear (1/3000–100 000 births). Equal sex ratio.
- ~10% of children have maternal UPD7.
- Genetically heterogenous condition characterized by intrauterine and postnatal growth retardation, with short stature and FTT. Typically, babies have disproportionately large head (OFC usually 3rd–25th centile), triangular facies, down-turned mouth, and some asymmetry of limbs.
- About 30–50% of cases will show hypomethylation of the paternal chromosome at the imprinting centre 1 (IC1) on 11p15.5.

Cornelia de Lange syndrome

- Rare; incidence ~1/50 000 live births.
- Intrauterine and postnatal growth impairment, limb anomalies, microcephaly, hirsutism, and distinctive facial features (neat, arched eyebrows; short, upturned nose; thin lips with down-turned corners of the mouth).
- ~60% of affected children have mutations in the gene *NIPBL* on chromosome 5p13.

Short stature

Turner's syndrome

(See also Ɔ Turner's syndrome, p. 443.)
- Affects ~1/2500 ♀.
- Most girls have a single X chromosome (45, X), usually due to non-disjunction.
- As well as short stature, the typical phenotype includes: neck webbing, ptosis, wide carrying angle at elbows (cubitus valgus), widely spaced hypoplastic nipples, low posterior hairline, and excessive pigmented naevi. Puffiness of the hands and feet is a common neonatal finding.
- Associated abnormalities include: CHD (15–50%), especially CoA and VSD; structural renal anomalies (~30%), e.g. horseshoe kidney or unilateral renal agenesis; and hypoplastic 'streak' ovaries (primary amenorrhoea and infertility).
- The phenotype can be subtle and is easily missed, and so chromosome analysis is advisable in girls with unexplained short stature.

Tall stature

Marfan's syndrome
(See ➔ Marfan's syndrome, p. 876.)

Obesity

Bardet–Biedl syndrome
- Rare condition; incidence in the UK population <1/100 000.
- Genetically heterogenous with multiple causal genes. In the majority of families, inheritance is AR.
- Features include: pigmentary retinopathy, post-axial polydactyly, obesity, cognitive impairment, and renal defects.
- Be aware that polydactyly can simply present as a tiny 'nubbin' on the lateral aspect of the fifth finger.

Prader–Willi syndrome
- Affects ~1/10 000 individuals.
- Caused by disruption to the paternally derived imprinted domain on 15q11–13.
- Babies are floppy with feeding difficulties and may fail to thrive in infancy. There is rapid weight gain between the ages of 1 and 6y.
- Older children have truncal obesity, mild/moderate learning difficulties, and short stature. Typically, children have an insatiable appetite with food foraging and other behavioural problems.
- Diagnosis is by molecular genetic analysis [small nuclear ribonucleoprotein polypeptide N (SNRPN) methylation assay].

Overgrowth

Beckwith–Wiedemann syndrome
- Incidence ~1/14 000.
- >10 times higher in children conceived by assisted reproduction.
- Genetic basis is complex—it is caused by disruption of the imprinted region on chromosome 11p15.
- Usually presents in the perinatal period with macrosomia. Birthweight is usually >97th centile and length is usually > +2 SD. Polyhydramnios or preterm delivery commonly occur.
- Associated congenital anomalies: exomphalos, umbilical hernia, dysmorphic features (e.g. earlobe creases, helical pits, facial haemangioma, macroglossia, visceromegaly, hemihypertrophy).
- Neonates are at risk of hypoglycaemia and should be monitored.
- Macrosomia continues through early childhood and then becomes less dramatic with increasing age.
- Some children are at ↑ risk of Wilms' tumour. Regular US surveillance is often warranted up to age 6y.
- In ~50%, diagnosis can be confirmed by molecular genetic testing. Uniparental disomy 11p15 analysis requires blood testing of child and both parents.

Sotos syndrome
- Incidence ~1/15 000 children.
- Due to mutation or deletion in the *NSD1* gene on chromosome 5q35. Most are isolated *de novo* mutations, but familial cases occur.
- Characterized by prenatal overgrowth (birthweight ~4200g in ♂; ~4000g in ♀), which persists in childhood, especially through the preschool years. Final adult height is often in the upper normal range. OFC is also ↑ and bone age is advanced. Affected children typically have a tall skull with a prominent broad forehead and a pointed chin. Developmental delay is almost always present but varies from mild to severe. Some children have seizures.

Macroglossia

Tongue enlargement that leads to functional and cosmetic problems. Although it is a relatively uncommon disorder, it may cause significant morbidity. Macroglossia may be congenital or acquired in origin.

Congenital
- Down's syndrome (see → Down's syndrome, pp. 872–3).
- BWS (see → Beckwith–Wiedemann syndrome, p. 885).
- MPS (see → Chapter 12).

Acquired
- Congenital hypothyroidism (see → Congenital hypothyroidism, p. 410).

In infants, macroglossia poses early difficulty with feeding, and in the longer term, children may need assistance with speech and language therapy.

Skeletal dysplasias

Achondroplasia

- *Macrocephaly*, alongside short stature (OFC >98th, birth length <5th).
- *Limb shortening* is symmetrical. All limbs are affected and the shortening is predominantly rhizomelic (affects the most proximal elements—humerus and femur).
- *Trunk* looks proportionately elongated.
- Occasional association with acanthosis nigricans.
- Characteristic radiological features.
- Associated with older fathers (>45y).
- >98% are due to one of two point mutations within the *FGFR3* gene.
- Clinical risk of cord compression by narrow foramen magnum and associated neurological decompensation.

The condition is generally easy to diagnose clinically. Confirm radiologically in discussion with an experienced paediatric radiologist. Molecular confirmation is then simply for completeness.

Miscellaneous genetic conditions

(See Table 24.1.)

Table 24.1 Miscellaneous genetic conditions

Syndrome	Features	Inheritance	Chromosome	Gene
Apert	Craniostenosis, beaked nose, cleft palate, severe syndactyly ('mitten hand'), ↓ IQ	AD	10q26	FGFR2
CHARGE	Coloboma, congenital Heart disease, choanal Atresia, Retarded growth (short stature), hypoGenitals, external Ear abnormality and deafness	AD (usually *de novo*)	8q12	CHD7
5p– (cri du chat)	Hypoplastic larynx (cat-like cry), small stature, microcephaly, micrognathia, low-set ears, hypertelorism, ↓ IQ	Sporadic	5p deletion (5p–)	
Crouzon	Craniostenosis, brachycephaly, prominent forehead, proptosis, beaked nose	AD	10q26	FGFR2
Holt–Oram	Hypoplastic thumbs ± radius, ASD, VSD	AD	12q	TBX5
Primary AR microcephaly	Sloping forehead, OFC << 0.4th centile (<4 SDs), moderate mental retardation	AR	Various	MCPH1
Smith–Lemli–Opitz	Ptosis, anteverted nostrils, narrow frontal region, hypospadias, toe syndactyly, ↓ IQ	AR	11q12–13	DHCR7
Thanatophoric dysplasia	Large head, small thorax, short limbs, lethal	Sporadic	4p16	FGFR3
Treacher Collins	Malar hypoplasia, micrognathia, down-slanting eyes, ear malformations, deafness, lower eyelid coloboma	AD	5q32	TCOF1
Zellweger	Prominent forehead, large fontanelles, flat facies, hypotonia, stippled epiphyses, nystagmus, hepatomegaly	AR	Various	PEX1-14

Miscellaneous congenital malformations

(See Table 24.2.)

Table 24.2 Miscellaneous congenital malformations

Condition	Features	Cause
Amniotic bands	Congenital facial clefts, limb constrictions, amputations, syndactyly or talipes	Annular amniotic bands
Diabetic embryopathy	Macrosomia, organomegaly (particularly heart and liver), polycythaemia, caudal regression syndrome (sacral and femoral agenesis or hypoplasia), transient hypertrophic cardiomyopathy, neural tube defects, pre-axial polydactyly of the foot	Maternal diabetes mellitus
Fetal compression syndrome	Joint contractions/dislocation, talipes, micrognathia, cleft palate, skull deformity	In utero compression, e.g. maternal pelvic abnormality
Fetal alcohol syndrome	IUGR, hirsutism, microcephaly, mid-face hypoplasia, short palpebral fissures, long smooth philtrum, ↓ IQ, low weight for height. Occasional agenesis of the corpus callosum	Excessive maternal alcohol ingestion in pregnancy
Fetal anticonvulsant syndrome	2–3 times increase in major malformations, growth retardation, mid-face hypoplasia, ↓ IQ. Maternal valproate causes a 10-fold ↑ incidence of neural tube defects	Maternal anticonvulsant therapy in pregnancy
Goldenhar syndrome	Asymmetric facial hypoplasia, eye coloboma/dermoid, ear hypoplasia, pre-auricular skin tags, vertebral defects, cardiac defects (ToF, VSD)	Unknown. Usually sporadic
Klippel–Feil syndrome	Cervical vertebral fusion, low hairline, webbed neck, torticollis, kyphoscoliosis, deafness	Usually sporadic
Moebius syndrome	Immobile face, strabismus, limb defects, syndactyly	Usually sporadic, possibly reflecting vascular compromise. Associated with cocaine use, misoprostol, and vasoconstriction
Pierre–Robin sequence (see ⊃ p. 809)	Micrognathia, glossoptosis, cleft palate	Unknown (need to exclude del22q11). Usually sporadic

(Continued)

Table 24.2 (Contd.)

Condition	Features	Cause
Potter's sequence	Depressed nasal bridge, crumpled low-set ears, talipes equinovarus, joint contractures, lung hypoplasia, and respiratory failure. Lethal	Severe oligohydramnios due to renal or urethral abnormalities
VATER association (see ⮩ Box 22.1)	Vertebral defects, Anal atresia, Tracheo-oEsophageal fistula, Renal defects (VACTERL = additional cardiac and radial limb defects)	Unknown. Usually sporadic

References

1. Firth HV, Hurst JA. *Oxford Desk Reference: Clinical Genetics and Genomics*, second edition. Oxford University Press, Oxford; 2017.

Further reading

The human genome contains 725 000 genes, so the few common genetic disorders in this section are a very tiny sample from an enormous range of genetic disorders. Other useful resources for information include the following.

General text

Cassidy SB, Allanson JE (eds). *Management of Genetic Syndromes*, third edition. Wiley, New York, NY; 2010.

For specific clinical signs, see Reardon W. *The Bedside Dysmorphologist: A Guide to Identifying and Assessing Congenital Malformations*, second edition. Oxford University Press, New York, NY; 2016.

Jones KL. *Smith's Recognizable Patterns of Human Malformation*. WB Saunders, Philadelphia, PA; 2005.

Reardon W. *The Bedside Dysmorphologist: A Guide to Identifying and Assessing Congenital Malformations*, second edition. Oxford University Press, New York, NY; 2016.

Web-based resources

Contact a Family (UK). Available at: ℬ http://www.cafamily.org.uk.

GeneReviews (now active as the amalgamation of GenClinics and GeneTests). Available at: ℬ https://omictools.com/genereviews-tool.

Genetic Alliance UK. *NHS genetic services in the UK*. Available at: ℬ https://geneticalliance.org.uk/information/services-and-testing/nhs-genetic-services-in-the-uk/.

National Organization for Rare Disorders (US). Available at: ℬ http://www.rarediseases.org.

Online Mendelian Inheritance in Man (OMIM). Available at: ℬ http://www.ncbi.nlm.nih.gov.

Orphanet. Available at: ℬ http://www.orpha.net.

Community child health

Voluntary and charitable organizations

Many different services are available and there is often a close connection between these and statutory agencies, particularly for children with disabilities.

- *Homestart:* volunteers offer support in the family's own home to families who have children aged <5y.
- *Mencap:* long-established national charity for learning disabilities—all ages and causes.
- *Scope:* national charity with focus on CP.
- *National Autistic Society.*
- *Contact a Family:* advice for families with disabled children.

Organizations and structures

The following agencies are responsible for the organization and delivery of child health services in the community.

Primary health care team

- The GP.
- Practice nurses.
- Midwives.
- Health visitor and community nursery nurses.
- School nurses for mainstream and special schools.
- District nurses.

The local authority

The local authority has responsibilities for the administration and delivery of education and social care.
- The *Children Act 2004* requires that local authorities have a director for children's services and a lead member responsible for children.
- In the UK, *central government* is responsible for national policies and guidance and for overseeing standards via various means of inspection, but local needs determine what services are available.

Education

In the UK, there are two levels of services:
- *Central and administrative level* (local authority departments):
  - Provide support to schools (includes educational psychology, specialist teachers for learning, behaviour, senses, and educational welfare).
  - Responsible for initiation, coordination, and provision of statement of special educational needs, according to the 2001 Special Educational Needs and Disability Act.
- *Schools and nurseries:*
  - Are directly managed by their governing body.
  - Have a special educational needs coordinator (SENCO).
  - Are allocated some funds to support children with special needs.
  - Have access to specialist educational services.
  - Are given extra resources, as specified in statements of special educational needs, for individual children within the school.

Specialist paediatric services

Include paediatricians in hospital and the community, as well as:
- *Specialist nurses:* e.g. diabetes, epilepsy, asthma.
- *Community paediatric nursing teams:* who provide nursing care at home and in other settings for children with complex needs.

Health surveillance and promotion

Disease prevention includes the following:
- *Primary prevention:* immunizations, accident prevention, dental.
- *Secondary prevention:* screening for inherited conditions.
- *Tertiary prevention:* reducing impairments and disabilities (e.g. hip dislocation in CP, hypothyroidism and hearing problems in children with Down's syndrome).

Primary prevention programmes

These are designed to reduce the number of new cases of disease and disorder presenting within the community.

> **Examples of primary prevention programmes**
> - Reducing the incidence of infectious diseases—immunization programme (see ⊃ Immunization, p. 652).
> - Reducing the risk of sudden infant death.
> - Reducing parental smoking.
> - Preventing accidents and poisonings.
> - Improving nutrition—breastfeeding promotion.
> - Preventing dental disease.
> - Promoting child development.
> - Preventing child abuse.

A range of early intervention programmes are designed to promote child development, reduce the risks of child abuse and accidental injury, and improve parents' mental health. Children's centres provide a variety of services to preschool children and their families, and often are a base for different organizations and services. Programmes for:
- *Parents and family:* primary prevention aimed at parents and the family (e.g. poor housing, poverty, illness, disability).
- *At-risk groups:* target at-risk groups (e.g. LBW babies, mothers with postnatal depression, families in poverty).
- *Young first-time mothers:* group parenting support focusing on behaviour management, some given by skilled professionals.

Secondary prevention

These programmes reduce the prevalence of disease:
- *Child Health Promotion Programme (UK):* remit of primary care, with government guidance recommending universal focus, with additional services for those with specific needs and risks.
- *Antenatal screening:* very important component of secondary prevention, beginning in early pregnancy and is universal at 28wk gestation with an ↑ focus on those women at higher risk or families requiring extra support or services (see Table 25.1).

Table 25.1 An approach to child health surveillance

Age	Screening procedure
Soon after birth	General examination and emphasis on eyes, heart, and hips
5–6 days	Blood spot test (see ⊃ Newborn screening, p. 511)
6–8wk old	Examination with emphasis on eyes, heart, and hips
By 1y	Health review
24–30mth	Review and promotion of development
4th to 5th birthday	Orthoptist assessment of vision to be phased in
School entry	Measurement of height and weight; hearing screening
Primary school	No further screening programme
Secondary school	No universal screening

Other opportunities for health professional contact include immunizations. Early detection of health problems is achieved by:
- Follow-up of babies at risk (e.g. LBW, premature).
- Follow-up of children with neurological problems or post-trauma.
- Targeted observation or follow-up of children with a strong family history of genetic disorders, e.g. hearing, vision, dislocated hips, learning difficulties, familial hypercholesterolaemia.
- Detection by parents or health professionals (i.e. neglect).
- Detection by professionals in the course of their work (particularly playgroup, nurseries, and schools, as well as health professionals).

Within each district, the preschool programme will vary according to what families need and will be targeted to those who are 'high risk'.

Particular concerns for preschool programmes
- First pregnancies and first-time mothers.
- Isolated mothers.
- Mother with postnatal depression.
- Unsupported young parent living in poverty.
- Domestic violence; drug or alcohol abuse.
- Parents with learning disability.
- Concern about child neglect or abuse.
- Infant with difficult feeding, sleeping, or temperament.
- Premature baby or child who is disabled.
- Refugee families.
- Smoking (pregnancy or postnatal).
- Obesity in parents.
- Poor attachment and inconsistent care.

Special educational needs

Twenty per cent of children have special educational needs at some time (see Box 25.1). Only 2% have a *statement of special educational needs*.

Box 25.1 Reasons for children having problems at school

- GDD (severe, detected preschool) (see ➲ Global neurodevelopmental delay, p. 733).
- General learning difficulties (see ➲ Learning difficulties/disabilities, p. 734).
- Specific learning difficulties (e.g. dyslexia, dyscalculia) (see ➲ Specific learning difficulties, p. 900).
- DCD (i.e. dyspraxia) (see ➲ Developmental coordination disorder, p. 900).
- Behavioural problems (see ➲ Operational defiant and conduct disorder, p. 755).
- Asperger's syndrome/high functioning autism (see ➲ Autism spectrum disorders, p. 757).
- Emotional difficulties (family, bullying, school phobia) (see ➲ Absence from school, p. 904).
- Depression in adolescents (see ➲ Depression, p. 744).
- Physical illness and disability.
- Chronic fatigue (see ➲ Chronic fatigue syndrome, p. 902–3).

Statutory UK assessment of special educational needs

The *Disability Discrimination Act* (1995) and amendments legislate no discrimination against people with disabilities. Schools implemented this Act in 2002. The *Special Educational Needs and Disability Act* (2001) requires:
- Promotion of the inclusion of such pupils in mainstream schools.
- A graduated response to assessment and help.
- Advice from other professionals, including health and education before statutory assessment.

Statutory assessment under the *Education Act*—UK

The assessment under the *Education Act* includes advice from:
- Parents and child.
- Health: a community paediatrician—'designated medical officer for education'; collates all medical and therapy advice.
- Education and educational psychology.
- Social services.

A provisional statement by the Education Department is seen by the parents before it is finalized (see ➲ Children with disabilities, p. 899). The annual review is required to ensure that targets and needs have not changed.

Children with disabilities

This includes children with physical and/or learning disabilities. Multi-agency assessments, including medical information and a management plan, are required.

- *'Key' worker* for these families should be identified in order to minimize disruption and coordinate care.
- *Early Support* is a national programme that has been developed to facilitate this process, and there is a wide range of information available for families and professionals to access.
- *Statement of special educational needs:* used in many severely disabled children—is an individual educational plan to identify targets and a means of achieving them, which is regularly reviewed.
- *Health needs:* other agencies, including therapists and doctors, must ensure that health needs are met. Therapy advice and targets are given to teachers and school support staff and are incorporated into the child's daily curriculum.

The UK *Children's Act* stipulates that children with disabilities may require additional services, e.g. social care and respite for the family.

Particular issues for families

- Home adaptations.
- Specialist equipment provision: standing frames, mobility, feeding, bathing, toileting.
- Augmentative communication: signing, symbols, speech aids, speech therapy.
- Financial support—may be eligible for:
  - Disability Living Allowance (not means-tested).
  - Invalid Carer's Allowance (dependent on income).
  - Mobility Allowance (related to level of physical and learning difficulty).
- Learning disabilities and challenging behaviours (common).
- Multiplicity of appointments.
- Lack of coordination of care.

Specific learning difficulties

Dyslexia

Children of normal intelligence who have not learnt to read despite exposure to adequate instruction:

- Aetiology uncertain; often family history; ♂:♀ 4–8:1.
- Cognitive processes involved include decoding (converting letter strings into sound sequences), encoding (spelling), and linguistic comprehension.
- Diagnosis is educational, but a child may have language difficulties and/or coordination difficulties.
- If severe, can lead to low self-esteem and school refusal.
- Dyslexia support societies (national and local) are often helpful.
- Specialist advice and support required from education.
- Paediatrician's role is limited to considering the diagnosis and excluding other conditions.

Dyscalculia

A specific learning disability affecting the acquisition of arithmetic skills. Less commonly recognized than dyslexia. Can coexist with writing difficulties and DCD.

Developmental coordination disorder

Previously referred to as dyspraxia or clumsy child syndrome. Defined as marked impairment in the development of motor abilities not explained by mental retardation and not due to a physical disorder. The diagnosis is only made if this impairment interferes with academic achievement or with activities of daily living:

- Prevalence: 10% of 8–12y olds; 1–3% of all children; ♂:♀ 4:1.
- For presenting features and signs, see Box 25.2.
- Characterized by perceptual difficulties that impede academic progress, e.g.:
  - Poor motor planning.
  - Poor visual–perceptual skills (discrimination, memory, visuospatial).
- Clinical assessment:
  - Neurological examination to exclude other conditions (mild CP, muscle disease).
  - Overlapping with other conditions, including autism and social skills problems.
  - May have additional learning difficulties.
- Treatment:
  - PT.
  - OT.
- Advice to school, as well as parents, is vital.

Box 25.2 Presenting features and signs of DCD

Presentation
- Poor motor skills.
- Difficulty using cutlery.
- Difficulty dressing and riding bike.
- Poor attention and organization.
- Problems with school progress (reading, copying, maths).
- Behaviour problems (disruptive, low self-esteem).

Signs
- Muscle tone may be low to normal.
- Poor balance.
- Poor coordination.
- Excess of overflow movement on effort.
- Persistence of primitive reflexes.
- Associated sensory difficulties: hypo-/hypersensitive to touch, sound, light, taste, and smell.

Chronic fatigue syndrome

CFS is defined as generalized fatigue persisting after routine tests and investigations have failed to identify an underlying cause. The fatigue in CFS may be associated with other symptoms:

- Difficulty in concentrating, cognitive dysfunction.
- Disturbed sleep.
- Fatigue (both mental and physical) exacerbated by effort.

The diagnosis should be made as soon as it is clear that the symptoms are causing functional impairment and no alternative explanation has been found (3mth in children).

Investigations

Routine investigations need to be undertaken to rule out plausible alternative causes. Second-line investigations are only undertaken if symptoms/signs or investigations suggest a particular diagnosis.

> **Investigations for chronic fatigue syndrome**
> - FBC and film, ESR.
> - Glucose, biochemistry, CK (muscle), LFTs.
> - TFTs.
> - Urine to exclude renal disease.
> - Screening tests for gluten sensitivity.
> - Assessment of ferritin levels.
> - EBV or viral tests only if history indicates recent infection.

An assessment of psychological well-being is essential and psychiatric disorders need to be excluded. Psychological morbidities, such as anxiety and depression, are common and important to recognize.

Management

There is no one single approach for all patients with CFS, but as a minimum, the following should be addressed.

Activity management

Establish baseline level and gradually increase as appropriate. Referral to PT and OT to supervise programme and treat symptoms. It is widely assumed that the correct approach is the use of graded activity and CBT, as supported by the literature in adults. However, some patients find it unacceptable to use psychological treatments and have found that any exercise is to be avoided. Parental mental illness, especially depression and anxiety, should be assessed. Treating these presentations may be important in a holistic treatment plan.

Other management
- Symptomatic treatment for pain and sleep.
- Dietary advice (e.g. poor appetite or weight gain due to immobility).
- Treatment for depression and mood disorders—need referral to child psychiatry team.

CFS and education

CFS causes significant disruption to school. The length of absence from school depends on severity and will range from part-time attendance to home tuition for many years. Liason with the school is essential in order to formulate a plan for return. Support in school may be needed for mobility or learning, and for some, a statement of special educational needs will be required. If the child is too unwell to attend school, home tuition can be organized with support from the paediatrician, but the maximum per week is usually a few hours and the child's needs should be monitored closely.

Prognosis

Severe or very severe CFS (housebound or bedridden ≥3mth) on rare occasions requires admission to hospital. In some cases, the condition persists for many years. Generally, though, outcome is favourable.

Absence from school

This may be due to long-term illness (10%). In many situations, absence from school may be the result of poor provision of extra support in class and/or information and training of the school staff. CFS is an important cause of school absence (see ➲ Chronic fatigue syndrome, pp. 902–3). Absence due to school refusal has a wide range of contributory factors (see Box 25.3).

> **Box 25.3 Factors contributing to refusal to go to school**
> - School phobia.
> - Anxiety concerning:
>   - Peers (bullying).
>   - Teachers.
>   - Difficulties with home life.
>   - Emotional problems.
> - Poor academic progress for whatever reason.
> - Truancy and antisocial behaviours.
> - Distressing symptoms such as soiling or wetting.

In most cases, a thorough medical assessment is needed to ascertain the cause of chronic or recurrent school absence. When it is thought appropriate, home tuition can be provided until the child returns to school.

Constipation and soiling

(See also ➔ Constipation, pp. 274–5.)

This is a common problem in childhood. Critical periods occur at around the time of infant weaning, toilet training, and starting school. Constipation may follow a period of dehydration, leading to hard stools that become painful to pass. The child therefore holds onto stool. Secondary soiling (overflow) is common and leads to anxiety at school that may lead to school refusal. It is important to review the past medical history for possible underlying reasons and causes of constipation.

Taking the history

Find out when the problem first arose. In infants, ask about:
- Delay in passage of meconium.
- Abdominal distension in early infancy.
- Explosive stools.

These are possible indicators of underlying HSD or short segment bowel (see ➔ Hirschsprung's disease, p. 832). Also ask about:
- Possible precipitants.
- Current diet and fluid intake.
- Psychological factors.
  - Coercive or chaotic toilet training.
  - Fear of toilet.
  - Parental neglect/discord/illness.
  - Environmental stressors.

Examination and investigations

Examination
- Inspect the anus for:
  - Fissures.
  - Infection.
  - Skin disease—excoriation/fistula.
  - Dilatation.
- Palpate the abdomen.
- General examination of the child, including growth—rarely presentation of hypothyroidism.

Investigations
- AXR (to demonstrate faecal loading)—not routinely needed for diagnosis; may be required for resistant constipation.
- Bloods:
  - FBC.
  - TFTs.
  - Coeliac screen.

Management

Throughout this time, parents and child will need considerable support from the nursing team (i.e. health visitor/school nurse/specialist nurse).

Short-term constipation with no soiling

- Soften retained stool, e.g. PO macrogols/Movicol®, lactulose, or docusate.
- PO colonic stimulant, e.g. PO senna. Continue until bowel pattern regular and then decrease.

Long-term and soiling

- Soften retained stools for at least a week, e.g. lactulose, docusate, macrogols/Movicol®.
- PO colonic stimulant, e.g. senna, single daily dose until stool passed.
- If no stool passed, consider using:
  - PO bowel evacuation preparation.
  - Enema.
  - Manual evacuation as a last resort (necessary if evidence of impaction).

Maintenance treatment

- Increase dietary fibre and fluid.
- Regular bulk laxative.
- Regular colonic stimulant.
- Persist with medication for at least 6mth.
- Behaviour management may be needed to establish toilet routine.
- Assessment by a clinical psychologist and family therapist if there is a degree of family discord.
- In resistant cases, treatment will need to be continued for longer.

Enuresis

Enuresis is involuntary emptying of the bladder. Although children may 'wet' themselves by day or night, the term enuresis is applied to nocturnal enuresis. When it occurs during the day, while awake, it is known as diurnal enuresis. Nocturnal enuresis is commoner.

In order to learn bladder control, the young child needs to overcome the infant automatic pattern of voiding. For the young child, conscious awareness of fullness and the ability to postpone voiding by suppressing the urge to void are not perfect. This response is first learnt for daytime control. Eventually, bladder control becomes automatic and does not require a conscious act. Night-time bladder control requires that the brain, during sleep, suppresses the automatic emptying reflex. Learning bladder control at night occurs gradually, and in some children and families, it takes much longer than average.

Girls achieve bladder control earlier than boys. Enuresis is defined as continued wetting in girls aged >5y and in boys >6y.

Enuresis may be primary, with children not having established an appropriate period of adequate bladder control in early childhood, or secondary occurring after a period of established bladder control.

Primary enuresis

- A strong family history.
- Boys more commonly than girls (ratio 2:1).
- 15% of 5y olds, 5% of 10y olds, and 1% of 16y olds have not established total bladder control and wet the bed once a week or more.
- Majority of cases have no underlying organic cause and it is thought to be due to delayed maturation of bladder control mechanisms.

Secondary enuresis

- Needs careful history and investigations because of probable organic cause.

Possible organic causes of secondary enuresis

- Renal tract: UTI.
- Neurological: spina bifida, spinal tumour.
- Endocrine: diabetes mellitus, DI.
- Behavioural problems.
- Abuse.
  Daytime wetting is usually caused by bladder detrusor instability.

History and investigations

History

Assess pattern and types of drink consumed:
- Often limited fluid in the day.
- Drink after school and evening.
- May have sugary drinks.

Voiding habits:
- Infrequent (<4 daily).
- Frequent (>7 daily).
- Dysfunctional/inappropriate place of voiding.

Investigations
- Urine testing for MC&S and glucose.
- USS of the renal tract: assess pre- and post-micturition bladder urine residual volume; any underlying anatomical abnormalities.

Treatment

Primary (nocturnal) enuresis
- Encourage regular drinks (water), but restrict in last hour before bed.
- Give drinking/voiding chart.

If primary nocturnal enuresis is associated with arousal from sleep or disturbance, then an enuresis alarm should be considered. This requires careful discussion with families. Compliance is often an issue and the family and child need to be motivated. If enuresis is associated with a small bladder, 'bladder training' exercises is the first-line approach. Also consider using bladder-stabilizing drugs (e.g. oxybutynin). If nocturnal enuresis and urine output exceeds bladder capacity, consider using desmopressin (ADH) and limit fluid intake 1h before bedtime.

If the problem is resistant to the above treatments, other pathologies need to be considered:
- Urinary outflow obstruction in boys.
- Chronic constipation.
- Neurodevelopmental problems.
- Psychological problems.

Further reading

General review

Hall DMB, Elliman D (eds). *Health for All Children*, fourth edition. Oxford University Press, Oxford; 2003.

Olds DL. The Nurse–Family Partnership: an evidence-based preventive intervention. *Infant Ment Health J* 2006; **27**: 5–25.

Acts

Department of Health. *The Child Health Promotion Programme*. London: Department of Health, London; 2008.

UK guidance

ERIC, The Children's Bowel and Bladder Charity. Includes enuresis and soiling information for parents and children, and useful for health professionals. Available at: ℞ https://www.eric.org.uk.

National Institute for Health and Care Excellence. (2007). *Chronic fatigue syndrome/myalgic encephalomyelitis (or encephalopathy): diagnosis and management*. Clinical guideline [CG53]. Available at: ℞ https://www.nice.org.uk/guidance/cg53.

National Institute for Health and Care Excellence. (2010). *Constipation in children and young people: diagnosis and management*. Clinical guideline [CG99]. Available at: ℞ https://www.nice.org.uk/guidance/cg99.

Chapter 26

Child safeguarding

Definitions

Child protection
The decisive action taken to safeguard children from harm.

Child abuse
This is defined as either:
- Deliberate infliction of harm to a child, or
- Failing to prevent harm to a child.

Children may be abused in the family home, in an institutional setting, or occasionally by a stranger. Most young people who are abused know their abuser. It is estimated that 1–2 children die each week due to abuse. Child abuse may be categorized as:
- Neglect.
- Physical (see ➲ Physical abuse, pp. 914–15).
- Sexual (see ➲ Sexual abuse, p. 916).
- Emotional (see ➲ Emotional abuse, p. 917).

Neglect
This is defined as a persistent failure to meet a child's basic physical or psychological needs that is likely to result in serious impairment of the child's health and development. Neglect may occur during pregnancy as a result of maternal substance abuse. Once a child is born, it may involve:
- Failing to provide adequate food.
- Failing to protect from physical harm or danger.
- Failure to access appropriate medical care or treatment.
- Failure to ensure adequate supervision.

Presentation
- FTT.
- Consistently unkempt and dirty appearance.
- Repeated failure by carers to prevent accidental injury.
- Lack of social responsiveness and/or developmental delay when there are other concerns about the environment at home.
- Medical advice is not sought, which compromises the health of the child, including if they are in ongoing pain.

Illness fabricated or induced by carers

This is an unusual form of child abuse. It was previously referred to as Munchausen syndrome by proxy. The salient feature is that the child is harmed by being presented for medical attention with symptoms or signs that have been falsified by the carer.
- The child is the victim of the abuse and the perpetrator is the person who fabricates the illness.
- Existing mental health difficulties in the perpetrator (child's natural mother in 90% of cases) have been described but are not essential for the diagnosis.

Presentation

There is a wide spectrum of severity of presentation of harm:
- False medical story.
- Fabrication of signs, e.g. blood on clothing or nappy, or sugar in urine specimen.

The most serious presentations include fabrication of illness induced by poisoning or suffocation.

Symptoms

Children may present with one or more of a range of symptoms:
- Seizures, collapse, coma.
- Apnoea.
- Vomiting and diarrhoea.
- FTT.
- Polyuria and polydipsia.
- Purpura.
- Recurrent fever.

Diagnosis

- It is important to realize that the medical profession may potentially harm children because unnecessary investigations are undertaken.
- The diagnosis can be established when the child is separated from the perpetrator or observed in the hospital environment and should be considered when other investigations are persistently normal.
- Very careful attention should be paid to the medical history, particularly as to who witnessed events and when they occurred.

Seek an opinion from an experienced colleague, who should arrange a strategy meeting between health care professionals to decide on what further action is necessary.

Physical abuse

Physical abuse involves any activity that causes physical harm to a child (e.g. hitting, shaking, burning, suffocating). Fabricated illness is also usually included in this category (see ⊃ Illness fabricated or induced by carers, p. 913).

> ## Typical presentations of physical abuse
>
> Any serious or unusual injury with an absent or unsuitable explanation.
>
> *Bruises*
> - Symmetrical bruised eyes.
> - Bruising of soft tissues of the face, especially in small babies. *Pre-mobile babies should not get bruises* or other injuries.
> - Bruising of the mouth or ears.
> - Finger marks on legs, arms, or chest (the latter may have associated rib fractures).
> - Bruising of different ages.
> - Linear bruising on buttocks or back.
> - Distinct patterns of bruising (e.g. handprint marks, implements, kicks).
> - Uncommon sites for accidents (e.g. stomach, chest, genitalia, neck).
>
> *Burns or scalds*
> - Typically with clear outlines or shape of an implement (e.g. cigarette burns, iron).
> - Soft tissue areas that are unusual (e.g. back of hands, sole of feet).
> - Forced immersion (e.g. glove-and-stocking distribution).
>
> *Fractures*
> It is rare for a child <1y of age to sustain an accidental fracture. Bone disorders (e.g. OI) are rare (see ⊃ Osteogenesis imperfecta, p. 688). Consider the following:
> - Long bones (arms/legs) in infants or non-mobile children; ribs.
> - Multiple fractures in various bones—almost always abuse.
> - Fractures of different ages.
>
> *Bite marks*
> - Adult or child marks can be determined by forensic dentistry.
>
> *Scars*
> - Especially if concurrent bruising present.
>
> *Poisoning*
> May be accidental (as a consequence of neglect) or deliberate (as in fabricated illness). An example of deliberate poisoning is salt intoxication, which may prove fatal. This should be considered when severe, recurrent symptoms or signs, such as coma, seizures, or severe GI upset (vomiting or diarrhoea), remain unexplained.

Investigations

Skeletal survey and other imaging

Infants do not localize pain. Hence, injuries of differing ages may be missed. X-rays must be planned with the radiology team, and the correct views carried out. A second skeletal survey is performed 1–2wk later as fractures are often not apparent initially, appearing later with callous formation on the second survey.

- *X-rays:* particularly in children aged <2y and for some older children.
- *Bone scan:* if X-rays inconclusive. Useful for rib fractures, but not for metaphyseal or skull fractures.
- *CT or MRI scan of brain:* in infants and young children who present with irritability or coma, but also recommended empirically to screen for head injury in infants with unexplained injuries. (See also ➲ Subdural haemorrhage, pp. 394–5.)

Clotting screen

Perform tests if extensive or unusual bruising or unexplained cerebral haemorrhage. *Obtain and discuss abnormal tests with a haematologist.* The first-line recommended tests are:

- PT.
- APTT.
- TT.
- Fibrinogen.
- FBC and film.
- Factor VIIIc, vWF (antigen and activity).

Ophthalmology examination

By an experienced ophthalmologist to look for evidence of retinal haemorrhages. The latter are suggestive of non-accidental head injury (see ➲ Inflicted abusive head injury, p. 987).

Sexual abuse

(See also ➔ About sexual abuse, p. 743.)

Forcing or enticing a child/young person to take part in sexual activities, whether or not the child is aware of it. This may include physical contact and penetrative or non-penetrative acts. It may also involve non-contact (e.g. looking at, or being involved in, pornography) or other sexual activities and includes abuse via the Internet.

Presentation

- STI: gonorrhoea, chlamydia, *Trichomonas vaginalis*.
- Pregnancy, vaginal bleeding in pre-pubertal girls.
- Genital or peri-anal injury with an absent or unsuitable explanation.
- Behavioural changes:
  - Self-harm, withdrawal, aggression, sexualized behaviour.
  - Unexplained deteriorating school performance.
- Disclosure by the child.
- Wetting and/or faecal soiling.

Signs

Few signs are diagnostic and 50–90% may not have findings.

Acute signs

NB: these signs may disappear rapidly.
- *Girls*: acutely—tears in hymen, vaginal bleeding, bruising around genital area, and 'hand' grip marks.
- *Boys*: bruising to genital area, urethral injury, penile torn frenulum.
- *Anal signs*: anal fissure, gaping anus, swelling of anal margin.

Chronic signs

These signs are more difficult to interpret. *In girls*, the following may be suggestive of previous repeated penetrative trauma:
- Scar in posterior fourchette, old tear or scar of the hymen.
- Complete absence of tissue at posterior hymen.

In both sexes: anal fissure/scars when other causes excluded.

Work-up

Refer to a sexual abuse centre and the police who will perform the necessary examinations and investigations.

Notes to bear in mind post-sexual assault

- *HIV prophylaxis* must be given ≤72h of assault.
- *Pregnancy prevention* with emergency contraception:
  - ≤72h with levonorgestrel.
  - 3–5 days using ulipristal acetate, copper-bearing intrauterine device.
- *Forensic samples*: collection recovery windows are 7 days for vaginal intercourse, 12h for digital penetration, and 3 days for anal intercourse.

Emotional abuse

Persistent, emotional ill treatment of a child that results in severe impairment in emotional development. This may involve:
- Conveying to children that they are worthless or unloved.
- Imposing age- or developmentally inappropriate expectations.
- Causing children to frequently feel frightened and threatened.
- Seeing or hearing the ill treatment of another, as in domestic violence.

This form of abuse often coexists with other forms of ill treatment.

Presentation

Symptoms are largely behavioural and may include:
- Being excessively clingy.
- Attention-seeking behaviour.
- Overly anxious.
- Overly serious.
- Being anxious to please.

Parental behaviours are a clue to the diagnosis. Any of these must be persistent and severe and have a major impact on the child in order to reach the threshold for emotional abuse:
- Persistently –ve view of the child.
- Inconsistent and unpredictable responses.
- Expectations that are very inappropriate.
- Induction of a child into bizarre parental beliefs.

Medical involvement in child protection

All health professionals have a role in ensuring that children and families receive the care, support, and services they need in order to promote child health and development. It is likely that health professionals will be the first to have contact with children or families in difficulty. Participation in child protection encompasses a range of activities.

- Recognizing children in need of support or protection, and parents who may need extra help in bringing up their children.
- Contributing to enquiries about a child or family.
- Assessing the needs of children and the capacity of parents to meet their children's needs.
- Planning and providing support for vulnerable children and families.
- Participating in child protection conferences.
- Planning support for children at risk of significant harm.
- Providing therapeutic help to abused or neglected children and parents under stress (usually the remit of the child and adolescent mental health team).
- Contributing to case reviews.

Initial concerns

Where there are concerns about a child, and when there is reasonable belief that a child is at serious risk of immediate harm, doctors should act immediately to protect the interests of the child, and this will almost always involve contacting one of the statutory bodies with responsibilities in this area:

- Social care.
- Police.

A full report of concerns will be required. The precise action taken should be governed by the procedures set out by the *Local Safeguarding Children Boards* (see also ➔ Referrals to other agencies p. 919; ➔ Medical assessment, pp. 920–1; ➔ Assessment by social care, pp. 922–3; ➔ Confidentiality and disclosure of medical information to other agencies, p. 959).

Referrals to other agencies

An experienced/senior member of the medical team must be involved when there are child protection concerns.

Agencies

- *Social care*: lead agency for investigation of child abuse.
- *Police service*: frequently involved in the initial joint investigation or when criminal prosecution is likely.

Referral procedure

- Inform parents, unless likely to result in further harm to the child.
- Referral does not need parental permission.
- Specific concerns should be clearly stated.
- Telephone referrals should be confirmed in writing.
- All referrals should be followed up if no acknowledgement is received or action taken.
- Follow local referral protocols.

The child's safety is of equal importance to their medical treatment. If hospitalization for medical treatment is not indicated, then the child should not be discharged without a clear plan and decision about a place of safety and future follow-up. This will be the joint decision and responsibility of the multidisciplinary agencies (medical, social care, and police). The police should be immediately informed if the parents/carers attempt to remove the child from hospital before these decisions are made.

Medical assessment

The purpose of the medical assessment is to:
- Assess whether the child has been injured and/or whether there are any other medical or developmental concerns.
- Provide appropriate investigations and treatment for the child.
- Provide an opinion about possible cause.

When assessing a child who may have been the victim of child abuse, it is important to inform and involve senior colleagues at an early stage. The assessment should be carried out (along with an experienced/senior colleague, if possible) in an environment that provides a sufficient degree of comfort for the child and their parents/carers, as well as sufficient access and lighting for examination. It is good practice to have a nurse or other health professional present at the time of history taking and examination.

History

Take a thorough history:
- *The presenting problem* should be documented chronologically, outlining the sequence of events and circumstances leading up to the presentation and referral.
- The *family history, past medical history* (e.g. clotting defects, bone disorders, psychiatric), and *social history* should be detailed.

Examination

This should include a general examination of all the systems.
- Weight, OFC, and height should be plotted on a growth chart.
- Neurodevelopmental assessment is appropriate in infants/toddlers.
- External injuries should be recorded in detail, including their location, size/dimensions, and appearance.
- Photographs should be taken (see ➲ Record keeping, p. 921).

Examination of children with suspected sexual abuse should only be undertaken by designated/trained professionals (e.g. the named child protection lead or police surgeon).

Child protection plan

- Where there are concerns about a child, enquiries should be made to social care (see ➲ Assessment by social care, pp. 922–3).
- A *child protection plan* is drawn up by professional staff working together with the parents and carers and the child (where old enough). Children with a child protection plan have a social worker who is responsible for coordinating work with the child and the family. The family must have a clear understanding of the planned outcomes and that they are willing to work to these within a specified time frame.
- A child will be the subject of a child protection plan until it is believed that the child is safe from any future harm. Regular meetings are held with the parents/carers and child to review the work being done and progress made.
- If a child moves out of one area, if they are the subject of a child protection plan, the information must be passed on to the new local authority area.

Consent

This is an important consideration that needs to be taken into account before proceeding with the medical assessment of any child. If the child is deemed to have sufficient understanding to make an informed decision, consent should be obtained from them. This principle is commonly referred to as 'Gillick competency', although now we think in terms of *Fraser competency* (see ⊃ Assent and consent, pp. 956–7). Children of sufficient understanding cannot be medically examined without their consent, even when an emergency protection order has been made.

Record keeping

Clear, detailed note-keeping is required.
- *Written notes:* keep full and contemporaneous notes, including comments made by the parents and the child. All notes must be signed and dated, with the doctor's name printed underneath each entry.
- *Diagrams:* particularly body maps to illustrate the location of injuries.
- *Photographs:* may be helpful; they should be dated and signed or requested from medical photography with parental consent.

Assessment by social care

Social care and the police will undertake an assessment. Referrals may result in:
- No further action being taken.
- Provision of support and help for the child and their family.
- A fuller assessment of the needs and circumstances of the child.

Strategy meeting

This is a meeting between professionals from all the relevant agencies (social services, police, education, health) to decide on the next action or steps.

Child protection conference

This will be convened if there are concerns about significant harm. The timing will vary and may be after discharge from hospital as long as the child is in a place of safety. A plan is needed to ensure the child's welfare and safety are addressed. When a child is considered at risk, then following the conference:
- He/she will be the subject of a child protection plan (see ⊃ Medical involvement in child protection, p. 918).
- A more comprehensive assessment (core assessment) will be arranged and undertaken.
- A key worker will be appointed.
- A review conference will be arranged within 3mth.

  Children not considered at risk have:
- A support plan organized.
- Follow-up between the family and other professionals arranged.

Report writing for child protection conferences

(See also ⊃ Confidentiality and disclosure, pp. 958–9.) Those members of the medical team directly involved in the initial assessment and/or subsequent management of the child should write a medical report. Parents have the right to see reports before a case conference. There are a number of important key points in writing these reports:
- They should distinguish fact from observation and allegation.
- Relevant information should be used from current and past records.
- Medical terms should be explained for the benefit of laypersons.
- Include observations and relevant statements from child and carer.
- Clearly state if injury is unexplained or inconsistent with history.
- State medical opinion only.

Confidentiality and disclosure of medical information

(See also ➔ Confidentiality and disclosure of medical information to other agencies, p. 959.) Guidance regarding confidentiality and information disclosure is provided by the UK *General Medical Council* (GMC). There are various reports that can be found on the GMC website (see ℘ http://www.gmc-uk.org/). In addition, there is a useful consultation document that can be downloaded called *Protecting children and young people: the responsibilities of all doctors* (2011).

- Information can be disclosed without consent in cases of serious crime (including child abuse).
- If information is not disclosed, the doctor should be prepared to justify their decision.
- In the absence of consent, confidential medical information about parents or third parties should be shared when relevant and necessary to protect the safety and welfare of the child. The more sensitive this information is, the greater the child's needs must be to justify disclosure.
- Normally permission from parents should be obtained, unless it is reasonable to conclude that this would hinder enquiries or place the child at greater risk.

Role of social care in prevention

Most children referred to social care will be those in need, rather than those requiring protection. Children in need are defined as those whose vulnerability is such that they are unlikely to reach or maintain a satisfactory level of health or development without the provision of support services. The role of social care in prevention is to undertake an initial core assessment and to implement a plan to maximize the child's health and development, including:

- Referral to universal support services, e.g. health visitors, parenting groups, school nurses, nursery placement, home support.
- Referral to specialist services, e.g. mental health (adult or child), paediatrics.

Further reading

General texts

Royal College of Paediatrics and Child Health (RCPCH). *Child Protection Companion 2013*, second edition. RCPCH, London; 2013 (latest version available on the Paediatric Care Online app— register with RCPCH membership number).

Safeguarding and abuse

Department of Education. (2010). *Working Together to Safeguard Children: A guide to inter-agency working to safeguard and promote the welfare of children*. Available at: ℘ https://www.education. gov.uk/publications/standard/publicationdetail/page1/DCSF-00305-2010.

National Institute for Health and Care Excellence. (2009). *Child maltreatment: when to suspect maltreatment in under 18s*. Clinical guideline [CG89]. Available at: ℘ http://www.nice.org.uk/CG89.

Royal College of Paediatrics and Child Health. (2008). *Physical signs of child sexual abuse: evidence-based review*. Available at: ℘ http://www.rcpch.ac.uk/csa (an updated 2012 summary can be downloaded and the hardcopy ordered).

Responsiblities of doctors

General Medical Council (GMC). There are various reports that can be found on the GMC website (see ℘ http://www.gmc-uk.org/).

General Medical Council. (2012). *Protecting children and young people: the responsibilities of all doctors*. Available at: ℘ https://www.gmc-uk.org/ethical-guidance/ethical-guidance-for-doctors/ protecting-children-and-young-people (useful consultation document that can be downloaded from the GMC website).

Chapter 27

Pharmacology and therapeutics

Prescribing for children

Licensing

Many medicines used in children are not licensed for such use. This does not mean that they should not be used, but that the pharmaceutical company has not sought a licence from the regulatory authorities. Hence, many medicines in children are used off-label, i.e. they are used at a different dose, route, age, or indication than specified within the product licence. It is important that medicines are used in children in relation to the scientific evidence available. In certain circumstances, this may involve off-label use.

Disease states

Certain diseases (e.g. CF) or clinical conditions (e.g. shock) may affect drug metabolism. Both liver and renal failure delay drug elimination and so require dosage reduction.

Breastfeeding

Most medicines taken by a breastfeeding mother are safe for her infant. Mothers should not be discouraged from breastfeeding because of uncertainty about possible toxic effects. The *British National Formulary for Children* gives detailed information regarding which medicines to avoid.

Medication errors

Medication errors are significant in children. In particular, tenfold errors have been associated with significant mortality and morbidity, especially in the very young. *All health professionals will commit a medication error during their career!* Medication errors include:

- *Incorrect dose:* commonest error and also the type most likely to be associated with a fatality. Knowledge of the child's actual weight and checking of dose calculation are vital, especially on the neonatal unit and with parenteral medicines.
- *Incorrect drug:* second commonest type of error and also associated with significant fatalities.
- *Incorrect route:* this is a particular problem with intrathecal drugs. This is a procedure for specialists and great care should be taken when drugs are to be given this way!
- *Other errors:* include incorrect rate of administration, duplicate dosing, and administration of the drug to the wrong patient.

Adverse drug reactions

One in ten children in hospital and one in 100 outpatients will experience an adverse drug reaction (ADR). One in eight will be severe. ADRs are responsible for ~2% of child admissions. ADRs in children are as varied as in adults. Children, because of growth and development, also suffer from specific ADRs. Differences in drug metabolism make some ADRs a greater problem in children (e.g. valproate hepatotoxicity) or a lesser problem (e.g. paracetamol hepatotoxicity following an overdose). The mechanisms of ADRs affecting children are illustrated below.

Mechanisms of ADRs

Impaired drug metabolism

Chloramphenicol, when first used in neonates → development of grey baby syndrome (vomiting, cyanosis, cardiovascular collapse, and, in some cases, death). Newborns metabolize chloramphenicol more slowly than adults, and so require lower antibiotic dosing. Reduction in dosage prevents grey baby syndrome.

> Children, particularly neonates, are more likely to have a reduced capacity to metabolize drugs than adults. Therefore, lower doses are usually required.

Altered drug metabolism

Children may have reduced activity of major hepatic enzymes associated with drug metabolism. To compensate, they may use other enzyme pathways, which is thought to be a factor contributing to ↑ risk of hepatotoxicity in children <3y who receive sodium valproate. This risk is raised by concurrent anticonvulsants which cause enzyme induction of certain metabolic pathways.

> Sodium valproate should not be used as a first-line anticonvulsant in children <3y of age.

Protein-displacing effect on bilirubin

The sulfonamide sulfisoxazole in sick neonates in the 1950s was associated with fatal kernicterus due to drug displacement of protein-bound bilirubin into blood because of its higher binding affinity to albumin. Ceftriaxone also is highly protein-bound and will displace bilirubin in sick neonates.

> The protein-displacing effect of medicines should be considered in sick preterm neonates.

Percutaneous absorption

Percutaneous toxicity can be a significant problem in the neonatal period because of their higher BSA:weight ratio (compared with children and adults). An example is the use of antiseptic agents (e.g. hexachlorophene) that are associated with neurotoxicity.

Drug interactions
Ceftriaxone and Ca^{2+}-containing solutions when used together in neonates may result in the precipitation of ceftriaxone–Ca^{2+} salt in the lungs. This drug interaction can result in fatalities, and therefore, ceftriaxone should be avoided in neonates. This interaction has only been reported in infants aged <3mth.

Ceftriaxone should be avoided in neonates.

Unknown
There are several examples of major ADRs that occur in children for which we have no mechanism. Salicylate given during a viral illness increases risk of *Reye-like illness* in children of all ages. Since salicylates have been avoided in children ≤12y, the incidence of Reye-like illness has dramatically reduced. Propofol has minimal toxicity when used in GA, but when used as a pro-longed sedative in critically ill children, it is associated with metabolic acid-osis, arrhythmia, and death (>10 children in the UK alone). The propofol infusion syndrome is related to the total dose of propofol infused.

Propofol should not be used as a sedative in critically ill children.

Suspect ADRs
One should always consider the possibility of an ADR being responsible for a child's symptoms. Table 27.1 lists some of the serious ADRs associated with widely used medicines.

Table 27.1 Serious ADRs associated with medicines

Drug	ADR
Corticosteroids	Adrenal insufficiency/sepsis
Cytotoxics	Neutropenia
Carbamazepine	SJS
NSAIDs (including ibuprofen)	GI haemorrhage
Opiates	Respiratory depression
Sodium valproate	Hepatotoxicity

Preventing ADRs
Recognizing which patients are at greater risk of ADRs can help reduce overall incidence. Health professionals should follow guidelines.

Reporting ADRs
Suspected ADRs should be reported to the regulatory authorities (i.e. *yellow card* scheme in the UK).

Pharmacokinetics

Pharmacokinetics defines the relationship between drug dose and its concentration in different parts of the body (usually plasma) in relation to time. This relationship is measured and defined numerically. Knowledge of several key terms is needed to understand the pharmacokinetic principles.

* *Absorption:* if a drug is given IV, 100% of the dose enters the bloodstream. If a drug is given PO, only a fraction is absorbed and the term bioavailability is used to describe the percentage of the drug administered that reaches the systemic circulation. Absorption is often reduced following PO administration in the neonatal period.

* *Volume of distribution (V_d):* this is not a physiological volume, but rather an apparent volume into which the drug would have to distribute to achieve the measured concentration. Water-soluble drugs, such as gentamicin, have a V_d that is similar to extracellular fluid volume. Drugs that are highly bound to plasma proteins have a low V_d. Children differ from adults because of their body composition (neonates and young children have higher total body water) and lower plasma protein concentrations.

* *Clearance:* describes the removal of a drug from the body and is defined as the volume (usually of plasma) that is completely cleared of drug in a given time. In adults, clearance is described in relation to volume/time (mL/min). In children, clearance is described in relation to body weight (mL/min/kg). Clearance is usually reduced in the neonatal period but may be higher in infants and young children than in adults.

* *Elimination half-life:* the time taken for the concentration of a drug (usually plasma) to fall to half its original value. It is inversely related to clearance. Therefore, 50% of the dose will be eliminated in one half-life; 97% of a drug will be eliminated after five half-lives. This is also the time required for steady state to be achieved following initial administration of the drug.

Mathematical formulae are available in standard texts that describe the interrelationship between clearance, V_d, and elimination half-life.

Drug metabolism

The major pathways involved in drug metabolism are divided into these reactions:
• Phase I: oxidation, reduction, hydrolysis, and hydration.
• Phase II: glucuronidation, sulfation, methylation, and acetylation.

As a general rule, clearance of drugs in the neonatal period is reduced. For many drugs, adult clearance values are reached by 2y.

Phase I pathways

The major pathway is oxidation which involves the cytochrome P450 enzymes (CYP). The major CYP enzymes are CYP3A4 and CYP1A2.
• CYP3A4: responsible for the metabolism of many drugs (e.g. midazolam, ciclosporin, fentanyl, nifedipine). CYP3A4 activity is reduced in the neonatal period and early infancy. Enzyme activity between individuals varies considerably → large range of plasma concentrations after the same dose of an affected drug.
• CYP1A2: accounts for 13% of total hepatic enzyme activity. Caffeine and theophylline are metabolized via the CYP1A2 pathway. Enzyme activity is reduced in neonates and then increases, such that by 6mth, activity approaches that of older children and adults.

Phase II pathways

Glucuronidation and sulfation are the two major pathways. Glucuronidation is reduced in the neonatal period and there is compensatory sulfation. The development of glucuronidation varies for different drugs. For example, children who are 2y old have rates of glucuronidation for morphine similar to those in adults, while for paracetamol, adult rates of glucuronidation are not reached until puberty.

Pain management

(See also ➔ Palliative care, pp. 618–19; ➔ Chronic pain in children, pp. 718–21; ➔ Postoperative care: analgesia, p. 849.)

Assessment

Always consider the possibility of a child being in pain, as a result of either their disease or the interventions that are required. Accurate assessment requires an age-appropriate, validated pain assessment scale. Self-reporting is the ideal, but the child needs to be ≥3y old to be able to do this. Do not use pain scales validated for acute pain to assess chronic pain.

- *Self-report scales:* usually involves the child pointing to a photograph of a child in pain (the *Oucher*) or a diagram of a child in pain (*Bieri Faces Pain Scale* or *Wong–Baker Faces Pain Scale*). The Oucher has been validated in children as young as 3y of age, whereas the Bieri Faces Pain Scale has only been validated in children aged ≥6y. The Wong–Baker Faces Pain Scale is more reliable in children aged 8–12y than in the 3–7y age group. The *Adolescent Paediatric Pain Tool* is for children aged 8–17y.
- *Behavioural pain scales:* rely on the child's behaviour. Validated for children aged 1–5y. Examples include the *Toddler—Preschooler Postoperative Pain Scale* (TPPPS) and the *Children's Hospital of Eastern Ontario Pain Scale* (CHEOPS). The *Face, Legs, Activity, Cry, Consolability* (FLACC) scale has been validated for children aged 2mth to 7y.
- *Neonatal pain scales:* examples include CRIES, Neonatal Facial Coding System (NFCS), Neonatal and Infant Pain Scale (NIPS), and Premature Infant Pain Profile (PIPP). These rely on behavioural observations and some include pulse, BP, and SpO_2. It is important to use a scale validated for the infant's gestation (e.g. is it valid only in full-term neonates?)

Management

It is best to consider pain as being mild, moderate, or severe.

- *Mild pain:* paracetamol is the safest analgesic available and is the first-line drug to be used for mild pain in all ages.
- *Moderate pain:* children unresponsive (or unlikely to respond) to paracetamol should receive an NSAID (e.g. ibuprofen or diclofenac).
- *Severe pain:* morphine is the drug of choice. Give IV (including PCA), intranasally, or PO.
- *Procedural pain:* for certain painful procedures (e.g. dressing change in burns patients), it may be better to use inhaled Entonox®. This is an effective and safe analgesic with a short duration of action, which the child can control themselves.

Sedation

There are two main areas where sedation is required—during procedures and while receiving paediatric intensive care.

Procedural sedation

There are many sedative agents available. All sedative agents decrease conscious level and thereby can have significant toxicity. The choice of sedative agent depends upon local experience and how quickly and for how long sedation is needed. Sedation for painful procedure should include adequate analgesia. If a child is likely to be difficult to sedate, then consider whether a short-acting GA, administered by a paediatric anaesthetist, is safer and kinder to the child.

Prolonged sedation (critical care)

The purpose of sedation in PICU is to help the child, not the health professional. IV midazolam has been the drug of choice on admission—but practice is changing because of risk of delirium. Once NG feeds are tolerated, clonidine, chloral hydrate, and promethazine are used, rather than midazolam. Propofol is contraindicated for prolonged use in PICU—with the exception for procedures (e.g. MRI scan)—because of the risk of *propofol infusion syndrome*.

Fever

Fever is a sign of an underlying illness. It is more important to treat the underlying illness than the fever itself. Fever is reduced to make the child more comfortable. The two most used antipyretics (paracetamol and ibuprofen) are also analgesics (see ➲ Antipyretics, p. 622).

Management

- *Paracetamol* is the drug of choice since it is less likely to be associated with significant ADRs than ibuprofen.
- *Ibuprofen* is appropriate as an antipyretic agent if paracetamol has failed. Although the safest of all NSAIDs, it should not be used in children with gastroenteritis or other GI symptoms. Ibuprofen should be avoided in children with chickenpox, gastroenteritis, or hypovolaemia, as it may predispose to sepsis, exacerbation of GI symptoms, or renal insufficiency, respectively.

Further reading

British National Formulary

Royal Pharmaceutical Society of Great Britain, British Medical Association. (2019). *British National Formulary for Children (BNFC) 2019–2020*. Available at: ℘ https://www.pharmpress.com/product/9780857113542/bnfc

International child health

Global childhood illness and survival

How many children die?

The world has made progress in reducing global child mortality rates. In 1990, there were 12.6 million child deaths worldwide (93 per 1000), with improvement to 5.6 million deaths by 2016. This rate of progress accelerated in the 2000–2016 period, compared with the 1990s—globally, the annual rate of reduction in mortality rate in <5y olds ↑ from 1.9% (1990–2000) to 4.0% (2000–2016).

Where do children die?

Progress in improving child mortality has been uneven, and a child's risk of death depends on where that child is born:

• ~80% of <5y olds mortality occurs in two regions: sub-Saharan Africa and Southern Asia.
• Six countries account for 50% of mortality in <5y olds: India, Nigeria, Pakistan, Democratic Republic of Congo, Ethiopia, and China.
• In 2016, sub-Saharan Africa had an average mortality rate in <5y olds of 79 deaths per 1000 live births, which translates to one in 13–15 times higher than in high-income countries.

Conflict, famine, and political instability exacerbate the risk of death for children. Among the ten countries with the highest mortality rate in <5y olds, seven are *fragile countries*. In addition to marked differences between countries in the rate of childhood mortality, there are huge inequalities within countries and children from poorer households remain disproportionately vulnerable. In 99 low- and middle-income countries, mortality in <5y olds amongst children born in the poorest households is, on average, twice that of children born in the wealthiest households.

Prevention is better than cure

Although doctors are focused on treatments and curing disease, the biggest impact on global child mortality, especially in the poorest settings, will come from improvements in the essential conditions of life.

The pathologies that result in proximate causes of childhood mortality are intricately linked to the underlying cause of these deaths, i.e. the inability of >1 billion people to access fundamental human rights such as shelter, clean water, sanitation, adequate nutritious food, education, and primary health care.

The structural violence implicit in the relationships between rich states and poorer ones, and between different social groups within nations, leads to people being excluded from their rights. The global health industry works to alleviate the end-result of such inequalities, but we also have a duty to address ourselves more clearly and systematically to the structural inequalities that produce suffering and death.

Major causes of childhood morbidity and mortality

Infectious diseases and neonatal complications are responsible for most mortality in <5y olds globally, and around half of those deaths occur in the neonatal period. Malnutrition is implicated in around half of post-neonatal deaths.

Neonatal deaths

A lack of, or suboptimal, antenatal care, a lack of skilled birth attendants, and the absence of essential care for the newborn are all implicated in the preventable deaths of babies around the world every year:

- *Marked disparities in neonatal mortality* exist across regions and countries, and rates are highest in sub-Saharan Africa and Southern Asia, each of which reported 28 deaths per 1000 live births. (The UK neonatal mortality rate is just under 3 per 1000.)
- *Many of these neonatal deaths could be prevented* if access to antenatal care were improved and safe practices followed during and after childbirth (see Box 28.1). Empowering mothers to make informed choices during pregnancy and childbirth can have a significant impact on mortality; scaling up community interventions could decrease mortality by 25%.
- The WHO and UNICEF's *Every Newborn Action Plan* recommends home-visiting programmes and participatory learning and action groups as strategies to improve maternal and newborn health.

Box 28.1 Safer delivery practices

- Appropriate antenatal care.
- Facility delivery.
- Use of a safe delivery kit.
- Handwashing by the birth attendant prior to delivery.
- Use of a sterilized instrument to cut the umbilical cord.
- Immediate wrapping of the newborn after delivery.
- Delayed bathing of the newborn.
- Early initiation of breastfeeding.
- Exclusive breastfeeding.

Diseases and status needing targeted intervention in global child health

Pneumonia
- The leading infectious cause of child mortality.
- Accounts for 1 million child deaths annually.
- Many of these deaths are caused by *Streptococcus pneumoniae*.
- Therefore, a substantial decrease in mortality could be achieved by expanding the coverage of childhood pneumococcal vaccination.
- At present, early treatment with PO antibiotics is not available for many children suffering from pneumonia in low-resource settings.

Diarrhoeal disease
- Although the safety and efficacy of treatment with oral rehydration was demonstrated in the 1970s, diarrhoea still kills around half a million children each year.
- Most of these cases are caused by microorganisms transmitted by dirty water.
- Worldwide, 780 million people have no access to improved drinking water, and 2.5 billion do not have access to improved sanitation.

Malaria
- An important cause of childhood illness and death for 50% of the world's population living in malaria-prone areas.
- The bedrock of attempts to reduce malaria transmission remains vector control, including use of insecticide-treated bednets and indoor insecticide residual spraying.
- The success of these tools has been challenged in recent years by growing resistance amongst mosquitoes to insecticide agents.

Malnutrition
- Worldwide, malnutrition has a role in ~50% of mortality in <5y olds.
- Smaller children depend on parents for food, who may not have access to enough or may not know how to prepare the best nutrition.
- Aggressively marketed low-quality foods may be substituted for local staples → lack of protein/micronutrients needed for growth.
- The most severely malnourished children are at high risk of death, and published in-hospital case fatality rates for children admitted with severe acute malnutrition vary between 20% and 30%.
- In the long term, malnourished children are at risk of stunting, slower/poorer intellectual development, and opportunistic infections, because their nutrition compromises immune function.

Trauma
- In 2016, trauma was the cause of 6% of child deaths globally.
- Around 10% of these deaths are caused by road traffic accidents or drowning, and stronger public health measures are urgently required to reduce these deaths around the world.
- While local causes of childhood injury vary, another constant theme is violence against children. In a rich country like the UK, estimates of the number of child deaths caused each year by abuse or neglect vary between 50 and 80. These estimates rise much higher in settings with fewer financial and infrastructural resources.
- In 2006, the Office of the United Nations High Commissioner for Human Rights commissioned a report on violence against children around the world, which developed 12 overarching recommendations to reduce the burden of violence. Although advocacy organizations, such as the Global Partnership to End Violence Against Children and the Global Initiative to End All Corporal Punishment of Children, have strongly promoted this agenda, progress remains slow.

Children on the move status
Worldwide, 65.6 million people have been forcibly displaced by persecution and violence; 22.5 million of these have sought sanctuary in another country and been granted refugee status, while ~40 million have been displaced within their own country (so-called 'internally displaced people') and often face ongoing threats from forces that originally set out to persecute them.
- The overwhelming majority of the forcibly displaced live in the global south. People subject to forced migration are often held in camps when they arrive in a new territory, and this situation can be prolonged for months or years.
- Sometimes children are born, grow up, and reach adulthood inside refugee camps.
- The health challenges of camp life are profound, with large groups of children living close together, with varying levels of vaccine coverage and disease exposure.
- The food supply in camps is often insufficient and sometimes subject to pilfering and corruption, and malnutrition is an important problem for children living in this setting.
- Medical care is also often limited in quality and scope, and the governments providing the space for camps are often dependent on organizations such as *Médecins Sans Frontières* or *Médecins du Monde* to provide frontline medical services.
- *Children on the move* have often made pragmatic decisions to make the best of their situation and display ingenuity and tenacity in so doing, but they may often be exposed to some of the biggest risks of any group of young people.

The Sustainable Development Goals

The *Millennium Development Goals* (MDGs) were developed at a United Nations summit in 2000 to set targets for state governments and international institutions for improvements in the conditions of life for people around the world, to be met by 2015. These goals were wide-ranging and ambitious, and several included a focus on child health. However, these goals were not enough to prompt the desired progress. For example, MDG 4 targeted a reduction in mortality rate in <5y olds by two-thirds. Despite improvements in this statistic, this goal was not achieved.

Recognizing the progress that had partly been inspired and driven by the MDGs, but also acknowledging that a lot of work remained to be done, a new set of goals was agreed as a replacement for the MDGs after they expired in 2015. The *Sustainable Development Goals* (SDGs) aimed to build on the momentum created by the MDGs, while trying to minimize the strain on resources and the environmental impact of the efforts undertaken to improve human health and well-being.

SDG 3 provides targets for child mortality:
- All countries aim to reduce neonatal mortality to at least as low as 12 deaths per 1000, and mortality in <5y olds to at least as low as 25 deaths per 1000.
- If every country achieves these targets by 2030, an additional 10 million lives of children aged <5y will be saved during 2017–2030, with ~50% of them being newborns.

While progress demonstrated since 1990 shows that change is possible, in the context of many of the poorest countries in the world, these targets are enormously ambitious. If these goals are to be met, the world will need the right commitments, concerted efforts on the part of donors, implementing ministries and agencies, and, most importantly, the political will of national governments to make change happen.

Building effective health care systems

Health services require a system that has a strategy and is adequately funded and appropriately staffed, but this can be difficult to achieve with limited resources.

Primary care

Effective health services are built on primary care. Local services are essential to meeting the needs of poor populations, especially for mothers and small children, who have greater difficulty travelling to urban hospitals. The 1978 *Declaration of Alma-Ata International Conference on Primary Health Care* affirmed that 'all countries should cooperate in a spirit of partnership and service to ensure primary health care for all people . . . ' This reflected a new mood that 'vertical' programmes targeting specific diseases had not had sufficient impact, and debate between advocates for comprehensive, intersectoral health planning and supporters of short-term, targeted interventions continues today.

Decentralization and empowering communities

Health systems have been further improved by programmes emphasizing decentralization and empowering of communities to take responsibility for health care, particularly through structures employing community health workers.

Task-shifting

Task-shifting has also produced important benefits in hospital medicine, with professionals other than doctors taking on tasks that had previously been regarded as exclusively medical such as undertaking anaesthesia or performing Caesarean sections.

Essential provision for health workers

No amount of tinkering with the system will succeed, however, if the essential materials for a health system are not available. Health workers need access not only to skills and information, but also to medicines and equipment to treat patients. The basic building blocks of a functional health system have been summarized by *Health Information For All* in the acronym SEISMIC (see Box 28.2).

Box 28.2 SEISMIC: essential provision for health workers

- Skills.
- Equipment.
- Information.
- Systems support.
- Medicines.
- Incentives (including a decent salary).
- Communication facilities.

Paying for health care

The efficacy of any health care system depends on the ability of people to access it. In many countries, vertical programmes provide antimalarial drugs and insecticide-treated bednets free of charge. However, amoxicillin that would treat a child's pneumonia is often not funded, and many of the families whose children die of neonatal sepsis, pneumonia, and diarrhoea do not have the financial resources to pay for initial antibiotic therapy, let alone a course of hospital treatment.

To address this challenge, some countries have introduced free health insurance for children or free health services for mothers and children. These programmes often increase children's access to health care, although implantation may often be dogged by difficulties related to ↑ demand and the challenges of administering such large and bureaucratically complex schemes.

In this context, the UK's National Health Service (NHS) is an important international example. As one of the few comprehensive health services provided via national taxation, the NHS demonstrates what can be achieved through state provision of universal health coverage.

Global programmes to improve practice: IMCI and ETAT

Worldwide, every day, millions of parents across a plethora of settings seek assessment and treatment for their child's health.

Health workers, many of whom have undergone limited amounts of formal training, undertake to provide assessment and treatment for these patients. In most cases, these health workers lack access to diagnostics, including laboratory investigations and radiology, and provide only basic interventions. Providing accurate and effective treatment based on history and examination only can be challenging and can lead to substantial variation in approaches and increase in the costs of assessment and treatment.

The *Integrated Management of Childhood Illness* (IMCI) is a strategy developed by the WHO and UNICEF to standardize the approach to childhood illness in primary care settings, to bring together preventive and curative interventions, and to minimize the time taken to refer the sickest children for hospital care. The IMCI handbook is adapted for the needs and disease profile of each country where the strategy is implemented, leading to a set of country-specific guidelines. The IMCI has three main aims:

• To improve case management skills of health care staff.
• To improve overall health systems.
• To improve family and community health practices.

A recent review of the implementation of IMCI showed that the strategy improves quality of care, reduces the cost of treatment, and can reduce child mortality, if implemented well.

Emergency Triage, Assessment, and Treatment (ETAT) is used at the secondary care level. Substantial improvements in quality of care and mortality have been demonstrated with this strategy that focuses on initial assessment, treatment, and care. As a large proportion (often as high as 50%) of paediatric deaths in hospital occur within 24h of admission, focusing attention on accurate triage of the sickest patients and timely assessment and treatment of common problems, such as hypoxaemia, hypovolaemia, anaemia, and hypoglycaemia, can have important benefits. As with IMCI, the standard WHO training manual should be adapted for each country context. Training to develop skills in triage, assessment, and treatment should be combined with a quality improvement process to optimize the space where children are assessed and treated and the availability of testing and treatments.

Working in international child health

Five reasons to work overseas

Work where you are needed the most

Working in a low-resource setting offers the opportunity to practise medicine where there are few clinicians and a large burden of disease; you use your expertise to address the greatest need.

Challenge the boundaries of your clinical knowledge

You will experience new diagnostic and therapeutic conundrums, encountering new pathogens and unfamiliar presentations of familiar diseases and making you a more rounded and thoughtful clinician.

Develop confidence in looking after sick children

Children presenting to hospital in low-resource settings are more unwell than those presenting to UK hospitals, and managing them with few diagnostic resources can help you to become more confident and resourceful.

Address logistical and organizational challenges

Health systems in low-resource settings face substantial difficulties due to staff shortages, lack of diagnostics, equipment, and medications, and poor infrastructure. As a fresh pair of eyes and an extra pair of hands, you can work with colleagues to develop improved efficiency and outcomes.

Bring new insights back to the NHS

The fresh perspective afforded by working in a different setting can give you insights that are transferable to your work in the NHS.

Training and electives in international child health

If you are interested in working in low-resource settings, it is worthwhile using your *medical school elective* to gain experience. Many hospitals in low- and middle-income countries offer electives for medical students, and it is good to explore your sub-specialty interest and to begin to understand the challenges involved in different settings.

Before undertaking a *professional placement* in a low-resource setting, it is worthwhile undertaking a course of further study. Diplomas in tropical medicine and health (DTM&H) are offered by:

- The London School of Hygiene and Tropical Medicine (in London and East Africa).
- The Liverpool School of Tropical Medicine.
- The Institute of Tropical Medicine, Lima, Peru.

Some organizations require a DTM&H before placing you. For example, *Médecins Sans Frontières* require this qualification in their volunteers. The DTM&H takes 9–13wk to complete, but longer courses are available, often as a 1y MSc course.

Practical suggestions for working in a low-resource setting

Calibrate your expectations
It is essential to review carefully the details of the placement you plan to undertake, the logistical arrangements, and the level of support and supervision that you will receive. Assess whether the organization has clear, appropriate, and achievable goals. Programmes and organizations can often be keen to recruit staff and that enthusiasm may outweigh the assessment of your knowledge and experience. It is your responsibility to ensure that you are not taking on too much—realizing when you are in the country is too late!

Plan ahead
Make your plans well in advance, and make sure that you have covered all the basics, including relevant vaccines, malaria prophylaxis where appropriate, water purification, and emergency lighting solutions for blackouts. Review the IMCI and ETAT standard guidance and revise the local guidelines for common conditions. It is also worth contacting the hospital or organization where you will be working to find out whether you can bring specific teaching materials or equipment that will be useful.

Learn every day; teach when you can
As a guest in a new institution and a new country, you will have enormous amounts to learn and this is a tremendous opportunity. Be humble, be gracious, and be thoughtful, and you will usually be offered the same in return. Seek out learning opportunities, and you will also find where there are knowledge gaps. As a specialist physician, you will often have knowledge that you can share with your colleagues; take the opportunity to teach, and this can be one of the most rewarding aspects of your placement.

Malnutrition
Under-nutrition contributes to as many as 50% of deaths in low-resource settings, and in-hospital case fatality rates for severe acute malnutrition (SAM) is still between 20% and 30%. However, with prompt recognition and sequential management of the most important physiological derangements, this toll can be dramatically reduced—in some studies, mortality from SAM was reduced to <5%.

Quality improvement
While institutions in low-resource settings face many challenges, working within them can provide opportunities for creative thinking and innovative solutions. You can be a catalyst for +ve change if you are able to build partnerships with your colleagues and develop approaches that recognize and address the difficulties faced by different members of the team. Change is hard in any context, and this is particularly true when members of staff have many other burdens. Be prepared for your work to be frustrating at times and for the pace of change to be slow.

Paediatrics, ethics, and the law

Ethics

Ethical frameworks have a history as long as medicine itself. Today, ethical traditions are broadly categorized into three traditions:
- Virtue ethics.
- Deontology.
- Consequentialism.

More recently, principlism has been proposed as a unifying approach.

Virtue ethics

Often associated with Aristotle's tradition and emphasizes the character and moral behaviour of the person or agent. Aristotle's nine virtues are:
- Wisdom.
- Prudence.
- Justice.
- Fortitude.
- Courage.
- Liberality.
- Magnificence.
- Magnanimity.
- Temperance.

Deontology

Most commonly associated with Immanuel Kant who formulated the concept of the categorical imperative. The tradition emphasizes individual dignity, truth telling, non-maleficence, beneficence, and autonomy. The good will and motive of the individual determine the rightness of the act.

Consequentialism

In contrast to deontology, consequentialism emphasizes that the rightness of an action is determined by its consequences. The tradition is often associated most with utilitarians such as Jeremy Bentham.

Principlism

Traces its origins to the *Nuremberg Code* (1948), the *Declaration of Helsinki* (1964), and the *Belmont Report* (1979), all of which focus on research on human subjects. Beauchamp and Childress have championed moral decision-making in medicine, based on principlism, emphasizing four moral attributes:
- Autonomy.
- Non-maleficence.
- Beneficence.
- Justice.

Common law

In England, the United States, Canada, Australia, India, and many other countries, the law has mainly developed from judges through case law or precedent, rather than statute or executive action. This system is known as 'common law'. In an idealized form, common law should mean similar cases are decided consistently and that the law will evolve when new circumstances require precedent to be created. Difficulties can present when two or more precedents suggest conflicting courses of action.

We all function within the legal framework of the state in which we live, and we will also have our own personal ethical views and ideas. All of these will have an impact on the way that doctors relate to their patients, colleagues, and everybody else with whom they interact in their professional lives.

As a paediatrician, you will need to do the following:
- *Identify the legal and ethical problems involving patients* that clinicians face most frequently. When might one anticipate the circumstances in which clinicians may require particular care in deciding a course of action?
- *Identify clearly the clinician's obligations* in each case. What duties does a clinician have when faced with a moral or ethical problem that affects the care for a patient?
- *Bring expert guidance, wisdom, and precedent* in complex situations. What resources can clinicians use to try to resolve legal and ethical problems effectively, so that care of the patient can be continued or altered appropriately?

Recognition of ethical issues in everyday clinical practice

Key areas and issues that arise frequently in paediatric practice are summarized in Box 29.1 and discussed in this Chapter.

Box 29.1 Key issues in paediatric practice

Consent
(See ➋ Assent and consent, pp. 956–7.)
- Age and Gillick/Fraser competence.
- Parental consent or refusal.
- Proxy consent.
- Refusal of treatment.
- Insistence on treatment.

Best interests
(See ➋ Withholding or redirecting treatment in children, pp. 960–1.)
- Aggressive treatment.
- Resuscitation and do-not-resuscitate orders.
- Refusal of treatment by doctors.
- Cultural factors (e.g. circumcision, blood transfusion in Jehovah's Witness).

Confidentiality
(See ➋ Confidentiality and disclosure, p. 958–9.)
- The doctor–patient relationship (see ➋ The doctor–child relationship, p. 952).
- Rights of minors with or without competence.
- Rights of the child versus the family.
- Rights of parents.

Neonatal and paediatric intensive care
(See ➋ Withholding or redirecting treatment in children, pp. 960–1.)
- Resuscitation.
- Withholding and withdrawing treatment and end-of-life decisions.

Child protection
(See ➋ Good ethical and legal practice in suspected child abuse, p. 962.)
- Duties of the doctor and breaching confidentiality.
- Conflicts of interest: GP's duties to the family.

Clinical case study

During clinical practice, as a postgraduate trainee or a medical student, there are many opportunities to consider some of the common ethical and legal issues at the core of paediatrics and child health. In order to help with consolidating this aspect of your learning, we suggest that you undertake this clinical case study. First, identify a case that has caused you to think. There are then four steps. In the first two, you note your initial thoughts. Step 3 is completed after a case discussion conference with your team and other learners. Step 4 is for your reflection. Write down a summary of each step—it will help to clarify your thoughts and you shouldn't need >250 words for each of the sections in Box 29.2.

Box 29.2 Steps in a clinical case study

Step 1: clinical vignette
Describe the key issues in your patient or scenario:
- The medical facts?
- Contextual factors?
- The patient's capacity?
- The child's preferences?
- Surrogate decision-makers?
- Competing interests?

Step 2: medical, ethical, and legal issues
- What problems are posed by the case or scenario?
- What options were there for resolution?

Step 3: clinical goal-setting and decision-making
After you have had an opportunity to discuss steps 1 and 2 in a group:
- Write down what you discussed in the group.
- Was there an answer or resolution to the problem?
- How was this achieved and what options or interventions were considered?

Step 4: implementation and evaluation
- How was the matter dealt with?
- Comment on whether the plan of action worked.
- In retrospect, do you think the problem could have been avoided or improved, etc.?

The doctor–child relationship

Involving children in decision-making about their own care presents some problems. The law in England is not clear and relies on the clinician exercising clinical judgement. In general, consider:

• Doctors should *act in partnership* with children, whenever possible.
• The *Children Act 1989* states children's views should be heard.
• The *United Nations Convention on the Rights of the Child* indicates that clinicians should give 'due weight to the views of the child according to age and maturity'.

The Children Act 1989

The legal framework within which action takes place to safeguard children. The key principles of this Act include:

• The welfare of the child is paramount.
• Children are best brought up in their own home and agencies should seek to work in partnership with parents.
• The social services authority has a duty to investigate the circumstances of individual children where there are reasonable grounds to believe that the child is at risk of suffering or suffers 'significant hardship'.

Note the following:

• 'Harm' is defined as ill-treatment (i.e. all forms of abuse) or impairment of health or development.
• 'Significant' is not defined in the Act but means considerable, noteworthy, or important.

The Children Act 1989 was added to the Children Act 2004 which gave legal underpinning to *Every Child Matters: Change for Children* (2004). From April 2006, education and social care services for children have been brought together under a director of children's services in each local authority. Closely linked to the Children Act are:

• Protection of Children Act 1999.
• Safeguarding Vulnerable Groups Act 2006.
• Children and Young Person Act 2008.
• Human Rights Act 1998.

Public authorities must act consistently with the *European Convention on Human Rights*. Most relevant are the following.

• Article 2: The right to life.
• Article 8: The right to respect for private and family life.
• Article 5: The right to liberty and security of person.
• Article 3: That no one shall be subjected to torture or inhumane or degrading treatment or punishment.

Parental responsibility

This is defined as 'all the rights, duties, powers, responsibilities, and authority which by law a parent has in relation to the child and his property'.

Parental responsibility (PResp) is allocated as follows:

- PResp is automatically given to the mother.
- The father has PResp if:
  - He and mother were married at the child's birth.
  - Unmarried, but name registered on birth certificate (after December 2003).
  - Unmarried and entered into a PResp agreement with the mother.
  - Unmarried and obtained a court order for PResp.
  - Unmarried and obtained a Residence Order.

In addition, unmarried fathers can acquire PResp by marrying the child's mother.

Parents cannot lose PResp, unless the child is freed for adoption [or awarded to local authority as part of an emergency protection order (EPO) or care order].

The doctor–parent relationship

Most professionals do not have any difficulty with the idea that competent adult patients must be involved in their treatment. In the case of children, parents are the proxy decision-makers and deemed to speak for the child's best interests. Since at least the 1600s in England and with a somewhat more developed legislative status in Australia and the United States, the state must, however, protect vulnerable citizens (*parens patriae*). Children in common law jurisdictions have therefore, for many centuries, not been the property of their parents or guardians as they had in previous legislative systems.

In this regard, the following must be considered.

• All doctors have a duty to *act in the best interests of their patients*. In the UK, the GMC requires this standard from medical practitioners.

• *Parents have the right to make decisions* about a procedure on behalf of their child.

• *Parents do not have the right to insist on a doctor doing something that they do not consider to be in the child's best interest*. Given this responsibility, there will be times when a doctor may be forced to act against the wishes of the parents, but in the interests of the child.

In 2017 and 2018, two tragic and internationally publicized cases in the UK of Charlie Gard and Alfie Evans illustrated the conflict that may arise where doctors and parents disagree about what is in a child's best interests. Striking in each of these cases was the role of social media in disseminating opinion and comment. The need for doctors to protect a child's right to confidentiality creates a specific need for sensitivity and resilience in handling such cases.

Assent and consent

(See also ➔ Consent for surgery, p. 847). In the United States, the term 'assent' in a child is used to distinguish valid 'consent' from a competent adult. The American Academy of Pediatrics (AAP) suggests that assent includes at least the following elements:

- *Helping the patient achieve a developmentally appropriate awareness:* of the nature of his or her condition.
- *Telling the patient what to expect:* with tests and treatment.
- *Making a clinical assessment of the patient's understanding of the situation:* the factors influencing how he or she is responding (including whether there is inappropriate pressure to accept testing or therapy).
- *Soliciting an expression of the patient's willingness to accept the proposed care:* do not solicit a patient's view without intending to weigh it seriously. Where the patient will have to receive medical care in spite of his/her objection, tell the patient that fact. Do not deceive them.

The AAP suggests that clinicians seek the assent of the school-age patient, as well as informed permission of the parent for procedures such as:

- Venepuncture for diagnostic study in a 9y old.
- Orthopaedic surgery device for scoliosis in an 11y old.

With regard to consent, the clinician must present information in a manner suited to the child's developmental level. Parents should be able to assist, but in some cases, they may be too close to the situation to assess the child's state accurately. Other professionals can provide important insight into a particular child's developmental level and comprehension of the information presented. In the process of consent, the child's situation influences each of these elements:

- Nature and purpose of the therapy.
- Risk and consequences of therapy, and of not having therapy.
- Benefits and probability that therapy will be successful.
- Feasible alternatives.

Consent

In the UK, consent must be sufficiently informed and freely given by the designated person who is competent to do so (see also ➔ Competence, p. 957).

- The adolescent if aged >16y.
- The adolescent if aged <16y and judged to be competent.
- Parents.
- Individual or local authority with parental responsibility.
- A court.

Competence

Defining whether an adolescent demonstrates competence can be difficult and may depend on the nature of the procedure, as well as the child. The adolescent must possess qualities associated with self-determination and self-identity, appropriate cognitive abilities, and the ability to rationalize and reason hypothetically. Understanding, intelligence, and experience are also important qualities that may determine competence.

Criteria for establishing competence

The patient must:
- Demonstrate an understanding of the nature, purpose, and necessity of the proposed therapy.
- Demonstrate an understanding of the benefits, risks, and potential consequences of not having the treatment.
- Understand that this information applies to him/her.
- Retain and use that information to make their decision.
- Ensure their decision is made without being pressurized.

Assessing competence is the legal responsibility of the patient's doctor or other designated health care professional. A patient's refusal to cooperate with competence assessment should not be regarded as demonstrating incompetence. In England, Wales, and Northern Ireland:
- Adolescents aged 16–18y can consent to treatment but cannot refuse treatment that is otherwise intended to prevent their serious harm or death.
- Adolescents aged <16y may legally consent to treatment if they fulfil the criteria for competence.

In Scotland, all children and adolescents may consent to treatment, irrespective of age, so long as they are deemed competent to do so.

Confidentiality and disclosure

- When should you tell the whole truth?
- What if you make a mistake?
- What do you say to the team?
- What will you say to the family?
- Will you disclose your error?
- Will you say you are sorry?
- How will you handle this in terms of your personal feelings?
- How will you feel about yourself?

These are questions we all have to think about—whatever our seniority and whatever our practice. The GMC provides guiding principles and responsibilities of the doctor in these situations. It should be remembered that deception or flawed disclosure may take many forms, e.g. presenting 'just the facts', or saying 'there's always hope', or thinking that 'you can't tell a patient everything', or omission, or evasion.

Confidentiality in regard to patients

The issue of confidentiality arises when the young person presents for certain types of advice or treatment (e.g. contraception, abortion, STIs, substance misuse, mental health issues, and family problems).

- The duty of confidentiality owed to a person <16y is the same as that owed to any other person.
- It is not absolute and may be breached where there is risk to the health, safety, or welfare of the young person or others.
- Disclosure should only take place after consulting the young person.
- The personal beliefs of a practitioner should not prejudice the care offered to a young person.

Objections to disclosure of information should be respected, although in certain situations, disclosure may be required by law for the purposes of protecting the adolescent or others from significant harm.

Breach of confidentiality and disclosure of information

It may be proven legal to breach confidentiality in the following situations:

- *Incompetent individual:* any situation in which there is a risk of harm to the adolescent or to others.
- *Competent individual:*
  - History of current or past sexual abuse.
  - History of current or recent suicidal thoughts or self-harm behaviour.
  - Homicidal intentions.
  - Where serious harm to the individual is likely to occur.

The patient should always be informed that the information will be disclosed and the reason why. Attempts should be made to encourage the patient to agree to disclosure. Legal guidance from professional bodies or from medicolegal services may need to be sought.

Confidentiality and disclosure of medical information to other agencies

(See also ➔ Confidentiality and disclosure of medical information, p. 923.) Improving children's well-being is dependent on agencies being able to share relevant information about them. The general rule is to seek consent to share information unless you believe it is contrary to the child's welfare. It is the parents (or whoever has parental responsibility) who can give consent.

In UK law, the parental right to determine whether a child aged <16y has medical treatment terminates if and when the child achieves sufficient understanding and intelligence to understand fully what is proposed. In practice, a young person <16y of age can consent to treatment, but if they refuse it, parents may override their decision. This is termed *Fraser or Gillick competence* (see ➔ Consent, pp. 956–7). Whether an adolescent is Fraser-competent depends on the complexity of their medical needs, as well as their emotional maturity and intellect.

Disclosing personal information and medical information about a child to other professionals (teachers, social worker, police, other health professionals) is not a problem if consent is given but should be proportionate.

- Judgement needs to be exercised and very personal medical information should only be shared if relevant and necessary to promote the child's well-being.
- Medical and other sensitive information about parents needs their permission to be divulged. Only share relevant facts when needed.
- If consent is not given, then it can be justified if:
  - There are very good reasons to do so (see ➔ Chapter 28); or
  - It is in the public's interest.
- Whatever decision is made, this must be in keeping with the Data Protection Act, the Human Rights Act, and the common law duty of confidence, and also guidance from the GMC (UK).

Withholding or redirecting treatment in children

There are situations when treatments used to keep a child alive neither restores them to nor provides any meaningful benefit. In these circumstances, MV, heart pumps, etc., may no longer be in the child's best interests.

Ethical framework

- *Duty of care and the partnership of care:* our duty as part of the health care team is to comfort and cherish our patient, the child, and to prevent them from experiencing pain and suffering. We undertake this in partnership with the child's parents or carers.
- *Legal duty:* all health care professionals are bound to fulfil their duty within the framework of the law. Any practice or treatment given with the intention of causing death is unlawful.
- *Respect for children's rights:* our treatments for children should have 'their best interests' as the main consideration.

Double effect

This is recognized in English and Scottish law (i.e. increasing doses of analgesia, necessary for the control of pain/distress, may shorten life). We use opiates to benefit the child during life and we do not use them to cause/hasten death, but this may result—the double effect. The principle has four frequently cited conditions:

- The action must be either morally good or neutral.
- The bad effect must not be the means by which a doctor achieves the good.
- The intention of the doctor must be the good effect.
- The good effect must be equivalent to, or greater than, the bad.

Euthanasia

Withholding or withdrawal of treatments (e.g. MV) often does not lead to death. It should be clear that active measures to shorten life are not appropriate or legal and that palliative care is to be continued.

Process of decision-making

Deciding about withholding or withdrawing life-sustaining treatment requires time. Involve the whole team and gain as much information about the child's condition as possible. The decision should go hand in hand with planning palliative care needs.

- *Process:* while decisions are being made, the child's life should be safeguarded in the best way possible.
- *Responsibility:* the clinical team has corporate moral responsibility for decision-making. The senior member of the team is the consultant in charge of the child's care and should lead decision-making process—s/he bears the final responsibility for the chosen course of action.
- *Family and parents:* the final decision about withdrawal of treatment is made with the consent of the parents. Good communication is essential, as is building a relationship based on trust.

- *Second opinions:* good practice to consider this option. Other consultants working within the team may have advice. However, additional input from experts in another hospital may be required. This is particularly useful in unusual circumstances when there is uncertainty about prognosis and the child's likely future impairments.
- *Legal input:* with time, effective communication, and support, decision-making in most cases can be brought to a resolution. There are instances where hospital legal advisers and court involvement are required, especially when there is disagreement between parents, or between parents and the medical team, about the way to proceed.

Professional framework

The Ethics Advisory Committee (EAC) of the RCPCH identified five situations when it may be ethical and legal to consider withholding or withdrawal of life-sustaining treatment (see Box 29.3). If there is disagreement, or when there is uncertainty over the degree of future impairment, the RCPCH advises that the child's life should always be safeguarded until these issues are resolved.

Box 29.3 EAC of the RCPCH recommendations[1]

- *Brain death:* MV in such circumstances is futile and withdrawal of PICU treatment is appropriate.
- *Permanent vegetative state:* this state, which has specific diagnostic criteria, follows brain insults (e.g. trauma, hypoxia). It may be appropriate to withdraw or withhold life-sustaining treatment.
- *No chance:* the child has such severe disease that life-sustaining treatment simply delays death, without significant alleviation of suffering. Treatment to sustain life is inappropriate.
- *No purpose:* the child may be able to survive with treatment, but the degree of physical or mental impairment will be so great that it is unreasonable to expect them to bear it.
- *Unbearable:* the child/family feel that, in the face of progressive and irreversible illness, further treatment is more than can be borne. They wish to have that treatment withdrawn or to refuse further treatment, irrespective of the medical opinion that it may be of benefit.

Good ethical and legal practice in suspected child abuse

(See also ➲ Chapter 26.) The crucial issue for doctors is the safety of the child and this overrides considerations such as confidentiality.

* *Reporting*: as soon as abuse is suspected, it is important to share this information with other clinicians and social services and the police.
* *Parents and carers* have parental responsibility. Share your concerns and course of action with them as far as is safe for the child.

Criminal proceedings

* Crown prosecution service decides whether to bring a criminal case.
* Burden of proof needed is 'beyond all reasonable doubt'.
* No hearsay evidence is permissible.
* Magistrates Court or Crown Court.

Civil proceedings

* Burden of proof needed is 'on balance of probability'.
* Magistrates Court, County Court, or High Court.
* Divorce and other civil matters included, as well as child abuse.

Court orders (Children Act 1989)

Police protection order
* Application: by the police in case of emergency.
* Duration: maximum 72h.
* Child removed to suitable accommodation or prevention of removal from a current location of safety (e.g. hospital ward).

Emergency protection order
* Duration: 8 days, but can extended to 7 days on one occasion only.
* Application: by anyone, but usually by social services.

Child assessment order
* Implemented when parents are uncooperative. In practice, little used and not if there are grounds for an EPO.
* Duration: 7 days.
* Application: by an authorized person, usually the local authority.

Interim care order
* Duration: maximum 8wk.
* Application: by the local authority usually [or National Society for the Prevention of Cruelty to Children (NSPCC)].
* Gives parental responsibility to social services care.

Supervision orders
* Duration: 12mth in the first instance.
* Application: by social services or NSPCC.

NB: courts have powers to authorize or prohibit medical examination of a child at the time the order is made or during the course of the order.

Serious case reviews

Following *Working Together to Safeguard Children* (2006), serious case reviews are commissioned in cases when a child dies or sustains serious injuries and abuse or neglect is known or suspected to be a factor. They were previously referred to as 'Part 8 reviews', as defined in Section 8 of *Working Together to Safeguard Children* (Department of Health, 1999).

The purpose of serious case reviews is to:

- Establish lessons to be learnt about the way in which local professionals and organizations work together to safeguard and promote the welfare of children.
- Identify what those lessons are, how they will be acted on, and what is expected to change as a result.
- Improve interagency working and better safeguard, and promote the welfare of children.

Manslaughter by gross negligence

Three recent high-profile cases in the UK and Denmark—David Sellu, Hadiza Bawa-Garba, and the Svendborg case—have drawn the attention of the media and medical community. Each case is distinct but resulted in the conviction of a doctor after the death of a patient. In the case of David Sellu, it resulted in a custodial sentence before the conviction was quashed by the Court of Appeal. Strikingly, the Svendborg case and Dr Bawa-Garba case involved junior doctors working in allegedly overstretched clinical environments. The potential for reflective learning material after serious untoward incidents (SUIs) and significant events (SEs) to be evidence against a doctor in training has come under scrutiny. The Academy of Royal Medical Colleges has issued interim guidance about the use of reflection and a template for reflective learning.

In the UK, there has been a documented continuing increase in convictions of doctors for gross negligence manslaughter that started in the early 1990s, although cases remain rare. The law was defined after the Adomako case by the House of Lords by the following criteria:

- The defendant owed the victim a duty of care.
- The defendant breached that duty.
- The breach caused (or significantly contributed to) the victim's death.
- The breach was grossly negligent.

In criminal proceedings, the standard of proof that the prosecution must demonstrate is beyond reasonable doubt, rather than the less stringent balance of probability applied to the family courts and the Medical Practitioners Tribunal Service.

In 2018, the UK government and the GMC each began reviews of how gross negligence manslaughter is applied to medical practice. In the rapid review commissioned by the Secretary of State for Health and Social Care, Professor Sir Norman Williams has recommended removing the right of the GMC to appeal the fitness to practise decisions of the Medical Practitioners Tribunal Service.

References

1. Larcher V, Craig F, Bhogal K, *et al.* Making decisions to limit treatment in life-limiting and life-threatening conditions in children: a framework for practice. *Arch Dis Child* 2015; **100** Suppl 2: s323. Available at: ℘ https://www.rcpch.ac.uk/resources/making-decisions-limit-treatment-life-limiting-life-threatening-conditions-children.

Further reading
End of life
Larcher V, Craig F, Bhogal K, *et al.* Making decisions to limit treatment in life-limiting and life-threatening conditions in children: a framework for practice. *Arch Dis Child* 2015; **100** Suppl 2: s323. Available at: ℘ https://www.rcpch.ac.uk/resources/making-decisions-limit-treatment-life-limiting-life-threatening-conditions-children.

Safeguarding
Department of Education. (2015). *Working together to safeguard children.* Available at: ℘ https://www.gov.uk/government/publications/working-together-to-safeguard-children--2.

Ophthalmology

Visual development and UK screening

Normal visual development

We rely on behavioural visual assessment in infants; visual acuity (VA measurement is possible at 2–3y. VA may be in Snellen or logMAR notation—Snellen VA of 6/6 (0.0 logMAR) is 'perfect' vision, and Snellen VA of 6/60 (1.0 logMAR) indicates that the child sees at target from 6m away what should be seen from 60m.

- *At birth:* babies can fixate lights and large targets (VA 6/200). Early variable angle squints are common and usually resolve as vision improves and binocular function develops.
- *At 6wk:* the baby should maintain eye contact and fix and follow a face or large toy. The eyes move in alignment.
- *At 3mth:* the baby smiles in response to a silent smile by the observer and will fix and follow small toys (VA is 6/60).
- *At 6mth:* the baby reaches for toys.

Visual neuroplasticity

Vision is poor at birth due to immaturity of the fovea and visual pathway. Normal development of the visual pathway depends on visual stimulation—absence of a focused image on the retina will result in an abnormal anatomical development of visual pathway and cortex, called *amblyopia*.

- The *critical period* of neuroplasticity is the *first 3mth of life*; untreated visual deprivation during this period, e.g. by severe cataracts or complete ptosis, will cause permanently poor vision.
- *Neuroplasticity* continues until at least 8y of age; any ocular abnormality acquired in this period will disrupt visual development.

Vision screening in the UK

National screening enables early detection of ocular problems within the period of neuroplasticity. Specialist screening is recommended for children at high risk (e.g. premature babies, children with a strong family history of eye conditions, a syndrome, SN hearing loss, or JIA).

Newborn and infant physical examination (NIPE)
<72h check

- *Assess risk factors:* family history of childhood eye disease.
- *General observation:* eyelids/eye symmetry, size, and appearance.
- *Red reflex assessment (with direct ophthalmoscope):*
  - Shadows in red reflex: cataracts/corneal opacities. The reflex may be absent with severe cataract (parents may notice a grey pupil).
  - White reflex: retinal malformations/retinoblastoma.

NIPE 6–8wk check
- Repeat above and assess visual behaviour.

School vision test
- VA test for children at 4–5y.

Findings on screening which should trigger urgent referral
- Abnormal/asymmetrical globe size; corneal opacity.
- Abnormally shaped or asymmetrical pupils; abnormal red reflex.
- Roving eye movements/nystagmus.
- Poor eye contact or squint at 12wk or older (see ➔ Squint (strabismus), p. 971).

Vision and eye assessment techniques

Visual acuity tests

Visual examination

- *6–8wk:* should fix and follow a bright target, and your face and smile in response to a silent smile.
- *4mth:* should not squint and should fix and follow toys.
- *6mth:* should reach out for toys.
- *6mth to 2y:* preferential looking techniques (specialist test).
- *2–3y:* picture/letter charts with matching cards (Kay iSight app).
- *4–5y:* letter charts (Snellen/logMAR or iChart2000 app).

Eye examination techniques

A relaxed child is much easier to examine; sit them on the carer's lap with a dummy, a bottle, or food.

Anterior segment examination

- *Cornea:* check the diameter of the corneas are equal and that light reflection from each is bright. Instil anaesthetic drops (proxymetacaine 0.5%, stings mildly for about 5s) before examination if the child is in pain. Look through the ophthalmoscope set on +20D for a magnified view of the cornea. If suspecting an ulcer or abrasion, instil a drop of fluorescein (does not sting) and use a blue torch or dial in the blue filter of the ophthalmoscope.
- *Red reflex examination:* dim the room lights. Look through the ophthalmoscope (set on zero) held about 25cm from the eye; hold the eyelids open with your other hand, if necessary. Suspect cataract if the red reflex is indistinct, asymmetrical, or irregular. A retinal abnormality or retinoblastoma can cause a white reflex (leukocoria). The red reflex is darker and can be more difficult to assess in non-Caucasian babies. Refer on if in doubt.

Posterior segment examination

Ask the child to look at an interesting target above your shoulder when trying to examine the optic disc with an ophthalmoscope.

Dilating drops (mydriatics) can be instilled safely to improve your chances but will interfere with neuro-observations for 24h—use 1% tropicamide in children over 1y, and 0.5% cyclopentolate if younger.

Examining eye movements and alignment

- *Eye movements:* using a toy fixation target, move the eyes in an 'H' to assess the action of each muscle (see Fig. 30.1).

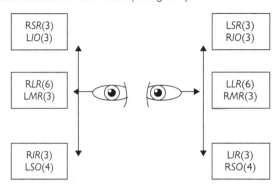

Fig. 30.1 Muscles (cranial nerves) controlling eye movements.

- *Ocular alignment:* compare the symmetry of the corneal reflections in each eye to a torch light held centrally in front of the child. The reflection will appear displaced in one eye if there is a manifest squint (see Fig. 30.2). Then hold up a toy target to attract attention; cover one eye, and look for movement in the uncovered eye to take up fixation (cover test). If no movement is seen, quickly move the cover from eye to eye and reassess for movement (alternating cover test for a latent squint).

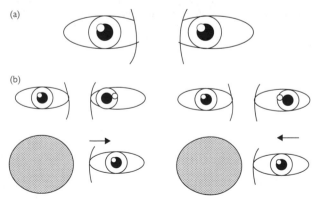

Fig. 30.2 Cover testing.

Disorders of visual development

Delayed visual maturation (DVM)

Some babies appear blind in the first few months, but their visual behaviour improves with age. There are three forms:

- *Isolated DVM:* there is no underlying pathology and there is rapid and full development of vision between 3 and 6mth of age. Motor development may also be delayed.
- *DVM associated with cerebral visual impairment:* e.g. infants with CP may initially appear blind. Vision usually improves over subsequent years but may be impaired.
- *DVM associated with ocular disease:* congenital ocular disease, e.g. cataracts and nystagmus, can interfere with early visual development. Vision improves over years, but with residual deficit.

Ametropia (refractive disorders)

To see clearly, the image must be focused on the retina. In myopia (short/near sight), the image is focused in front of the retina, and in hypermetropia (long/far sight), the image is focused behind the retina. Astigmatism results from uneven focusing power at different meridians, causing image blur. Children are usually born a little long-sighted and the refraction normalizes as the eyes grow. Ametropia may lead to squints and amblyopia. *Quick rule of thumb:* convex lenses (for long sight) magnify an image; concave lenses (for short sight) minify an image.

Amblyopia

A reduction in VA in one or both eyes due to abnormal cerebral visual development in the period of neuroplasticity; this may be due to visual deprivation from cataract or ptosis, visual blur due to refractive error, or visual suppression due to squint occurring before the age of 8y. Amblyopia is managed by correction of the refractive error, surgery to correct visual deprivation, e.g. early cataract surgery, and penalization of the better seeing eye, either with patches or with atropine drops.

Squint (strabismus)

A squint is a misalignment of the visual axes and affect 3% of children. If a squint develops in the period of neuroplasticity (i.e. <8y), it can reduce vision permanently in the squinting eye due to amblyopia.

Causes of squint

Concomitant squint

The commonest type of childhood squint. The angle of misalignment is similar in all directions of gaze.

- *Causes:* uncorrected refractive error (usually long-sightedness/ hypermetropia), disorders of accommodation (focusing), or poor vision in one or both eyes.
- *Manifest versus latent concomitant squint:* the eyes are kept in alignment by cerebral fusional processes. Many of us have a well-controlled latent squint, but fusion can break down with fatigue or illness, causing a latent squint to become manifest, i.e. the misalignment becomes noticeable and/or causes double vision.

Incomitant (paralytic) squint

Much less common in children. The angle of the squint is different, depending on the direction of gaze.

- *Causes:* cranial neuropathy (an intracranial cause must be excluded) or orbital disorders.

Management

The aims are to achieve good VA in each eye, improve binocular function, and squint cosmesis. This is done by correcting any refractive error with glasses, penalizing the better seeing eye with part-time occlusion or atropine drops, and improving the alignment with surgery. Some forms of squint can be improved with eye movement exercises. Management takes place in a hospital eye service and usually continues until the child is 8y old and visually mature.

Important: any child >12wk with an intermittent or constant squint, or with symptoms of double vision, should be referred to an ophthalmologist.

> ### Describing a squint using the following terminology
> - *Convergent (esotropia):* one eye turned inwards.
> - *Divergent (exotropia):* one eye turned outwards.
> - *Vertical (hyper-/hypotropia):* one eye appears higher than the other.
> - *Pseudosquint:* arises when wide epicanthic folds give the appearance of a squint, which is excluded on testing.

Nystagmus

Nystagmus is an involuntary rhythmic oscillation of one or both eyes (see Table 30.1). The direction of the fast phase and the frequency and amplitude of the nystagmus should be noted. Acquired nystagmus always requires investigation (neuro-imaging and/or electrophysiology). Nystagmus may also occur if there is muscle paralysis or weakness (e.g. secondary to myasthenia gravis) (see ➔ Neuromuscular junction disorders, p. 388).

Table 30.1 Types and patterns of nystagmus

Type	Pattern/cause
Congenital motor nystagmus	Horizontal jerk
Sensory nystagmus (poor vision)	Usually horizontal jerk
Vestibular nystagmus	Horizontal jerk
Neurological nystagmus: Gaze paretic Pendular Upbeat/downbeat See-saw	Jerk nystagmus beats towards and worse on lateral gaze High frequency, low amplitude, any direction. Seen in white matter disorders Seen in posterior fossa disorders, e.g. downbeat with Arnold–Chiari malformation One eye elevates, while the other depresses: midline disorders/parasellar masses
Opsoclonus/ocular flutter	Bursts of high-frequency saccades in all directions, e.g. opsoclonus–myoclonus syndrome

Visual impairment

One in 1000 children have VA worse than 6/18 (0.5 logMAR) in the UK, and 70% have an additional disability. Children may be registered as severely visual-impaired or partially sighted, based on a combination of their VA and peripheral vision; for instance, a child may have good central vision but be severely sight-impaired due to limited peripheral vision. Registration enables early specialist educational and mobility support. Most visually impaired children will have mainstream education using low-vision aids and magnifiers; a minority require Braille. In developed countries, only a third of blindness is preventable.

Causes of childhood visual impairment in the UK

Inherited/genetic (50%)
- Trisomy 21 (see ➔ Down's syndrome, pp. 872–3).
- CHARGE association (see ➔ Table 24.1).
- Congenital cataract (see ➔ Cataract, p. 978).
- Congenital glaucoma.
- Albinism.
- Retinal dystrophy.
- Retinoblastoma (see ➔ Retinoblastoma, p. 597).

Antenatal/perinatal factors (30%)
- Congenital infection, e.g. CMV, rubella (see ➔ Transplacental (congenital infection), p. 164).
- ROP (see ➔ Retinopathy of prematurity, p. 982).
- HIE/CP (see ➔ Cerebral palsy, pp. 392–3).
- Optic nerve hypoplasia.

Postnatal (20%)
- Visual pathway tumour (e.g. retinoblastoma, craniopharyngioma).
- Prolonged raised ICP.
- Accidental and inflicted head injury.
- Uveitis (e.g. associated with JIA (see ➔ Uveitis screening and treatment, pp. 698–9; ➔ Anterior uveitis, p. 977).

Infective/inflammatory disorders (1)

The red eye

Warning symptoms are pain, photophobia, and reduced vision. Evaluate with a direct ophthalmoscope set on +20D and a blue light to identify fluorescein staining.

Causes
- Subconjunctival haemorrhage.
- Conjunctivitis.
- Corneal pathology.
- Uveitis.
- Episcleritis and scleritis.

Differential diagnosis
- *With localized eyelid swelling and redness:*
  - Blepharitis: styes, lid cysts.
  - Painful swelling at nasal corner of the eye: lacrimal sac abscess.
- *With generalized eyelid swelling and redness:*
  - Preseptal or orbital cellulitis (see ⊃ Periorbital cellulitis, p. 628; ⊃ Periorbital cellulitis, p. 981).
  - Skin conditions, e.g. contact dermatitis, eczema.
  - Acute allergic or infective conjunctivitis.
  - Herpes simplex/herpes zoster ophthalmicus.
- *Associated with eye pain, photophobia, and epiphora:*
  - Corneal abrasion, subtarsal or corneal FB.
  - Viral (adenoviral or herpetic) keratitis (see ⊃ Keratitis, p. 977).
  - Bacterial, *Acanthamoeba*, or fungal keratitis.
  - Exposure keratitis.
  - Type IV hypersensitivity keratitis (atopy or secondary to blepharitis).
  - Anterior uveitis (iritis) (see ⊃ Anterior uveitis, p. 977).
  - Associated with dull ache worse on eye movement.
  - Episcleritis (mild), scleritis (severe).
- *Associated with discomfort and stickiness:*
  - Conjunctivitis: viral, bacterial, allergic, chemical (see ⊃ Childhood conjunctivitis, p. 976).
  - Neonatal conjunctivitis (see ⊃ Neonatal conjunctivitis, p. 976).

Corneal abrasion, subtarsal or corneal foreign body

Occasionally, an FB may stick onto the cornea or lodge underneath the tarsal plate of the upper eyelid, causing FB sensation and epiphora.
- If the child is in pain, instil proxymetacaine 0.5% (slight sting).
- Perform a VA check (where appropriate).
- Examine the ocular surface with a direct ophthalmoscope set on +20D.
- Use moistened cotton bud to remove FB if seen.
- Instil fluorescein (a drop or touch with dye strip).
- Inspect with blue torch or blue filter on ophthalmoscope.

Patterns of fluorescein staining include:
- Branch-like pattern: HSV.
- A round area: bacterial ulcer or corneal erosion.
- Staining on the inferior cornea: corneal exposure.
- Linear staining—if vertical in orientation, suspect a subtarsal FB. Evert the upper lid if necessary—ask child to look down, placing the cotton bud tip on the upper lid skin crease; apply downward pressure. Grasping the upper eyelid lashes, pivot the lid margin up and over the cotton bud. When everted, use the cotton bud to sweep along the exposed tarsal conjunctiva and remove the FB.
- Give chloramphenicol ointment tds for a week.

The conjunctiva is a mucous membrane lining the eyelids and covering the sclera. Its function is to lubricate the ocular surface. Inflammation of the conjunctiva causes 'pink eye' associated with mild discomfort and discharge. Tears are produced in the lacrimal gland and drained via the lacrimal punctae into the lacrimal sac, located near the nasal corner of the eye. Photophobia is an important symptom of corneal disorders or intra-ocular inflammation.

Infective/inflammatory disorders (2)

'Sticky eyes' of infancy

Mucoid discharge due to congenital nasolacrimal duct obstruction is common and causes mucus to collect in the lacrimal sac. If the eye is white, microbiological swabs are not necessary. Parents should massage the sac and clean discharge away with pads soaked in sterile water.

Neonatal conjunctivitis

This causes marked puffiness of the eyelids, conjunctival swelling and redness, and discharge in the first month of life. Viral, chlamydial, and bacterial swabs are required. Bacterial pathogens include *Staphylococcus aureus, Pseudomonas aeruginosa*, or streptococcal species.

- *Treatment*: refer for urgent specialist review; topical ofloxacin or azithromycin drops are started empirically until microbiological results are available.

Gonococcal conjunctivitis

Should be suspected if purulent discharge with swelling of the eyelids occurs within the first 48h of life. Can cause early corneal perforation.

- *Treatment*: IV ceftazidime or benzylpenicillin required.

Chlamydial conjunctivitis

Usually presents at the end of the first week of life.

- *Treatment*: 2wk course of PO erythromycin and topical azithromycin drops are required.

Herpes simplex infection

Look for blisters on the lids and corneal ulceration.

- *Treatment*: IV and topical aciclovir.

Childhood conjunctivitis

Viral conjunctivitis accompanies URTI and usually resolves within 7 days with conservative measures, including cold compresses, cleaning, and lubrication. Bacterial conjunctivitis is characterized by purulent discharge and should be treated empirically with topical antibiotics, e.g. chloramphenicol if severe. Conjunctivitis is contagious, so parents should be advised how to prevent spread of infection. If symptoms are severe or last >7 days, or the child becomes photophobic, perform bacterial and viral swabs.

Allergic conjunctivitis causes itchiness as the cardinal feature. An acute allergic response causes rapid-onset lid and conjunctival swelling. Seasonal/perennial forms present with other features of atopy. Topical mast cell stabilizers and antihistamines can improve symptoms.

Periorbital cellulitis

(See Periorbital cellulitis, p. 628; Periorbital cellulitis, p. 981.)

Keratitis (corneal infection/inflammation)

Keratitis can lead to corneal scarring and requires urgent specialist management. Symptoms include FB sensation, pain, and photophobia with a red eye.

- *Bacterial keratitis:* risk factors include contact lens wear, trauma, and corneal exposure. Ulceration can lead to corneal perforation.
- *Viral keratitis:* caused by adenovirus, HSV, and HZV, in conjunction with skin lesions or conjunctivitis.
- *Staphylococcal hypersensitivity:* a reaction to blepharitis.
- *Toxic epitheliopathy:* commonly seen with cytarabine chemotherapy.

Anterior uveitis (iritis)

Anterior uveitis is an acute or chronic inflammation of the uveal tract structures (i.e. iris, ciliary body, and choroid).

- *Acute anterior uveitis:* characterized by symptoms of eye ache, photophobia, epiphora, and blurred vision. Redness is concentrated around the corneal limbus. Most signs, such as cells in the anterior chamber and keratic precipitates, are only visible on biomicroscopy, but occasionally a pus level in the anterior chamber (hypopyon) may be visible. Mydriatic drops may reveal an irregular pupil due to posterior synechiae.
- *Chronic anterior uveitis:* often asymptomatic until vision is lost due to cataract or secondary macular oedema.

Causes
- Local infection: e.g. HSV/HZV.
- Trauma or surgery.
- Systemic disease:
  - Seronegative arthritides—HLA-B27 +ve, ankylosing spondylitis, Reiter's syndrome, psoriatic arthritis (see ➔ JIA subtypes, pp. 694–5).
  - IBD (see ➔ Inflammatory bowel disease, pp. 300–1).
  - JIA—screening required (see ➔ Uveitis screening and treatment, pp. 698–9).
  - Sarcoidosis.
  - Behçet's disease.

Management
Referral to the ophthalmologist and treatment with topical steroid drops/ointment and mydriatic agents are required.

Endophthalmitis

Intra-ocular infection may be *endogenous* (from sepsis) or *exogenous* (secondary to trauma or surgery) and causes a red, painful eye, photophobia, floaters, and loss of vision. A pus level within the anterior chamber (hypopyon) may be seen. Endophthalmitis requires emergency ophthalmic referral and management with systemic and intravitreal antibiotics, but despite this, there is poor prognosis for visual recovery.

Cataract

Lens opacities can be congenital or acquired and unilateral or bilateral, and vary in severity. Cataracts cause an absence of, or shadows on, the red reflex. A severe cataract will make the pupil look cloudy on torch light examination. Visually significant congenital cataracts occurring within the period of neuroplasticity can permanently reduce vision and require urgent referral.

Causes

(See also ➔ Chapter 12.)

Primary

- *Idiopathic.*
- *Developmental:* persistent intra-ocular fetal vasculature (PFV).
- *Inherited/genetic:*
  - Isolated genetic point mutations (AD, AR, X-linked recessive).
  - Aniridia.
  - Myotonic dystrophy.
  - Chromosomal disorders, e.g. trisomy 21,13, and 18.
- *Metabolic disorders:*
  - Galactosaemia.
  - Wilson's disease.
  - Lowe syndrome.
  - Fabry syndrome.
  - Zellweger syndrome.
  - Hallerman–Streiff–François syndrome.
  - Hypoglycaemia, hypocalcaemia.
- *Congenital infection:* e.g. rubella, HSV, VZV, toxoplasmosis (see ➔ Transplacental (congenital infection), p. 164).

Secondary

- *Inflammation:* e.g. from chronic anterior uveitis.
- *Iatrogenic:* from long-term steroids, radiotherapy, eye surgery.
- *Traumatic:* blunt or penetrating injury.

Management

Unilateral congenital cataracts are generally sporadic and not investigated. Bilateral cataracts require genetic investigation (congenital cataract gene panel), TORCH screen, and tests for urinary amino acids and reducing sugars.

Early lensectomy is indicated if the cataract is visually significant. The resultant aphakia is corrected with extended-wear contact lenses in infants. Intra-ocular lenses are usually implanted in a second procedure from 9mth of age. Occlusion therapy is required for unilateral or asymmetrical cataracts, even after lensectomy.

Glaucoma

Glaucoma is the loss of optic nerve axons associated with raised intra-ocular pressure. This is manifested by optic disc cupping and visual field loss. Unlike adults, the sclera in children <3y is stretchy, and raised eye pressure results in globe enlargement (buphthalmos, ox-eye), as well as cloudiness of the cornea due to oedema, photophobia, and excessive lacrimation. Globe enlargement may be bilateral or unilateral, causing asymmetry of size.

Causes

Congenital glaucoma is rare and usually sporadic. It usually occurs as an iso-lated abnormality of development of the eye. A port wine stain involving the eyelids in Sturge–Weber syndrome (see ➔ Sturge–Weber syndrome, p. 383) can cause unilateral glaucoma. Glaucoma may also complicate cata-ract surgery or anterior uveitis or develop with steroid therapy.

Management

Medical management
- Topical β-blockers: e.g. timolol 0.1% od.
- Topical prostaglandin analogues: e.g. latanoprost 0.05%.
- Topical miotics: pilocarpine 1%.
- Topical α2-agonist: apraclonidine 0.5%.
- Topical and PO acetazolamide.

Surgical management
- Goniotomy.
- Trabeculotomy.
- Trans-scleral laser ablation of the ciliary body.
- Trabeculectomy augmented with mitomycin.
- Tube drainage surgery.

Congenital glaucoma may require numerous operations in infancy, and des-pite this, visual impairment is common.

Orbit and eyelids

Blepharitis and meibomian cyst/chalazion

Blepharitis is a common chronic inflammation of the lid margin, which can result in recurrent styes, meibomian cysts, and occasionally keratitis. The eyelid margins are red and crusty.

Parents should clean their child's lid margins using a flannel soaked in a hand-hot mild baby shampoo solution at bath time. An antibiotic ointment, e.g. chloramphenicol, can then be applied to the lid margins with a fingertip. Styes and cysts often respond to this treatment too, but compresses need to be hot (40°C) to be effective. Chronic, hardened meibomian cysts may require incision and curettage under GA.

Congenital eyelid abnormalities

- True *entropion* (in-turned lid) or *ectropion* (out-turned lid) are extremely rare in children. Lower lid *epiblepharon* can resemble entropion since the lower lashes are in-turned due to a fold of skin close to the lid margin. This is seen more commonly in Asian children and resolves as the face grows; surgical correction is rarely required.
- Congenital *ptosis* due to dystrophy of the levator muscle can be unilateral or bilateral, and occasionally syndromic, e.g. NS. Asymmetrical pupil size (anisocoria) or restricted eye movements suggest a neurological cause requiring further investigation. If the lid covers the visual axis, amblyopia will rapidly ensue. Occlusion therapy may be required, but unless ptosis is severe, surgery is delayed until 4–5y.

Congenital nasolacrimal duct obstruction

This common condition causes stickiness and epiphora, but the eyes are white despite the copious discharge. Swabbing and topical antibiotics are not required. Most will resolve in the first few months of life; about 5% persist beyond 1y and require referral for syringing and probing of the duct.

Advise parents to massage the lacrimal sac (just below the nasal corner of the eye) firmly against the bone with a finger when the baby is feeding. This expresses the sac contents. The discharge can then be cleaned away with a pad soaked in cooled tap water. If the eyelid skin is sore due to overflow of tears, it can be waterproofed by application of petroleum jelly.

Capillary haemangioma of the lid

These may be deep and bluish in colour or be a superficial 'strawberry' naevus. Capillary haemangiomas can enlarge rapidly and cause amblyopia due to ptosis or induced astigmatism in the first years of life.

Occlusion therapy and spectacle correction are often necessary.

- PO propranolol is effective at shrinking the lesion and has replaced PO and steroid injections in the management of sight-threatening haemangioma.
- Exclusion of CHD and intracranial haemangioma associated with PHACES syndrome is necessary before propranolol therapy (see ➔ Vascular malformations and tumours, pp. 800–1).
- *Port wine stains* involving the eyelids may cause glaucoma on the affected side. Ophthalmic referral is required for screening.

Periorbital cellulitis

(See ➔ Periorbital cellulitis, p. 628.)

Periorbital cellulitis is an infection of the soft tissues around and in the orbit. The commonest organisms are S. aureus, β-haemolytic *Streptococcus*, and HiB (if not immunized). Anaerobic bacteria from the sinuses can be involved in teenagers, and fungal infection should be considered in immunosuppressed children. The cellulitis may be in the superficial tissues (preseptal) or involve the orbit. The proximity of the orbit to the brain makes this a potentially life-threatening infection.

Preseptal cellulitis

The infection may originate from skin wounds, e.g. from an infected insect bite or trauma, from periorbital tissues such as infected meibomian cysts or lacrimal sac abscess, or from paranasal sinuses.

- *Treatment:* if the child is systemically well and the eye is visible and has a full range of movement, the infection can be treated with PO antibiotics (co-amoxiclav) and regular review. Children with fever, lethargy, and anorexia or in whom the eye cannot be examined should be admitted and started on IV antibiotics.

Orbital cellulitis

The presence of proptosis, conjunctival swelling, or restricted eye movement signals infection and potentially an orbital abscess. If left untreated, optic neuropathy, intracranial abscess formation, meningitis, or cavernous sinus thrombosis may follow.

- *Treatment:* high-dose IV cephalosporin (and metronidazole if over 8y) is required without delay. Nasal decongestants are also indicated. A CT scan of the head and orbits is indicated to assess if orbital abscess drainage or sinus surgery is required, and multidisciplinary management with paediatrician, ophthalmologist, and ENT input is required.

Retinal problems

Retinopathy of prematurity

(See also → Retinopathy of prematurity, pp. 170–1.) This is a fibrovascular proliferative retinal disorder occurring in preterm, LBW infants. Normal vascularization of the fetal retina proceeds from the optic nerve anteriorly and is not complete until term. Premature birth and the requirement for O_2 supplementation drive abnormal neovascularization of the peripheral avascular retina which, if untreated, leads to inoperable retinal detachment. Although fewer than 5% of premature babies require treatment for ROP overall, the risks increase considerably the lower the gestational age and birthweight. ROP is responsible for 3% of UK childhood blindness despite screening.

ROP screening

All infants born <32wk gestation and/or weighing <1500g should be screened by an experienced ophthalmologist. Screening is initiated at 30–31wk post-menstrual age for babies of gestational age <27wk or 4–5wk postnatally for babies of 27–32wk gestational age. Regular screening is continued until the retina is sufficiently vascularized.

ROP treatment

ROP is classified by its severity (stages 1–5) and zone (zones I–III), with zone I (disease in the most posterior retina) most likely to result in sight loss. Plus-disease refers to engorgement and tortuosity of the retinal blood vessels and is a major sign of aggressive disease. Laser treatment is needed for all ROP with evidence of plus-disease (type 1 disease).

VEGF is a major driver of ROP. Intravitreal injection of an anti-VEGF agent (ranibizumab or bevacizumab) can be used in babies too unstable to tolerate laser treatment or as additional therapy in recalcitrant cases. However, the ocular and systemic long-term effects remain unknown.

Other medical conditions causing neovascular retinopathy

Sickle-cell disease

Deformed RBCs in SCD may cause retinal vascular occlusion or ischaemia. Proliferative retinopathy with new vessel formation or non-proliferative retinopathy with scarring and fibrosis may develop. Retinal screening for SC and SThal genotypes should begin at 9y, and SS genotype at 13y. Laser treatment may be required to prevent new vessel formation (see → Sickle crises and problems, pp. 550–1).

Diabetes mellitus

Diabetic retinopathy is rarely seen in children with T1DM or T2DM. Annual retinal photographic screening should start at 12y of age (see also → Retinopathy, p. 478).

Retinal dystrophies

This is a heterogenous group of disorders causing rod, cone, and/or inner retinal cell dysfunction. Retinal dystrophy may be isolated or part of a syndrome. Symptoms vary, depending on the photoreceptor—if cones are predominantly affected, central and colour vision will be poor; if rods are affected, there will be night blindness and loss of peripheral vision. Often there is a mixture of rod and cone involvement. The term *retinitis pigmentosa* refers to the typical pattern of 'bone spicule' pigmentation visible in the peripheral retina in many retinal dystrophies.

Syndromes associated with retinal dystrophies
- *Usher syndrome:* congenital deafness.
- *Bassen–Kornweig syndrome:* abetalipoproteinaemia, ataxia, and malabsorption.
- *Refsum's disease:* polyneuropathy, deafness, and cerebellar dysfunction.
- *Kearns–Sayre syndrome:* ophthalmoplegia, cardiac conduction defect.
- *BBS:* obesity, polydactyly, renal dysfunction.
- *Neuronal ceroid lipofuscinosis (Batten disease):* neurological deterioration, epilepsy.

All children with SN hearing loss should have an ophthalmic examination to detect visual/retinal abnormalities. Supportive help with optical and educational aids has been the mainstay of management in the past, but recent success with gene therapy gives us some optimism for future treatment.

Optic disc

Optic disc swelling

The term papilloedema is reserved for disc swelling due to raised ICP. In addition to headache and nausea, the child may have a whooshing tinnitus, visual obscurations (momentary loss of vision when leaning over or coughing), and diplopia secondary to bilateral cranial nerve VI paresis.

Causes of optic disc swelling with good visual acuity
• Early papilloedema (raised ICP).
• Malignant hypertension.
• Optic disc drusen.

Causes of optic disc swelling with poor visual acuity
• Prolonged papilloedema.
• Optic neuritis.
• Optic nerve compression (e.g. optic nerve glioma).
• Infiltration: e.g. leukaemia, sarcoid.
• Ischaemia.

Optic disc drusen
Calcific deposits in the optic nerve head, causing a swollen appearance. Optic nerve head imaging and ultrasonography (performed by an ophthalmologist) are useful in confirming the diagnosis and preventing unnecessary neurological investigation for papilloedema.

Optic neuritis/neuropathy

Inflammation, infiltration, or compression of the optic nerve cause early loss of central and colour vision. Assessment of optic nerve function should include:

- VA.
- Visual fields to confrontation (or perimetry if available).
- Colour vision (ask child to compare brightness of red target in one eye to the other).
- Pupil reactions: look for a relative afferent pupillary defect (see Fig. 30.3).
- Visualization of the optic disc—it may be swollen or atrophic.

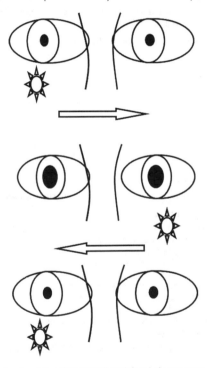

Fig. 30.3 Testing for relative afferent pupillary defect. Left optic neuropathy: both pupils constrict when light is shone in the right eye. When the torch is swung over to shine in the left eye, both pupils dilate (relative to the previous constriction).

Eye trauma

Chemical injury (alkali, acids, solvents, detergents, and irritants)

Start treatment immediately, unless penetrating eye injury is suspected.
- Instil topical anaesthesia (proxymetacaine 0.5%).
- Irrigate with copious saline for 30min.
- Wait 5–10min—ascertain nature of chemical.
- Check pH using litmus paper inside bottom lid.
- Continue irrigation until pH is 7.
- Sweep conjunctival fornices with moistened cotton bud.

Refer if severe injury and alkali involved; otherwise, give chloramphenicol ointment tds 2–3 days and SOS appointment.

Corneal abrasion and foreign bodies

(See ⊃ Corneal abrasion, subtarsal or corneal foreign body, pp. 974–5.)

Blunt trauma

Blunt trauma is common in older children (especially boys) due to their propensity for throwing things at each other! The child usually complains of achy pain and blurred vision.
- Instil anaesthetic to facilitate examination.
- Check VA.
- Compare pupil size: traumatic mydriasis may be seen.
- Examine with ophthalmoscope on +20D for hyphaema (blood in anterior chamber).
- Check red reflex.

Refer to the ophthalmologist if hyphaema/traumatic mydriasis is present.

Penetrating trauma

Suspect penetrating trauma if there is a history of the child falling onto a sharp object (e.g. pencil) or a history of high-velocity missile (e.g. air gun pellet). The severity of pain and reduction of vision is variable.
   Instil anaesthetic if the child is in pain.
- Check VA.
- Examine pupil reactions and look for symmetry.
- Signs of perforation/penetration include:
  - Subconjunctival haemorrhage.
  - Dark pigment on surface or under conjunctiva.
  - Distorted pupil and hyphaema.

Refer immediately; protect eye with hard eye shield, and keep nil by mouth.

Inflicted (abusive) head injury (NAI)

(See ➲ Subdural haemorrhage, pp. 394–5; ➲ Physical abuse, pp. 914–15.)

Severe shaking and shaking/impact injury in infants can cause the triad of subdural haemorrhages, encephalopathy, and retinal haemorrhages. The finding of multi-layered pan-retinal haemorrhages is not diagnostic for abusive head injury in these circumstances but is highly suggestive, following the exclusion of other metabolic or haematological causes.

Causes of retinal haemorrhage

- Abusive head injury.
- Severe accidental trauma.
- Leukaemia.
- Sepsis.
- Acute intracerebral haemorrhage (Terson's syndrome).
- GA1.
- OI.
- Viral retinitis.

Multi-layered haemorrhages include

- *Deep retinal haemorrhages* (blots and white-centred haemorrhages).
- Spindle-shaped *superficial nerve fibre layer retinal haemorrhages* (flame-shaped haemorrhages).
- *Sub-hyaloid haemorrhages* (often associated with a fluid level).

Typically, the haemorrhages increase in confluence towards the peripheral retina. Vitreous traction can cause peri-macular retinal folds and splitting (schisis) of the macular retina.

Retinal nerve fibre layer haemorrhages can disappear within days, but the deeper and sub-hyaloid haemorrhages can take months to resolve.

If inflicted head injury is suspected, mydriatic ophthalmoscopy should be performed by an ophthalmologist. Both this and subsequent wide angle retinal imaging are easier when the infant is sedated. Following detection and documentation of retinal haemorrhages, a senior ophthalmologist should be involved in multidisciplinary discussion regarding safeguarding. Often the visual prognosis in such cases is poor, not because of the retinal injury, but because of the associated brain injury which causes cerebral visual impairment.

Further reading

Online reference

UpToDate. *Pediatric ophthalmology*. Available at: ℜ https://www.uptodate.com/contents/table-of-contents/pediatrics/pediatric-ophthalmology.

Patient (and medical professional) online literature

Moorfields Eye Hospital NHS Foundation Trust. *Eye conditions*. Available at: ℜ https://www.moorfields.nhs.uk/listing/conditions.

NHS UK. *Eye tests for children*. Available at: ℜ https://www.nhs.uk/conditions/eye-tests-in-children/.

Index

Note: Tables, figures, and boxes are indicated by an italic *t*, *f*, and *b* following the page number.